MW01612800

Tumors of the Peripheral Nervous System

Atlas
of
Tumor Pathology

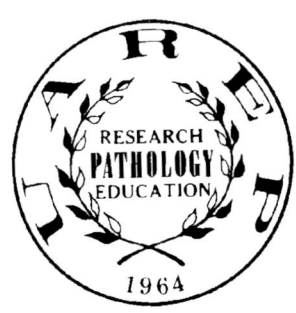

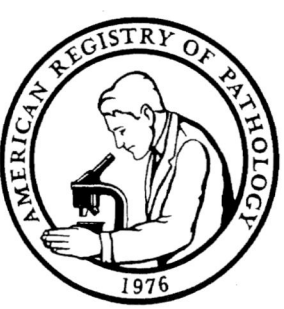

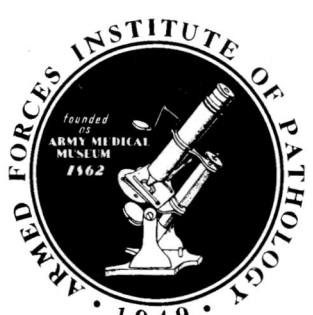

ATLAS OF TUMOR PATHOLOGY

Third Series
Fascicle 24

TUMORS OF THE
PERIPHERAL NERVOUS SYSTEM

by

BERND W. SCHEITHAUER, M.D.
Consultant in Pathology
Mayo Clinic
Professor of Pathology
Mayo Graduate School of Medicine
Rochester, Minnesota

JAMES M. WOODRUFF, M.D.
Attending Pathologist
Memorial Sloan-Kettering Cancer Center
Professor of Pathology
Cornell University Medical College
New York, New York

ROBERT A. ERLANDSON, Ph.D.
Attending Electron Microscopist
Memorial Sloan-Kettering Cancer Center
Associate Professor of Pathology
Cornell University Medical College
New York, New York

Published by the
ARMED FORCES INSTITUTE OF PATHOLOGY
Washington, D.C.

Under the Auspices of
UNIVERSITIES ASSOCIATED FOR RESEARCH AND EDUCATION IN PATHOLOGY, INC.
Bethesda, Maryland
1999

Accepted for Publication
1997

———————

Available from the American Registry of Pathology
Armed Forces Institute of Pathology
Washington, D.C. 20306-6000
ISSN 0160-6344
ISBN 1-881041-45-X

ATLAS OF TUMOR PATHOLOGY

EDITOR
JUAN ROSAI, M.D.
Department of Pathology
Memorial Sloan-Kettering Cancer Center
New York, New York 10021-6007

ASSOCIATE EDITOR
LESLIE H. SOBIN, M.D.
Armed Forces Institute of Pathology
Washington, D.C. 20306-6000

EDITORIAL ADVISORY BOARD

Jeffrey Cossman, M.D.   Georgetown University School of Medicine
Washington, D.C. 20007

Ronald A. DeLellis, M.D.   Cornell University Medical College
New York, New York 10021

Glauco Frizzera, M.D.   Cornell University Medical College
New York, New York 10021

Leonard B. Kahn, M.D.   Long Island Jewish Hospital/Hillside Medical Center
New Hyde Park, New York 11042

Richard L. Kempson, M.D.   Stanford University Medical School
Stanford, California 94305

Paul Peter Rosen, M.D.   Cornell University Medical College
New York, New York 10021

Robert E. Scully, M.D.   Harvard Medical School and Massachusetts General Hospital
Boston, Massachusetts 02114

Steven G. Silverberg, M.D.   University of Maryland School of Medicine
Baltimore, Maryland 21201

Sharon Weiss, M.D.   Emory University Hospital
Atlanta, Georgia 30322

EDITORS' NOTE

The Atlas of Tumor Pathology has a long and distinguished history. It was first conceived at a Cancer Research Meeting held in St. Louis in September 1947 as an attempt to standardize the nomenclature of neoplastic diseases. The first series was sponsored by the National Academy of Sciences-National Research Council. The organization of this Sisyphean effort was entrusted to the Subcommittee on Oncology of the Committee on Pathology, and Dr. Arthur Purdy Stout was the first editor-in-chief. Many of the illustrations were provided by the Medical Illustration Service of the Armed Forces Institute of Pathology, the type was set by the Government Printing Office, and the final printing was done at the Armed Forces Institute of Pathology (hence the colloquial appellation "AFIP Fascicles"). The American Registry of Pathology purchased the Fascicles from the Government Printing Office and sold them virtually at cost. Over a period of 20 years, approximately 15,000 copies each of nearly 40 Fascicles were produced. The worldwide impact that these publications have had over the years has largely surpassed the original goal. They quickly became among the most influential publications on tumor pathology ever written, primarily because of their overall high quality but also because their low cost made them easily accessible to pathologists and other students of oncology the world over.

Upon completion of the first series, the National Academy of Sciences-National Research Council handed further pursuit of the project over to the newly created Universities Associated for Research and Education in Pathology (UAREP). A second series was started, generously supported by grants from the AFIP, the National Cancer Institute, and the American Cancer Society. Dr. Harlan I. Firminger became the editor-in-chief and was succeeded by Dr. William H. Hartmann. The second series Fascicles were produced as bound volumes instead of loose leaflets. They featured a more comprehensive coverage of the subjects, to the extent that the Fascicles could no longer be regarded as "atlases" but rather as monographs describing and illustrating in detail the tumors and tumor-like conditions of the various organs and systems.

Once the second series was completed, with a success that matched that of the first, UAREP and AFIP decided to embark on a third series. A new editor-in-chief and an associate editor were selected, and a distinguished editorial board was appointed. The mandate for the third series remains the same as for the previous ones, i.e., to oversee the production of an eminently practical publication with surgical pathologists as its primary audience, but also aimed at other workers in oncology. The main purposes of this series are to promote a consistent, unified, and biologically sound nomenclature; to guide the surgical pathologist in the diagnosis of the various tumors and tumor-like lesions; and to provide relevant histogenetic, pathogenetic, and clinicopathologic information on these entities. Just as the second series included data obtained from ultrastructural (and, in the more recent Fascicles, immunohistochemical) examination, the third series will, in addition, incorporate pertinent information obtained with the newer molecular biology techniques. As in the past, a continuous attempt will be made to correlate, whenever possible, the nomenclature used in the Fascicles with that proposed by the World Health Organization's International Histological Classification of Tumors. The format of the third series has been changed in order to incorporate additional items and to ensure a consistency of style throughout. Close cooperation between the various authors and their respective liaisons from the editorial board will be emphasized to minimize unnecessary repetition and discrepancies in the text and illustrations.

To its everlasting credit, the participation and commitment of the AFIP to this venture is even more substantial and encompassing than in previous series. It now extends to virtually all scientific, technical, and financial aspects of the production.

The task confronting the organizations and individuals involved in the third series is even more daunting than in the preceding efforts because of the ever-increasing complexity of the matter at hand. It is hoped that this combined effort—of which, needless to say, that represented by the authors is first and foremost—will result in a series worthy of its two illustrious predecessors and will be a suitable introduction to the tumor pathology of the twenty-first century.

Juan Rosai, M.D.
Leslie H. Sobin, M.D.

PREFACE

This monograph describes the spectrum of neoplasms, hamartomas, hyperplasias, reactive lesions, and inflammatory pseudotumors arising from or associated with peripheral nerves. Included are lesions affecting spinal nerves and extradural portions of cranial nerves. Specifically excluded from this discussion are lesions of the optic nerve, a central nervous system structure.

Tumors affecting the substance of nerves, such as a) metastatic carcinoma, lymphoma, and melanoma; b) rare primary epineural tumors; and c) direct extensions from surrounding soft tissue neoplasms are also included. With the exception of carcinoma and neurotropic melanoma, such tumors often remain extrinsic to nerve fascicles or involve perineurium rather than exhibiting the endoneurial pattern of spread so characteristic of primary peripheral nerve sheath tumors.

Peripheral nerve tumors are generally classified as soft tissue tumors, but they differ significantly from most neoplasms in this category. Notable differences include the frequent association of nerve sheath tumors with genetic disorders and the origin of a majority of malignant nerve sheath tumors from neurofibroma, a benign precursor lesion. Furthermore, tumors of peripheral nerves are histologically diverse and arise in a complex tissue with distinctive anatomic compartments. Nerves consist not simply of axons but of specialized ensheathments and compartments. These include: 1) Schwann cells that enwrap axons and form the boundary for the inner limits of the endoneurium; 2) the endoneurium, which consists of capillaries, fibroblasts, macrophages, and mast cells; 3) a specialized barrier layer, the perineurium, that forms the outer limit of the endoneurium; and 4) the epineurium, an external layer of fibroadipose tissue. Vascular elements are present in all three layers. Hamartomas, hyperplasias, reactive lesions including true neuromas and inflammatory pseudotumors, as well as neurofibromas typically involve several if not all these components of peripheral nerve. Although, theoretically, neoplasms may arise from Schwann cells, perineurial cells, fibroblasts, and other cells comprising the nerve sheaths, most peripheral nerve neoplasms are in fact derived from Schwann cells. The latter are neuroectodermal cells of neural crest origin, ones unique to peripheral nerves. The histologic diversity so characteristic of peripheral nerve tumors is in large part attributable to the metaplastic repertoire of neoplastic Schwann cells which produce not only a variety of collagens and melanin, but display a remarkable capacity for divergent differentiation toward rhabdomyoblasts, chondroblasts, and epithelial cells of varying type. Also unique to peripheral nerves are perineurial cells, tumors of which are rare. Whereas vascular and adipose tumors of peripheral nerves have been reported, ones presumably derived from fibroblasts are not well defined.

The diagnosis and classification of nerve sheath lesions requires correlation with clinical and surgical data as well as considerable attention to the histochemical features. In many instances, immunohistochemistry and electron microscopy are also necessary. Although some authors have prematurely concluded that electron microscopy is no longer of diagnostic utility, we feel it plays an important role in surgical pathology, most notably for the classification of peripheral nerve tumors. For example, electron microscopy is useful for recognizing: 1) advanced schwannian differentiation in cellular schwannoma, a lesion that must be distinguished from S-100–positive malignant peripheral nerve sheath tumors which often demonstrate only minor degrees of Schwann cell differentiation; 2) the one third of malignant peripheral nerve sheath tumors that lack light microscopic or immunohistochemical evidence of nerve sheath differentiation; and 3) those perineurial neoplasms that may not express epithelial membrane antigen immunoreactivity. No doubt the application of new methods, including immunoelectron microscopy, in situ hybridization, and molecular genetics will further our understanding of nerve sheath neoplasia.

The publication of large clinicopathologic studies and the application of new investigative methods have advanced our understanding of the nature and behavior of nerve sheath tumors. In addition, they have permitted the recognition of entities described since the publication of the last Fascicle, and morphologic variants of those already well established. Among reactive processes, this includes inflammatory pseudotumor, pacinian neuroma, and palisaded encapsulated neuroma. Newly described malformative lesions include lipofibromatous hamartoma and neuromuscular choristoma, both of which exhibit highly distinctive morphologic features. With respect to benign neoplasms, the clinically most important development has been the recognition of cellular schwannoma, a lesion often mistaken for malignant peripheral nerve sheath tumor (MPNST). In addition, the spectrum of schwannomas has been further expanded to include plexiform schwannoma, a tumor with no hereditary disposition, and psammomatous melanotic schwannoma, one frequently occurring in the setting of Carney's complex. Newcomers to the category of benign nerve sheath tumors are neurothekeoma as well as intraneural and soft tissue perineurioma. Intraneural perineurioma, once considered a reactive lesion, has been found to be a neoplasm, a monoclonal proliferation cytogenetically similar to ordinary schwannoma. Lastly, the clinicopathologic spectrum of malignant peripheral nerve sheath tumor has been expanded to include postradiation examples as well as the very rare tumors that arise from schwannoma, ganglioneuroma, and pheochromocytoma.

ACKNOWLEDGMENTS

The authors wish to acknowledge the assistance of those who have contributed significantly to this work. We are grateful to Dr. Caterina Giannini of Mayo Clinic whose expertise in diseases of nerve particularly enriched the sections on normal anatomy and non-neoplastic diseases; Dr. Richard Kempson of Stanford University and Dr. Richard Reed of New Orleans, Louisiana for painstaking critiques of the initial version of this work; Dr. Hymie Gordon and Dr. Pamela Karnes of Medical Genetics, Mayo Clinic for sharing their invaluable illustrations and clinical perspective regarding neurofibromatosis; Dr. David Scollard of the GWL Hansen's Disease Center, Baton Rouge, Louisiana, for his assistance on leprous neuropathy; Dr. Doris Wenger, Diagnostic Radiology, Mayo Clinic, for contributing imaging studies; Dr. Takanori Hirose of Saitama Medical School, Saitama, Japan, Dr. John Kepes of the University of Kansas, Dr. Federico Roncaroli of the University of Bologna, Bologna, Italy, Dr. Helen Kourea of the University of Patras, School of Medicine, Patras, Greece, Dr. Ernest Lack of George Washington University, Dr. Mia MacCollin of Massachusetts General Hospital, and Mike Baser, Ph.D. of Los Angeles, California for their selected contributions as reviewers; Mr. John Hagen of Medical Illustrations, Mayo Clinic, for his exquisite artwork; and Mrs. Lori Riess of Secretarial Services, Mayo Clinic, for her tireless, cheerful service and attention to details.

Lastly, the first author wishes to acknowledge a former Mayo Clinic resident, Dr. Barbara Ducatman, for her youthful enthusiasm and hard work in early studies of the Mayo Clinic experience with malignant peripheral nerve sheath tumors.

B. W. Scheithauer, M.D.
J. M. Woodruff, M.D.
R. A. Erlandson, Ph.D.

Permission to use copyrighted illustrations has been granted by:

American Medical Association:
    JAMA 1962;180:521–24. For figure 3-25.

Lippincott-Raven:
    Am J Surg Pathol 1995;19:1325–32. For figure 10-9.
    Atlas of Neuropathology, 1988. For figures 3-4, 3-19A, 7-1C, 7-3C, 8-4, 8-14, 8-33B&C
        11-10A, 13-4, 13-8C&D, 13-20, 13-21A, and 13-22.

Williams & Wilkins:
    Mod Pathol 1997;11:1075–81. For figures 7-44 and 7-45.
    Neurosurgery 1994;35:127–32. For figures 6-3 and 6-5.

DEDICATION

To my parents, Walter Ernst Scheithauer (1913–1996),
who by his inquisitive nature and enthusiasm
for science sparked an interest, and
Renate Margarete Scheithauer whose drive
and confidence remains an inspiration.

B. W. Scheithauer, M.D.

To my wife, Corazon, who has the patience of a saint,
and to my sons, Dr. James N. Woodruff and
Dr. Prescott G. Woodruff, my pride and joy.

J. M. Woodruff, M.D.

To my wife, Elaine, and my devoted staff,
Ann Baren, Elizabeth Weiss, Kin Kong,
Loraine Biedrzycki, and Milagros Soto.

R. A. Erlandson, Ph.D.

Pioneers in Peripheral Nerve Pathology

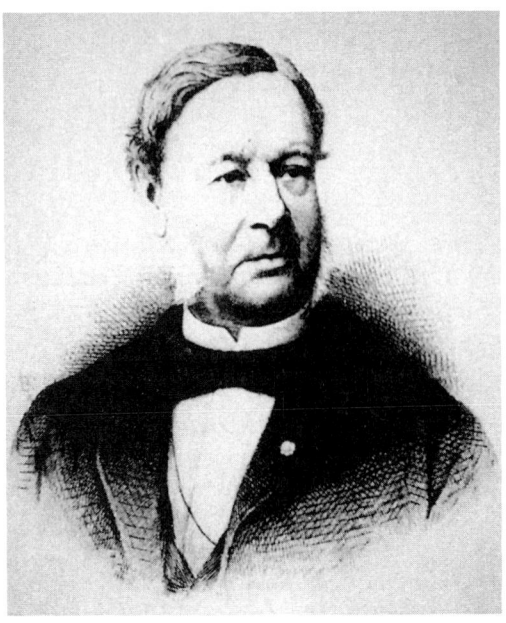

Theodor Schwann, 1810–1882

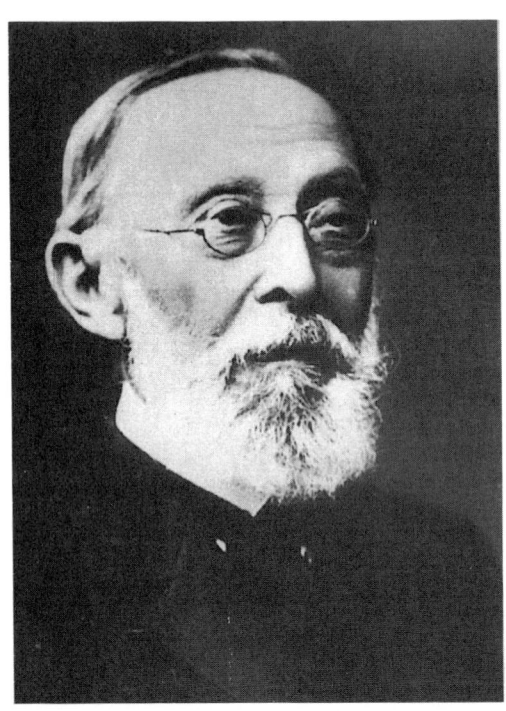

Rudolph Virchow, 1821–1902

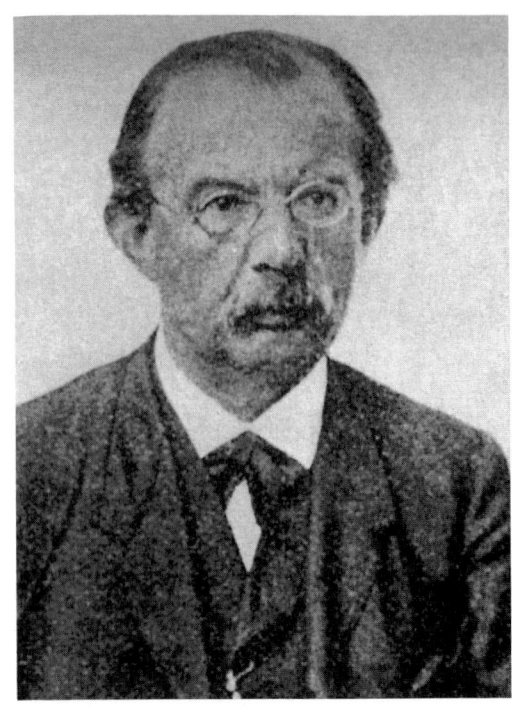

Friedrich von Recklinghausen, 1833–1910

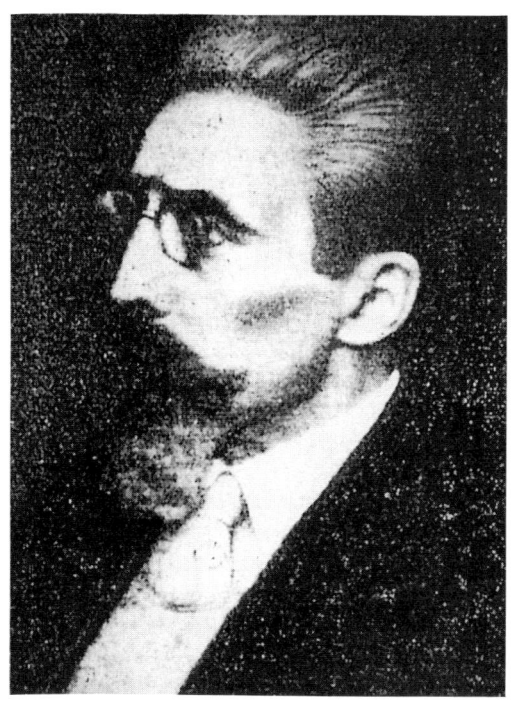

José Verocay, 1876–1927

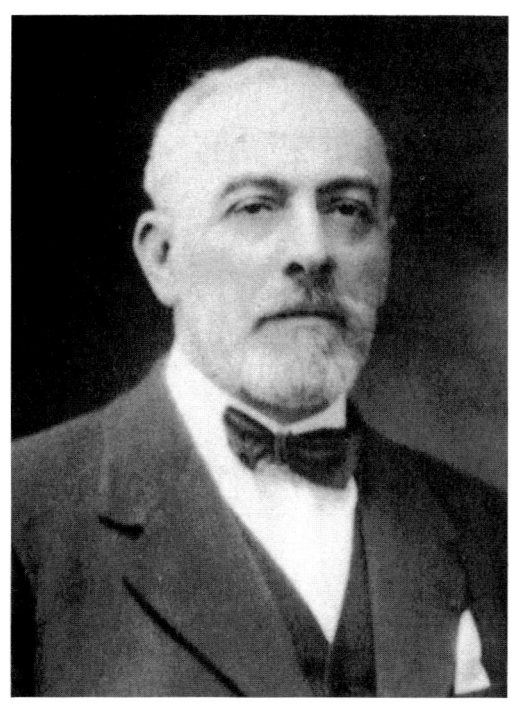

Pierre Masson, 1880–1959

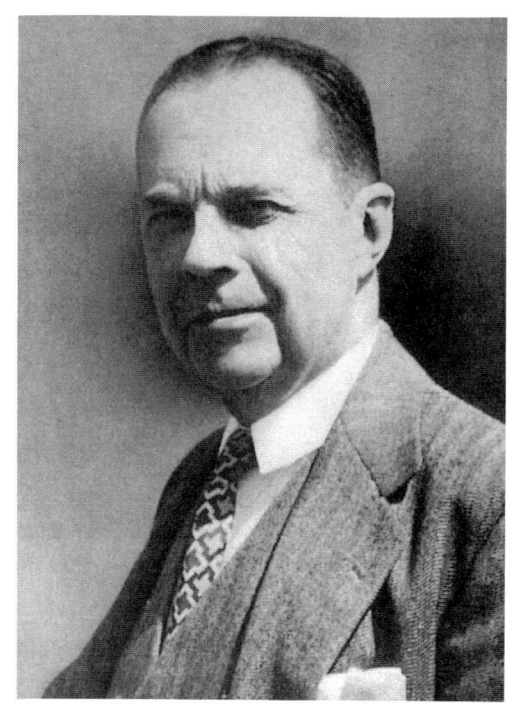

Arthur Purdy Stout, 1885–1967

Contents

TUMORS OF THE
PERIPHERAL NERVOUS SYSTEM

1
INTRODUCTION, OVERVIEW, AND SPECIMEN ASSESSMENT

INTRODUCTION

This monograph describes the spectrum of neoplasms, hamartomas, hyperplasias, reactive lesions, and inflammatory pseudotumors arising from or associated with peripheral nerves. Included are lesions affecting spinal nerves and extradural portions of cranial nerves. Specifically excluded from this discussion are lesions of the optic nerve, a central nervous system structure.

Tumors affecting the substance of nerves, such as metastatic carcinoma, rare examples of melanoma, and direct extensions from surrounding soft tissue neoplasms are also included. With the exception of carcinoma and neurotropic melanoma, such neoplasms are often extrinsic to nerve fascicles, or involve perineurium rather than exhibiting the endoneurial pattern of spread so characteristic of primary peripheral nerve sheath tumors.

Peripheral nerve tumors are generally classified as soft tissue tumors, but they differ significantly from most neoplasms in this category. Notable differences include the frequent association of nerve sheath tumors with genetic disorders and the origin of a majority of malignant nerve sheath tumors from neurofibroma, a benign precursor lesion. Furthermore, tumors of peripheral nerves are histologically diverse and arise in a complex tissue with distinctive anatomic compartments. Nerves consist not simply of axons but of specialized ensheathments and compartments. These include: 1) Schwann cells that enwrap axons and form the boundary for the inner limits of the endoneurium; 2) the endoneurium, which consists of capillaries, fibroblasts, macrophages, and mast cells; 3) a specialized barrier layer, the perineurium, that forms the outer limit of the endoneurium; and 4) the epineurium, an external layer of fibroadipose tissue. Vascular elements are present in all three

layers. Hamartomas, hyperplasias, reactive lesions including true neuromas and inflammatory pseudotumors, as well as neurofibromas typically involve several if not all these components of peripheral nerve. Although theoretically, neoplasms may arise from Schwann cells, perineurial cells, fibroblasts, and other cells comprising the nerve sheaths, most peripheral nerve neoplasms are in fact derived from Schwann cells. The latter are neuroectodermal cells of neural crest origin unique to peripheral nerves. The histologic diversity so characteristic of peripheral nerve tumors is in large part attributable to the metaplastic repertoire of neoplastic Schwann cells which produce not only a variety of collagens and melanin, but display a remarkable capacity for divergent differentiation toward rhabdomyoblasts, chondroblasts, and epithelial cells of varying type. Also unique to peripheral nerves are perineurial cells, tumors of which are rare. Whereas vascular and adipose tumors of peripheral nerves have been reported, those presumably derived from fibroblasts are not well defined.

The diagnosis and classification of nerve sheath lesions requires correlation with clinical and surgical data as well as considerable attention to their histochemical features. In many instances, immunohistochemistry and electron microscopy are also necessary. Although some authors have concluded that electron microscopy is no longer of diagnostic utility, we feel it plays an important role in surgical pathology, most notably in the classification of peripheral nerve tumors. For example, electron microscopy is useful in recognizing: 1) advanced schwannian differentiation in cellular schwannoma, a lesion that must be distinguished from S-100–positive malignant peripheral nerve sheath tumors which often demonstrate only minor degrees of Schwann cell differentiation; 2) the fully one third of malignant peripheral nerve sheath tumors that lack light microscopic or immunohistochemical evidence of nerve sheath differentiation; and 3) those perineurial neoplasms that may not express epithelial membrane antigen immunoreactivity. No doubt the application of new methods, including immunoelectron microscopy, in situ hybridization, and molecular genetics will further our understanding of nerve sheath neoplasia.

The publication of large clinicopathologic studies and the application of new investigative methods have advanced our understanding of the nature and behavior of nerve sheath tumors. In addition, they have permitted the recognition of new entities, described since the publication of the last Fascicle on peripheral nerve tumors, and morphologic variants of those already well established. Among reactive processes, this includes inflammatory pseudotumor, pacinian neuroma, and palisaded encapsulated neuroma. Newly described malformative lesions include lipofibromatous hamartoma and neuromuscular choristoma, both of which exhibit highly distinctive morphologic features. The clinically most important development in benign neoplasms has been the recognition of cellular schwannoma, a lesion often mistaken for malignant peripheral nerve sheath tumor (MPNST). In addition, the spectrum of schwannomas has been further expanded to include plexiform schwannoma, a tumor with no hereditary disposition, and psammomatous melanotic schwannoma, one frequently occurring in the setting of Carney's complex. Newcomers to the category of benign nerve sheath tumors are neurothekeoma as well as intraneural and soft tissue perineurioma. Intraneural perineurioma, once considered a reactive lesion, has been found to be a neoplasm, a monoclonal proliferation cytogenetically similar to ordinary schwannoma. Lastly, the clinicopathologic spectrum of MPNST has been expanded to include a postradiation type as well as the very rare examples that arise from schwannoma, ganglioneuroma, and pheochromocytoma.

OVERVIEW

The boundaries of the peripheral nervous system as they relate to this Fascicle include intradural and extradural nerve roots, ganglia, and peripheral nerves and their specialized sensorimotor endings. Also included are autonomic nerves and their paravertebral and visceral ganglia. On rare occasion, peripheral nerve sheath tumors arise not only within recognizable nerves but within viscera. Such lesions are treated in other Fascicles and are not covered here in depth.

Anatomy. Gross, light microscopic, immunohistochemical, and ultrastructural features of the peripheral and autonomic nervous systems are described. The discussion will be primarily limited to features of practical diagnostic significance to the surgical pathology of peripheral nerve sheath tumors (PNSTs).

Lesion Spectrum. The lesions discussed in this Fascicle are limited to those of reactive, hyperplastic, hamartomatous, and neoplastic (benign and malignant) nature. The limitations of a strictly benign/malignant approach are best illustrated by atypical and cellular neurofibromas, in which morphologic features such as pleomorphic cells and increased cellularity might suggest early malignant transformation. Such tumors must be recognized because they are typically cured by resection and show no tendency to metastasis. Unfortunately, the literature specifically referring to their biology is scant.

Hereditary disorders with peripheral nerve manifestations, including neurofibromatosis 1 and 2 and multiple endocrine neoplasia type IIb, are discussed, with emphasis placed upon peripheral and autonomic nerve lesions.

Nerve Sheath Tumor Classification. As much as possible, a classification of PNSTs is based upon the finding of specific features of cellular differentiation, be it schwannian, perineurial, fibroblastic, melanocytic, or divergent. An outline of the lesions to be discussed appears in the Table of Contents.

Etiology. Etiologic factors associated with PNST are briefly discussed with respect to individual lesions. These include genetic factors, radiation, and environmental factors.

Prognosis. Factors reportedly affecting prognosis are mentioned with regard to malignant PNST. These include the presence of phakomatosis, large tumor size, high tumor grade, DNA ploidy status, proliferation indices (mitotic counts, percent S-phase determinations by flow cytometry, and labeling indices for Ki-67 or MIB-1 and for proliferating cell nuclear antigen), and p53 protein immunoreactivity.

Diagnostic Approach and Specimen Handling. The Fascicle stresses a practical approach to diagnosis based on gross features, routine light microscopy, and immunohistochemistry featuring only well-characterized, readily available antibodies. Flow cytometry (ploidy and percent S-phase determination), proliferation marker data, and molecular diagnostic methods are also discussed. Electron microscopy is included where relevant to diagnosis. The discussion of malignant lesions touches upon the approach to the gross specimen, e.g., margin assessment including inking, adequate sampling of specimens, and intraoperative communication.

Grading. The status of histologic grading relative to malignant PNST is discussed. Because no established, formal grading scheme is available, and since the large majority show significant degrees of anaplasia, we emphasize a multifactorial approach to prognostication, based upon clinical factors, tumor size, relation to nearby structures (staging), extent of resection, and the pathologic factors previously mentioned.

Staging. The staging of the tumors discussed in this Fascicle will be covered in the Third Series Fascicle on tumors of the soft tissue, which is scheduled for publication in 1999, and is not separately discussed herein.

Differential Diagnosis. In text and table, processes entering into the light microscopic differential diagnosis of nerve lesions are discussed. Emphasis is placed on lesions having a distinctly different behavior from the tumor in question (see Table 1-1).

SPECIMEN ASSESSMENT

Peripheral nerve tumors present either as soft tissue tumors of unknown type, or as lesions clinically and grossly recognized as being of peripheral nerve origin. In either situation, the recommended initial steps are to: 1) record their gross appearance before dissection by taking color photographs; 2) measure in centimeters the specimen's three dimensions; and 3) accurately describe the gross appearance, particularly with regard to tumor configuration and the presence or absence of a nerve. Following these initial steps, if there is any question that the tumor might be malignant, the external surface of the specimen should be coated with India ink, thus permitting an accurate microscopic assessment of margins of resection.

To determine the shape, color, and texture of the lesion, the specimen is next cross-sectioned along its longest dimension (longitudinal section), preferably with a single stroke of a sharp knife. An exception is when the tumor has the shape of a long cylinder of relatively uniform diameter. In this situation, multiple cross sections along the shortest dimension of the tumor are as important as longitudinal sections. Cross sections assure the proper evaluation of lesions such as soft tissue perineurioma. The cut surface is then photographed and described. In order to prevent recording adventitious colors which invariably develop after exposure to air, photographs need to be taken within 3 minutes of dissecting the specimen. If the tumor is large, multiple cross sections are needed for adequate sampling. Comments regarding homogeneity of tumor tissue or lack thereof, and the presence or absence and percentage of necrosis are also noted. It is recommended that samples for microscopy should be taken from every centimeter of the tumor's greatest dimension and additional samples obtained from areas with unusual color or texture. Sections representing circumferential as well as proximal and distal margins of the specimen are also required. Inking is encouraged.

Whereas the above steps are essential in the evaluation of PNSTs, we consider it important to set aside a tumor sample in fixative for electron microscopy. Although preservation in either glutaraldehyde or Trump's fixative is optimal, even formalin fixation will suffice. In selected cases, submitting fresh tissue for cytogenetics, quick-freezing a sample in liquid nitrogen for molecular genetics, and saving a sample in an appropriate media, such as RPMI, for tissue culture or flow cytometry, is also useful.

Table 1-1

DIFFERENTIAL DIAGNOSIS OF PERIPHERAL NERVE LESIONS

Peripheral Nerve Tumors	Differential Diagnosis
1. Tumor-like lesions	
a. Reactive lesions	
1) Traumatic neuroma	Neurofibroma, palisaded encapsulated neuroma, mucosal neuroma
2) Localized interdigital neuritis	Traumatic neuroma
3) Pacinian neuroma	Nerve sheath myxoma
4) Nerve cyst	Nerve sheath myxoma, cystic schwannoma
5) Inflammatory pseudotumor	Infection, lymphoma
b. Inflammatory and infectious lesions	
c. Hyperplastic lesions	
1) Palisaded encapsulated neuroma (PEN)	Plexiform schwannoma, leiomyoma
2) Mucosal neuromatosis Ganglioneuroma/ganglioneuromatosis	Traumatic neuroma, PEN, ganglioneuroma (ganglioneuromatosis)
3) Localized hypertrophic neuropathy	Intraneural perineurioma
d. Hamartomas	
1) Fibrolipomatous hamartoma	Lipoma
2) Neuromuscular choristoma	Rhabdomyoma, benign and malignant "triton tumor"
2. Benign Tumors	
a. Schwannoma (neurilemoma)	Neurofibroma, leiomyoma, palisaded myofibroblastoma, PEN
1) Cellular schwannoma	Malignant peripheral nerve sheath tumor (PNST), fibrosarcoma, leiomyosarcoma
2) Plexiform schwannoma	Plexiform neurofibroma, plexiform fibrohistiocytic tumor
3) Melanotic schwannoma	Melanoma, pigmented dermatofibrosarcoma protuberans, melanotic neurofibroma
a) Psammomatous melanotic schwannoma	
b. Neurofibroma	
1) Diffuse (cutaneous)	Dermatofibroma, dermatofibrosarcoma protuberans, mucinosis, myxoid fibrous histiocytoma, spindle cell lipoma
2) Localized	Schwannoma, myxoma, ganglioneuroma
3) Plexiform	Plexiform schwannoma
4) Divergent differentiation (glandular, rhabdomyomatous, pigmented, etc.)	
c. Perineurioma	
1) Intraneural perineurioma	Localized hypertrophic neuropathy
2) Soft tissue perineurioma	Neurofibroma, meningioma, dermatofibrosarcoma, solitary fibrous tumor, myoepithelioma, fibroma, meningioma, low-grade fibrosarcoma, fibromyxoid sarcoma
d. Nerve sheath myxoma and neurothekeoma	Myxoid neurofibroma and schwannoma, soft tissue myxoma, myxoma, myxoid MFH; mucinosis
e. Granular cell tumor	Malignant granular cell tumor, granular epithelioid leiomyoma, hibernoma, rhabdomyoma, paraganglioma, alveolar soft part sarcoma
f. Ganglioneuroma	Schwannoma, neurofibroma
g. Miscellaneous lesions	
1) Meningioma	Soft tissue perineurioma
2) Paraganglioma (cauda equina)	Ependymoma (filum terminale)
3) Lipoma	Lipofibromatous hamartoma

Table 1-1 (continued)

DIFFERENTIAL DIAGNOSIS

Peripheral Nerve Tumors	Differential Diagnosis
4) Hemangioma	Angiomatosis
5) Angiomatosis of nerve	Hemangioma
6) Hemangioblastoma	Metastatic renal cell carcinoma
7) Adrenal adenoma	Metastatic renal cell carcinoma, granular cell tumor
3. Malignant Tumors	
a. Malignant peripheral nerve sheath tumors (MPNST)	Cellular neurofibroma, cellular schwannoma, fibro-sarcoma, leiomyosarcoma, monophasic synovial sarcoma, neurotropic melanoma, clear cell sarcoma
1) MPNST variants	
a. Epithelioid MPNST	Melanoma, carcinoma, rhabdoid tumor, clear cell sarcoma
b) MPNST with divergent (mesenchymal/epithelial) differentiation	Synovial sarcoma, rhabdomyosarcoma, osteosarcoma and chondrosarcoma, carcinoma
c) Schwannoma with malignant transformation	Cellular schwannoma, metastatic carcinoma, primitive neuroectodermal tumor (PNET)
d) MPNST arising from ganglioneuroma or ganglioneuroblastoma	
e) Malignant perineurioma	Conventional MPNST
b. Malignant tumors of possible peripheral nerve origin	
1) Primitive neuroectodermal tumor (peripheral neuroepithelioma)	Small cell carcinoma/sarcoma, lymphoma
2) Malignant granular cell tumor	Granular cell tumor, granular variant of leiomyo-sarcoma, alveolar soft part sarcoma, rhabdoid tumor
c. Secondary neoplasms	Carcinoma, sarcoma, neurotropic melanoma, lymphoma

2

THE NORMAL PERIPHERAL NERVOUS SYSTEM

DEVELOPMENT

Early in embryogenesis, the midline dorsal ectoderm gives rise to the neural plate which develops a longitudinal groove, the walls of which fold and fuse to form the neural tube. From the level of the diencephalon through the distal neuraxis, the lateral portions of the fold form the neural crest. Derivatives of the neural crest include sensory and autonomic nerves as well as their ganglia, Schwann cells and their variant satellite cells, and melanocytes. Not only are neural crest cells pluripotential, but their differentiation is affected by their milieu and by interaction with surrounding cells. For instance, neurite growth and its direction is in part genetically determined, but is also strongly influenced by Schwann cell growth factors and by trophic substances produced by target organs. Best known among these is nerve growth factor (NGF), a 14-kD polypeptide encoded on chromosome 22. Particularly during development, Schwann cells produce not only NGF but possess NGF receptors. Early neurotransmitter synthesis is also induced by NGF. By its chemotactic properties and action upon the cytoskeleton of receptor-bearing axons, NGF promotes growth cone mobility in growing axons. The latter, by way of receptors, also are affected by extracellular substances such as collagen, laminin, fibronectin, and entactin.

With a few exceptions, neurons giving rise to sensory nerves lie within either cranial nerve sensory ganglia or dorsal root ganglia. Dorsal root ganglion cells are round and are encircled by satellite cells, specialized cells indistinguishable from Schwann cells. The initially single process of a sensory ganglion cell divides in a T-fashion, sending a proximal axon into the substance of the spinal cord (efferent fiber) and another distally within the sensory nerve (afferent fiber). In contrast, motor neurons lie within the central nervous system, either in motor nuclei of the brain stem or in anterior horns of the spinal cord. They send a single process distal via a motor nerve root. The central portions of sensory and motor axons are ensheathed by "central myelin" formed by oligodendrocytes. In contrast, the distally directed processes of cranial and spinal sensory and motor axons are ensheathed by Schwann cell–derived "peripheral myelin."

Myelinization in the peripheral nervous system precedes that in the central nervous system. The process is initiated by axon-Schwann cell contact. Functionally, myelin serves as an insulator and allows rapid, saltatory conduction along the fiber. During development Schwann cells follow elongating axons and form concentric sheaths around them. Actual myelination begins by the 18th week of gestation. Large axons tend to be myelinated before and to a greater extent than smaller ones. Only a minor proportion of peripheral nerves are myelinated, but all axons, regardless of size, are encircled by Schwann cells. Although the term "nerve fiber" has been used to denote either the axon alone or the axon with its accompanying Schwann sheath, we adhere to the latter definition. The axon and Schwann sheath function as a unit, not only physiologically but also in response to injury. In myelinated fibers a single Schwann cell provides myelin for a segment of only one axon, whereas in unmyelinated nerves a number of axons are ensheathed by a single Schwann cell.

GROSS ANATOMY

Anterior (motor) and posterior (sensory) spinal nerve roots exit the spinal cord separately, traverse the subarachnoid space, and coalesce just proximal to the dorsal root ganglion. Here the roots form peripheral nerve trunks surrounded by a dural sleeve that continues into the intervertebral foramen (fig. 2-1). Proximally the sheath is also formed by arachnoid tissue which becomes confluent with the perineurium (fig. 2-2). Distal to the dorsal root ganglion, having traversed the intervertebral foramen, each spinal nerve trunk divides into dorsal and ventral rami, the former supplying the posterior portion of the body and the latter the anterior portion and limbs. Plexuses such as the brachial and lumbosacral are formed by fusion of the ventral rami of adjacent spinal nerves. Major peripheral

Figure 2-1
SCHEMATIC
REPRESENTATION OF THE
SENSORIMOTOR AND
AUTONOMIC NERVES
AND THEIR GANGLIA
RELATIVE TO THE SPINAL
CORD AND MENINGES

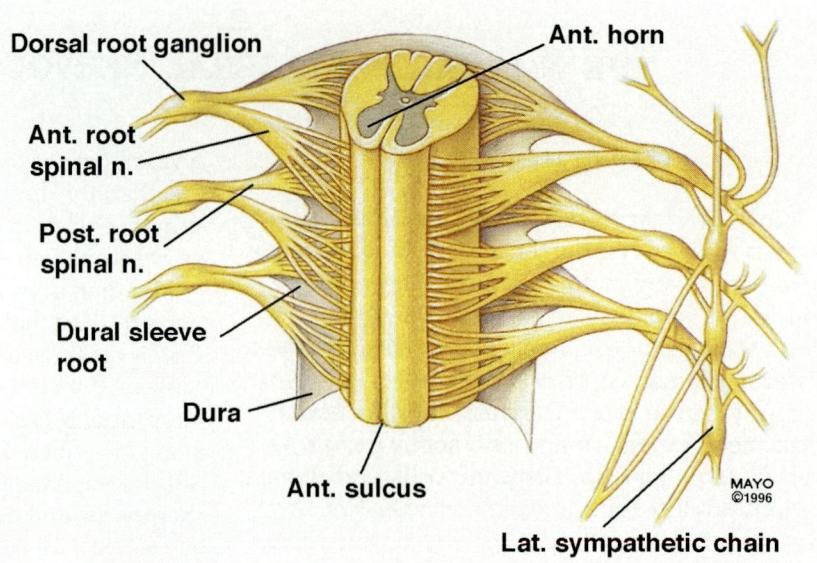

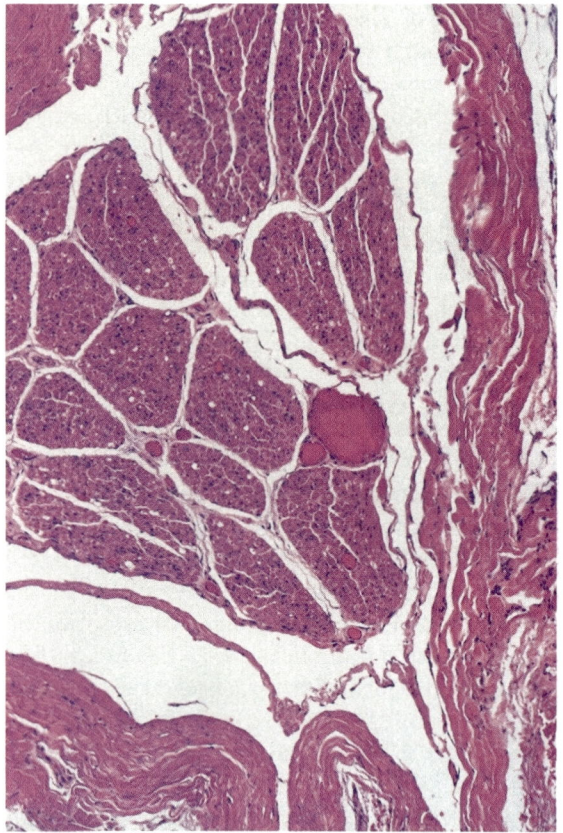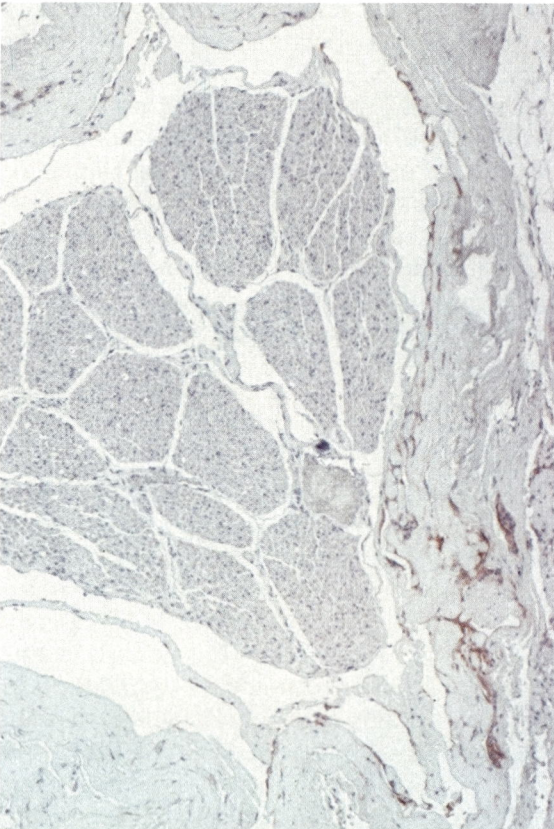

Figure 2-2
SPINAL NERVE TRUNK: RELATION OF PERINEURIUM TO MENINGES

Left: The relationship of the meninges to spinal nerve trunks is intimate.

Right: Note the delicate arachnoid membrane encircling and partly in continuity with the epithelial membrane antigen (EMA)-reactive perineurium surrounding nerve fascicles. Both are contained within the much thicker, collagen-rich dura.

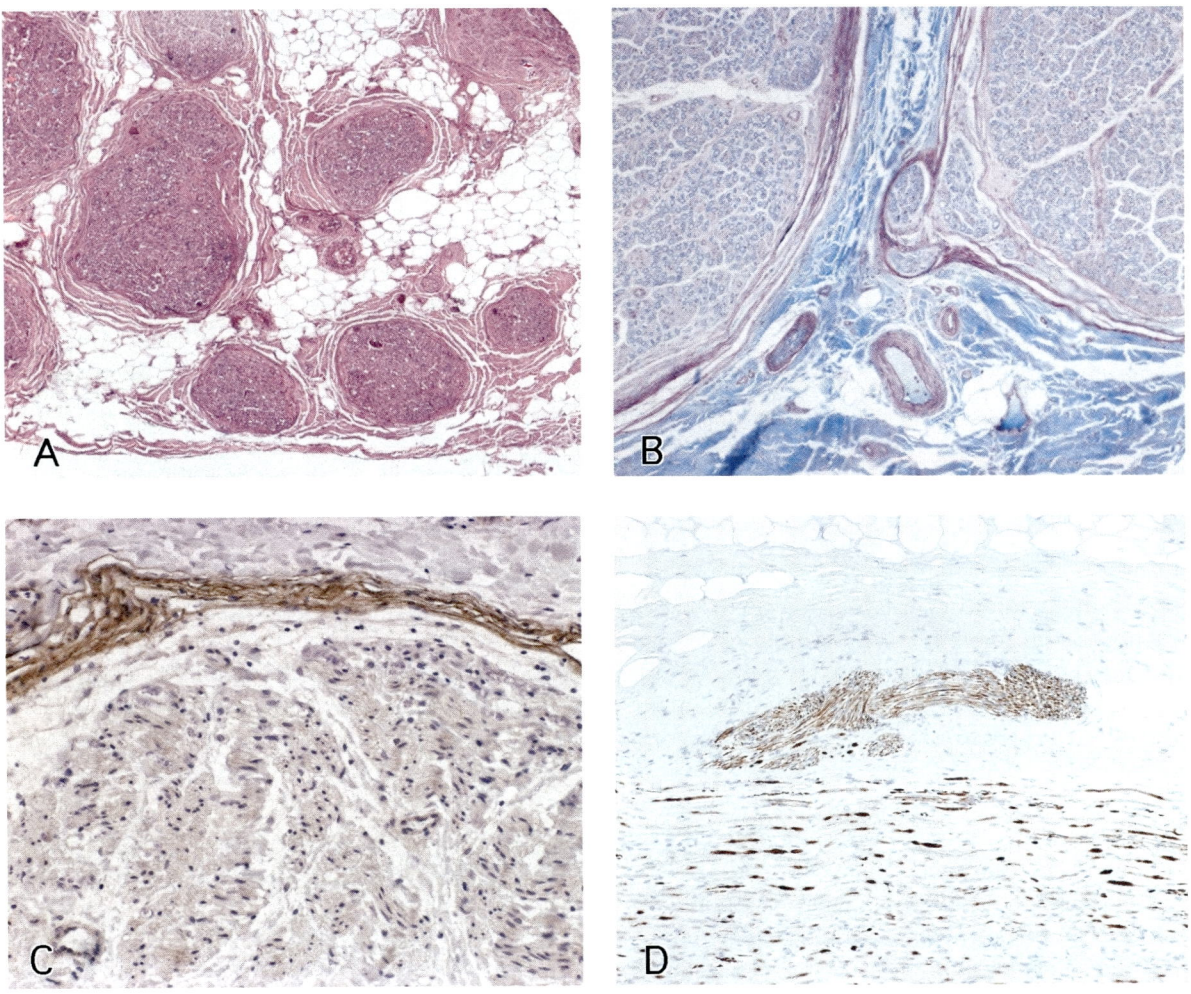

Figure 2-3
CROSS SECTION OF A NERVE

A: Seven fascicles are embedded in fibrofatty epineurial tissue.

B: On Luxol-fast blue–periodic acid-Schiff stain, two nerve fascicles are seen, each surrounded by PAS-positive perineurium. Note the vasa nervorum. The endoneurium contains numerous nerve fibers, each surrounded by a blue cylinder of myelin.

C: Epithelial membrane antigen stains the perineurium.

D: On occasion nerve fascicles may be seen to branch, here shown on neurofilament protein immunostain.

nerves originating from the plexuses thus receive fibers from multiple spinal cord segments. Peripheral nerves progressively divide into smaller nerves as, grouped or single, their fascicles sweep from them. The nerve fibers comprising a fascicle of a peripheral nerve do not necessarily remain with that parent fascicle. Instead, some bridge from one fascicle to another ("bridging fascicles") (fig. 2-3D). All peripheral nerves are compound in nature and consist of a variable admixture of motor, sensory, and autonomic nerve fibers. Motor nerve fibers terminate on somatic muscle end-plates, whereas sensory fibers terminate in specialized sensory structures or transducers in skin, muscle, and other organs (see below). Unlike spinal nerves, cranial nerves arise from the brain at irregular intervals and are not comprised of dorsal and ventral roots. Instead, the efferent and afferent fibers exit and enter the brain at the same site.

Autonomic nerves of parasympathetic and sympathetic type innervate viscera, blood vessels, and the smooth muscle of skin and eye. The preganglionic neurons of parasympathetic fibers

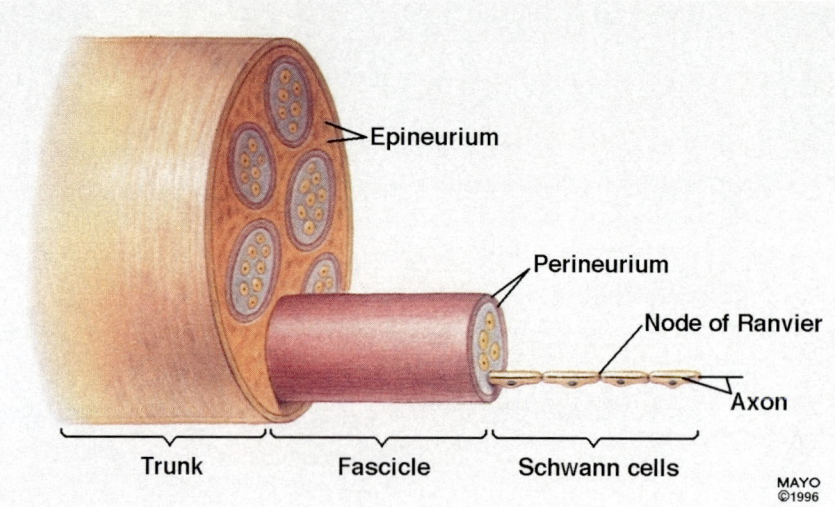

Figure 2-4
SCHEMATIC
REPRESENTATION OF
THE BASIC ARCHITECTURE
OF NORMAL NERVE

are cranial or sacral in origin, their nerve fibers exiting the brain stem in cranial nerves 3, 7, 9, 10, and 11 as well as in sacral ventral roots 2 and 3 or 3 and 4. The ganglion cells are located near or within the structures they innervate. Sympathetic preganglionic fibers, on the other hand, arise from the intermediolateral gray columns of the thoracolumbar spinal cord (T1-L2) and exit via anterior nerve roots. Such fibers are myelinated and terminate upon sympathetic ganglion cells in perivertebral or prevertebral locations.

For a more detailed discussion of the gross anatomy of the peripheral nervous system, the reader is referred to an authoritative text (7).

MICROANATOMY

Peripheral Nerves

The basic anatomy of peripheral nerves is schematically illustrated in figures 2-4 and 2-5. Normal peripheral nerves consist of shiny white bundles of fascicles surrounded and separated by fibrovascular stroma termed *epineurium,* a layer generally distinct from surrounding soft tissue. Epineurial tissue contains collagen types 1 and 3 as well as elastic fibers, the latter being most concentrated around nerve fascicles. The quantity of epineurial tissue varies and is more abundant in the vicinity of joints. Whereas large nerves have a well-developed epineurium consisting of adipose tissue as well as nutrient arteries, veins, and lymphatics, all of which follow

the course of the nerve (fig. 2-3A,B), minute nerves consisting of but one fascicle often possess little epineurial tissue. Mast cells in small number are also present in epineurium.

A functionally specialized structure, the *perineurium,* is contiguous with the arachnoid membrane (fig. 2-2) and ensheaths individual peripheral and autonomic nerve fascicles as well as their ganglia (figs. 2-3A–C, 2-6A,B). Although perineurial and arachnoidal cells share a common immunophenotype, they differ somewhat at the ultrastructural level (see below). The cytogenesis of perineurial cells, whether derived from the Schwann cell, fibroblast, or arachnoidal cell, remains unsettled (6). The terms "perineurial fibroblasts" and "perineurial epithelium" should therefore be avoided. Perineurium consists of layers of concentrically disposed, flattened, polygonal cells separated by thin layers of collagen (figs. 2-7, 2-8). The number of perineurial cells ensheathing any one fascicle varies in proportion to fascicle size. Distal nerve twigs often possess but a single layer of perineurial cells, whereas large fascicles may possess ten or more. At the termination of sensory nerves, perineurium becomes incorporated into the architecture of specialized sensory structures (see below). In motor nerves the perineurium ends in a funnel-like aperture capping the motor end-plate. Perineurial cells function as a diffusion barrier. In conjunction with the specialized vasculature of peripheral nerve, they help to maintain the physiologic milieu of the endoneurium.

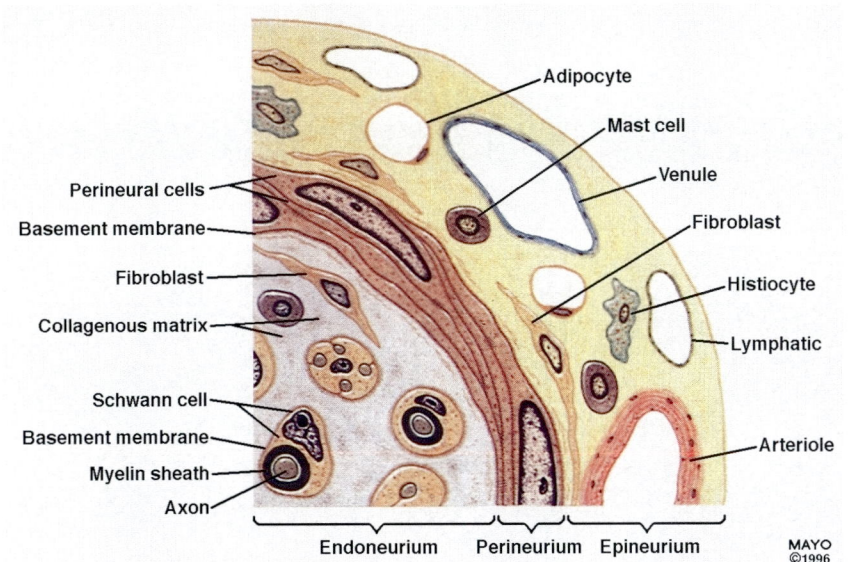

MAYO
©1996

Figure 2-5
THE ESSENTIAL
ELEMENTS OF
EPINEURIUM,
PERINEURIUM, AND
ENDONEURIUM

Contained within the encircling perineurium is the *endoneurium,* a compartment surrounding axons and accompanying Schwann cells, and wherein fibroblasts, macrophages, mast cells, and capillaries reside (figs. 2-4–2-7). The cellular constituents of the endoneurium are similar in spinal nerve roots and peripheral nerves. Approximately 20 to 30 percent of the endoneurium consists of endoneurial fluid and connective tissue matrix. Albumin is the major protein component of the endoneurial fluid and its transfer through the blood-nerve barrier may increase in pathologic conditions. The connective tissue matrix is composed of collagen fibrils, mainly of type 1, but also 2 and 3. Longitudinally oriented and in part closely ensheathing nerve fibers, they form what were once termed the sheaths of Plenk and Laidlaw, and of Key and Retzius. A distinct but inconspicuous feature of endoneurium is the finding of Renaut bodies, cylindrical hyaline structures lying on the inner aspect of the perineurium. They are collagen rich and Alcian blue positive, as is the remainder of the endoneurium. The function of Renaut bodies is uncertain, but their increased number near normal joints as well as in the setting of compressive neuropathies suggests that they may have a mechanical role as cushions.

The vasa nervorum, the vascular supply of peripheral nerves, is derived from regional arteries entering the epineurium, wherein they run longitudinally and form an anastomosing plexus (figs. 2-3A,B, 2-5, 2-6A,B). Arteriolar branches obliquely penetrate the perineurium to gain access to the endoneurial space. As they do, they carry with them a short sleeve of perineurium. The longitudinally oriented endoneurial capillary network is surrounded by pericytes. Its nonfenestrated capillary endothelium is in part the basis of the "blood-nerve barrier." This barrier is lacking in dorsal root and autonomic ganglia. Unlike epineurium, endoneurium lacks lymphatics.

Whether engaged in myelin production or not, *Schwann cells* ensheath axons of all sizes (figs. 2-5, 2-6C,D). The cytoplasm of the myelin-forming Schwann cells distributed along the length of axons is wrapped around them in a spiral fashion. In myelinated nerves only one Schwann cell ensheaths an axon segment. In unmyelinated fibers, portions of several axons are individually encased in a simple, cuff-like manner by a single Schwann cell. These relationships are schematically and ultrastructurally illustrated in figures 2-5, 2-7, 2-9, and 2-10. Although on transverse hematoxylin and eosin (H&E)–stained sections large axons may be recognized as eosinophilic dots at the center of myelin sheaths, they and their relation to the sheaths are more readily seen with special stains (fig. 2-6). In longitudinal sections, Schwann cell nuclei appear elongate and are serially arranged along the axon (fig. 2-11A,B). Their cytoplasm varies from pink to inconspicuous depending on

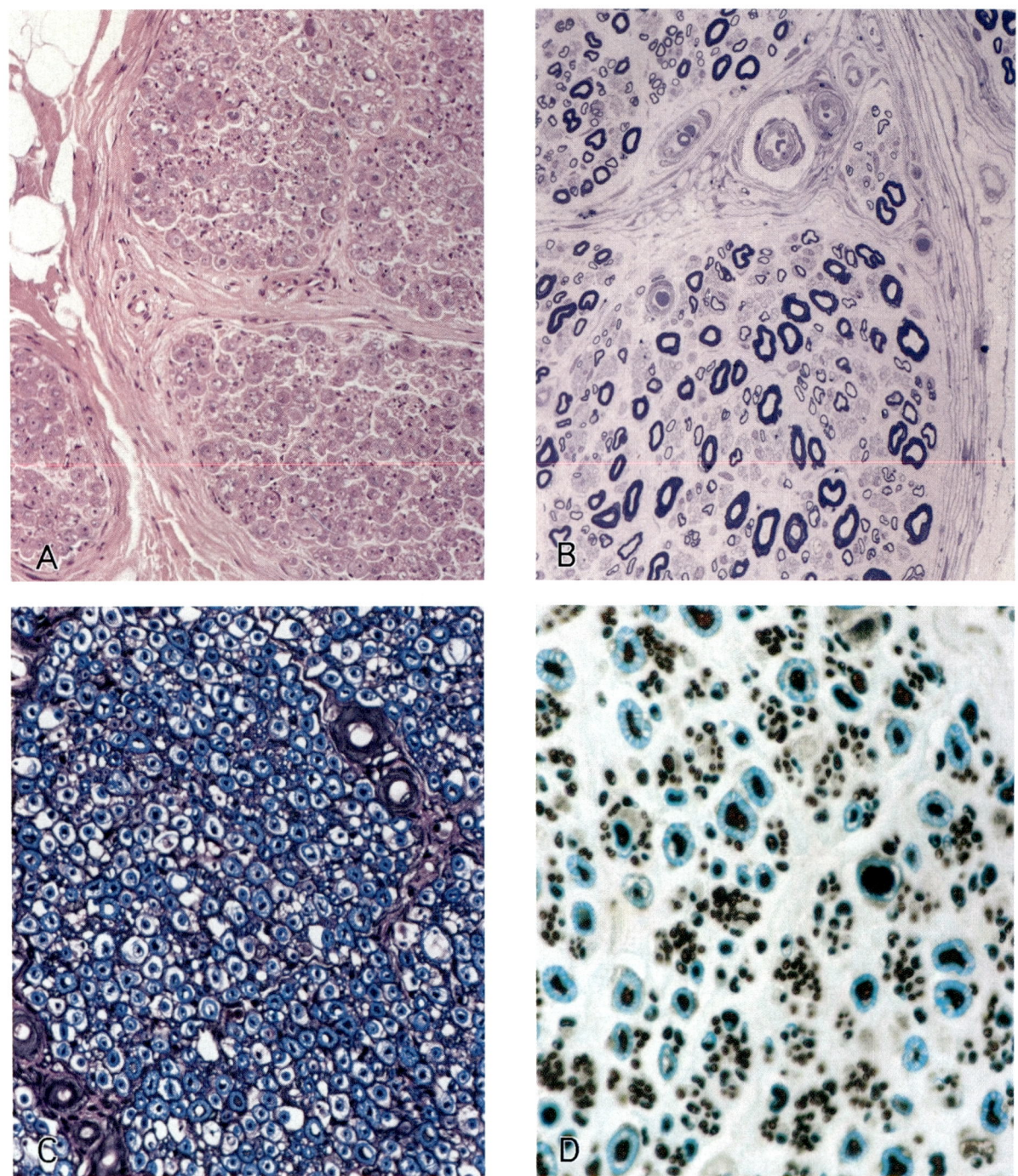

Figure 2-6
NORMAL NERVE IN CROSS SECTION

A: On H&E stain, a nerve fiber–filled fascicle is surrounded by perineurium. Myelinated axons are numerous and mainly appear as dots, each surrounded by a cuff of myelin. Unmyelinated axons are minute and inapparent.

B: The toluidine blue–stained semi-thin section shows these microanatomic features in greater detail, particularly the direct relationship between axon diameter and the thickness of myelin sheaths. An arteriole is present within a perineurial septum.

C: A Luxol-fast blue–periodic acid-Schiff–Bielschowsky stain shows myelin in sensorimotor nerves to be prominent when compared to largely unmyelinated autonomic nerves (see fig. 2-17B).

D: A combination immunostain (PGP 9.5) and LFB preparation underscores the considerable variation in axon and myelin sheath size. (B and D, courtesy of Dr. P. C. Johnson, Tucson, Arizona.)

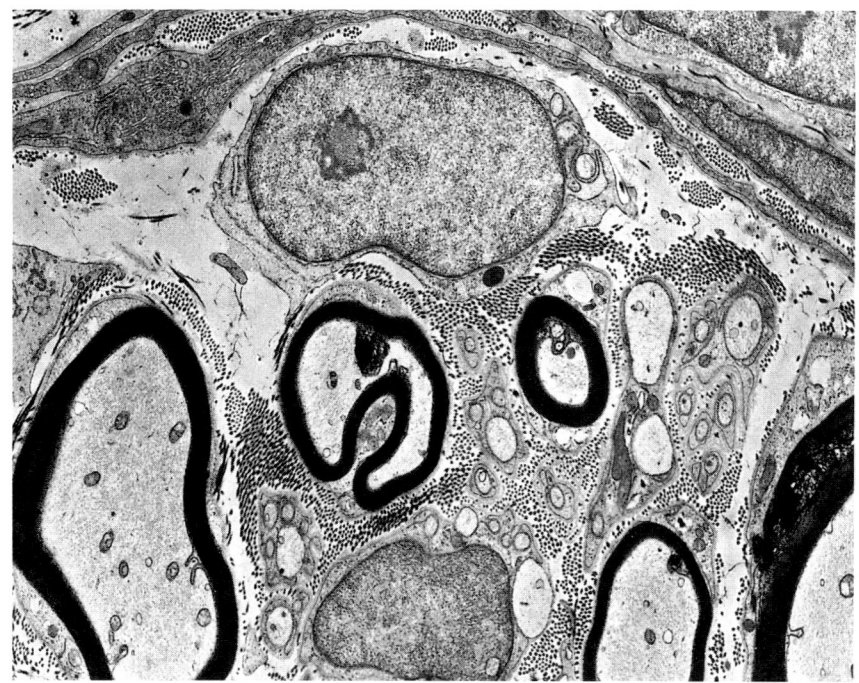

Figure 2-7
NORMAL
CUTANEOUS NERVE
Portion of a dermal nerve illustrating myelinated and unmyelinated axons and endoneurial collagen fibrils. A three cell thick sheath of perineurial cells, the perineurium, is present at the top (X10,600).

Figure 2-8
SURAL NERVE
PERINEURIAL SHEATH
Seven layers of perineurial cells are illustrated. The thin perineurial cell cytoplasmic processes contain prominent pinocytotic vesicles and are coated on both sides by a thick continuous basement membrane. Collagen fibrils are found in the intercellular matrix (X13,800).

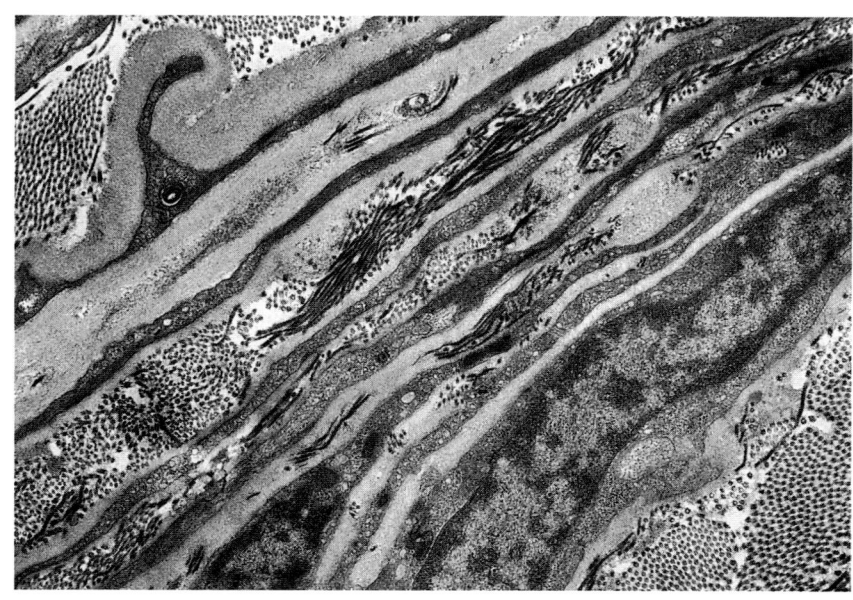

whether the nerve is myelinated or not. Axons are difficult to visualize, since in longitudinal section they typically enter and exit the visual plane. On routine H&E sections, only sizable myelinated axons are discernible. The visualization of axons is greatly enhanced, however, by silver impregnation methods (Bielschowsky or Bodian stain) and of course by immunostaining for neurofilament protein (fig. 2-11D,E). Some structures, such as nodes

of Ranvier, points of abutment between adjacent Schwann sheaths, are most clearly seen in plastic-embedded, semi-thin sections (fig. 2-12). At the light microscopic level, the intimate relationship between Schwann cells and axons is best appreciated on teased fiber preparations. Histochemically, Schwann cells exhibit pericellular reticulin staining which corresponds to the basement membrane, a structure composed of

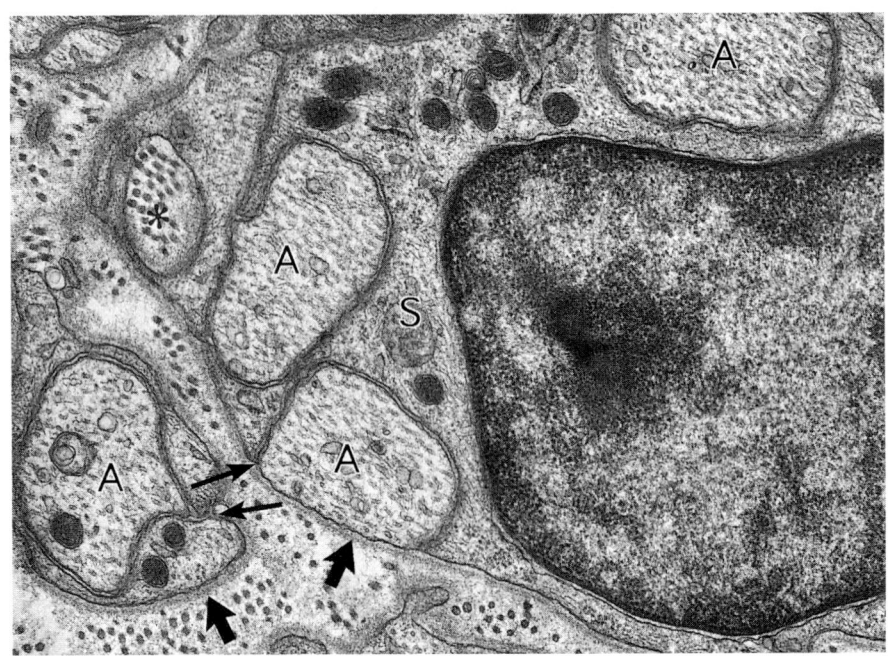

Figure 2-9
UNMYELINATED
NERVE FIBERS

This human sural nerve biopsy shows numerous unmyelinated axons (A) embedded within the surface of a single Schwann cell. The processes are entirely surrounded but no spiral of myelin is present. The Schwann cell nucleus is present at the right. A continuous basement membrane surrounds the entire Schwann cell (arrows). A "collagen pocket" is also noted (asterisk). This characteristic grouped arrangement of axons is known as a Remak bundle (X28,200). (Courtesy of Dr. G. Moretto, Verona, Italy.)

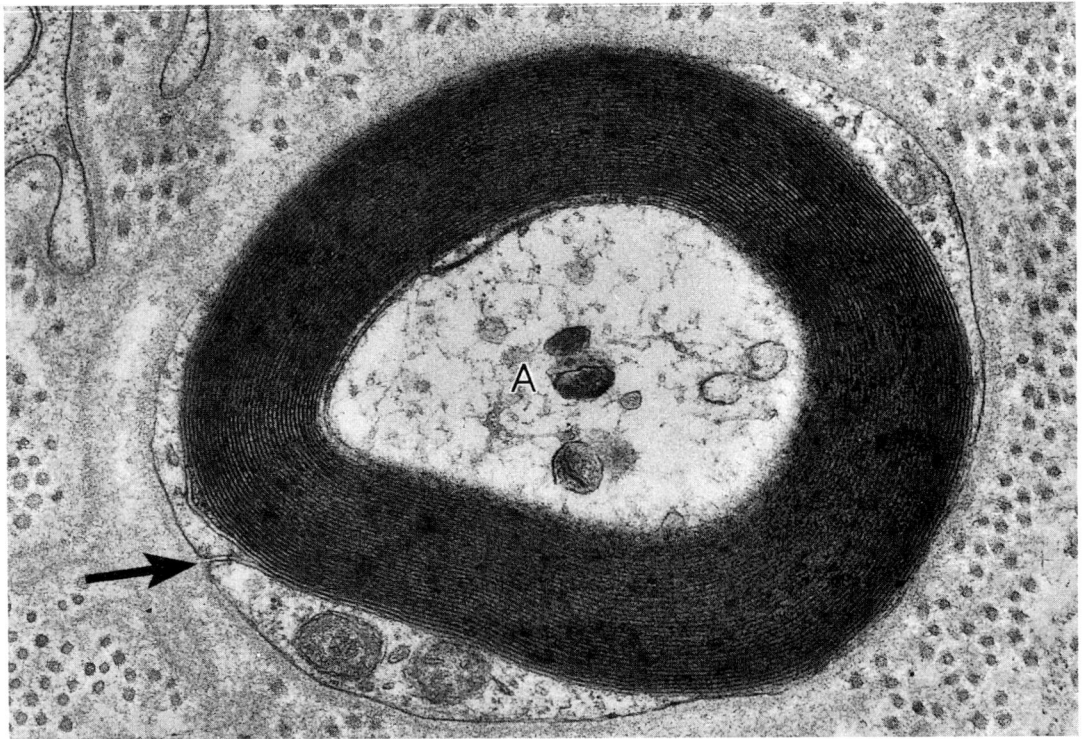

Figure 2-10
MYELINATED NERVE FIBER

This small myelinated fiber and its ensheathing Schwann cell are surrounded by a continuous basement membrane. The nucleus of the Schwann cell is not present at this level. The axon (A) contains neurofilaments, microtubules, and a few smooth endoplasmic reticulum profiles. The characteristic periodicity of the myelin sheath is apparent, with clearly visible major dense lines. Inner mesaxon formation is seen at the inner aspect of the myelin sheath in the adaxonal space. The external mesaxon is obliquely cut but can be clearly identified (arrow). The Schwann cell cytoplasm at this level contains relatively abundant rough endoplasmic reticulum, glycogen, and a small, spherical Elzholz body (X36,000). (Courtesy of Dr. G. Moretto, Verona, Italy.)

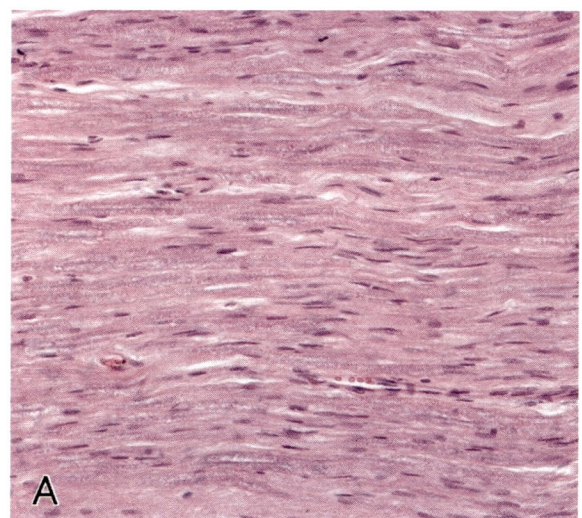

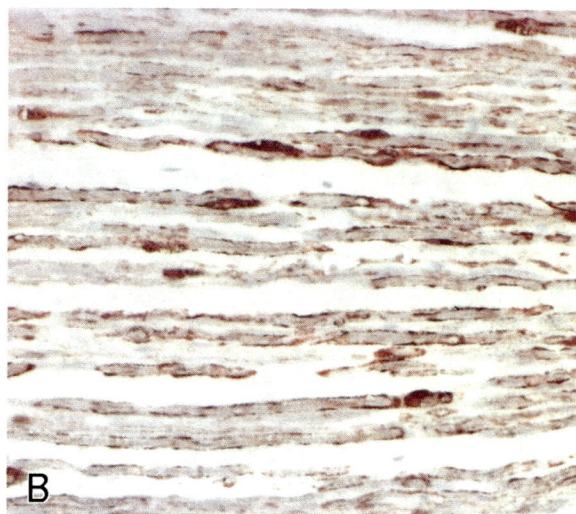

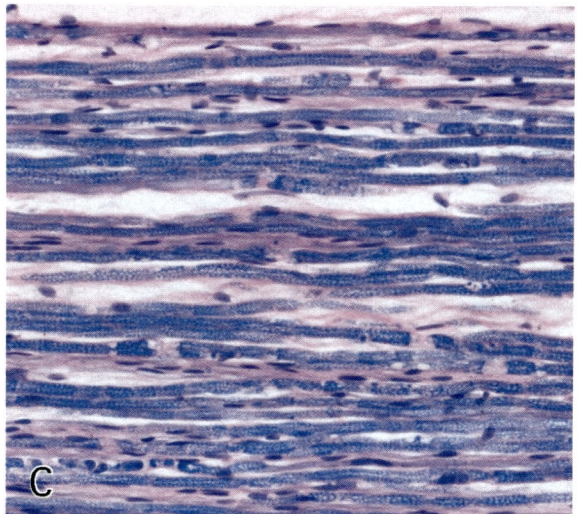

Figure 2-11
NORMAL PERIPHERAL NERVE: LONGITUDINAL
SECTION OF A SINGLE NERVE FIBER

A: On H&E stain, axons are barely discernible as delicate gray threads obscured by myelin and Schwann cells.

B: The latter, particularly their nuclei, are best seen on S-100 protein immunostain.

C: Myelin is most apparent with the LFB-PAS stain.

D: Axons are identified with silver stains, such as the Bielschowsky preparation.

E: Neurofilament protein immunostains more reliably demonstrate axons than do silver impregnations.

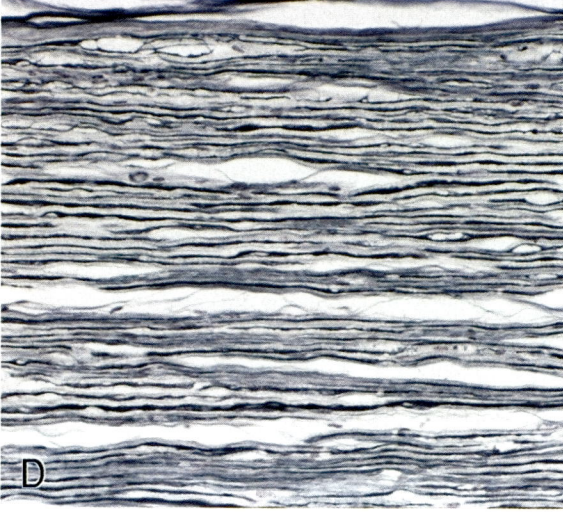

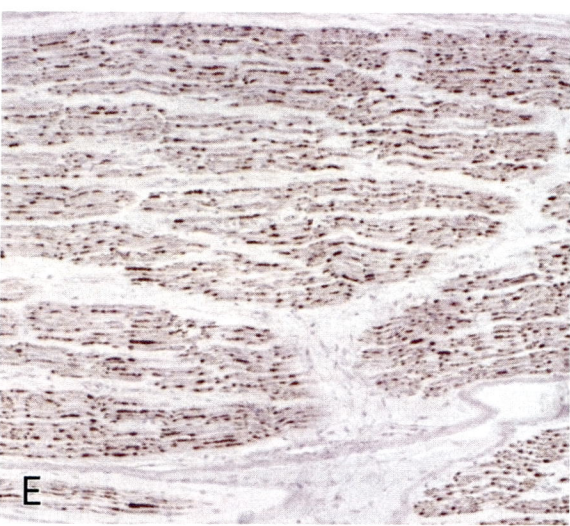

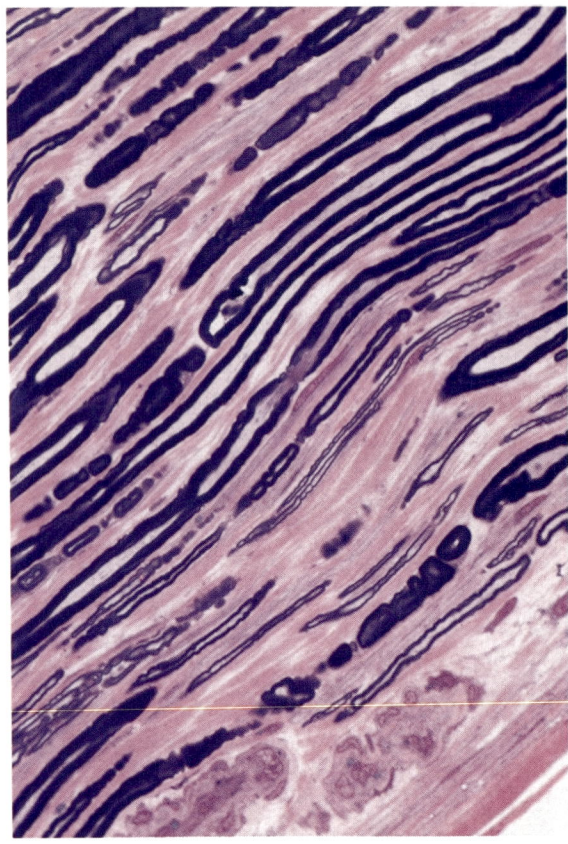

Figure 2-12
MYELINATED PERIPHERAL NERVE IN A
SEMI-THIN, OSMIUM- AND EOSIN-STAINED SECTION
Note the node of Ranvier (center), the juncture of two myelin
sheaths. (Courtesy of Dr. P. C. Johnson, Tucson, Arizona.)

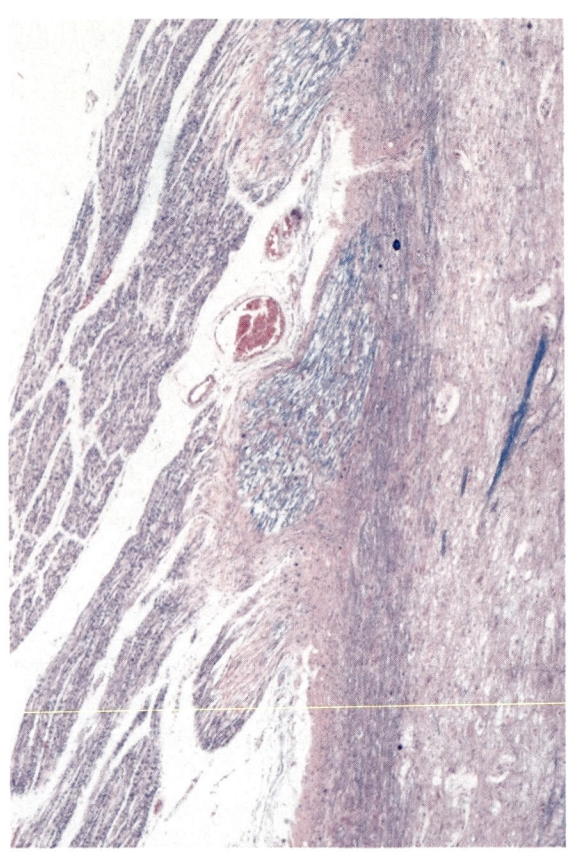

Figure 2-13
NORMAL SPINAL CORD AND NERVE ROOT
IN LONGITUDINAL SECTION
This LFB-PAS stain shows the transition zone between
the central and peripheral nervous systems. Note the lighter
staining of central, oligodendrocyte-derived myelin of the
spinal cord (right) as opposed to peripheral or Schwann cell
myelin in nerve roots (left).

laminin, fibronectin, entactin, heparin sulfate, and collagen, primarily of type 4.

Myelin is a complex substance consisting in large part (75 percent) of lipids, including cholesterol, sphingomyelin, and galactolipids, and to a lesser extent (25 percent) of protein. In the peripheral nervous system, the greater part of the protein consists of glycoprotein Po, a substance lacking in central myelin. This appears to underlie the differing antigenicity and perhaps the tinctorial characteristics of central and peripheral myelin (fig. 2-13). Myelin-associated glycoprotein (MAG) also plays an important role in myelination, being present in myelin-forming Schwann cells but not in those accompanying unmyelinated fibers.

Peripheral nerve fibers are classified by neurophysiologists according to their diameters, which are directly related to their conduction velocity.

Myelinated fibers conduct more rapidly than do nonmyelinated fibers. Peripheral nerve fibers within most nerves are of both myelinated and unmyelinated type (figs. 2-5, 2-7, 2-9, 2-10). Their relative frequencies can only be assessed by counting them at the ultrastructural level. Although myelinated fibers are readily evident in epoxy-embedded, toluidine blue–stained sections (fig. 2-6B), unmyelinated fibers are not. Longitudinal sections of peripheral nerve are less informative than are cross sections, not only in demonstrating variations in fiber type or abnormalities, such as axonal degeneration or demyelination, but in revealing the architectural features peculiar to reactive processes and some neoplasms, e.g., intraneural perineurioma.

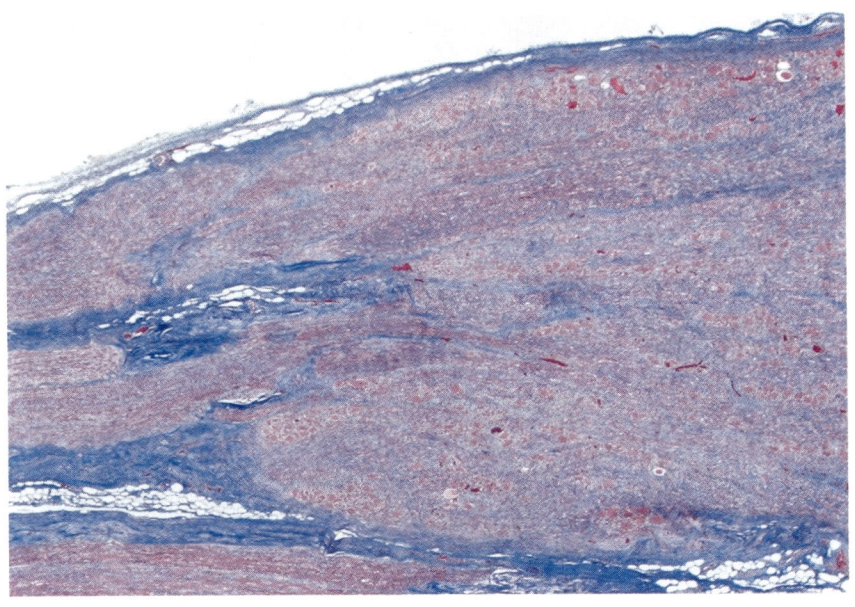

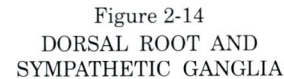

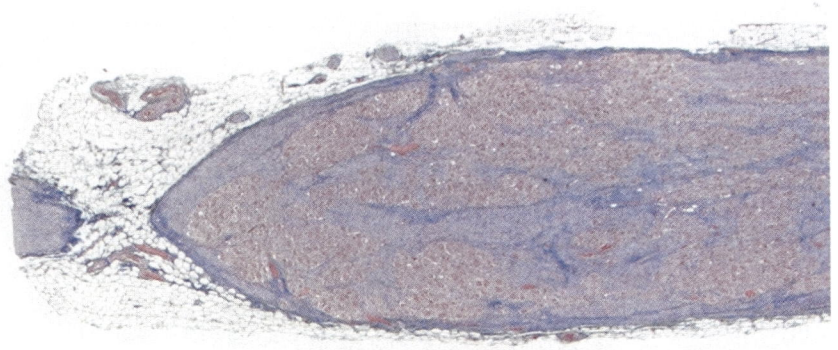

Figure 2-14
DORSAL ROOT AND
SYMPATHETIC GANGLIA
Dorsal root (top) and sympathetic ganglia (bottom), at the same magnification and stained with Masson's trichrome stain, differ markedly in size but exhibit basic architectural similarities. These include a delicate fibrous capsule, traversing bundles of afferent and efferent nerve fibers, and clustering of ganglion cells, a feature most apparent in dorsal root ganglia.

Sensory and Autonomic Ganglia

Despite significant differences in their size, the general architectural features of ganglia, be they spinal or autonomic, are similar (fig. 2-14).

Sensory Ganglia. As previously noted, fibers giving rise to sensory nerves originate either in cranial nerve sensory ganglia or in dorsal root ganglia. Aside from differences in their size and content of cytoplasmic Nissl substance, no significant differences exist between their ganglion cells. All possess centrally situated round nuclei with ve-

sicular chromatin and prominent nucleoli. Ensheathed by perineurial cells and dura, the ganglia consist of often clustered cell bodies separated by bundles of myelinated dorsal root fibers (fig. 2-15). The neurons or ganglion cells in dorsal root ganglia are of two types, small and large. These vary in terms of their neurotransmitter content and are functionally distinct. Individual ganglion cells are surrounded by specialized Schwann cells (satellite or capsular cells). In dorsal root ganglia, these totally surround ganglion cells and possess delicate overlapping cytoplasmic processes. The

17

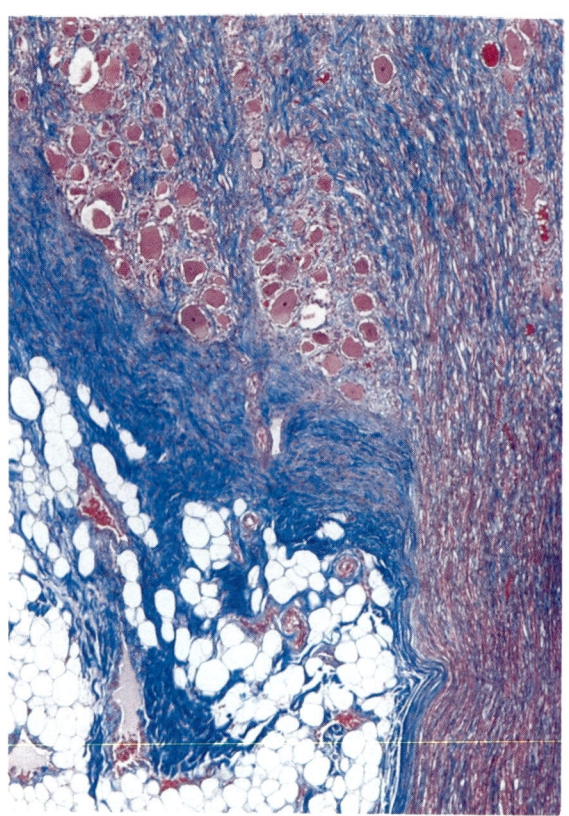 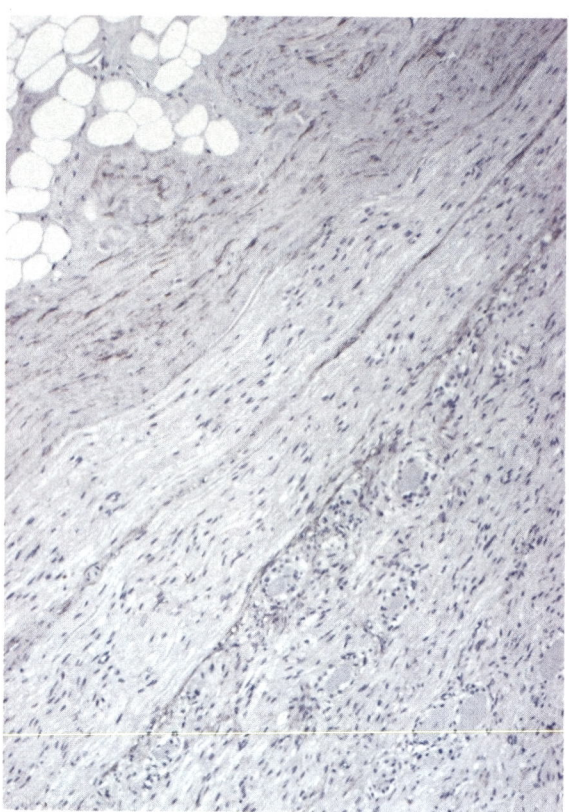

Figure 2-15
DORSAL (SENSORY) ROOT GANGLION
Left: On trichrome stain, the ganglion is seen to be surrounded by a collagenous capsule.
Right: The connective tissue capsule surrounding the ganglion contains perineurial cells as evidenced by epithelial membrane antigen (EMA) staining (upper left).

cellular ensheathment is invested by basement membrane. As expected, special histochemical and immunocytochemical stains clearly distinguish the satellite and other Schwann cells of ganglia from ganglion cells and their processes (fig. 2-16). No synapses are present in dorsal root ganglia. Although ganglion cells do possess proximal and distal processes, these result from branching of a short, initially unipolar and highly coiled process termed the glomerular segment. Lastly, in an ill-defined region of transition proximal to the ganglion, Schwann cells are replaced by oligodendrocytes on centrally directed processes (fig. 2-13). The extent of this transition zone may be somewhat variable and does not strictly correspond to the anatomic limit between a nerve root and the spinal cord surface.

Autonomic Ganglia. Ganglia are also found in the sympathetic and parasympathetic divisions of the autonomic nervous system. The structure of *sympathetic* and *dorsal root ganglia* are very similar (figs. 2-16, 2-17). Both are invested by a fibrous tissue capsule contiguous with epineurium. Their ganglion cells are surrounded by satellite or capsular cells although, unlike in dorsal root ganglia, the investment is often incomplete. In further distinction, autonomic ganglion cells are multipolar and receive synapses from preganglionic fibers. The majority of these synapses are to dendrites. As in dorsal root ganglia, autonomic ganglion cells are not uniform: some are relatively large with eccentric nuclei, vesicular chromatin, prominent nucleoli, and abundant Nissl substance. Dense core granule–containing, these cells are adrenergic. In many sympathetic ganglia a second, minor population of smaller ganglion cells is identified, the nuclei of which are often ovoid or convoluted and contain

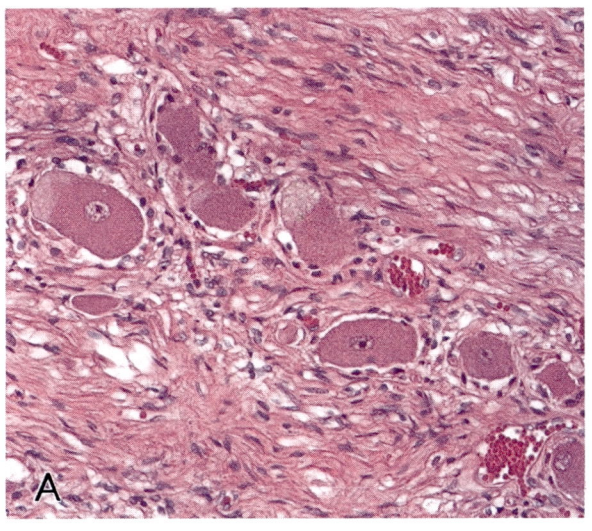

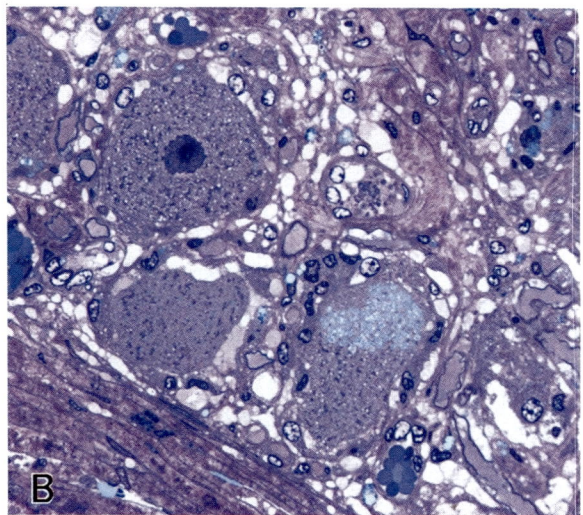

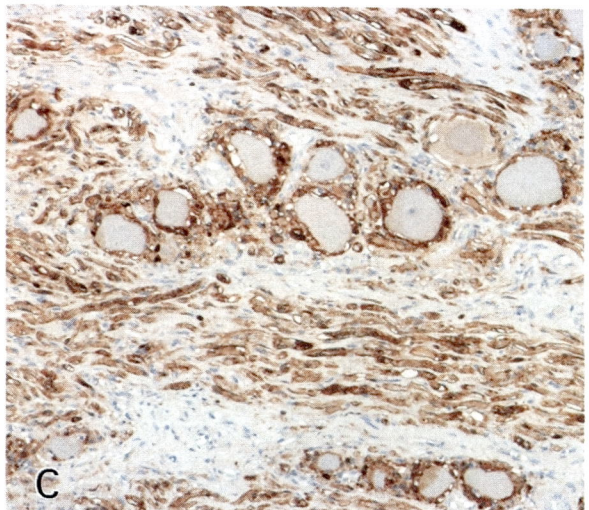

Figure 2-16

DORSAL (SENSORY) ROOT GANGLION

A: The clustered ganglion cells lie separated by bundles of their nerve fibers.

B,C: The ganglion cells with their centrally situated nuclei are surrounded by satellite cells best seen on toluidine blue stained semi-thin sections (B) and on S-100 protein immunostain (C).

D,E: Myelinated nerve fiber bundles traversing the ganglion are seen with LFB-PAS-Bielschowsky's stain (D) as well as with neurofilament protein immunostain (E).

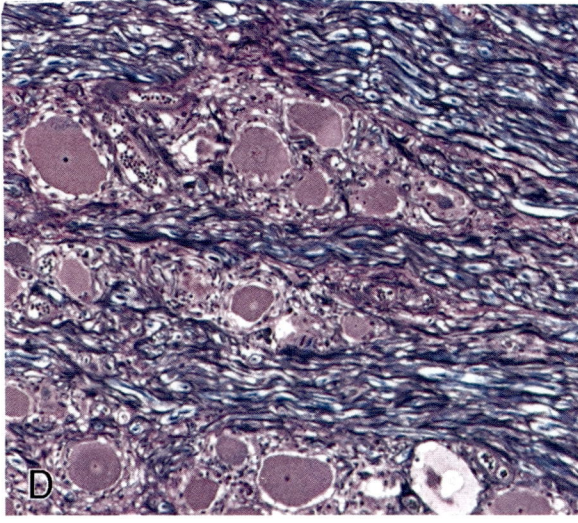

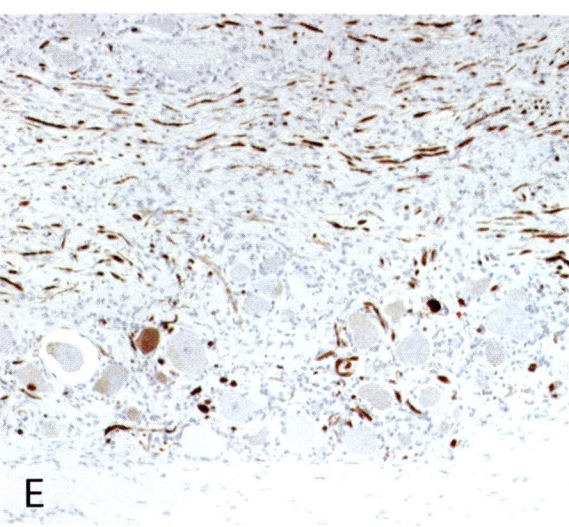

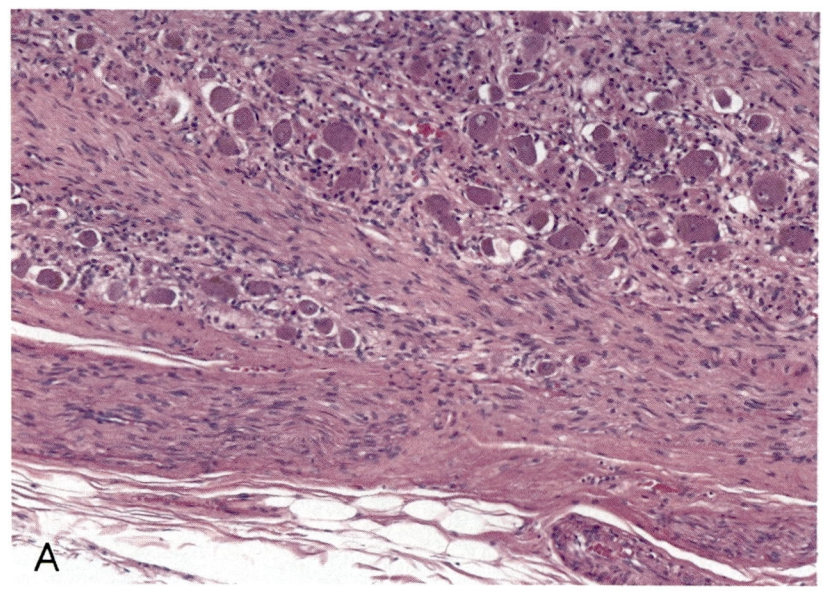

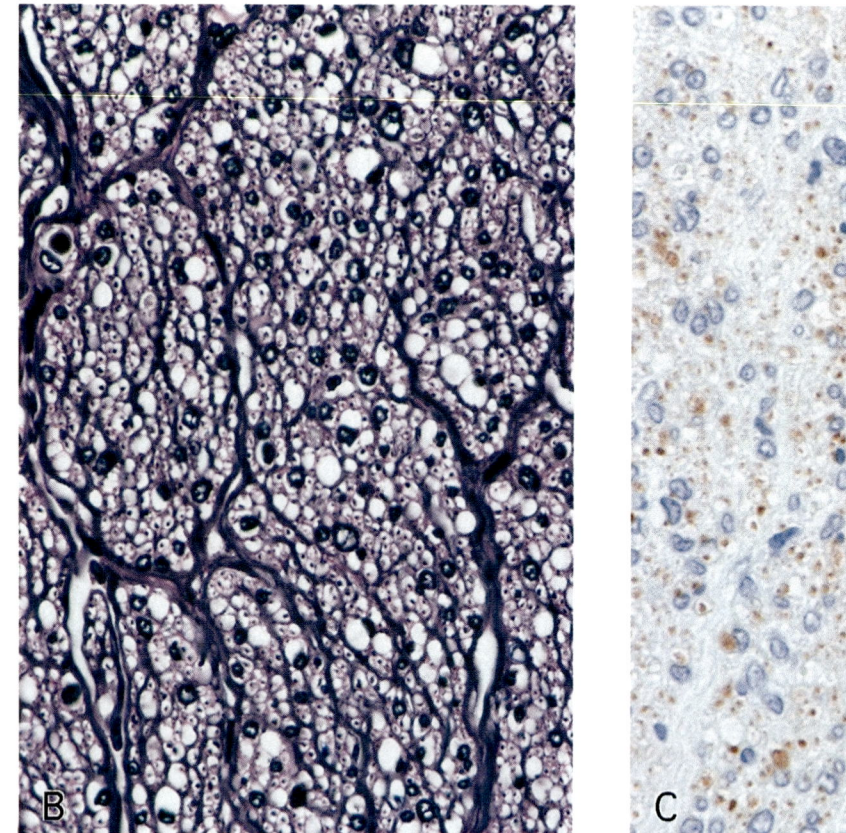
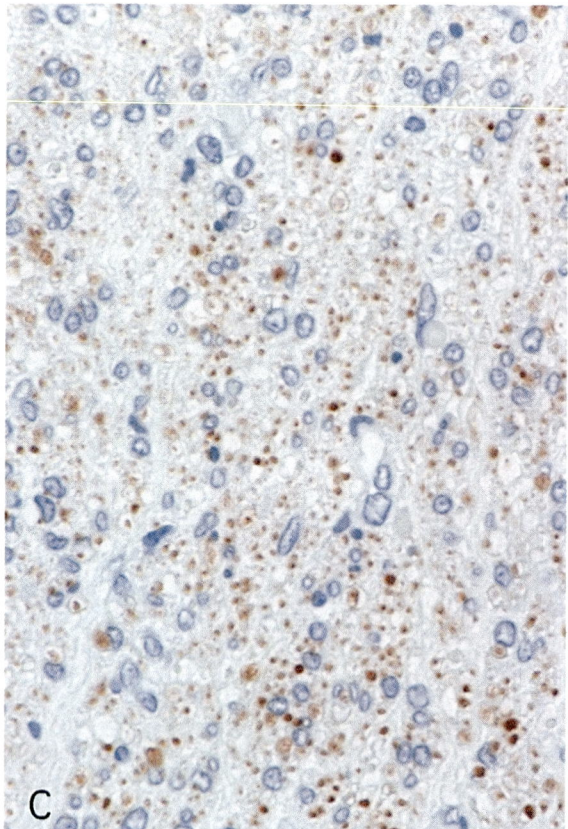

Figure 2-17
CERVICAL SYMPATHETIC GANGLION AND NERVE

Although these ganglia closely resemble dorsal root (sensory) ganglia (fig. 2-12), at least three differences (A) are apparent. Sympathetic ganglia appear more cellular, and their neurons are both smaller and feature eccentric nuclei. On LFB-PAS-Bielschowsky's stain (B), sympathetic nerves are seen to be largely unmyelinated and to contain minute axons. The small size of these axons is best seen on neurofilament protein immunostains (C).

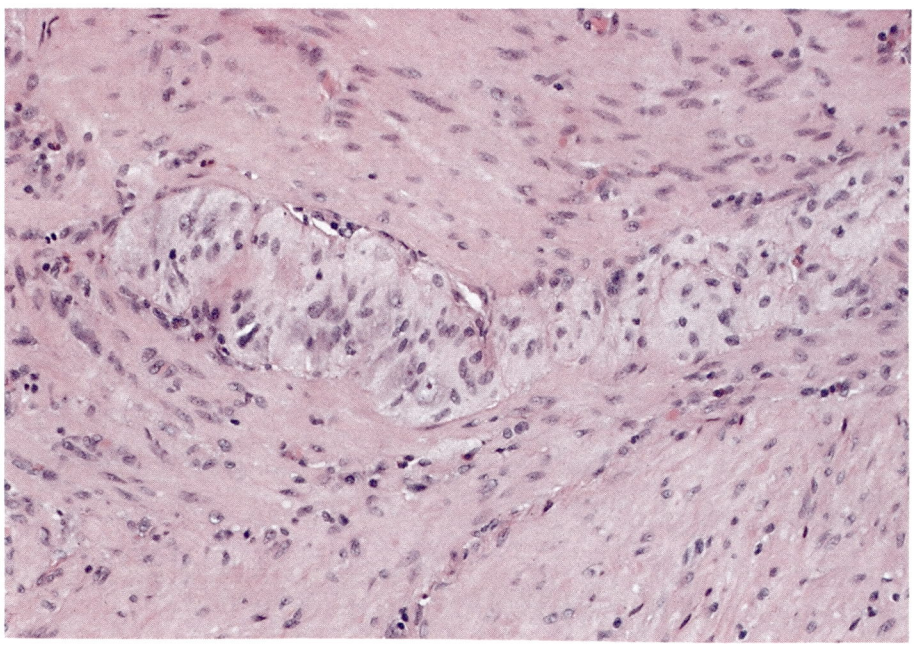

Figure 2-18
PARASYMPATHETIC GANGLIA OF COLON
The myenteric plexus consists of ganglia and nerves distributed as a circumferential layer between inner and outer muscle coats.

more heterochromatin. These cells contain large dense core granules and are dopaminergic.

Of *parasympathetic ganglia,* those arising in the gastrointestinal tract are most relevant to the surgical pathology of the peripheral nervous system (fig. 2-18). They lie within the wall of the gut, connected with nerves derived from the vagus nerve and the sacral outflow. Such intramural ganglia occur in two locations, the submucosa (Meissner's plexus) and between the layers of the muscularis propria (Auerbach's or myenteric plexus). Surrounded by satellite or capsular cells, the ganglion cells possess many dendrites and typically have eccentrically situated nuclei, again of vesicular type with prominent nucleoli. Parasympathetic nerves of the gut are cholinergic. They contain not only acetylcholine, but also vasoactive intestinal polypeptide, a gut hormone. A number of other peptides have also been identified in parasympathetic nerves and ganglia. Stimulation of parasympathetic nerves generally increases muscular activity, circulation, and secretion. In contrast, these activities are decreased by stimulation of the sympathetic nerves, the ganglia of which lie outside the gut.

The principal histologic stains useful in the study of peripheral nerve pathology are summarized in Table 2-1.

Specialized Nerve Endings

Because non-neoplastic lesions may affect specialized nerve endings, and since a variety of peripheral nerve neoplasms may mimic the architecture of sensory endings, a brief discussion is in order (5,10,15).

Nerve endings, among which sensory ones are most numerous, include free nerve endings, expanded tip endings, and encapsulated tip endings. *Free nerve endings* are unassociated with specialized receptor structures and subserve pain, touch, and temperature sensation. Their fibers usually measure less than 1 mm in diameter and lose their Schwann sheaths near their terminations. Such receptors are most numerous in epidermis and cornea, about tendons, and within soft tissue. *Expanded tip endings* are characterized by bulbous terminations. Principal among them are Merkel's touch corpuscles which consist of 10-mm nerve terminals forming a flat disk upon the Merkel cells

Table 2-1

HISTOLOGIC TECHNIQUES FOR PERIPHERAL NERVES

General Stains

Hematoxylin and eosin	Detection of inflammation including vasculitis, fibrosis; myelin and axons
Reticulin	Basement membrane surrounding Schwann cells in normal nerve are barely evident, but are more readily demonstrated in nerve sheath tumors
Masson trichrome	Fibrosis; fibrinoid necrosis in vasculitis; myelin, red
Alcian blue	Glycosaminoglycans, blue
Toluidine blue	Mast cells, metachromatic; general stain for semi-thin resin sections

Stains for Myelin

Luxol-fast blue	Myelin, blue; can be combined with silver stains for axon
Periodic acid–Schiff	Degenerating myelin and macrophages; perineurium
Osmium	Myelin, black
Congo red	Amyloid

Stains for Axons

Bodian, Bielschowsky, or Palmgren (silver stains)	Axons, black

Immunocytochemistry

S-100 protein	Schwann cells, normal and neoplastic
Leu-7 (CD56)	Schwann cells, normal and neoplastic
Glial fibrillary acidic protein	Some Schwann cells and Schwann cell tumors
Myelin basic protein	Myelin
Epithelial membrane antigen	Perineurial cells
Synaptophysin	Axons, neurons
Neurofilament protein	Axons, neurons
Collagen 4, laminin	Basement membranes

of skin receptors involved in pressure sensation. Expanded nerve terminals for cold sensation terminate upon basal epidermal cells. *Encapsulated tip endings* are among the most frequent of sensory endings encountered in peripheral nerve pathology. These include Meissner corpuscles, pacinian corpuscles, and muscle spindles.

Meissner Corpuscles. These receptors sense low frequency vibrations and touch, and are most numerous in glabrous skin of the fingertips, palms, and soles, as well as in sensitive mucosal surfaces. They measure 50 to 150 μm and are small in comparison to pacinian corpuscles. Meissner corpuscles are laminated structures (fig. 2-19) composed of flattened layers of Schwann cells oriented across the long axis of one or several nerve fibers entering one end of the corpuscle. Having lost their myelination, such fibers branch or spiral in a zigzag fashion, making contact with the specialized Schwann cells throughout the corpuscle. As expected, the

layered Schwann cells are S-100 protein immunoreactive and the axons stain for neurofilament protein (fig. 2-19B,C) (15). Normal Meissner corpuscles lack EMA reactivity (16).

Pacinian (Vater-Pacini) Corpuscles. These structures were the first receptors to be recognized and have been particularly well studied (5). They are fully differentiated in the 20-cm fetus and function as pressure or tension receptors capable of sensing high frequency vibrations. It is thought unlikely that stimulation of pacinian corpuscles produces subjective sensations. They are most numerous in the deep dermis of the hands and feet. To underscore their frequency, a single finger may contain up to 350 such corpuscles (5). Their well-documented association with arteriovenous anastomoses of the skin suggests that pacinian corpuscles also have a vasoregulatory role. Such corpuscles are also found in the vicinity of joints, tendons, periosteum and perimysium, as well as within mesentery and

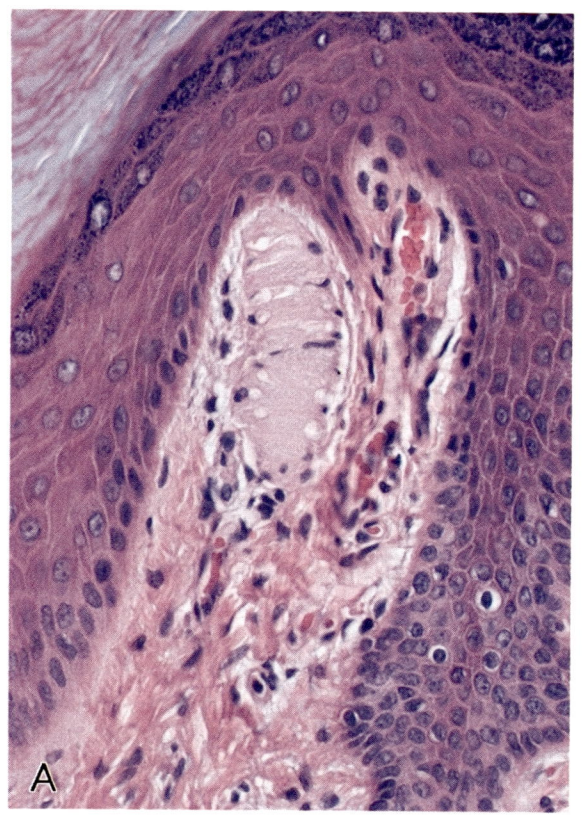

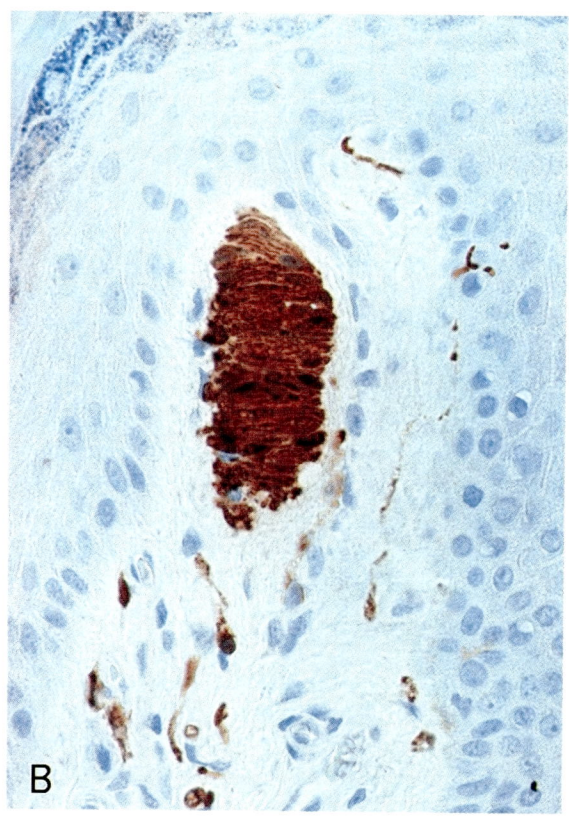

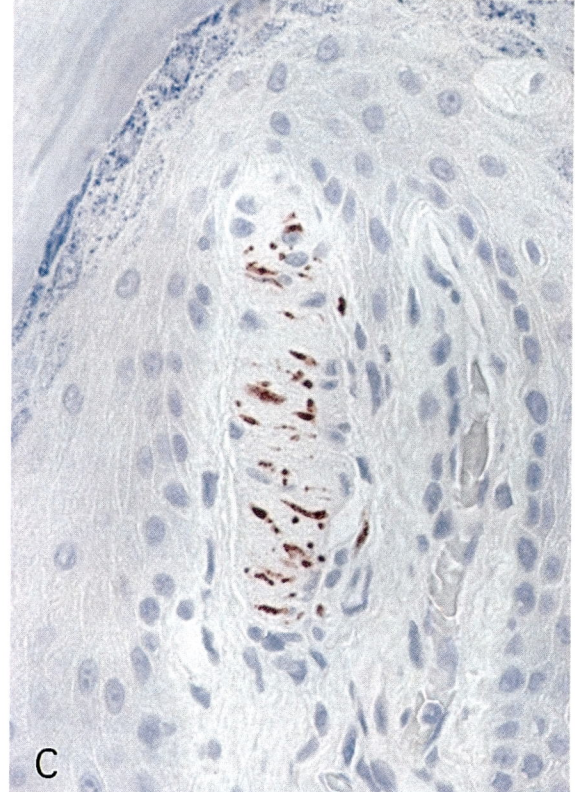

Figure 2-19
MEISSNER CORPUSCLES
These tactile bodies lie within the papillary dermis (A) and consist of stacked lamellae of S-100 protein–positive Schwann cells (B) between which are interposed neurofilament protein–positive axons (C).

sensitive mucosal surfaces. They are also found in association with large vessels where they appear to act as pressor receptors. Single or occasionally paired, pacinian corpuscles are connected to their parent nerve by a myelinated nerve fiber. Less often they are more intimately associated with the parent nerve, lying either within the epineurium or near the perineurium.

Pacinian corpuscles represent the largest of sensory receptors, measuring less than 1 mm in maximal dimension at birth and up to 4 mm in adulthood. Their structure and function is the basis of a recent review (4). Distributed singly or in groups (see fig. 3-15), these oval or occasionally folded, rice grain-like structures are surrounded by a collagenous capsule and consist of an outer and inner bulb (fig. 2-20A,B). The outer bulb is composed of 20 to 60 onion-like lamellae of flattened perineurial cells with scant intervening collagen fibrils (fig. 2-20B,C). Each layer measures approximately 1 μm in thickness and is epithelial membrane antigen immunopositive (fig. 2-20D) (15). A sizable artery enters the mid-portion of the corpuscle, its capillaries ramifying within the interlamellar spaces. At the avascular center of the corpuscle, the inner bulb, lies a large, neurofilament protein–positive (fig. 2-20E) nerve fiber which has lost its myelin sheath to become flattened, branched, and coiled. Its spray of knob-like terminal endings occupies the center of the corpuscle and is surrounded by multiple lamellae of S-100 protein–immunoreactive Schwann cells (fig. 2-20F). Pacinian corpuscles grow by the addition of lamellae and by retrograde extension along their nerve. In the process, their myelinated nerve fibers come to lie more deeply within the corpuscle. With age, the corpuscles exhibit regressive changes, become smaller and irregular in configuration, and undergo interlamellar and pericorpuscular fibrosis.

Muscle Spindles. These highly specialized receptors are involved in proprioception. Although present in all striated muscles, they are most numerous in those involved in delicate movements of the eye, hand, and neck. Muscle spindles consist of 3 to 20 modified striated muscle fibers ranging from 1 to 5 mm in length and up to 0.2 cm in diameter. Termed intrafusal fibers, they are smaller than normal skeletal muscle fibers. Intrafusal fibers include one or two long, thick fibers with central aggregated nuclei (nuclear bag

fibers) as well as more numerous short, thin fibers in which nuclei are arranged longitudinally (nuclear chain fibers). Both exhibit cross striations. Myelinated motor and sensory nerve fibers enter the muscle spindle to branch and spiral among the muscle fibers at its center. The nerves maintain tone within the spindle and sense its degree and rate of stretch. Analogous structures also occur in tendons (tendon spindles of Golgi). For a more detailed discussion of the microanatomy of the muscle spindle, the reader is referred to authoritative texts (13,14).

IMMUNOCYTOCHEMISTRY

Familiarity with the immunoreactivities of nerve is important to understand nerve sheath tumors. Schwann cells are characterized by strong staining for vimentin and S-100 protein, an acidic protein of unknown function. Both Schwann cells engaged in myelin formation and those in nonmyelinated nerves are immunoreactive. Leu-7, an antibody directed against human killer T cells, also stains Schwann cells by recognizing a carbohydrate epitope on myelin-associated glycoprotein (MAG) (12). Some but not all Schwann cells stain for glial fibrillary acidic protein (GFAP), the principal component of glial fibrils in both astrocytes and ependymal cells (8). This antigen seems to be present mainly in Schwann cells not engaged in myelin formation (9). As previously noted, pericellular basement membrane contains laminin, fibronectin, entactin, and various collagens, mainly type 4. Thus immunoreactivity for collagen 4 and laminin is of diagnostic use for the demonstration of Schwann cell–associated basement membranes. MAG plays a role in myelination, being present in the membranes of Schwann cells engaged in myelination but lacking in those accompanying nonmyelinated axons. Perineurial cells also exhibit vimentin staining but unlike Schwann cells, lack immunoreactivity for S-100 protein, Leu-7, and GFAP (11,12). Perineurium and arachnoid membrane (2,11) share some similarities in that both are reactive for epithelial membrane antigen (EMA), a group of carbohydrate-rich, protein-poor, high molecular weight substances present in nearly all epithelia and in plasma cells. Nerve sheath fibroblasts are immunoreactive for vimentin alone.

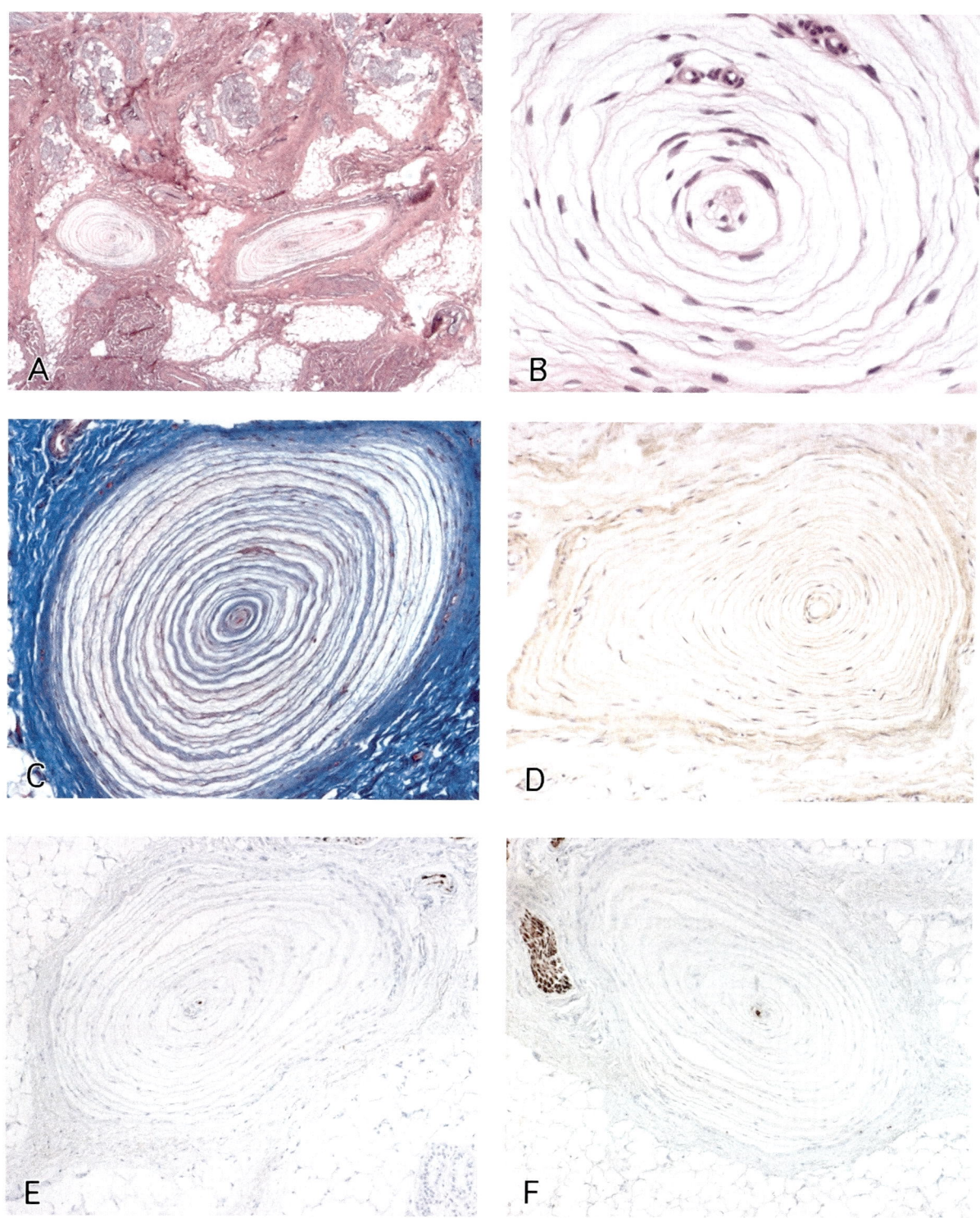

Figure 2-20
PACINIAN CORPUSCLES

These specialized receptors, here seen at the dermal-subcutaneous junction (A), consist of an outer core composed of spherical laminae of perineurial cells (B) with interposed delicate collagen (C, trichrome). The perineurial cells stain for epithelial membrane antigen (D). The delicate central nerve fiber and accompanying Schwann sheath that comprise the inner core are best seen on neurofilament protein (E) and S-100 protein immunostains (F).

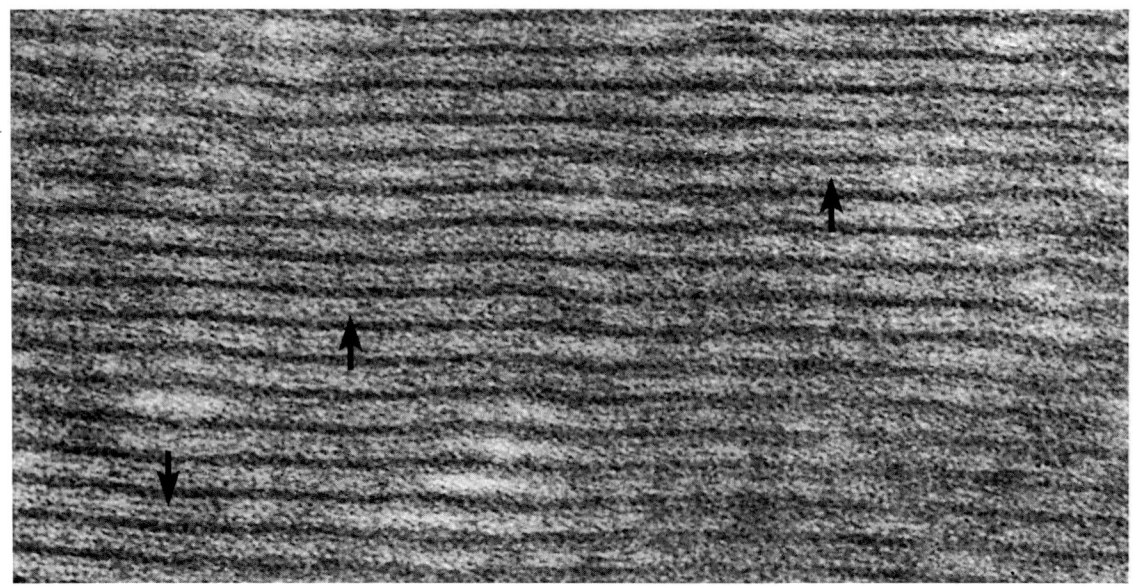

Figure 2-21
MYELIN SHEATH
Detail of the myelin sheath of a medium-sized myelinated nerve from the parotid gland. The myelin sheath consists of alternating major dense lines with a periodicity of approximately 12 nm and two intraperiod lines with a 2-nm intraperiod gap. The double intraperiod lines are seen in favorable planes of section (arrows) (X210,000).

ULTRASTRUCTURE

The cellular composition and fine structural features of peripheral nerves are readily apparent on transmission electron microscopy (fig. 2-7). As previously noted, unmyelinated axons in varying number are enclosed by the cytoplasm of a single Schwann cell (fig. 2-9). Axons are readily recognized by the presence of numerous, fairly evenly spaced microtubules having an average diameter of 25 nm, as well as of 10-nm neurofilaments. Occasional mitochondria and ribosomes also are found within axoplasm.

Unlike unmyelinated nerve fibers, more than one of which may be embedded within the surface of a single Schwann cell, myelinated examples appear as a single axon surrounded by a myelin sheath formed by concentric wrappings of the Schwann cell membrane (fig. 2-10). The space formed by the outer invaginating Schwann cell membranes is called the *external mesaxon* (fig. 2-10), whereas the junction where the membranes separate to surround the axon is sometimes referred to as the *internal mesaxon*. Ultrastructural studies show the *myelin sheath* to be formed of uniform, multilayered, spiral wrappings of the Schwann cell membrane which at high magnification appear as 3-nm thick major dense lines alternating with an intraperiod line doublet separated by a space known as the intraperiod gap (fig. 2-21) (1). The periodicity of the major dense lines is approximately 12 nm.

The outer Schwann cell membrane of both myelinated and unmyelinated axons is separated from the endoneurial matrix by a continuous *basement membrane* (figs. 2-9, 2-10). The endoneurial matrix is electron lucent and contains primarily collagen fibrils. Cellular constituents of *endoneurium* include fibroblasts containing often branching rough endoplasmic reticulum, endothelial cells and pericytes of small blood capillaries, mast cells, and macrophages.

The endoneurium is surrounded by the *perineurial sheath* (fig. 2-7), which on cross section consists of multiple layers of elongated perineurial cells bounded on their inner and outer aspect by a continuous, irregularly thick basement membrane and a matrix consisting mainly of collagen fibrils (fig. 2-8). Perineurial cells with their elongate, blunt-ended nuclei are characterized by long, thin, bipolar cytoplasmic processes, the cell membranes of which exhibit pinocytotic vesicles.

Such vesicles are also evident in the cytoplasm of perineurial cells (fig. 2-8). Organelles are sparse although diffuse arrays of both actin microfilaments and vimentin intermediate filaments may be prominent. For a more detailed discussion of the fine structure of peripheral nerves, the reader is referred to several authoritative texts (1,14).

REFERENCES

1. Angevine JB. The nervous tissue. In: Bloom and Fawcett. A textbook of histology. New York: Chapman and Hall, 1994:309–64.

2. Ariza A, Bilbao JM, Rosai J. Immunohistochemical detection of epithelial membrane antigen in normal perineurial cells and perineuriomas. Am J Surg Pathol 1988;12:678–83.

3. Barker D, Bank R. The muscle spindle. In: Engle A, Armstrong F, eds. Myology: basic and clinical. New York: McGraw-Hill, 1994:333–56

4. Bell J, Bolanowski S, Holmes MH. The structure and function of pacinian corpuscles—a review. Prog Neurobiol 1994;42:79–128.

5. Cauna N, Mannan G. The structure of human digital pacinian corpuscles (corpuscula lamellosa) and its functional significance. J Anat 1958;92:1–20.

6. Erlandson RA. The enigmatic perineurial cell and its participation in tumors and in tumor-like entities. Ultrastruct Pathol 1991;15:335–51.

7. Gardner E, Bunge RP. Gross anatomy of the peripheral nervous system. In: Dyck PJ, Thomas PK, eds. Peripheral neuropathy. 3rd ed. Philadelphia: W.B. Saunders Co., 1993:8–27.

8. Gould VE, Moll R, Moll I, Lee I, Schwechheimer K, Franke WW. The intermediate filament complement of the spectrum of nerve sheath neoplasms. Lab Invest 1986;55:463–74.

9. Gray MH, Rosenberg AE, Dickersin GR, Bhan AK. Glial fibrillary acidic protein and keratin expression by benign and malignant nerve sheath tumors. Hum Pathol 1989;20:1089–96.

10. Malinkovsky L. Sensory nerve formations in the skin and their classification. Microsc Res Tech 1996;34:283–301.

11. Perentes E, Nakagawa Y, Ross G, Stanton C, Rubinstein LJ. Expression of epithelial membrane antigen in perineurial cells and their derivatives: an immunohistochemical study with multiple markers. Acta Neuropathol (Berlin) 1987;75:160–5.

12. Perentes E, Rubinstein LJ. Recent applications of immunoperoxidase histochemistry in human neuro-oncology. An update. Arch Pathol Lab Med 1987;111:796–812.

13. Poppele RE. The muscle spindle in peripheral neuropathy. In: Dyck PJ, Thomas PK, eds. Peripheral neuropathy. Philadelphia: W.B. Saunders Co., 1993:121–40.

14. Thomas PK, Berthold CH, Ochoa J. Microscopic anatomy of the peripheral nervous system. In: Dyck PJ, Thomas PK, eds. Peripheral neuropathy. Philadelphia: W.B. Saunders Co., 1993:28–92.

15. Vega JA, Haro JJ, Del Valle ME. Immunohistochemistry of human cutaneous Meissner and pacinian corpuscles. Microsc Res Tech 1996;34:351–61.

3
REACTIVE LESIONS

The non-neoplastic lesions discussed herein are included in this Fascicle because they clinically, radiographically, or histologically mimic neoplasms. Of these, traumatic and pacinian neuromas are "true neuromas," hyperplastic lesions composed of both axons and nerve sheath elements. The term is also applied to mucosal neuromas (see chapter 5), some but not all of which have a genetic basis, and to palisaded encapsulated neuroma, a hyperplastic lesion of unknown etiology (see chapter 5). Other reactive lesions, such as interdigital neuritis (Morton's neuroma), nerve cysts, and neuritis ossificans are accompanied by degeneration of nerve fibers. Thus, the spectrum of reactive change varies, as does the etiology.

TRAUMATIC NEUROMA

Definition. This is a non-neoplastic, disorganized proliferation of axons, Schwann cells, and perineurial cells, all in a fibrocollagenous stroma and forming a mass at the site of partial or complete transection of a nerve. Traumatic neuroma is also known as *amputation neuroma*.

General Comments. Although normal peripheral nerve is the site of intense physiologic activity, it is quiescent in terms of cell turnover. No Schwann cell multiplication is evident. Injury is required to prompt proliferative changes in nerve sheath cells. The most commonly encountered example of a reparative proliferation affecting nerve is traumatic neuroma, the prototypic "true neuroma." An understanding of this lesion requires familiarity with the sequence of events occurring in experimental nerve transection (2,5,7). Successful reinnervation of the distal stump requires: 1) relative proximity of the injury to the end organ; 2) proximity of the severed proximal and distal nerve segments; and 3) no obstruction to the path of regenerating axons. With reference to the distal segment, complete degeneration of residual axons and myelin sheaths (wallerian degeneration) is required to prepare the nerve for ingrowth by proximal neurites. The process is readily apparent at 24 hours when fiber fragmentation is underway.

Lysosomal enzymes alter the degenerating myelin with resultant loss of its birefringence and characteristic tinctorial properties. Thus, normally Luxol-fast blue–positive myelin is transformed into periodic acid–Schiff (PAS)-, sudanophilic oil red O-, and Marchi-positive debris. By 4 weeks Schwann cells and macrophages will have removed most axonal and myelin debris. In its place, cords or tubes of basement membrane–enshrouded Schwann cells (bands of Büngner) await the ingrowth of regenerating proximal axons. In the absence of the latter, the bands atrophy (4).

Alterations occurring proximally affect both the cell body and axons. The cell body shows chromatolysis, a decrease in prominence of Nissl substance and a manifestation of intense synthetic activity. The severed axon undergoes dramatic changes as well. Between 1 and 3 weeks after transection the proximal axonal stump forms an organelle-rich, 50- to 100-μm diameter expansion. Neurites emerge from the expansion under the influence of nerve growth factor, a substance elaborated by surrounding Schwann cells, as well as trophic factors secreted by macrophages. Growing 1 to 2 mm per day, the new axons cross the trauma-induced gap, reach the distal nerve segment, and colonize the bands of Büngner. Fibers regenerate down the bands, mature and, if possible, reconnect with their original or with a different, but meaningful, target. If misdirection occurs and connections cannot be established, fibers atrophy.

When effective regeneration is thwarted because the outgrowing axons are too removed from the distal stump or encounter scar tissue, the result is a traumatic neuroma. The lesion essentially represents a frustrated attempt at re-establishment of nerve continuity and consists of massive, disorganized tangles of microfascicles, each a crude caricature of a nerve, replete with axons, Schwann sheaths, and a perineurial investment.

Clinical Features. Following nerve injury, either transection or crush, the previously described degenerative and reparative changes

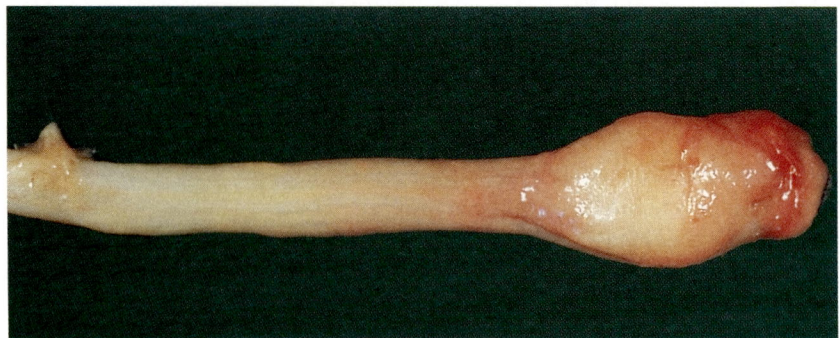

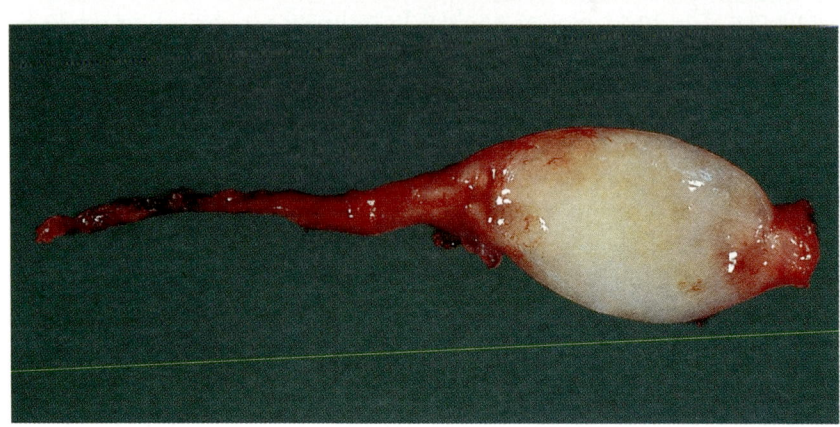

Figure 3-1
TRAUMATIC NEUROMA
Top: This intact lesion forms a localized bulbous expansion at the distal end of a once transected nerve.
Bottom: On cut section, neuromas appear as localized, gray-tan and translucent masses.

ensue. The growth of new axons from the proximal nerve stump begins even before degeneration of distal axons is complete. The lesion resulting from unsuccessful regeneration presents as a firm, often tender or painful nodule. Whereas the majority of traumatic neuromas arise in the postsurgical setting, in some instances they follow seemingly insignificant injury. A rare form occurs in utero after auto-amputation of a supernumerary digit (8,11); such lesions usually appear on the proximal, ulnar aspect of the hand. Traumatic neuromas also occur at visceral sites, particularly the gallbladder (3) and bile ducts (9,12). Most, but not all (6), occur months to years after cholecystectomy or in association with lithiasis. Occasional examples are polypoid (10).

Gross Findings. Traumatic neuromas are somewhat circumscribed, gray-white, nodular masses which occur either at the proximal stump of a transected nerve (fig. 3-1) or along the course of an incompletely transected or otherwise traumatized nerve (fig. 3-2). In the case of a nerve plexus, severe injury may result in the formation of multiple neuromas (fig. 3-3). Nearly all traumatic neuromas are less than 5 cm in maximal dimension.

On longitudinal section the proximal portion of the nerve is seen to splay and to disappear into a firm, fibrous mass. These features are best seen in whole mount sections (figs. 3-2, 3-4A,B).

Microscopic Findings. The essential features of traumatic neuroma include haphazard tangles of regenerated axons accompanied by ensheathing Schwann cells. As previously noted, the process is unencapsulated and consists of nerve fibers organized into microfascicles of varying size (figs. 3-2, 3-4C,D). The fibers are far less myelinated than are those in the parent nerve (fig. 3-5A). Microfascicles vary in size and appearance. When well formed and captured in cross section, they are surrounded by a perineurial membrane (fig. 3-5D). On occasion, circumferential proliferation of nerve fibers may also be seen about parent nerve fascicles (fig. 3-6). Proliferating nerve fibers and fascicles may be surrounded by a mucoid matrix (fig. 3-7A), but in well-established neuromas they lie enmeshed in fibrocollagenous tissue (fig. 3-7B). Extension into adipose tissue or even nearby skeletal muscle fibers is less often seen (fig. 3-7C,D). Mild chronic inflammation and focal foreign body reaction is uncommon (fig. 3-8).

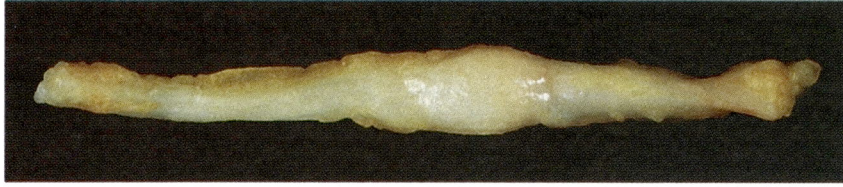

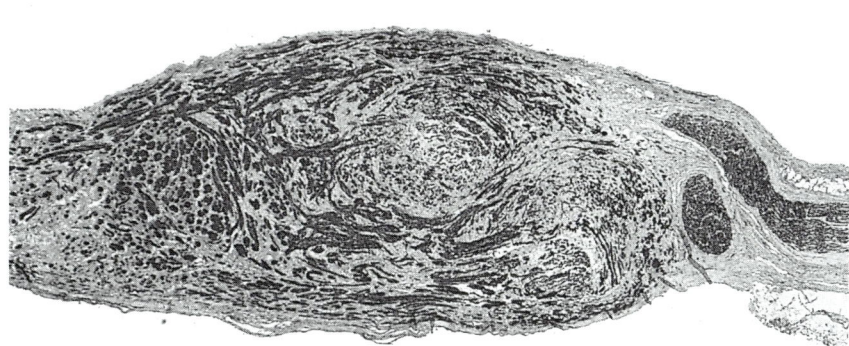

Figure 3-2
TRAUMATIC NEUROMA
Top: This example formed after trauma without complete division of the nerve. As a result, the nerve is still in continuity.
Bottom: On Bielschowsky stain, tangled, newly formed microfascicles are seen to comprise the bulk of the lesion. Note the large entering nerve fascicles (right) and only small fascicles within the lesion (left).

Immunohistochemical Findings. All the immunoreactivities of normal nerve are encountered in traumatic neuromas. Axons are positive for neurofilament protein (fig. 3-5B), Schwann cells react for S-100 protein (fig. 3-5C) or Leu-7, and perineurial cells surrounding microfascicles stain for epithelial membrane antigen (fig. 3-5D).

Ultrastructural Findings. In early phases of regeneration, axons are often unmyelinated, being surrounded by the cytoplasm of Schwann cells (fig. 3-9). With time, limited myelin formation results from Schwann cell wrappings about axons and microfascicles become surrounded by perineurium.

Differential Diagnosis. In that traumatic neuromas occur at almost any site, the differential diagnostic considerations are relatively broad. Simulators include *localized interdigital neuritis* (LIN; Morton's neuroma), palisaded encapsulated neuroma, mucosal neuromatosis, schwannoma, and neurofibroma.

As a response to chronic nerve injury, LIN is etiologically related to traumatic neuroma. Given the stereotypic clinical setting and anatomic location of LIN, the two lesions are usually readily distinguished. With rare exception, LIN is limited to the feet and to females. Both lesions, but particularly LIN, affect grossly recognizable nerves. Unlike traumatic neuroma, which is a proliferative,

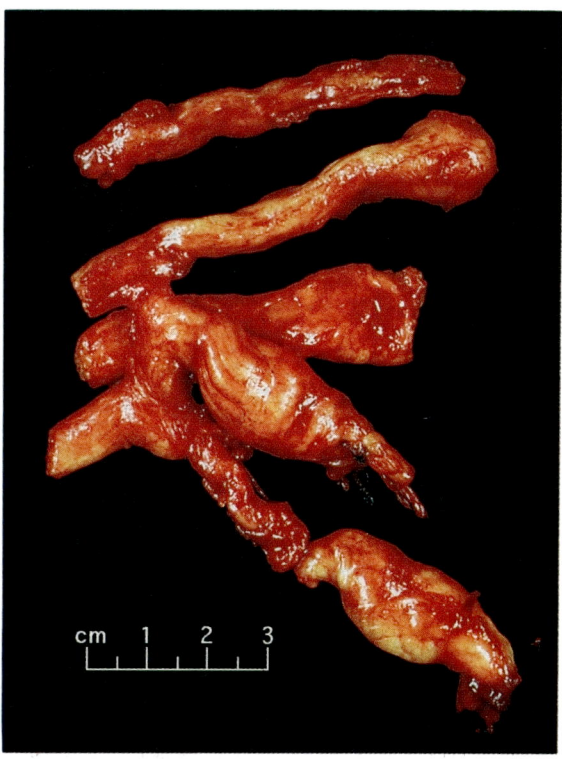

Figure 3-3
TRAUMATIC NEUROMA
In severe injuries, such as this example of avulsion of the brachial plexus, traumatic neuromas are multiple, involving several nerve trunks.

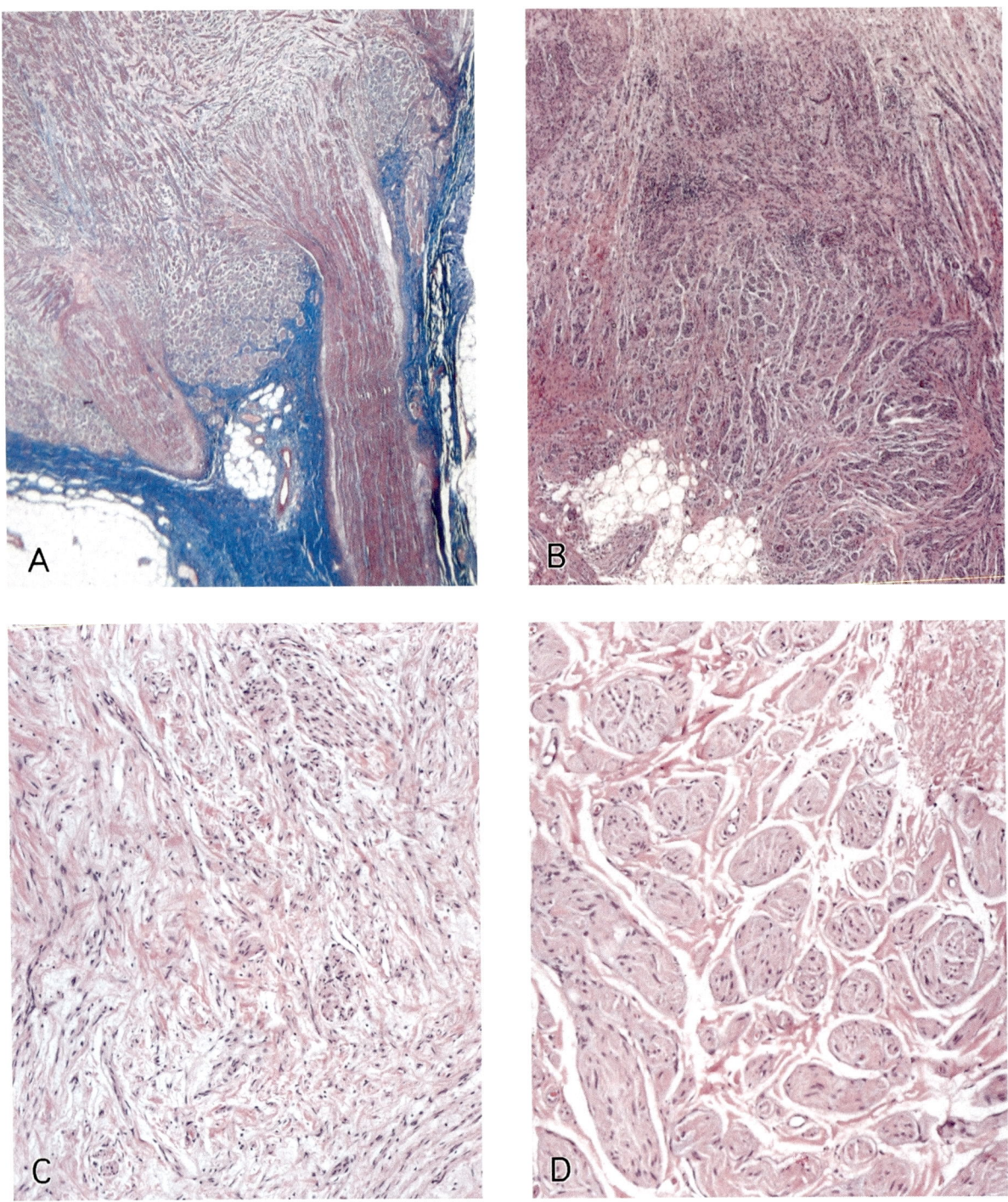

Figure 3-4
TRAUMATIC NEUROMA

A: A whole mount section demonstrates a globular example associated with a small myelinated nerve (lower left). Transition of the nerve to neuroma is clearly seen. Despite apparent circumscription, these lesions lack a capsule. Instead, this trichrome preparation highlights associated perilesional fibrosis. (Fig. 3.402 from Okazaki H, Scheithauer BW. Atlas of neuropathology, 1988. With permission from the Mayo Foundation.)

B: Another example illustrates the manner in which the neuroma (center and right) erupts from the parent nerve (left).

C,D: Varying in size from small and disorganized (C) to larger and better defined (D), newly formed microfascicles make up the substance of traumatic neuroma.

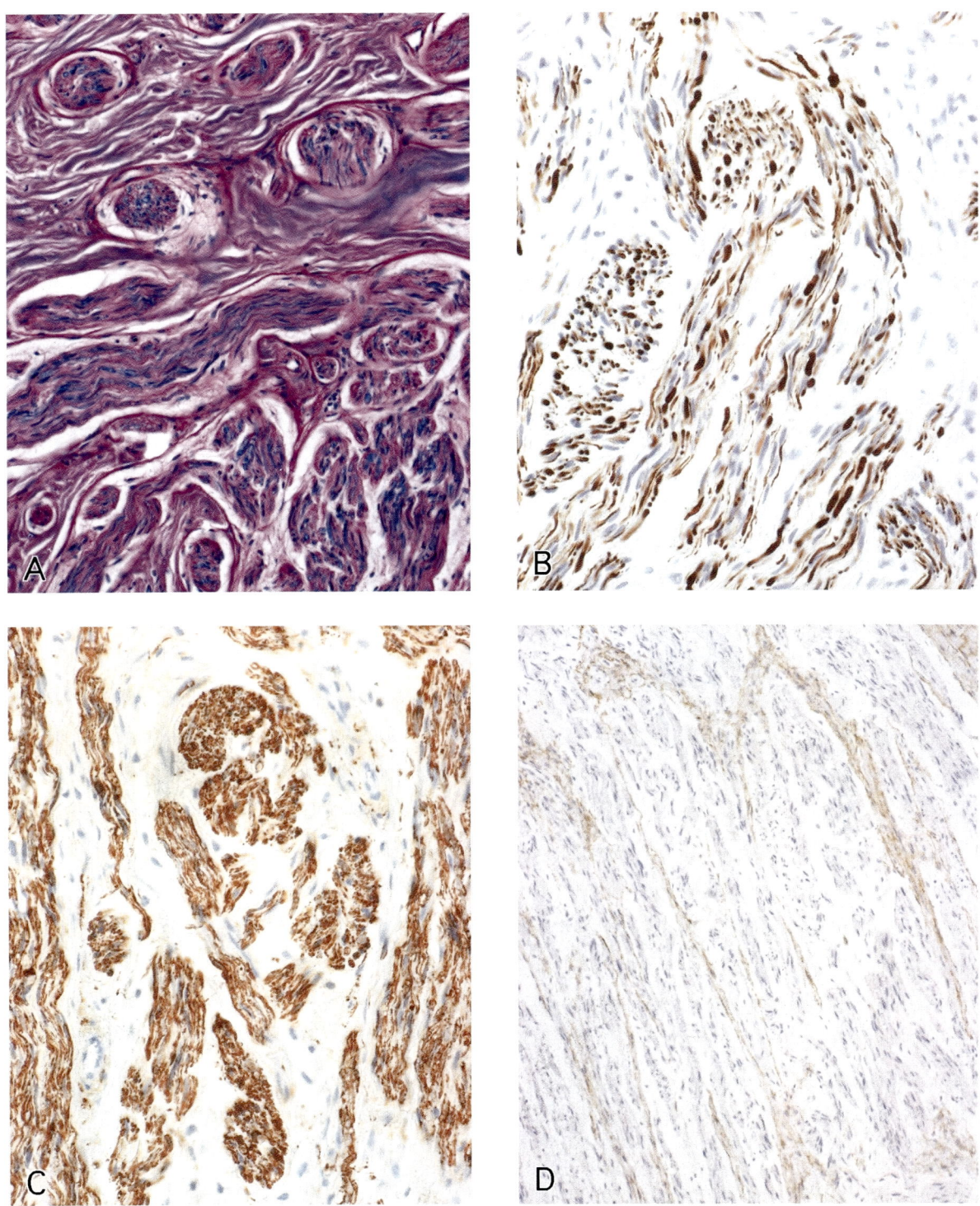

Figure 3-5
TRAUMATIC NEUROMA

A: Regenerating nerve fiber bundles (microfascicles) become arranged in relatively uniform, tangled bundles which on Luxol-fast blue–PAS stain are seen to be composed of variably myelinated nerves.

B,C: A delicate collagenous stroma separates the fascicles. Immunostains for neurofilament protein and S-100 protein highlight their axons and Schwann sheaths, respectively.

D: A perineurial investment, best seen here on epithelial membrane antigen immunostain, surrounds the microfascicles.

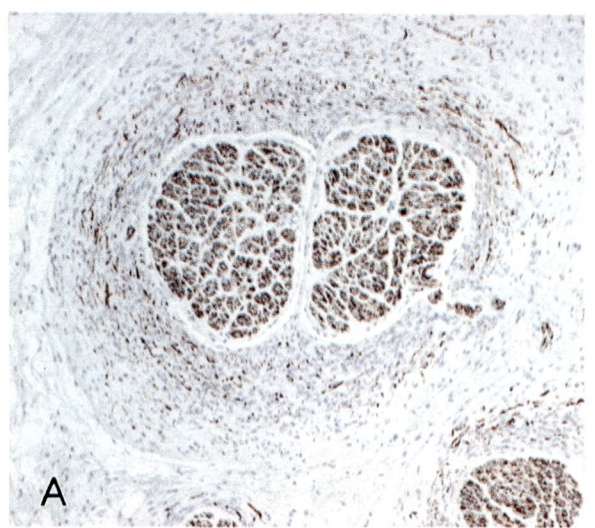
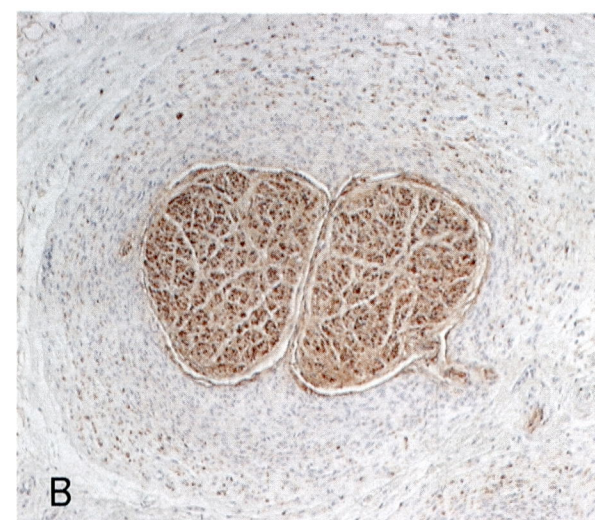
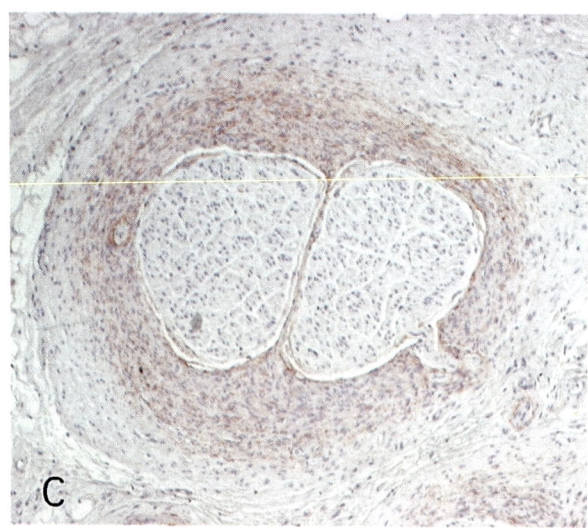

Figure 3-6
TRAUMATIC NEUROMA
An unusual finding is proliferation of axons (A), accompanying Schwann cells (B), and perineurial cells (C) in a circumferential pattern about the parent nerve fascicles (A, NF protein; B, S-100 protein; C, EMA immunostains).

reparative lesion composed of microfascicles of axons with accompanying Schwann cells, LIN consists of a recognizable nerve with marked degenerative changes affecting epineurium, perineurium, and endoneurium. Schwann cell, myelin, and axonal loss typify the condition. What remains within the endoneurium are aligned, albeit diminished numbers of axons and Schwann cells. Due to preservation of architectural features, LIN is more orderly than the random meandering of new microfascicles that characterizes traumatic neuroma. Lastly, LIN features perineurial fibrosis and elastic tissue deposition as well as perineural vascular thrombosis and sclerosis.

A number of features aid in the distinction of *palisaded encapsulated neuroma* (PEN) from traumatic neuroma. Unlike the latter, PENs occur primarily in females, are superficially situated, and are usually found in skin rather than deep soft tissue. Traumatic neuromas are more frequently associated with a recognizable nerve and are usually microscopically less circumscribed than are PENs. Although both lesions consist of axons and of Schwann and perineurial cells, traumatic neuroma represents a more orderly physiologic response, featuring axons uniformly ensheathed by Schwann cells as well as microfascicle formation, replete with perineurial ensheathment. In contrast, PEN consists in greater part of Schwann cells; orderly ensheathment of axons and well formed microfascicle formation are lacking. Instead, a delicate perineurium often surrounds all but the most superficial portions of PEN.

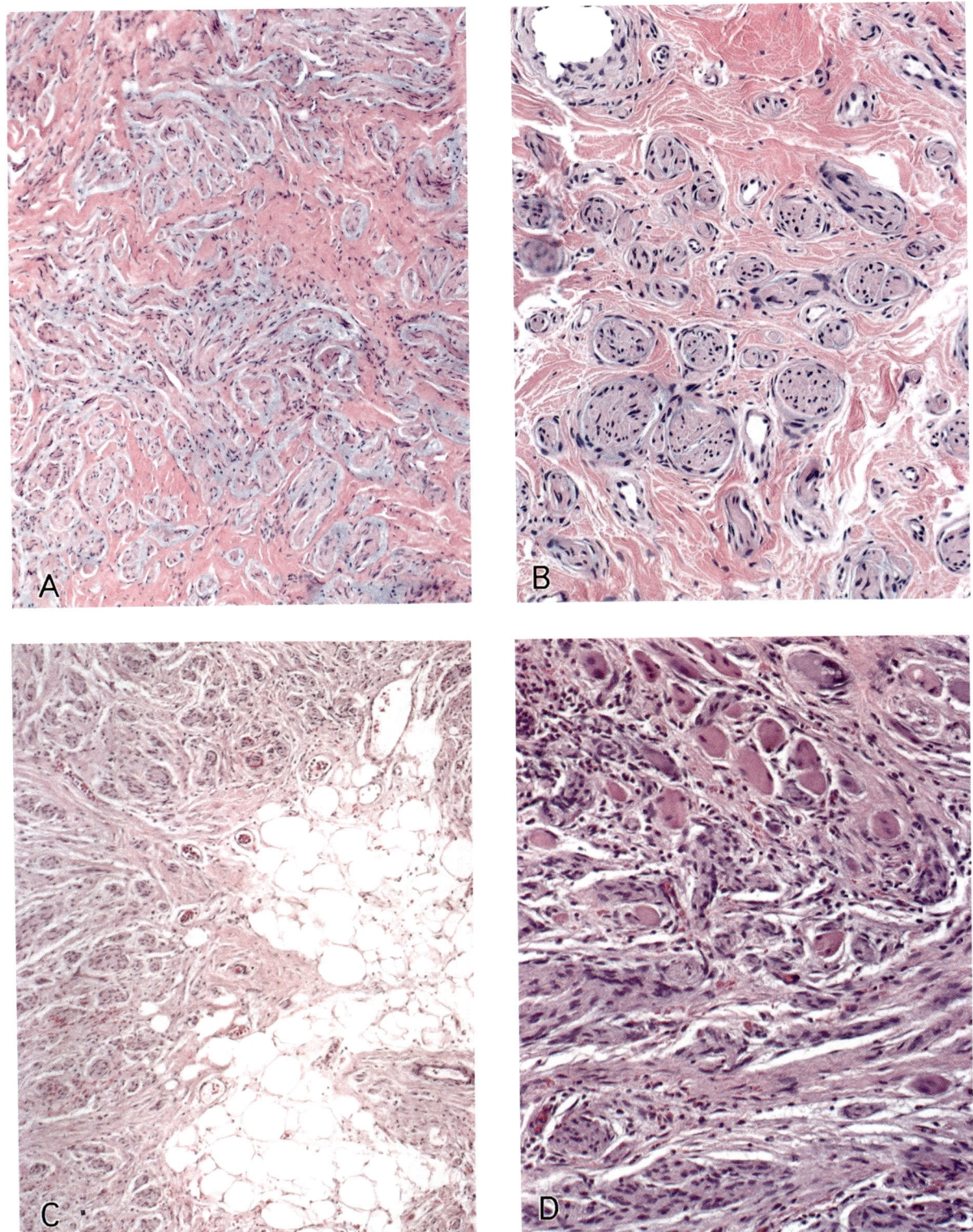

Figure 3-7
TRAUMATIC NEUROMA

The stroma of such lesions varies from partly mucinous (A) to dense fibrous connective tissue (B). Some lesions, due to their loose texture, or to extension into surrounding fibroadipose tissue (C) or muscle (D), superficially resemble neurofibroma.

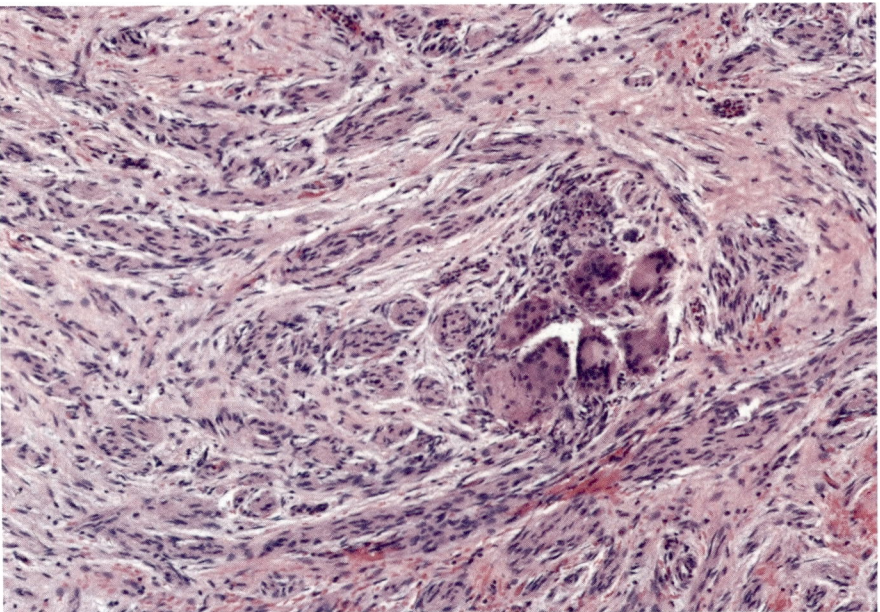

Figure 3-8
TRAUMATIC NEUROMA
Chronic inflammation and foreign body reaction related to the original trauma, although an uncommon finding, may be a hint to the diagnosis.

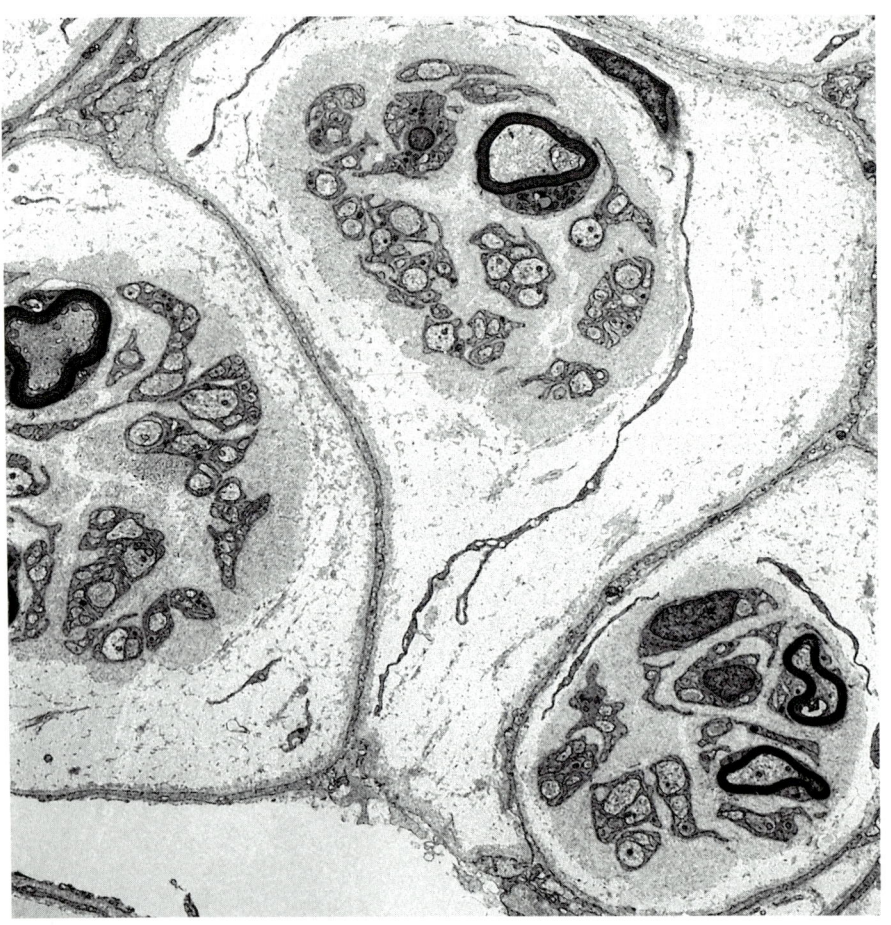

Figure 3-9
TRAUMATIC NEUROMA, ULTRASTRUCTURE
Resected 8 years after traumatic amputation of the lower leg, this stump neuroma arising from a small nerve shows three microfascicles, each composed largely of unmyelinated axons, to be surrounded by a delicate perineurium (X1,800).

Also in the differential diagnosis of traumatic neuroma is *mucosal neuroma*. When multiple and consisting of well-formed nerves, as in multiple endocrine neoplasia (MEN) IIb, the distinction is easy. On the other hand, solitary mucosal neuromas such as those of the biliary system, duodenum, and appendix may closely resemble traumatic neuroma. In fact, we believe the two lesions may be etiologically related (see figs. 5-12, 5-13).

Particularly in cases in which biopsies are small and nonrepresentative, schwannoma enters into the differential diagnosis. Unlike traumatic neuroma, schwannomas are unassociated with antecedent trauma. Whereas traumatic neuromas are solid, gray-white, ill-defined, complex lesions composed of regenerating axons with accompanying Schwann and perineurial cells, schwannomas are encapsulated, often partially cystic, tan or yellow lesions composed only of Schwann cells. Features typical of schwannoma, including Antoni A and B patterns as well as Verocay bodies, are lacking in traumatic neuroma. The maximal size of traumatic neuroma is approximately 5 cm, but schwannomas are often considerably larger. Whereas Schwann cell–ensheathed axons are present throughout traumatic neuromas, the parent nerve is usually eccentric to schwannomas, essentially being displaced by the proliferation. As a result, neurofilament protein stains only infrequently show small numbers of entrapped axons within the subcapsular region. Furthermore, schwannomas exhibit S-100 protein reactivity but lack epithelial membrane staining. Fibrosis, granulation tissue, and focal inflammation, common features of traumatic neuroma, are not seen in small schwannomas. At the ultrastructural level, axons are usually not encountered in schwannomas.

Soft tissues are a common site of *neurofibromas*. Both lesions vary in gross appearance, being localized or less defined. Soft tissue infiltration may be widespread in neurofibroma but is limited in traumatic neuroma (fig. 3-7C,D). Due in large part to the presence of a mucopolysaccharide matrix in neurofibroma, the latter appears less cellular than does traumatic neuroma. This matrix is often conspicuous within the "worm-like" branches of plexiform neurofibromas. As a result, they differ in appearance from the far smaller, complex microfascicles of traumatic neuroma. Histochemical stains and immuno-stains show the microfascicles of traumatic neuroma to be rich in axons, whereas they are generally dispersed in neurofibroma.

Treatment and Prognosis. The treatment of fully developed traumatic neuroma is simple excision. Their formation may be avoided if, at the time of nerve injury, the ends of traumatized nerves are optimally approximated to facilitate orderly regeneration. Graft placement may be required when proximity cannot be achieved.

Resection may not only be required for traumatic neuromas associated with pain or dysesthesia, but also to distinguish them from recurrent neoplasm in the setting of prior cancer surgery (1). Excision of the traumatic neuroma and embedding of its proximal nerve stump into normal soft tissue is sufficient treatment.

LOCALIZED INTERDIGITAL NEURITIS

Definition. This is a non-neoplastic, localized, degenerative lesion usually affecting a plantar digital nerve and characterized by axon and myelin loss with accompanying fibrosis. Synonyms include *Morton's neuroma, plantar neuroma, Morton's toe,* and *Morton's node.*

General Comments. Localized interdigital neuritis (LIN) is attributed to chronic, repetitive nerve trauma as well as to ischemia resulting from vascular and perivascular fibrosis (16). A vascular role is supported by the observation, in early cases, of fibrodegenerative alterations surrounding the neurovascular bundle (15).

Clinical and Radiographic Features. The clinicopathologic features of LIN, a common lesion, have been well studied (17). Although its precise incidence is unknown, LIN affects primarily, but not exclusively, the feet of adult females. The process is usually unilateral. Fully 90 percent of patients present with moderate to severe, paroxysmal pain beneath the metatarsal arch between the third and fourth toes. The second and third interspaces may also be affected. Point tenderness is noted on compression over the interspace. Pain has often been present for weeks to years and is typically exacerbated by exercise and relieved by rest. The condition is usually attributed to the compressive effects of ill-fitting shoes. On occasion, a similar lesion affects the hands, usually of males with chronic, repetitive occupational trauma.

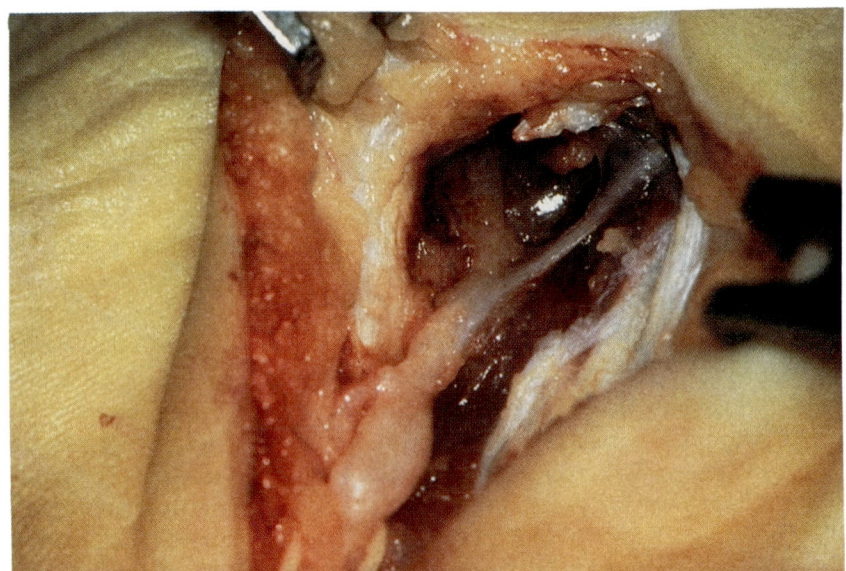

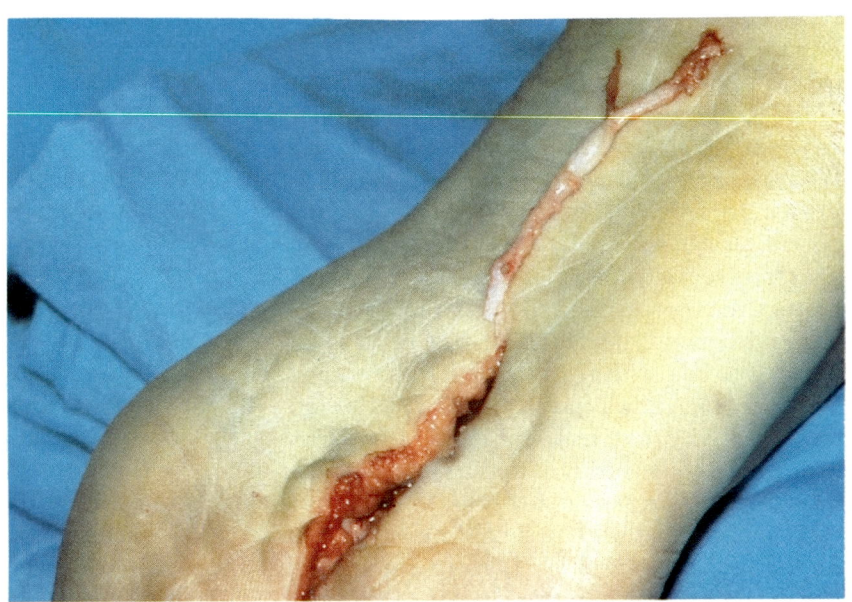

Figure 3-10
LOCALIZED
INTERDIGITAL NEURITIS

Top: This sequence of intraoperative photographs demonstrates the neuroma as a firm, gray, fusiform to somewhat nodular expansion of the digital plantar nerve.

Bottom: Still in situ, the size of the lesion (bottom) is contrasted with the normal-appearing remainder of the nerve (upper right).

Gross Findings. LIN presents as a localized, fusiform, firm expansion, usually at the bifurcation of the fourth plantar digital nerve (fig. 3-10). In well-established cases the nerve sheath is often adherent to the intermetatarsal bursa and the adjacent digital artery. Most lesions are small, measure less than 1 cm in size, and grossly resemble either traumatic neuroma or neurofibroma. On cut section they appear gray-tan and fibrous.

Microscopic Findings. Despite obvious enlargement of the plantar digital nerve, LIN is primarily a degenerative rather than a proliferative process. All compartments of the nerve are involved, but basic architectural features are preserved. Epineurial tissue is often extensively fibrotic (fig. 3-11A,B). Vessels, including the digital artery, are hyalinized (fig. 3-11A) and frequently thrombosed. The perineurium appears thickened (fig. 3-11B), more so on collagen than PAS stain (fig. 3-11C). Mucinous degeneration is present in early cases (fig. 3-12), but over time gives way to fibrosis. Laminated collagenous

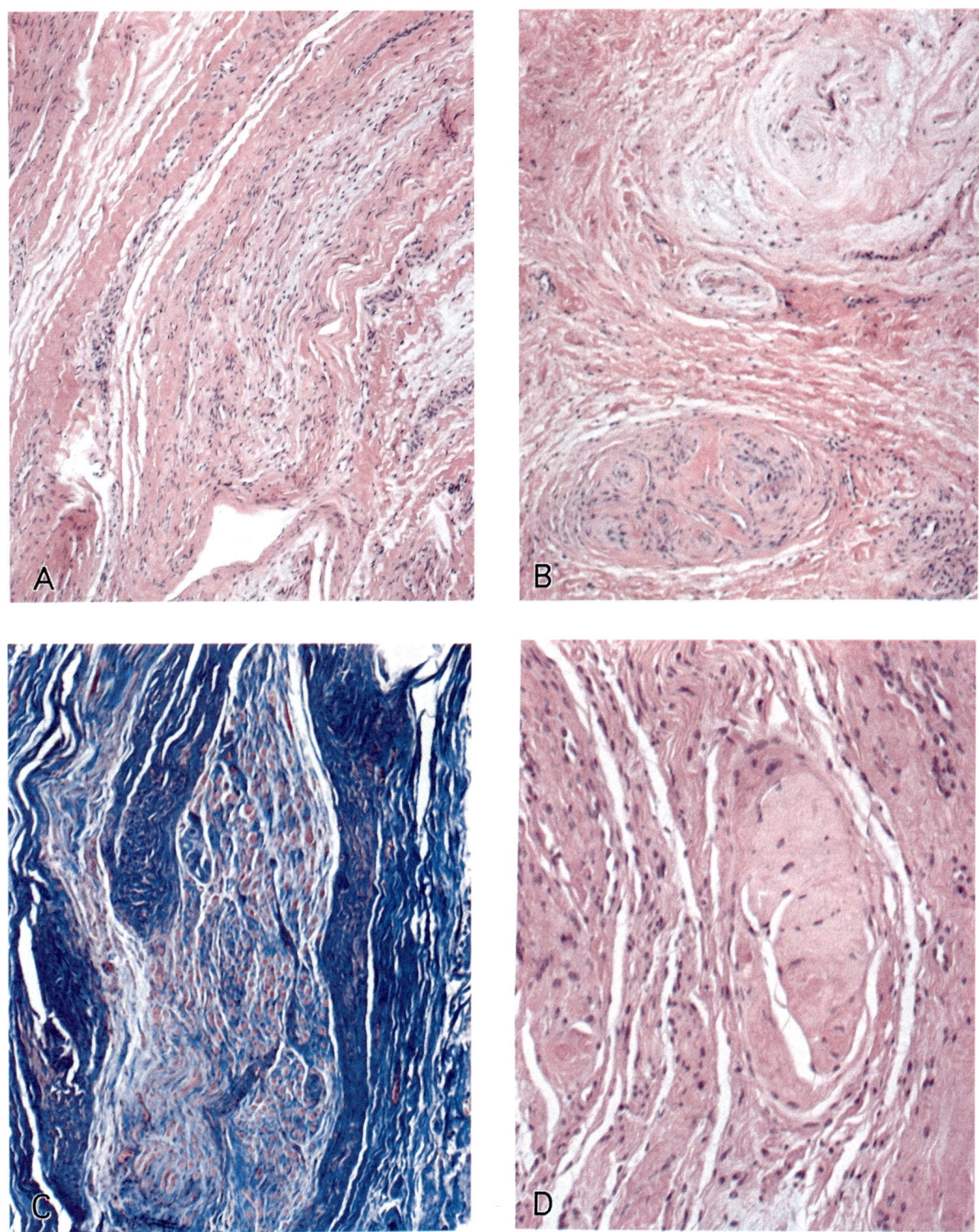

Figure 3-11
LOCALIZED INTERDIGITAL NEURITIS
At low magnification, the digital nerve, its perineurium and epineurium, as well as surrounding vasculature are fibrotic (A,B). These changes are most conspicuous on trichrome stain (C). Intraneural collagenous nodules are also a feature of some examples (D).

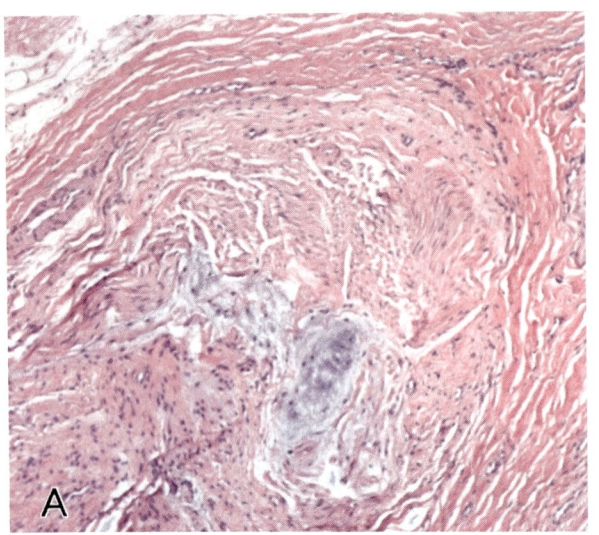

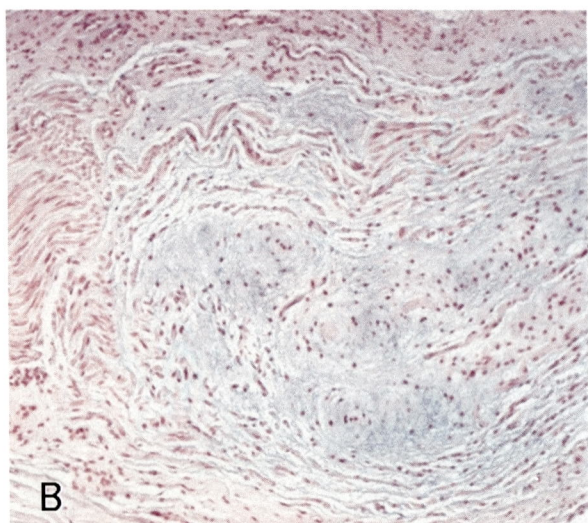

Figure 3-12
LOCALIZED INTERDIGITAL NEURITIS
Endoneurial mucin accumulation may be seen (A), and is
most apparent on Alcian blue stains (B). In many instances,
elastosis is also evident (C, Elastic Van Gieson).

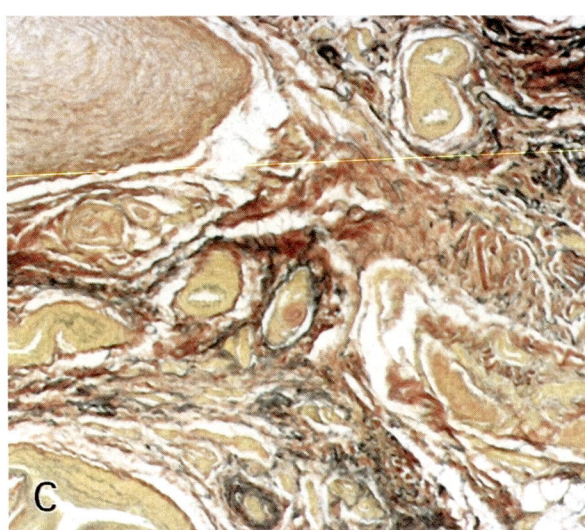

nodules, a nonspecific feature, may be seen within the endoneurium (fig. 3-11D). Stromal deposition of elastic tissue (elastofibrositis) is a late-stage feature (fig. 3-12C) (15). Although special stains are generally not required to make a diagnosis of localized interdigital neuritis, silver stains for axons as well as stains for myelin typically show a reduction of both (fig. 3-13). Loss of axons and Schwann sheaths is also evident with immunostains (fig. 3-14). In keeping with the chronic nature of LIN, the changes are unaccompanied by obvious wallerian degeneration or Schwann cell hyperplasia. No significant inflammation is seen, although fibrin deposits are common and nearby synovium included in an occasional biopsy may show mild nonspecific chronic inflammation.

Immunohistochemical Findings. Residual axons are seen on neurofilament stain but are reduced in number. S-100 protein stains show a proportionate reduction in Schwann cells. Epithelial membrane antigen preparations highlight the abnormal architecture of the hyalinized perineurium.

Ultrastructural Findings. Aside from fibrosis of extraneural tissues, electron microscopy reveals a variety of changes in the digital nerve, including endoneurial vessel thickening due to multilayering of basement membrane, edema and sclerosis of endoneurium with collagen fibril deposition, thickening of the perineurial sheath, degenerative changes in nerve fibers, and myelin loss (14).

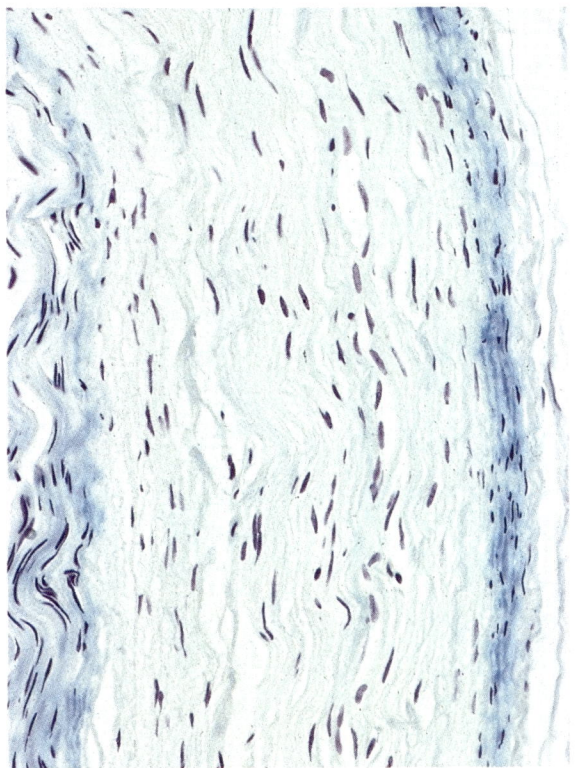 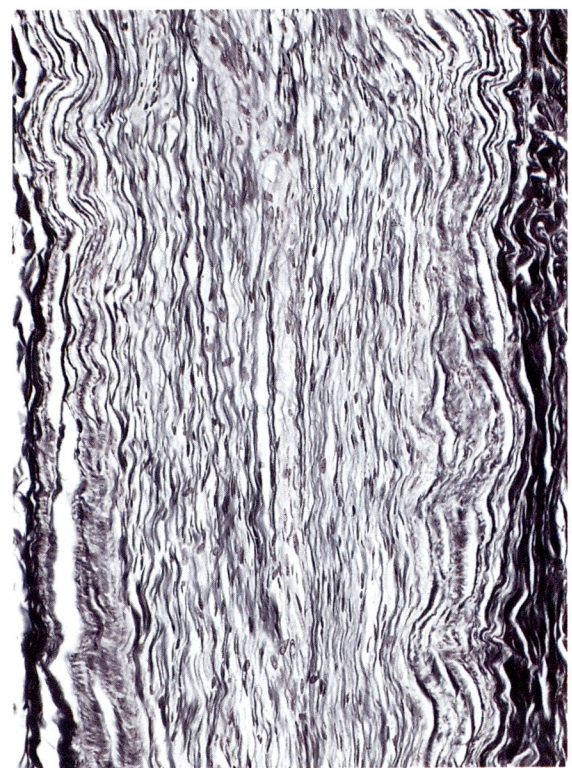

Figure 3-13
LOCALIZED INTERDIGITAL NEURITIS
Reduction in axons and myelin loss are apparent on silver impregnation for axons (left) and on myelin stain (right). (Left, Bielschowsky; right, Luxol-fast blue–PAS.)

Differential Diagnosis. The clinical and morphologic features of LIN are so characteristic that few lesions enter into the differential diagnosis. Unlike *traumatic neuroma,* a proliferative process, the nerve is intact and lacks the low-power, tangled, microfascicular architecture of that lesion. LIN is degenerative in nature: the axons are decreased in number and aligned rather than regenerating and haphazardly arranged.

Treatment and Prognosis. Although a change of footwear or steroid/anesthetic injection may alleviate symptoms (13), resection may be required. The failure rate of neurectomy is approximately 10 percent. This is due, in nearly all instances, to the formation of a traumatic neuroma, the resection of which is curative (18).

PACINIAN NEUROMA

Definition. This neuroma results from hypertrophy or hyperplasia of pacinian corpuscles, with or without associated degenerative changes. It is also known as *pacinian corpuscle neuroma, pacinian corpuscle hyperplasia,* and *pacinioma.*

General Comments. The basic anatomy and physiology of pacinian corpuscles as well as their immunohistochemical and ultrastructural features are described in chapter 2. Briefly, pacinian corpuscles are mechanoreceptors which are most numerous in deep layers of the skin of hands and feet, but also occur in the walls of viscera, in mesentery, and within the adventitia of vessels. In the hands, the site most often affected by pacinian neuroma, corpuscles are preferentially situated in palmar fat beneath the level of sweat glands, near the periosteum on the lateral aspects of the proximal and middle phalanges, between flexor tendons and periosteum, and at the bases of proximal phalanges (28). At surgery, their characteristic locations serve as anatomic landmarks for nerves. It is of note that pacinian

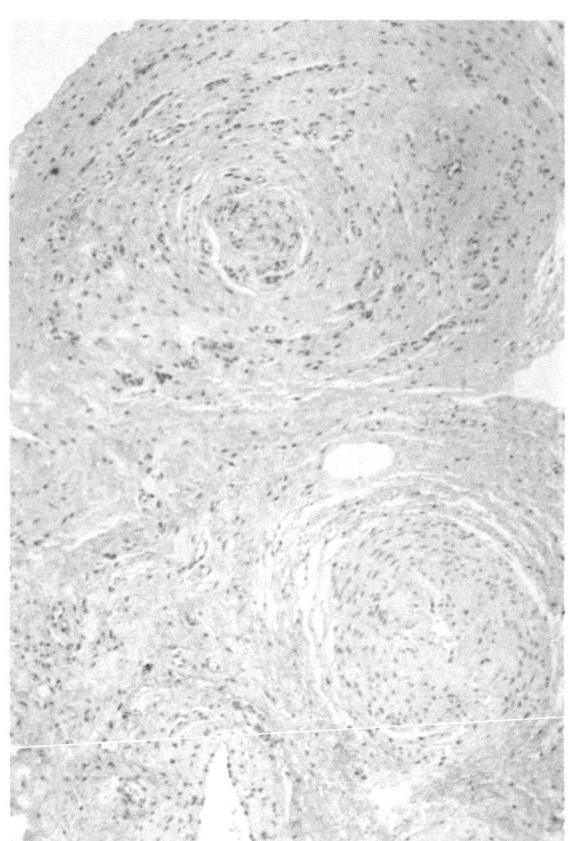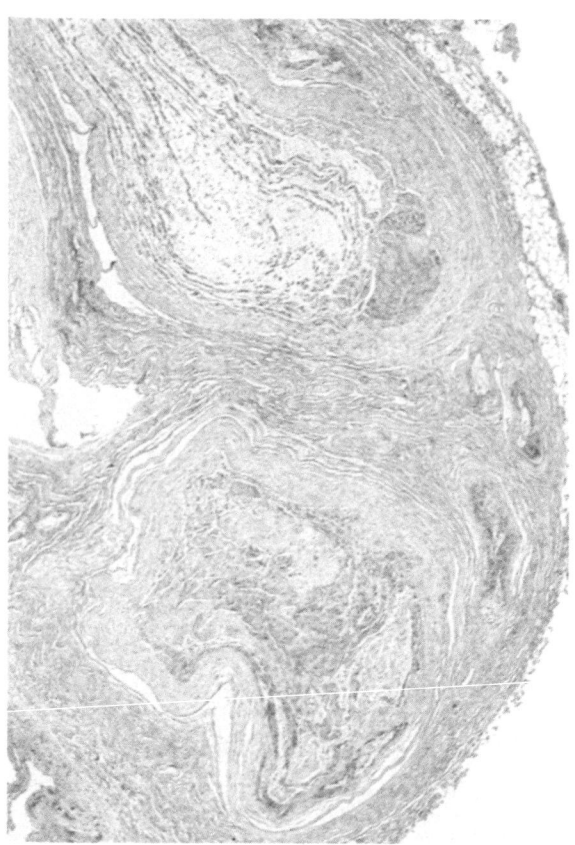

Figure 3-14
LOCALIZED INTERDIGITAL NEURITIS
The effects of degenerative changes upon the architecture of the digital nerve are best appreciated on neurofilament protein (left) and S-100 protein immunostains (right) which show nerve fibers and Schwann sheaths to be reduced in number, dispersed, and distorted.

corpuscles undergo morphologic changes in response to trauma or physiologic stimuli. In both animals (29) and man (44), they are capable of regeneration from terminations of their nerves. Given the frequent association of pacinian neuroma with prior trauma (see below) and the near normal morphology of many examples, we view them not as neoplasms but as a form of true neuroma (68). A diagnostic word of caution is in order. In view of the frequent operative finding of a sizable corpuscle(s) in the absence of an alternative explanation for a patient's symptoms, pacinian neuromas are no doubt overdiagnosed.

Clinical Features. Pacinian neuromas occur most frequently in the hands and are important in the differential diagnosis of digital pain. The English-speaking literature contains in excess of 20 reported cases affecting the hands (23,26,27, 33–36,38–40,47,49,53,54,56,58,69). Pacinian neu-

romas affecting the feet may be associated with a compression syndrome resembling localized interdigital neuritis (37,65). With the rare exception of two extremely longstanding and perhaps congenital examples (33 [case 1], 49), both bilateral and affecting the thumbs, most pacinian neuromas occur in adults in the fifth and sixth decades. Females are twice as often affected. The majority of lesions are associated with a history of prior direct or nearby trauma with an interval to clinical presentation of weeks to years. Pacinian neuromas occurring in the hands are all related to digital nerves. Nearly all occur in fingers, primarily the index and middle, or rarely in the palm (34). Unusual patterns of disease include involvement of multiple digits (33 [case 1],36,49) and of two nerves of the same digit (26,39,40,69). Erosion of adjacent bone is an uncommon feature (36,47). Pain is present in nearly all cases and sensory loss in a

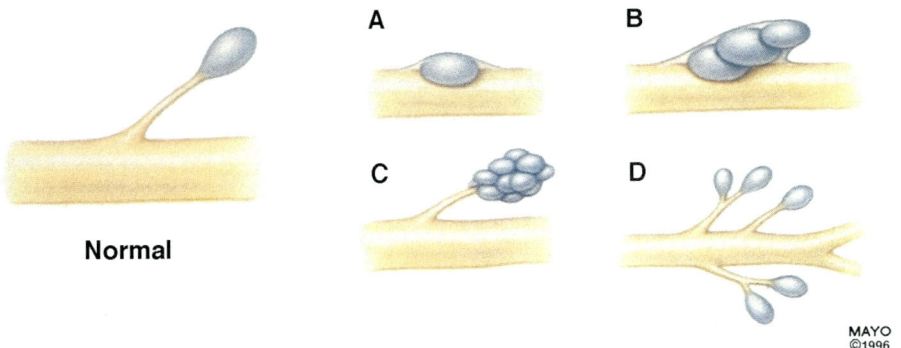

Figure 3-15
PACINIAN NEUROMA
Schematic representation of the most common growth patterns. Modified from Rhode and Jennings (36).

few. Asymptomatic lesions incidentally encountered at surgery are uncommon (34,49).

On rare occasion pacinian neuromas occur within the abdomen. Specific locations have included the pancreatic region (59), mesentery (62), and aortic adventitia (30). Most such neuromas have occurred at a site of prior surgery. Some have been associated with spinal dysraphism (21,22).

Gross Findings. Pacinian neuromas do not form a tumor-like mass. Whether hypertrophic or of relatively normal size, single or multiple, the constituent corpuscles appear as rice-like, pearl gray, often ovoid nodules embedded in fibroareolar tissue. Their entering nerves may be sufficiently prominent or numerous as to make multiple corpuscles appear interconnected. Pacinian neuromas vary considerably in terms of surgical anatomy. Based upon the number of constituent corpuscles, their spatial distribution, and their relation to the parent nerve, Rhode and Jennings developed a simple four-tier classification of pacinian neuromas (fig. 3-15) (54). Their categories include: type A, a single enlarged subepineural corpuscle; type B, enlarged corpuscles arranged in tandem beneath the epineurium; type C, a grapelike cluster of pacinian corpuscles of normal size attached to the digital nerve by a fine filament; and type D, multiple hyperplastic corpuscles arranged along the length of the affected nerve. Unfortunately, the application of this scheme is predicated upon data obtained only by detailed or extensive dissection. Overall, the majority of pacinian neuromas are of type B, whereas lesions

of types C and D are rare. Normal corpuscles as well as most hypertrophic and hyperplastic examples are attached to a digital nerve by a minute nerve fiber. On the other hand, some examples (type A pattern) are actually situated within the perineurium (23,26,35,54,69). Although not always apparent at surgery, nerve compression is considered to be the basis of symptoms. As a rule, no gross nerve injury is seen.

Microscopic Findings. Pacinian neuromas consist of enlarged or multiple pacinian corpuscles (fig. 3-16), some associated with fibrosis. When aggregated in a mass, their smooth contoured profiles lie jumbled in fibroareolar tissue but not surrounded by a fibrous capsule. The corpuscles may vary in shape (fig. 3-17, left) or appear to be "budding." Hypertrophic corpuscles generally measure more than 1.6 mm in greatest dimension (34) and most exhibit greater than 20 concentric lamellae (40 to 60 in some cases). Degenerative changes are commonly seen and include capsular and interlamellar collagen deposition (fig. 3-17, left) as well as perineural and endoneurial fibrosis of nerves entering the corpuscles (fig. 3-17, right). Capsular elastosis is an uncommon finding, even in neuromas of the feet, a site at which elastic fibers are normally found within corpuscle capsules (50). In some cases fibrosis is marked (fig. 3-18, left) and the inner core lacks a nerve fiber (fig. 3-18, right).

Given the frequent association of pacinian neuromas with antecedent injury, it is not surprising that an occasional example is accompanied by a traumatic neuroma (33 [case 3]). Also, given the normal association of pacinian corpuscles with

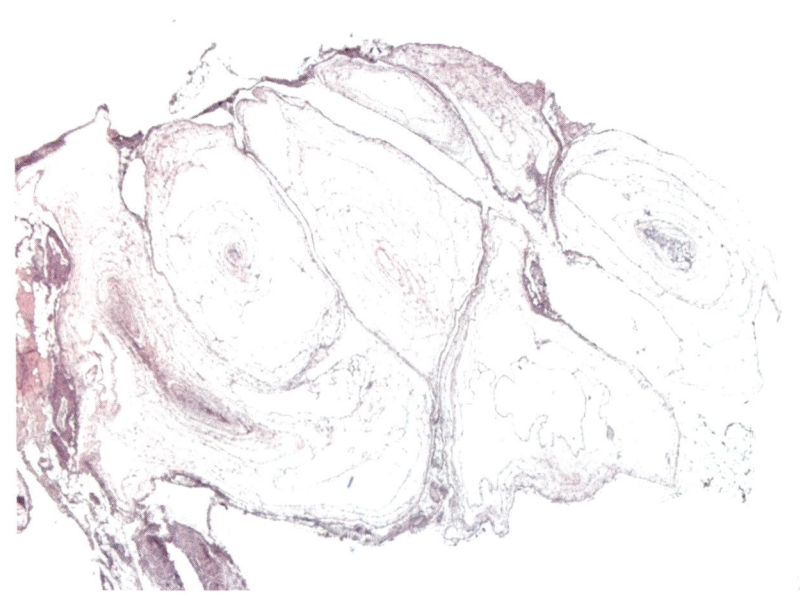

Figure 3-16
PACINIAN NEUROMA
Clustering of corpuscles (Rhode and Jennings pattern C), as in this example from the transverse mesocolon, represents a common form of pacinian neuroma.

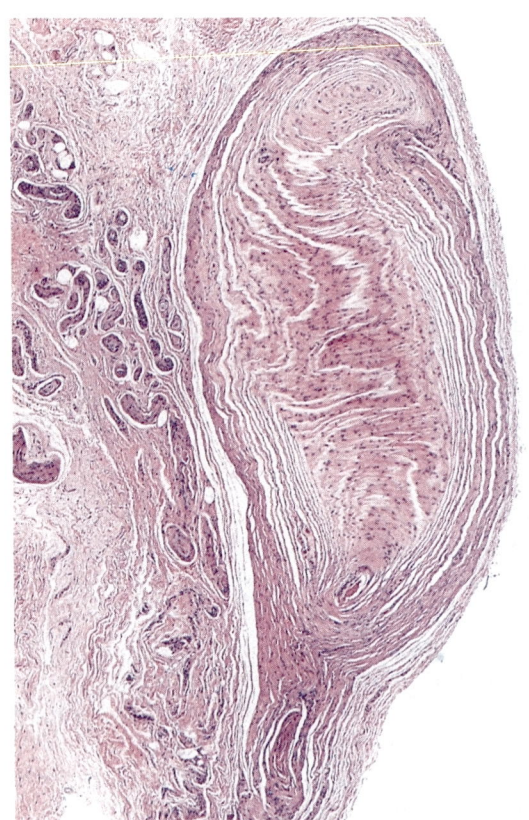

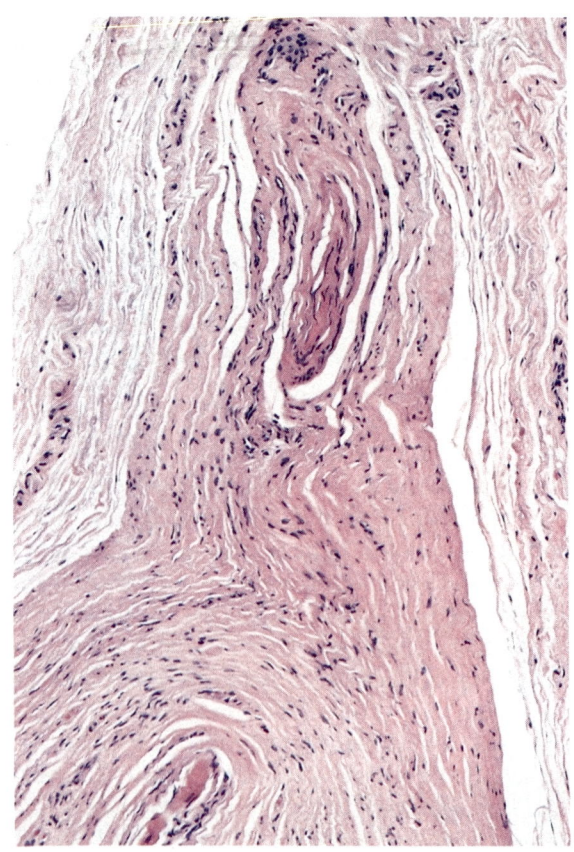

Figure 3-17
PACINIAN NEUROMA
These micrographs show a pacinian neuroma of irregular contour with thickening of its capsule and somewhat disordered, sclerotic lamellae in the outer core (left). Its entering nerve is also affected (right).

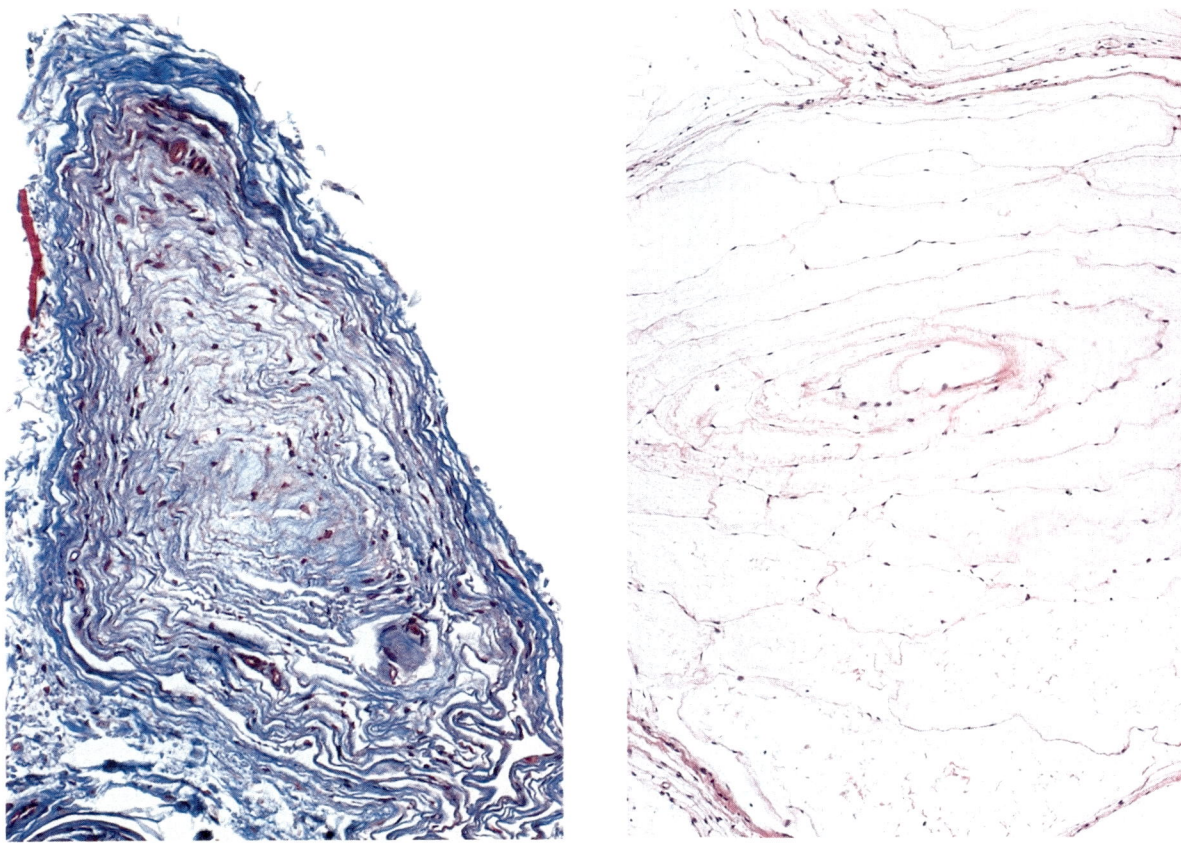

Figure 3-18
PACINIAN NEUROMA
Advanced degenerative changes include dense sclerosis of the entire corpuscle, a change best seen on trichrome stain (left), as well as loss of the nerve fibers within the inner core (right).

arteriovenous anastomoses, pacinian neuromas occur in association with contiguous or spatially separate glomus tumors (38).

Immunohistochemical Findings. The immunoprofile of pacinian neuroma is that of normal pacinian corpuscles. The perineurial cell lamellae comprising the outer core are epithelial membrane antigen positive, whereas Schwann cells and axons within the inner core are reactive for S-100 protein and neurofilament protein, respectively (20,27,63).

Ultrastructural Findings. Electron microscopic studies have shown that the outer lamellae of the pacinian corpuscle consist of long, thin perineurial cell processes with prominent pinocytotic vesicles (see chapter 2). Since these outer lamellae are immunoreactive for epithelial membrane antigen (see below), and the pacinian-like structures found in pacinian neurofibro-

mas have the immunohistochemical and ultrastructural features of perineurial cells (57,61, 67), it can be assumed that the lamellae of the hyperplastic pacinian corpuscles composing pacinian neuromas also exhibit these features.

Differential Diagnosis. Pacinian neuromas may be confused with *normal pacinian corpuscles* or with neurofibromas containing tactile body-like structures, so-called pacinian neurofibromas. Since the resection of pacinian neuromas does not always result in relief of digital pain, questions may arise as to the nature of pacinian corpuscles commonly found in resection specimens. Findings favoring a diagnosis of pacinian neuroma over an incidentally discovered pacinian corpuscle include: 1) a history of local trauma; 2) point tenderness and palpability of a lesion; 3) the operative findings of nodule(s) variously related to a peripheral nerve; 4) corpuscle abnormalities such as large size, increased number, and abnormal shape; 5) microscopic abnormalities or degenerative changes such as fibrosis or loss the inner core of the corpuscle(s); and 6) postoperative resolution of pain.

Of tumors exhibiting tactile corpuscle-like differentiation, the one most often linked to pacinian neuroma is the so-called *pacinian neurofibroma*. The term has been loosely applied to palpable masses of varied histology occurring at a variety of sites, usually ones only rarely affected by pacinian neuroma. Such tumors bear no resemblance to pacinian neuromas as discussed here. In retrospect, a number of reported pacinian neurofibromas can be reclassified as dermal nerve sheath myxoma (32,45,48) and neurothekeoma (51 [case 1]). Of the remainder, the numerous corpuscle-like structures are either unaccompanied by an underlying lesion (24, 43) or occur in association with proliferations resembling large nevi (25,46), neurofibromas (31, 57,61,64,67), schwannoma (52), possible traumatic neuroma (19), or unclassifiable lesions (51 [case 2]). The distinction of these processes from the fully differentiated pacinian neuroma with its characteristic morphology and anatomically appropriate localization generally poses no problem. Morphologically, the tactile corpuscle-like differentiation most often seen in neurofibroma closely resembles that of Wagner-Meissner corpuscles (41,42,66). Whether considered to be pacinian or Wagner-Meissner in type, their features are similar (42,61,66,67), exhibiting perineurial-like ultrastructure despite expression of S-100 protein immunoreactivity (60,66). Thus, such cells show hybrid features and resemble the perineurial-like cells often seen in neurofibromas. We agree with Fletcher and Theaker (33) that true pacinian differentiation has never been convincingly demonstrated in benign or malignant nerve sheath neoplasms. Pacinian body–like structures have also been demonstrated in experimentally induced nerve sheath tumors (55).

Treatment and Prognosis. Although initial excision is curative, the symptoms of pacinian neuroma occasionally persist and are only relieved after additional resection of corpuscles not found at first surgery (39). Care must be taken to spare the parent nerve, particularly in cases in which corpuscles lie within the epineurium.

NERVE CYST

Definition. These are solitary or multifocal, often mucin-filled, nonepithelial-lined, uniloculate or multiloculate cysts involving a peripheral nerve. Synonyms include *nerve ganglion, pseudocyst of nerve,* and *mucinous ganglion cyst.*

General Comments. Cysts involving peripheral nerve are rare and occur in two principle forms, solitary and multiple. The relation of the two is unclear. Most are fibrous-walled and are situated in the vicinity of a joint. The nature and origin of nerve cysts is unsettled. Their location in areas subject to mechanical stress favors a traumatic etiology (97). In our experience, many arise from a joint, in which case they secondarily attach themselves to or extend into epineurium. Yet others originate within nerve sheath. The most frequent location of nerve sheath cysts is the common peroneal nerve near the head of the fibula (72, 87,90). In one review, this nerve was affected in 86 percent of cases (94). Other sites include the ulnar nerve at the wrist (70,78,85), the median nerve (79,84), and the posterior interosseous (80), radial (95), suprascapular (83), tibial (76), lateral popliteal (92), and sural (81) nerves.

As noted above, the majority of nerve cysts arise near a joint, either from its capsule (figs. 3-19, 3-20) or rarely, from underlying bone (74,90). The presence of a pedicle connecting the lesion with the tibiofibular joint (94) in almost half of the peroneal nerve cysts provides supportive evidence for an extrinsic origin of many such examples (92,93). Still other nerve cysts, particularly multifocal-appearing examples (fig. 3-21), originate in nerve sheath as a degenerative change.

Clinical Features. Patients with nerve cysts range in age from 4 to 74, with a mean of 34, years (89,90). Pediatric examples are uncommon (90). Approximately 80 percent are males (94). The cysts cause nerve compression with resultant motor dysfunction, pain, or sensory loss (94). Peroneal nerve cysts may cause atrophy of the muscles of the anterior compartment of the leg, a steppage gait, and pain on the anterolateral surface of the leg and dorsum of the foot (90). As a rule, sensory loss is slight (90). A tender and fluctuant mass is often present on palpation. Percussion of the lesion often elicits a positive Tinel's sign, i.e., tingling sensation radiating distally in an extremity upon percussion of a nerve

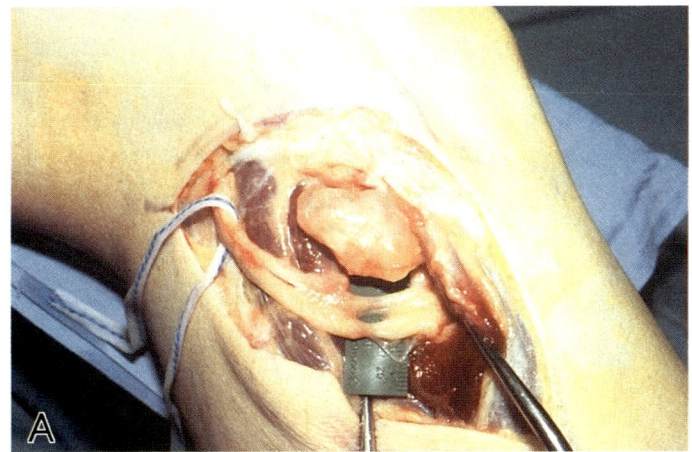

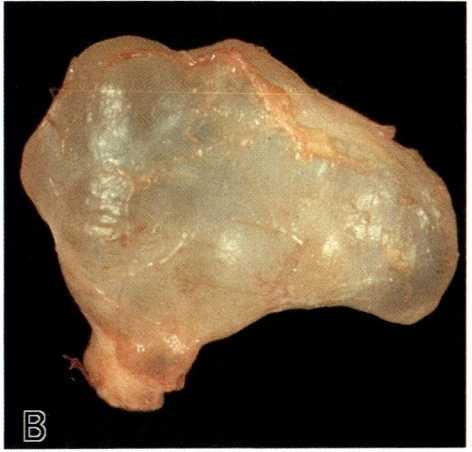

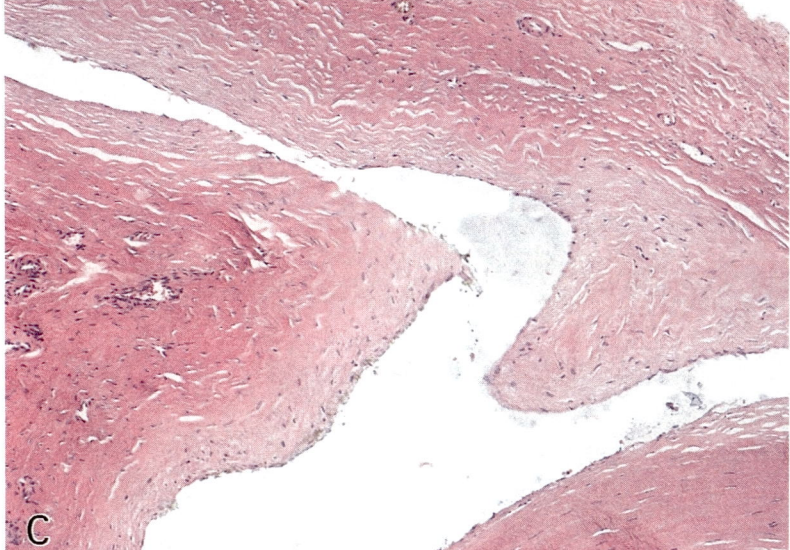

Figure 3-19
NERVE CYST

The peroneal nerve is the most common site of nerve cysts. This example was related to local trauma 8 months prior. At surgery (A) the cyst was found to arise from the tibiofibular joint to which it was connected by a stalk. The anterior tibial nerve lies inferior to the cyst; markedly compressed and displaced, it was contiguous with the capsule. Grossly, the cyst contained clear fluid and appeared thin-walled, distended, and translucent (B). Microsections of another example show typical features of a ganglion (C). (A,B: Figs. 3.406 and 3.407 from Okazaki H, Scheithauer BW. Atlas of neuropathology, 1988. With permission from the Mayo Foundation.)

lesion. The diagnosis may be suspected on ultrasonography or magnetic resonance imaging (77,88). Electromyograms demonstrate a neuropathy. On imaging scans the configuration of the cysts may suggest either a cystic nerve sheath tumor or, in the case of multifocal cystic change, a plexiform neurofibroma.

Gross Findings. At surgery (fig. 3-19) the nerve is variably affected, being either locally displaced and compressed by a uniloculate cyst (fig. 3-19) or misshapen by multiple cysts along its length (fig. 3-20). The lesions, measuring up to 10 cm in greatest dimension, may be either lobulated or fusiform, and uniloculate or multiloculate ("daughter cyst" formation). Gentle dissection shows nerve sheath cysts to either originate from a nearby joint through a stalk which

appears to serve as a "ball valve" (fig. 3-19A,B) or within epineurium as a beaded multilocular lesion involving a nerve segment (fig. 3-20). The lesions typically displace nerve fascicles and when ruptured, drain a clear fluid. In the case of joint-associated examples, this may be yellow and more viscid than normal joint fluid.

Microscopic Findings. Microscopically, nerve cysts somewhat resemble ordinary ganglion cysts because of the fibrous wall and lack of an epithelial lining (fig. 3-19C). The walls of cysts occasionally contain distorted nerve fascicles (fig. 3-21, left) or abut the perineurium of ones adjacent (fig. 3-21, right). Loose-textured mesenchymal cells comprise early examples (fig. 3-22, left), whereas abundant collagen and occasionally plump cells simulate a lining in chronic

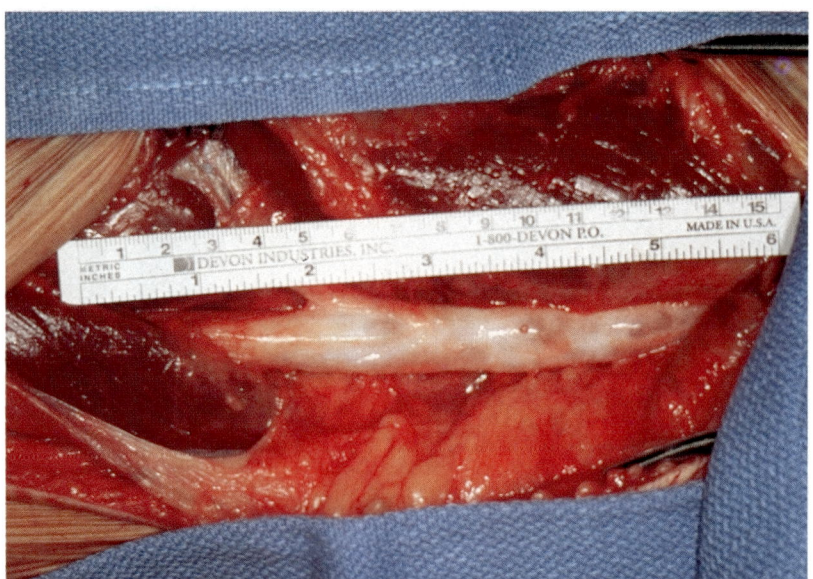

Figure 3-20
NERVE CYST
Top: This tibial nerve example showed multiple cysts to be distributed within a segment of epineurium.

Bottom: A longitudinal section of another example shows multiple cysts and segments of nearby, displaced nerve fascicles.

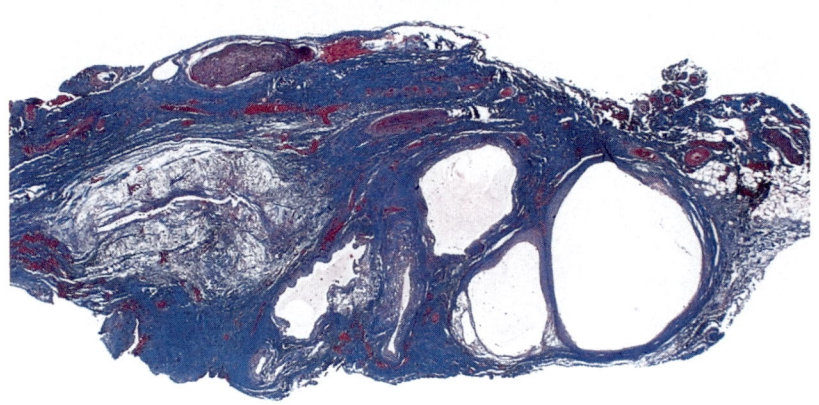

lesions (fig. 3-22, right). Occasional vacuolated cells or histiocytes may be present within the mucoid or proteinaceous material that fills the cyst cavity. Accumulation of mucin may sometimes be seen in endoneurium (fig. 3-23).

Immunohistochemical Findings. Lacking the characteristics of nerve sheath, the cells comprising the nerve cyst wall stain for vimentin and perhaps actin, but are nonreactive for S-100 protein (fig. 3-21, right) (90) and epithelial membrane antigen.

Ultrastructural Findings. One ultrastructural study of the wall of a nerve cyst found the constituent cells to be myofibroblasts rather than synovial cells (94).

Differential Diagnosis. A markedly *cystic schwannoma* with involvement of a grossly recognizable nerve is readily distinguished from a nerve cyst of the large, uniloculate type, given the absence in nerve cyst of a biphasic Antoni A and B pattern, Verocay bodies, and reactivity for S-100 protein. *Ganglion* and *synovial cysts* of the spine frequently compress nerve roots (82,86). A ruptured Baker's or synovial cyst, as occurs in rheumatoid synovitis, can also cause nerve entrapment or compression and may, therefore, clinically simulate a nerve cyst (71,73,75).

Treatment and Prognosis. Although the treatment of nerve cysts is operative intervention, there is currently no uniform surgical approach.

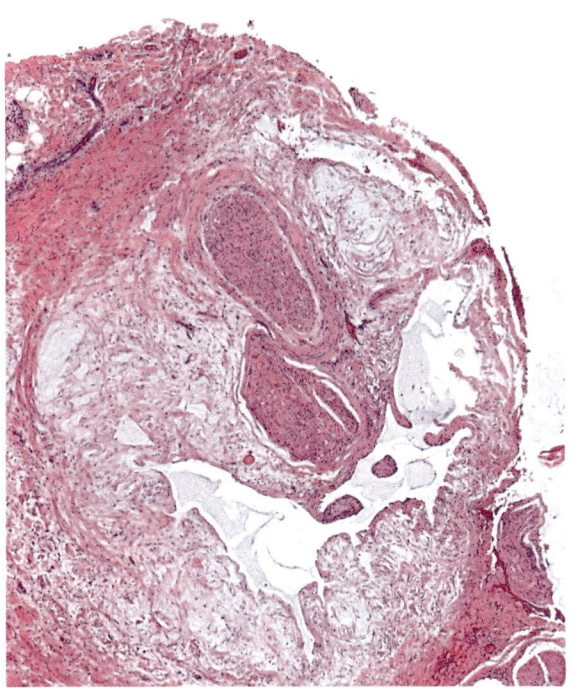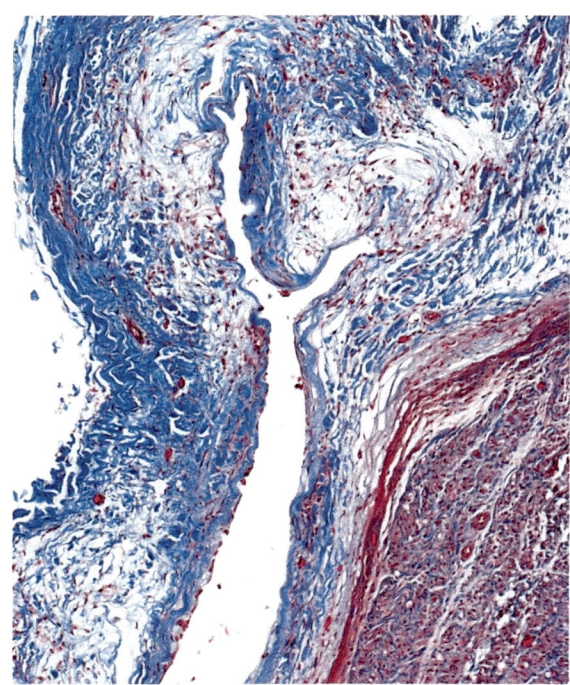

Figure 3-21
NERVE CYST
On cross section, several nerve fascicles seem to lie within (left) or to abut the cyst (right).

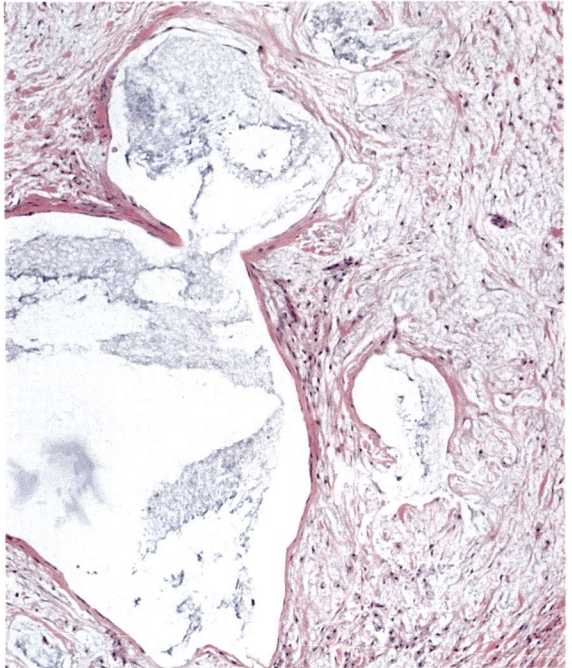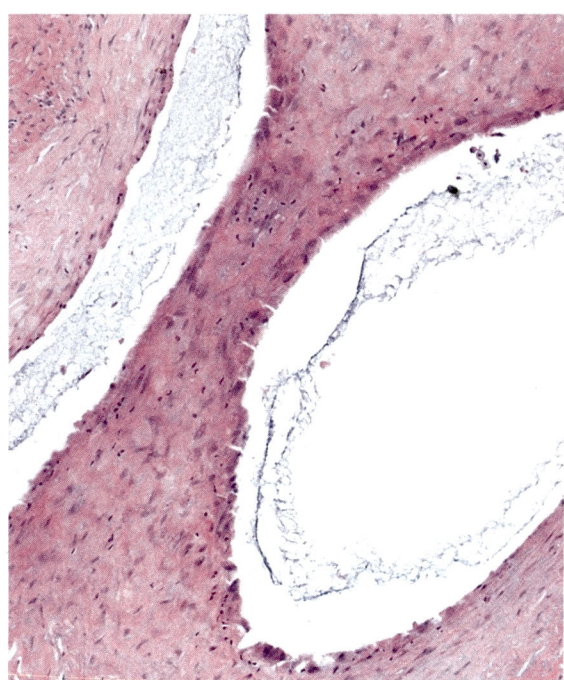

Figure 3-22
NERVE CYST
Left: In early phases of cyst development, the lining is thin.
Right: With time, fibrosis ensues and its inner aspect may assume a pseudoepithelial appearance.

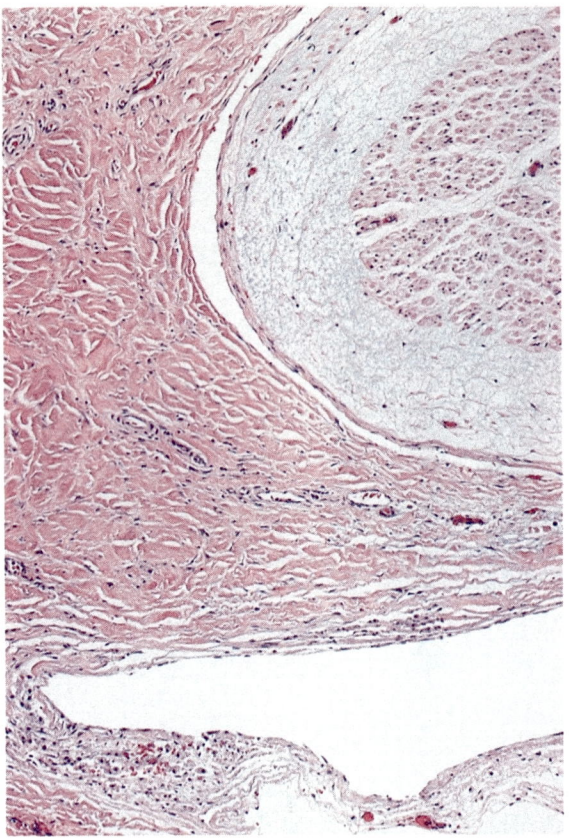

Figure 3-23
NERVE CYST
Fascicles nearby a cyst may show endoneurial accumulation of mucinous fluid.

Treatment varies from simple drainage to marsupialization or subtotal excision of the cyst. The latter is favored by those who view total excision as damaging to nerve or detrimental to neurologic function. Alternatively, some believe that use of an operating microscope permits total removal of nerve cysts without significant damage to nerve fibers (90). Whereas simple drainage is often followed by cyst recurrence, complete excision sometimes results in severe or complete nerve deficit (90). A 1982 literature review (96) found 65 percent of surgically treated patients to have complete return of nerve function after surgery; the remainder experienced residual paresis or paralysis. The overall rate of recurrence of nerve cysts reportedly varies from 7 (93) to 23 percent (91).

ENDOMETRIOSIS OF SCIATIC NERVE

Clinical Features. Although the most common cause of sciatic pain is vertebral disk prolapse, when cyclic in nature and occurring in reproductive-age females, the differential diagnosis includes endometriosis. To date, only 9 cases of endometriosis affecting the sciatic nerve have been reported (101). In early cases, the diagnosis had been suspected (100), but it was not until 1955 that the first biopsy-proven example of nerve involvement was reported (98). Symptoms typically include pain, sensory motor deficits, and occasionally foot drop. In classic cases, sciatica just precedes menses and persists several days after cessation of flow. With time, the asymptomatic interval often becomes shorter, and in some instances pain becomes constant. The right sciatic nerve is most often affected, since the position of the sigmoid colon prevents implantation of endometriosis deposits on the left pelvic side wall.

The diagnosis of endometriosis is suggested by the cyclic nature of the pain and may be confirmed by relief of symptoms with hormone suppression treatment. A negative gynecologic examination is the rule and does not exclude the diagnosis. Electromyography may help localize the lesion by distinguishing nerve root from peripheral nerve involvement. In the majority of cases, neuroimaging of the pelvic peritoneum demonstrates a characteristic "pocket sign" (99), a peritoneal evagination containing a mass of ectopic endometrial tissue (figs. 3-24, 3-25). It is unclear whether the pocket represents a fully developed preexisting structural abnormality (fig. 3-24) in which endometrial implants come to lie, or whether the implant and resulting tissue traction promote its formation. In any event, careful intraoperative examination usually demonstrates such a pocket as well as endometrial tissue compressing or involving the epineurium of the sciatic nerve or its roots (fig. 3-26).

Treatment and Prognosis. Definitive therapy consists of total abdominal hysterectomy with bilateral salpingo-oophorectomy. On the other hand, in patients wishing to preserve reproductive function, conservative treatment consists of meticulous resection of deposits from the sciatic nerve or its roots. Radiation therapy is also reportedly curative. Hormonal suppression therapy has had only limited success (101).

HETEROTOPIC OSSIFICATION OF NERVE (NEURITIS OSSIFICANS)

General Comments. This rare lesion is akin to myositis ossificans. A similar process follows trauma or burns.

Clinical Features. To date, only one well-documented example has been reported (102). It presented as a palpable mass in a female with a 9-year history of sensory abnormalities referable to an ulnar nerve, but no prior trauma. At surgery the hard, calcified mass was situated entirely within intact epineurium, separating but not directly involving fascicles. Interfascicular neurolysis led to sacrifice of only a number of small fascicles and resulted in no appreciable neurologic deficits. We have observed an identical lesion involving the tibial nerve of a 16-year-old male with a 4-week history of acute onset of painful pseudoparalysis and sensory loss. There was no history of prior trauma or of familial neurologic or metabolic disease. Partly calcified on plain X rays and measuring 4 cm, the lesion lay entirely

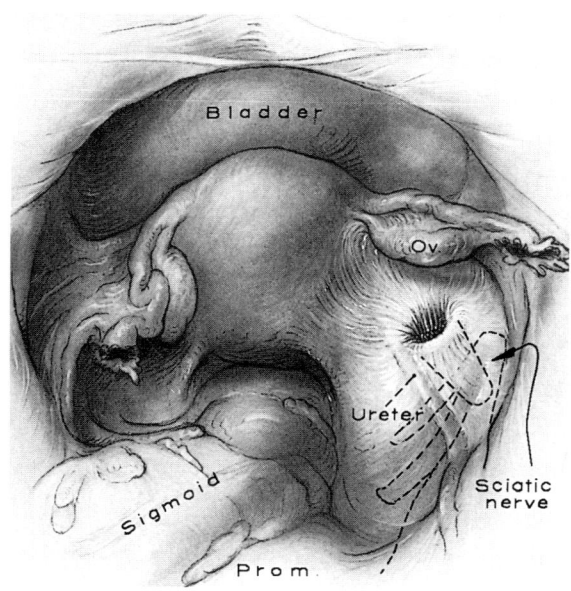

Figure 3-24
EVAGINATION OF PERITONEUM OF
RIGHT BROAD LIGAMENT ("POCKET SIGN")

(Fig. 1 from Head HB, Welch JS, Mussey E, Espinosa RE. Cyclic sciatica: report of a case with introduction of new surgical sign. JAMA 1962;180:521–4.)

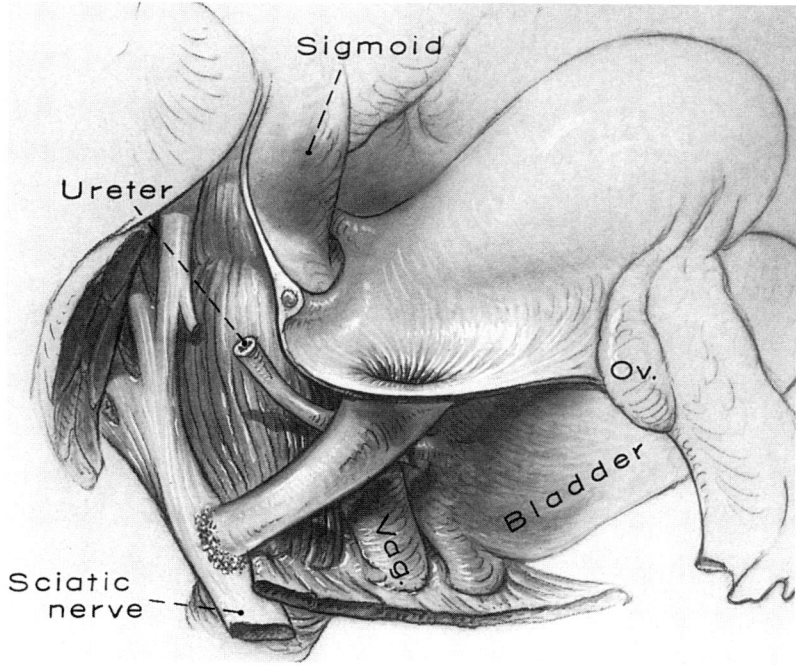

Figure 3-25
SCHEMATIC REPRESENTATION OF THE "POCKET SIGN"
WITH ENDOMETRIOSIS AND SCIATIC NERVE INVOLVEMENT

Note evagination of the pelvic peritoneum with endometriosis at its base and in intimate association with the sciatic nerve. (Fig. 2 from Head HB, Welch JS, Mussey E, Espinosa RE. Cyclic sciatica: report of a case with introduction of new surgical sign. JAMA 1962;180:521–4.)

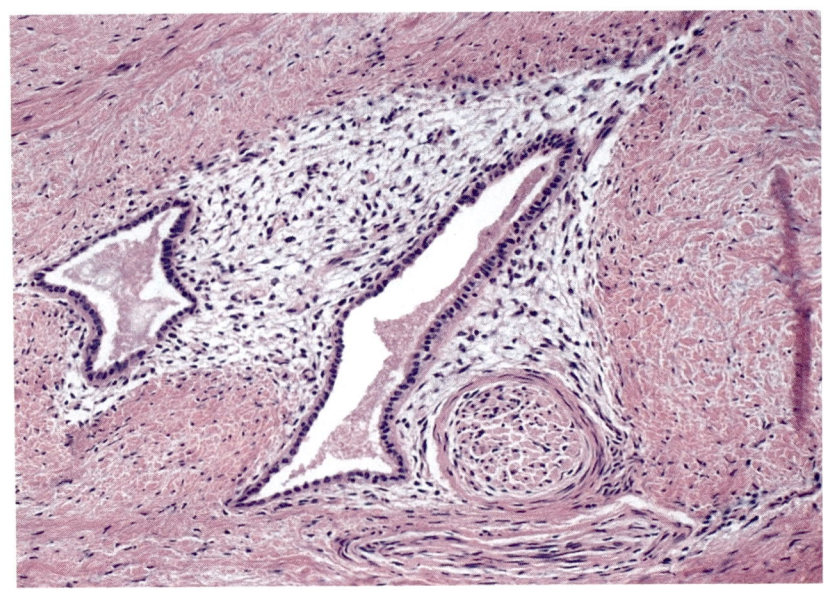

Figure 3-26
ENDOMETRIOSIS
OF SCIATIC NERVE
This typical deposit lay within the sciatic nerve epineurium. Note the association of endometriotic tissue with minute nerve branches.

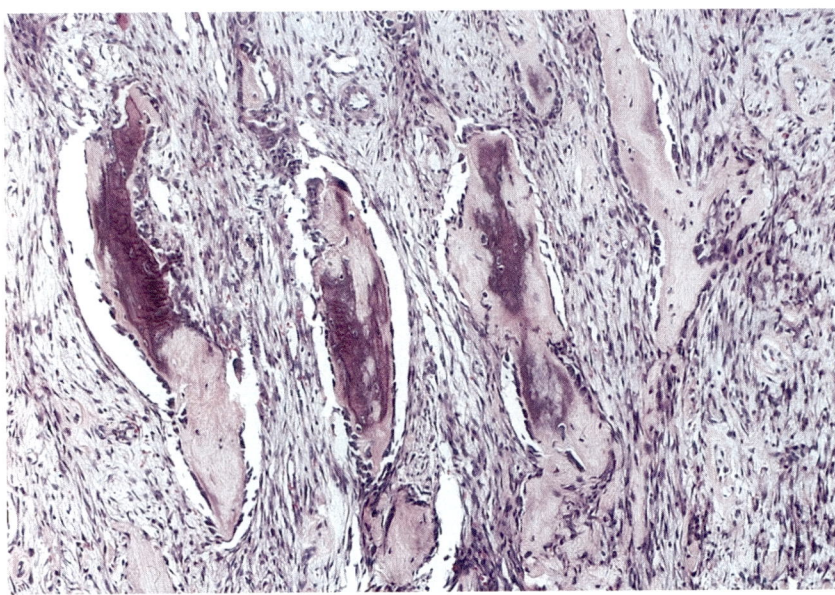

Figure 3-27
NEURITIS OSSIFICANS
The periphery of this epineurial lesion occurring in a 16-year-old male without a prior history of trauma shows an organized lamellar pattern of bone formation resembling that seen in myositis ossificans.

within the nerve and was associated with edema of surrounding nerve and soft tissue. Lobulated and peripherally ossified, its resection resulted in sacrifice of one third of the nerve fascicles, but only minimal sensory and motor loss. The histologic features were similar to those of myositis ossificans (fig. 3-27).

Although, as is often the case in myositis ossificans, no history of injury was elicited in the above-noted cases, we suspect that neuritis ossificans is a reaction to local trauma. This is

supported by the rare occurrence of somewhat similar, post-traumatic processes (103,104) that vary in extent. Such lesions include: 1) localized plaque-like ossification of nerve sheath; 2) segmental ossification of nerve and an adjacent but separate major artery (103); 3) shell-like perineural ossification adherent to nerve; and 4) destructive lesions in which ossification and fibrosis replaced an entire segment of nerve with no fascicles remaining. Short of one reported case (103) in which mature lamellar bone was enmeshed among fascicles of the median nerve, many of these lesions feature central ossification, often with bone marrow formation and surrounding reactive fibrosis. The preoperative evolution of this spectrum of post-traumatic ossifications extended from as little as 7 months to 12 years. Heterotopic bone formation, typically with encasement of the ulnar nerve, also occurs as a complication of severe burns in the region of the elbow (109).

Differential Diagnosis. The differential diagnosis of neuritis ossificans is limited and includes ossification in a lipofibromatous hamartoma of nerve (106) and perhaps of a peripheral nerve tumor. The latter is rare and usually occurs in "ancient" schwannomas (108). Calcification of perineurium as a consequence of metabolic disease, particularly diabetes (105), and the CREST syndrome (calcinosis, Reynaud's phenomenon, esophageal motility disorders, sclerodactyly, and telangiectasia) poses no problem in differential diagnosis (107).

Treatment and Prognosis. The favorable outcome of neuritis ossificans in which the nerve is intact and unaffected by major trauma (102) is attributable to a conservative, nerve sparing, microsurgical approach to therapy.

REFERENCES

Traumatic Neuroma

1. Das Gupta TW, Brasfield RD. Amputation neuromas in cancer patients. NY State J Med 1969;69:2129–32.
2. Dyck PJ, Giannini C, Lais A. Pathologic alterations of nerves. In: Dyck PJ, Thomas PK, eds. Peripheral neuropathy. 3rd ed. Philadelphia: WB Saunders Co., 1993:514–96.
3. Elhag AM, Al Awadi NZ. Amputation neuroma of the gallbladder. Histopathology 1992;21:586–7.
4. Giannini C, Dyck PJ. The fate of Schwann cell basement membranes in permanently transected nerves. J Neuropathol Exp Neurol 1990;49:550–63.
5. Lundborg G. Nerve regeneration and repair. A review. Acta Orthop Scand 1987;58:145–69.
6. Matsuoka J, Tanaka N, Kojima K, et al. A case of traumatic neuroma of the gallbladder in the absence of previous surgery and cholelithiasis. Acta Med Okayama 1996;50:273–7.
7. Nadim W, Anderson PN, Turmaine M. The role of Schwann cells and basal lamina tubes in the regeneration of axons through long lengths of freeze-killed nerve grafts. Neuropathol Appl Neurobiol 1990;16:411–21.
8. Reed RJ, Harkin JC. Tumors of the peripheral nervous system. Atlas of Tumor Pathology, 2nd Series. Fascicle 3, Supplement. Armed Forces Institute of Pathology, 1983.
9. Rush BF Jr, Stefaniwsky AB, Sasso A, Dumitrescu I, Wexler D. Neuroma of the common bile duct. J Surg Oncol 1988;39:17–21.
10. Sano T, Hirose T, Kagawa N, Hizawa K, Saito K. Polypoid traumatic neuroma of the gallbladder. Arch Pathol Lab Med 1985;109:574–6.
11. Shapiro L, Juhlin E, Brownstein MH. Rudimentary polydactyly: an amputation neuroma. Arch Dermatol 1973;108:223–5.
12. Shumate CR, Curley SA, Cleary KR, Ames FC. Traumatic neuroma of the bile duct causing cholangitis and atrophy of the right hepatic lobe. South Med J 1992;85:425–7.

Localized Interdigital Neuritis

13. Bennett GL, Graham CE, Mauldin DM. Morton's interdigital neuroma: a comprehensive treatment protocol. J Foot Ankle Surg 1995;16:760–3.
14. Lassmann G, Lassmann H, Stockinger L. Morton's metatarsalgia: light and electron microscopic observations and their relation to entrapment neuropathies. Virchows Arch [A] 1976;370:307–21.
15. Reed RJ, Bliss BO. Morton's neuroma: regressive and productive intermetatarsal elastofibrositis. Arch Pathol 1973;95:123–9.
16. Scotti TM. The lesion of Morton's metatarsalgia (Morton's toe). Arch Pathol 1957;63:91–102.
17. Wu KK. Morton's interdigital neuroma: a clinical review of its etiology, treatment, and results. J Foot Ankle Surg 1996;35:112–9.
18. Young G, Lindsey J. Etiology of symptomatic recurrent interdigital neuromas. J Am Podiatr Med Assoc 1993;83:255–8.

Pacinian Neuroma

19. Altmeyer P. Histologie eines rankenneuroms mit vater-pacini-lamellenkörper-èhnlichen strukturen. Der Hautarzt 1979;30:248–52.
20. Ariza A, Bilbao JM, Rosai J. Immunohistochemical detection of epithelial membrane antigen in normal perineurial cells and perineurioma. Am J Surg Pathol 1988;12:678–83.
21. Bale PM. Sacrococcygeal developmental abnormalities and tumors in children. Perspect Pediatr Pathol 1984;8:9–56.
22. Bale PM. Sacrococcygeal paciniomas. Pathology 1980;12:231–5.
23. Bas L, Oztek I, Numanoglu A. Subepineural hyperplastic pacinian corpuscle: an unusual cause of digital pain. Plast Reconstr Surg 1993;92:151–3.
24. Bennin B, Barsky S, Salgia K. Pacinian neurofibroma. Arch Dermatol 1976;112:1558.
25. Brögli M. Ein Fall von Rantenneurom mit Tastkörperchen. Frankf Z Pathol 1931;41:595–610.
26. Brynildsen PJ. Painful digital subepineural pacinian corpuscles [Letter]. Plast Reconstruct Surg 1985;75:929–30.
27. Calder JS, Holten I, Terenghi G, Smith RW. Digital nerve compression by hyperplastic pacinian corpuscles. A case report and immunohistochemical study. J Hand Surg 1995;20:218–21.
28. Cauna N, Mannan G. The structure of human digital pacinian corpuscles (corpuscula lamellosa) and its functional significance. J Anat (London) 1958;92:1–20.
29. Davydow. Materialien zur Kenntnis der Entwicklung des peripheren Nerven-systems, Dissert., Moskow, 1903. (Cited by Keibel F, Mall FP. Manual of human embryology. In: Keibel F, Mall FP, eds. Vol. 2. Philadelphia: JB Lippincott, 1912:180–1.)
30. Dembinski AS, Jones JW. Intra-abdominal pacinian neuroma: a rare lesion in an unusual location. Histopathology 1991;19:89–90.
31. Enzinger FM, Weiss SW. Benign tumors of peripheral nerves. In: Soft tissue tumors. St. Louis: CV Mosby, 1983:580–624.
32. Fletcher CD, Chan JK, McKee PH. Dermal nerve sheath myxoma: a study of three cases. Histopathology 1986;10:135–45.
33. Fletcher CD, Theaker JM. Digital pacinian neuroma: a distinctive hyperplastic lesion. Histopathology 1989;15:249–56.
34. Fraitag S, Gherardi R, Wechsler J. Hyperplastic pacinian corpuscles: an uncommonly encountered lesion of the hand. J Cutan Pathol 1994;21:457–60.
35. Friedman HI, Nichter LS, Morgan RF, Edgerton MT. Subepineural pacinian corpuscle: a cause of digital pain. Plast Reconstr Surg 1984;74:699–703.
36. Gama C, Mattosinho Franca LC. Nerve compression by pacinian corpuscles. J Hand Surg 1980;5:207–10.
37. Goldman F, Garner R. Pacinian corpuscles as a cause for metatarsalgia. J Am Podiatry Assoc 1980;70:561–7.
38. Greider JL Jr, Flatt AE. Glomus tumor associated with pacinian hyperplasia—case report. J Hand Surg 1982;7:113–7.
39. Hart WR, Thompson NW, Hildreth DH, Abell MR. Hyperplastic pacinian corpuscles: a cause of digital pain. Surgery 1971;70:730–5.
40. Jones NF, Eadie P. Pacinian corpuscle hyperplasia in the hand. J Hand Surg 1991;16A:865–9.
41. Jurecka W. Tactile corpuscle-like structures in peripheral nerve sheath tumors in plastic embedded material. Am J Dermatopathol 1988;10:74–9.
42. Jurecka W, Lassmann H, Lassmann G, Matras H, Watzek G, Hollmann K. Tactile corpuscle-like structures in a case of plexiform neurofibromatosis. Arch Dermatol Res 1979;266:43–50.
43. Levi L, Curri SB. Multiple pacinian neurofibroma and relationship with the finger-tip arterio-venous anastomoses. Br J Dermatol 1980;102:345–9.
44. Levi S. Osservazioni sullo sviluppo delle terminazioni nervose intraepiteliali, corpuscoli del Meissner e corpuscoli del Pacini. Arch ital di anat e di embriol 1933;32:149–70.
45. MacDonald DM, Wilson-Jones E. Pacinian neurofibroma. Histopathology 1977;1:247–55.
46. McCormack K, Kaplan D, Murray JC, Fetter BF. Multiple hairy pacinian neurofibromas (nerve-sheath myxomas). J Am Acad Dermatol 1988;18:416–9.
47. McPherson SA, Meals RA. Digital pacinian corpuscle neuroma eroding bone: a case report. J Hand Surg 1992;17A:476–8.
48. Owen DA. Pacinian neurofibroma [Letter]. Arch Pathol Lab Med 1979;103:99–100.
49. Patterson TJ. Pacinian corpuscle neuroma of the thumb pulp. Br J Plast Surg 1956;9:230–1.
50. Pease DC, Quillam TA. Electron microscopy of pacinian corpuscles. J Biophys Biochem Cytol 1957;3:331–42.
51. Prichard RW, Custer RP. Pacinian neurofibroma. Cancer 1952;5:297–301.
52. Prose PH, Gherardi GJ, Coblenz A. Pacinian neurofibroma. Arch Dermatol 1957;76:65–9.
53. Reed RJ, Harkin JC. Tumors of the peripheral nervous system. Atlas of Tumor Pathology, 2nd Series, Fascicle 3, Supplement. Washington, D.C.: Armed Forces Institute of Pathology, 1983.
54. Rhode CM, Jennings WD Jr. Pacinian corpuscle neuroma of digital nerves. South Med J 1975;68:86–9.
55. Rigdon RH. Neurogenic tumors produced by methylcholanthrene in the white pekin duck. Cancer 1955;8:906–15.
56. Sandzen SC, Baksic RW. Pacinian hyperplasia. Hand 1974;6:273–4.
57. Schochet SS Jr, Barrett DA II. Neurofibroma with aberrant tactile corpuscles. Acta Neuropathol (Berl.) 1974;28:161–5.
58. Schuler FA III, Adamson JE. Pacinian neuroma: an unusual cause of finger pain. Plast Reconstr Surg 1978;62:576–9.
59. Sellyei M, Balo J. Pathologic changes in the pacinian corpuscles around the pancreas. Acta Morphol Acad Sci Hung 1964;13:75–82.
60. Shiurba RA, Eng LF, Urich H. The structure of pseudo-meissnerian corpuscles. An immunohistochemical study. Acta Neuropathol 1984;63:174–6.
61. Smith TW, Bhawan J. Tactile-like structures in neurofibromas. An ultrastructural study. Acta Neuropathol 1980;50:233–6.
62. Stouder DJ, McDonald LW. Enlarged intra-abdominal pacinian corpuscles simulating tumor implants. Am J Clin Pathol 1968;49:79–83.
63. Theaker JM, Fletcher CD. Epithelial membrane antigen expression by the perineurial cell: further studies of peripheral nerve lesions. Histopathology 1989;14:581–92.

64. Toth BB, Long WH, Pleasants JE. Central pacinian neurofibroma of the maxilla. Oral Surg 1975;39:630–4.

65. Toth SP. Vater-pacinian corpuscle: a case report. J Am Podiatry Assoc 1975;65:247-9.

66. Watabe K, Kumanishi T, Ikuta F, Oyake Y. Tactile-like corpuscles in neurofibromas: immunohistochemical demonstration of S-100 protein. Acta Neuropathol 1983;61(3–4):173–7.

67. Weiser G. An electron microscope study of "pacinian neurofibroma." Virchows Arch [A] 1975;366:331–40.

68. Woodruff JM. Tumors and tumorlike conditions of peripheral nerve. Contemp Surg Pathol 1991;18:205–28.

69. Zweig J, Burns H. Compression of digital nerves by pacinian corpuscles: a report of two cases. J Bone Joint Surg 1968;50:999–1001.

Nerve Cyst

70. Bowers WH, Doppelt SH. Compression of the deep branch of ulnar nerve by an intraneural cyst. J Bone Joint Surg 1979;61:612–3.

71. Chang LW, Gowans JD, Granger CV, Millender LH. Entrapment neuropathy of the posterior interosseous nerve. A complication of rheumatoid arthritis. Arthritis Rheum 1972;15:350–2.

72. Cobb CA III, Moiel RH. Ganglion of the peroneal nerve. Report of two cases. Neurosurgery 1974;41:255–9.

73. DiRisio D, Lazaro R, Popp AJ. Nerve entrapment and calf atrophy caused by a Baker's cyst: case report. Neurosurgery 1994;35:333–4.

74. Donahue F, Turkel DH, Mnaymneh W, Mnaymneh LG. Intraosseous ganglion cyst associated with neuropathy. Skeletal Radiol 1996;25:675–8.

75. Fernandes L, Goodwill CJ, Srivatsa SR. Synovial rupture of rheumatoid elbow causing radial nerve compression. Brit Med J 1979;2:17–8.

76. Friedlander HL. Intraneural ganglion of the tibial nerve. A case report. J Bone Joint Surg 1967;49:519–22.

77. Ghossain M, Mohasseb G, Dagher F, Ghossain A. Compression du nerf sciatique poplite externe par un kyste synovial. Neurochirurgie 1987;33:412–4.

78. Gurdjian ES, Larsen RD, Linder DW. Intraneural cyst of peroneal and ulnar nerves. Report of two cases. J Neurosurg 1965;23:76–8.

79. Hartwell AS. Cystic tumor of median nerve. Operation: restoration of function. Boston Med Surg J 1901;144:582–3.

80. Hashizume H, Nishida K, Nanba Y, Inoue H, Konishiike T. Intraneural ganglion of the posterior interosseous nerve with lateral elbow pain. J Hand Surg 1995;20:649–51.

81. Herrin E, Lepow GM, Bruyn JM. Mucinous cyst of the sural nerve. J Foot Surg 1986;25:14–8.

82. Hsu KY, Zucherman JF, Shea WJ, Jeffrey RA. Lumbar intraspinal synovial and ganglion cysts (facet cysts). Ten-year experience in evaluation and treatment. Spine 1995;20:80–9.

83. Iannotti JP, Ramsey ML. Arthroscopic decompression of a ganglion cyst causing suprascapular nerve compression. Arthroscopy 1996;12:739–45.

84. Jaradeh S, Sanger JR, Maas EF. Isolated sensory impairment of the thumb due to an intraneural ganglion cyst in the median nerve. J Hand Surg 1995;20:475–8.

85. Jenkins SA. Solitary tumors of peripheral nerve trunks. J Bone Joint Surg 1952;34:401–11.

86. Kornberg M. Nerve root compression by a ganglion cyst of the lumbar anulus fibrosus. A case report. Spine 1995;20:1633–5.

87. Krucke W. Pathologie der Peripheran Nerven. In: Olivecrona H, Tonnis W, Krenkel W, eds. Handbuch der Neurochirurgie; Vol 7, Pt 3. Berlin: Springer-Verlag, 1974.

88. Masciocchi C, Innacoli M, Cisternino S, Barile A, Rossi F, Passariello R. Myxoid intraneural cysts of external popliteal ischiatic nerve. Report of two cases studied with ultrasound, computed tomography and magnetic resonance imaging. Eur J Radiol 1992;14:52–5.

89. Nicholson TR, Cohen RC, Grattan-Smith PJ. Intraneural ganglion of the common peroneal nerve in a 4-year-old boy. J Child Neurol 1995;10:213–5.

90. Nucci F, Artico M, Santoro A, Bardella L, Delfini R, Boseo S. Intraneural synovial cyst of the peroneal nerve. Report of two cases and review of the literature. Neurosurgery 1990;26:339–44.

91. Orf G. Intraneurale ganglienzysten. Schweizer Arch Neurol Neurochirug Psychiatr 1972;110:55–67.

92. Parkes AR. Intraneural ganglion of the lateral popliteal nerve [Abstract]. J Bone Joint Surg 1960;42B:652.

93. Robert R, Resche F, Lajat Y, Thoulouzan E, De Kersaint-Gilly A, Descuns P. Kyste synovial intraneural du sciatique poplite externe. A propos d'un cas. Neurochirurgie 1980;26:135–43.

94. Scherman BM, Bilbao JM, Hudson AR, Briggs RT. Intraneural ganglion. A case report with electron microscopic observations. Neurosurgery 1981;8:487–90.

95. Seddon HJ. Surgical disorders of the peripheral nerves. 2nd edition. Edinburgh: Churchill Livingstone, 1975:124–6.

96. Sotelo D, Frankel VH. Intraneural ganglion of the peroneal nerve. A cause of peripheral neuropathy. Bull Hosp Joint Dis Orthop Inst 1982;42:230–5.

97. Weller RO, Cervos-Navarro J. Pathology of peripheral nerves. London: Butterworth, 1977:153–4.

Endometriosis of Sciatic Nerve

98. Denton RO, Sherrill JD. Sciatic syndrome due to endometriosis of sciatic nerve. South Med J 1955;48:1027–31.

99. Head HB, Welch JS, Mussey E, Espinosa RE. Cyclic sciatica: report of case with introduction of a new surgical sign. JAMA 1962;180:521–4.

100. Schlicke CP. Ectopic endometrial tissue in the thigh. JAMA 1946;132:445–6.

101. Torkelson SJ, Lee RA, Hildahl DB. Endometriosis of the sciatic nerve: a report of two cases and a review of the literature. Obstet Gynecol 1988;71:473–7.

Heterotopic Ossification of Nerve (Neuritis Ossificans)

102. Catalano F, Fanfani F, Pagliei A, Taccardo G. Sur un cas d'ossification intraneurale primitive du nerf cubital. Ann Chir Main Memb Super 1992;11(2):157–62.

103. Dal Monte A, Zanoli S. Su di un caso di ossificazione dell'arteria omerale e del nervo mediano. Chir Org Mov 1959;47:465–71.

104. Gui L. Ossificazioni post-traumatiche dei nervi periferici. Chir Org Mov 1948;32:241–70.

105. King RH, Llewelyn JG, Thomas PK, Gilbey SG, Watkins PJ. Perineurial calcification. Neuropathol Appl Neurobiol 1988;14:105–23.

106. Louis DS, Dick HM. Ossifying lipofibroma of the median nerve. J Bone Joint Surg 1973;55A:1082–4.

107. Polio JL, Stern PJ. Digital nerve calcification in CREST syndrome. J Hand Surg 1989;14A:201–3.

108. Sarma DP, Robichaux J, Fondak A. Ossified neurofibroma. J La State Med Soc 1983;135:22–3.

109. Vorenkamp SE, Nelson TL. Ulnar nerve entrapment due to heterotopic bone formation after a severe burn. J Hand Surg 1987;12A:378–80.

4

INFLAMMATORY AND INFECTIOUS LESIONS
SIMULATING TUMORS OF NERVE

On rare occasion, non-neoplastic conditions result in variable enlargement of nerve. This chapter focuses upon: inflammatory pseudotumor, a rare lesion; sarcoidosis, the nature of which is unsettled; and leprosy, the most common infection of nerve. We have seen examples of inflammatory pseudotumor and of leprosy that clinically simulated a neoplasm. Although sarcoidosis and leprosy generally produce only limited, localized enlargement of nerve, both are discussed for the sake of completeness.

Nerves may also become secondarily entrapped within benign fibroproliferative lesions, such as with extra-abdominal fibromatosis; idiopathic processes, including mediastinal fibrosis, retroperitoneal fibrosis, and Riedel's thyroiditis; or tumefactive fibroinflammatory lesions of the head and neck (5,10–12).

INFLAMMATORY PSEUDOTUMOR OF NERVE

Definition. This is an idiopathic, localized, tumefactive inflammatory process of nerve which is typically composed of chronic inflammatory and reactive mesenchymal cells. Synonyms include *lymphoid hyperplasia, plasma cell granuloma,* and *inflammatory myofibroblastic tumor.*

General Comments. The term inflammatory pseudotumor has been used to denote a heterogenous group of tumor-like lesions of wide distribution with no known etiology (2). Composed of chronic inflammatory and fibrohistiocytic cells, examples at non-neural sites include nodular lymphoid hyperplasia, plasma cell granuloma, and fibrous xanthoma. The varied designations applied to these lesions reflect their broad range of appearance and cellular composition (2). Inflammatory pseudotumors have been described in a number of locations including lung (8), lymph node (3), brain (6), orbit (4), and soft tissues. Many present as mass lesions clinically suggestive of malignancy.

Clinical Features. To date, only four cases of inflammatory pseudotumor originating in nerve have been reported, one each involving the facial, sciatic, and radial nerves, and the greater auricular nerve (1,7,9). In lieu of a detailed discussion of this small number of cases, their essential clinicopathologic features are summarized in Table 4-1. Also uncommon is mononeuropathy due to secondary involvement of nerve by fibroinflammatory processes in surrounding soft tissues (11,12).

Gross Findings. Affected nerves are segmentally enlarged and are either fusiform or nodular (fig. 4-1). In reported cases, the process has been limited to epineurium; the perineurium and endoneurium are spared.

Microscopic Findings. Aside from the presence of chronic inflammation, the histologic features of reported cases have varied greatly, ranging from patchy chronic lymphoplasmacellular inflammation with a variable fibrous reaction (fig. 4-2) through dense nodular lymphoid hyperplasia (fig. 4-3). One unusual example was composed primarily of uninucleate and multinucleate histiocytes (fig. 4-4). By definition, special stains for microorganisms, e.g., bacteria, tubercle bacilli, lepra bacilli, and fungi, are negative.

Immunohistochemical Findings. In three reported cases (1,9) the lymphocytes were polyclonal and predominantly of T-cell type. In one case (figs. 4-1, 4-2; Table 4-1, case 2) lymphocyte subtyping showed the infiltrate to be composed of a mixture of T and to a lesser extent B cells of normal phenotype. As expected, the histiocytes and giant cells occasionally seen are immunoreactive for macrophage markers (fig. 4-4) and lack both S-100 protein and CD1A reactivity.

Differential Diagnosis. Although a clinical consideration, the histologic distinction of inflammatory pseudotumor from benign and malignant peripheral nerve sheath tumors poses no problem. With the exception of schwannomas, which in our experience may show appreciable capsular and perivascular lymphocytic infiltrates in approximately 5 percent of cases, peripheral nerve tumors are infrequently inflamed. For unknown reasons, schwannomas also rarely exhibit multiple foci of

Table 4-1

INFLAMMATORY PSEUDOTUMOR OF NERVE: LITERATURE SUMMARY

Authors	Age/ Sex	Nerve	Clinical	Gross/Operative Finding	Surgery	Pathology	Follow-Up
Keen et al. (7)	41/M	Right facial n. and geniculate ganglion	Two episodes Bell's palsy 5 yrs. and 4.5 mos. prior. Initial bout responsive to steroids and stellate ganglion block	Hard, vascular mass involving geniculate ganglion, facial n., and tensor tympani muscle	Resection mass and nerve	Epidural lesion. Nerve surrounded by fibrotic granulation tissue with chronic inflammation	Total facial n. palsy at 6 mos. nerve function < 5% at 2 yrs.
Weiland et al. (9; case 1)	35/M	Sciatic n.	Two yr. progression of idiopathic right lower leg weakness, numbness, and pain, through atrophy to total sensorimotor loss in peroneal, tibial, sural nerves	Fusiform 16 x 2 cm enlargement of right sciatic n. (see fig. 4-1)	Resection of epineurial mass encompassing the sciatic n.	Epineurial T- and to a lesser extent B-lymphocyte infiltrate with fibrosis and loss of myelinated nerve fibers (see fig. 4-2)	Diminution in pain but persistent total sensorimotor loss. No recurrence at 4 yrs.
Weiland et al. (9; case 2)	18/F	Radial n.	Three mos. painful enlargement right distal radial n. with associated radiation and dysesthesia to thumb, index, and middle fingers	Ovoid, lipomalike, 2.5 cm lesion involving right radial n.	Resection of epineurial based lesion with sparing of nerve fascicles	Epineurial infiltrate of histiocytes, giant cells, and predominantly T lymphocytes (see fig. 4-4)	Neurologic recovery and no evidence of recurrence at 3-mos. follow-up
Beer et al. (1)	41/M	Left greater auricular n.	One yr. painful, mobile right neck mass. Associated dental carries	Mass affecting left greater auricular nerve. Intact fascicles traversed the lesion	Resection with segment of nerve	Follicular lymphoid hyperplasia with primarily perifascicular growth. Extension into one fascicle noted (see fig. 4-3)	Hypoesthesia of left face

noncaseating granulomatous inflammation (see fig. 7-22). In such instances, stains for organisms are negative and the neoplastic nature of the underlying lesion is readily apparent.

The distinction of inflammatory pseudotumor from infection is based on negative histochemical stains for organisms as well as cultures. A discussion of the differential diagnosis with lymphoma is beyond the scope of this work but, to date, the lymphocytes of inflammatory pseudotumors have lacked atypia and have been polytypic. Neither Langerhans' histiocytosis nor Rosai-Dorfman disease have been reported to cause tumor-like enlargement of nerve; unlike inflammatory pseudotumors rich in histiocytes, both these lesions are immunopositive for S-100 protein, the former also being CD1A reactive.

Treatment and Prognosis. Timely biopsy and nerve-sparing microsurgical resection afford a maximal chance of cure without neurologic deficit. We have observed only one instance of recurrence: regrowth of a lesion of the auricular nerve affecting proximal and distal nerve stumps 2 years after gross total resection.

SARCOIDOSIS OF PERIPHERAL NERVE

Definition. Sarcoidosis is a systemic disorder characterized by idiopathic noncaseating granulomatous inflammation.

General Comments. Sarcoidosis clinically affects the nervous system in approximately 5 percent of patients (15). In many instances, involvement is largely or entirely of either the

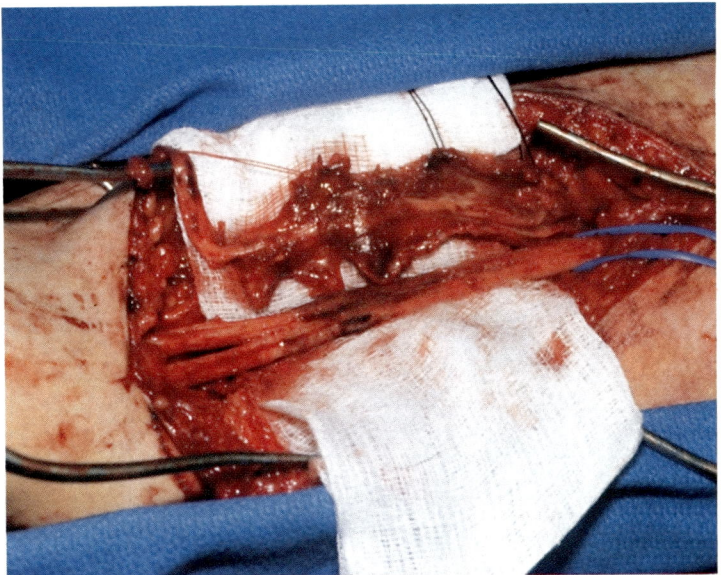

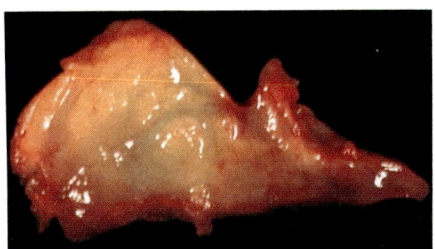

Figure 4-1
INFLAMMATORY PSEUDOTUMOR

Left: The operative photograph of a reported case (ref. 7, Table 4-1, case 1) shows the intact, grossly normal sciatic nerve as well as the pseudotumor, a layer of fibroinflammatory epineurial tissue (above) which was dissected free of the nerve.

Above: The thick shell of affected epineurium, seen in cross section, had chronically compressed the nerve with resultant near-total loss of neurologic function. (Figures 4-1 and 4-4 are from the same case.)

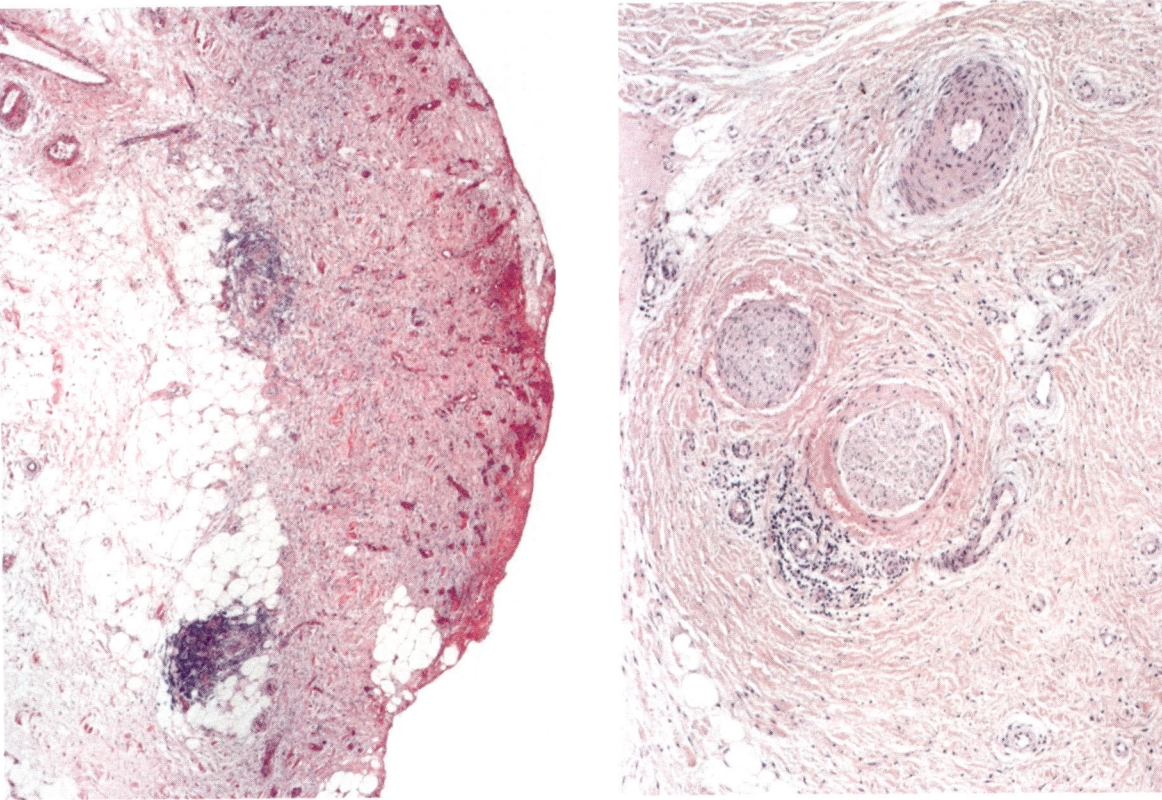

Figure 4-2
INFLAMMATORY PSEUDOTUMOR

The surgical specimen consisted of inflamed epineurial fibroadipose tissue. At low magnification and in cross section (left), the markedly thickened epineurium (same case as fig. 4-1) shows extensive fibrosis and chronic inflammation. The smooth contour (left) represents the perimeter of the epineurium. Composed of benign lymphocytes and occasional plasma cells, the inflammatory infiltrate entraps minute, otherwise normal-appearing nerve fascicles (right).

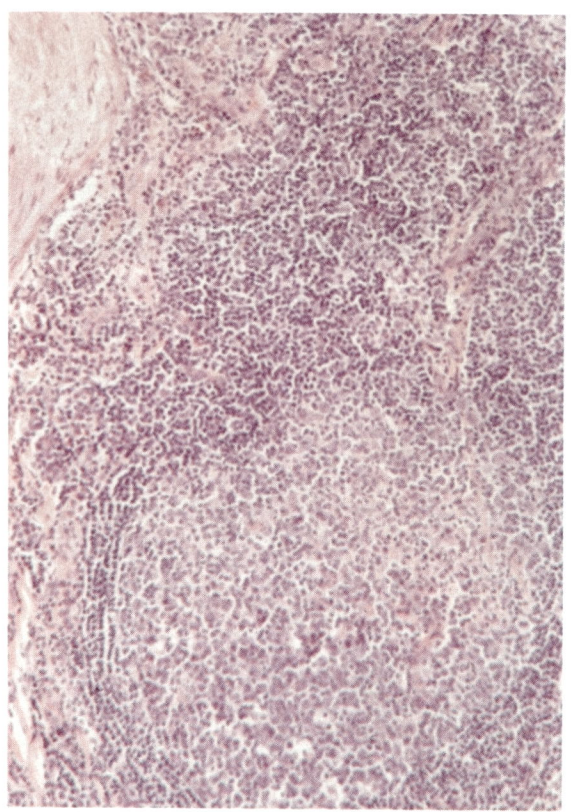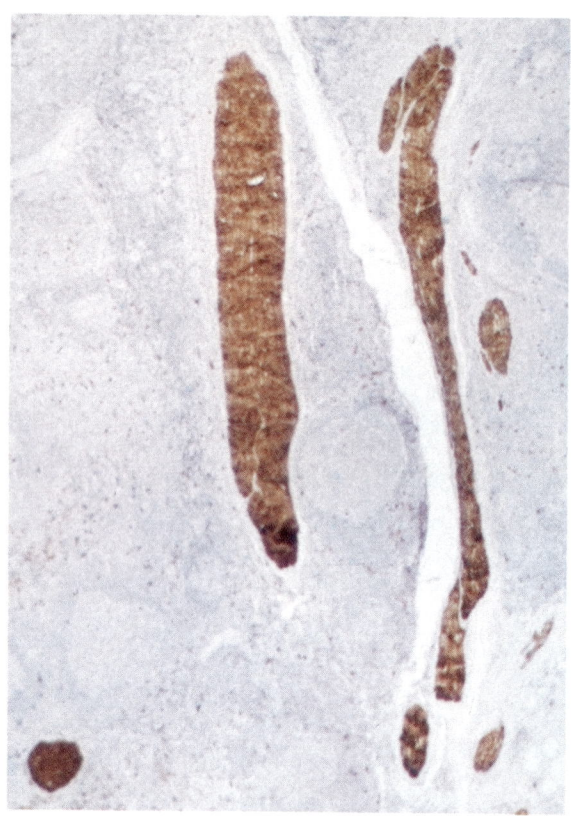

Figure 4-3
INFLAMMATORY PSEUDOTUMOR

This example, occurring in the greater auricular nerve of 41-year-old male, featured nodular lymphoid hyperplasia limited to epineurium. Note encirclement of the intact, S-100 protein-positive nerve fascicles (right). Intrafascicular growth was a focal finding. (Courtesy of Dr. T. Beer, Gosport Hants, UK.)

peripheral or central nervous system. In a majority of cases, the peripheral nervous system is affected, most often the 7th cranial nerve (19). Patient age at the onset of peripheral neurosarcoidosis ranges from the second to the eighth decade. Females are more often affected. The disorder occurs in all races but shows a proclivity for blacks.

Clinical Features. Peripheral neurosarcoidosis may present in one of three forms: multiple mononeuropathy, radiculopathy, and polyneuropathy. Inasmuch as significant nerve enlargement or hypertrophy is not a clinical feature of sarcoidal neuropathy, the lesions do not clinically mimic neoplasms. Sarcoidosis may affect cranial and spinal nerves. Cranial polyneuritis is characterized by the occurrence of multiple fluctuating and remitting cranial nerve palsies, usually in young to middle-aged women, and may be associated with the uveoparotid form of sarcoid-

osis. Systemic symptoms are generally minimal. The facial nerve is most frequently affected. Lesions are often bilateral but are usually asynchronous. Although cranial and spinal nerves can be involved in isolation, these lesions frequently coexist. Often affected nerves include the peroneal, median (16), radial (14), and phrenic nerves (18), as well as cauda equina nerve roots (13). Sarcoidal polyneuropathy may be acute and indistinguishable from Guillain-Barré syndrome, or may present as a slowly progressive sensorimotor neuropathy. No specific clinical features distinguish progressive sarcoidal polyneuropathy from other forms of peripheral neuropathy.

A diagnosis of sarcoidosis may be made on biopsy of any accessible lesion, such as of skin, lymph node, muscle, scalene fat pad, gingiva, conjunctiva, bronchus, or liver. It may also be facilitated by a careful ophthalmologic examination, as well

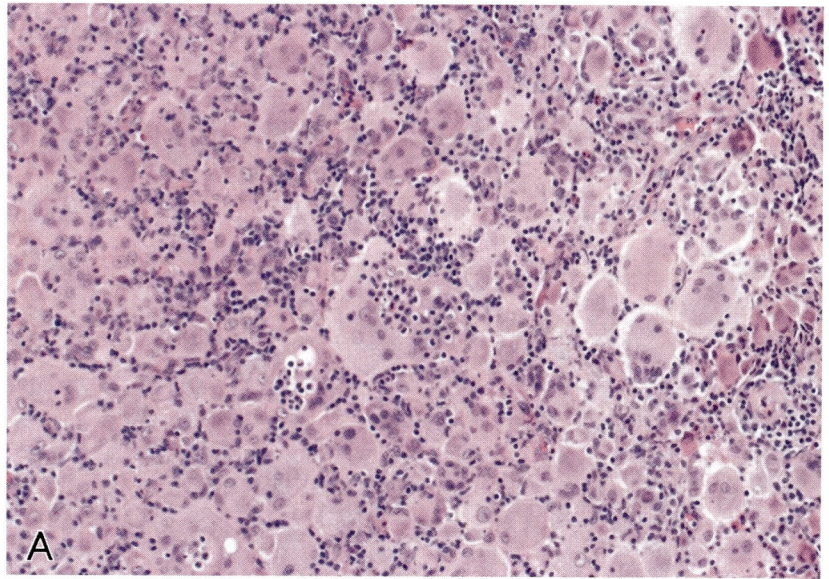

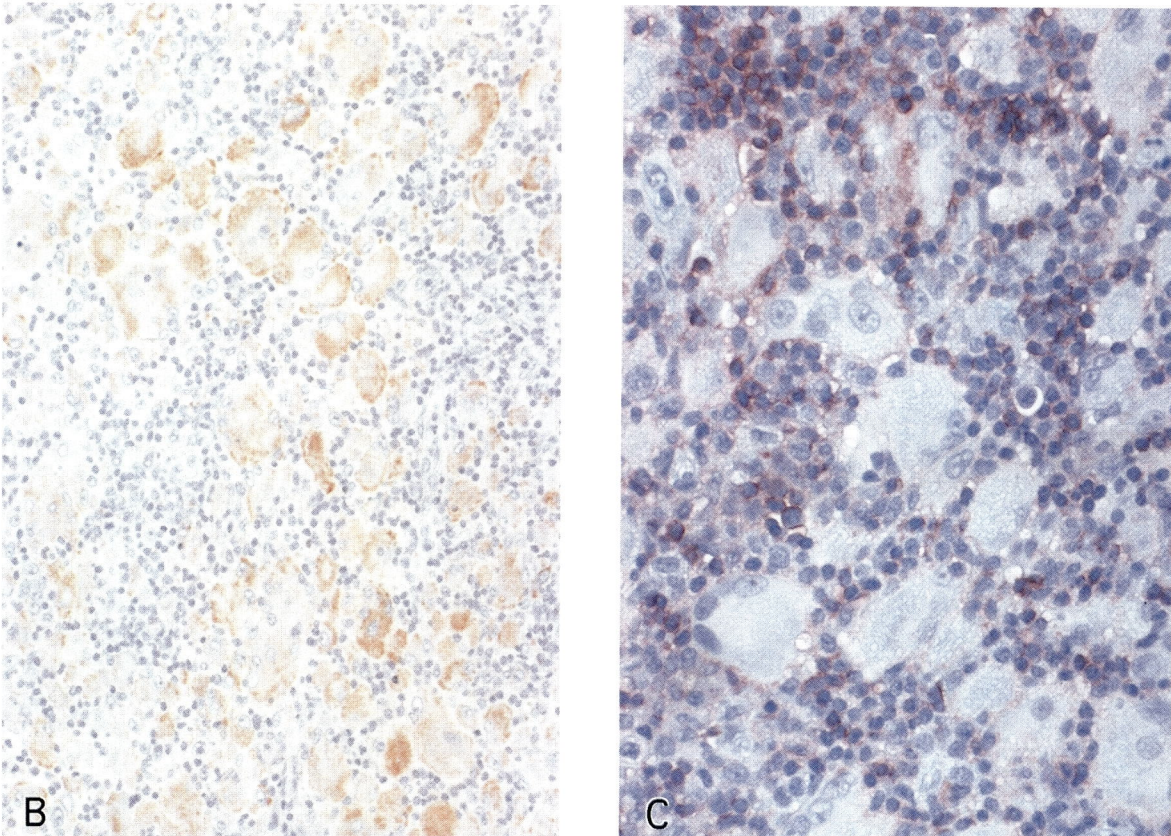

Figure 4-4
INFLAMMATORY PSEUDOTUMOR
This reported example (case 2 [9]), a lesion of the radial nerve epineurium (A), consisted of KP1-positive multinucleate giant cells (B), small CD46-reactive lymphocytes (C), and occasional eosinophils.

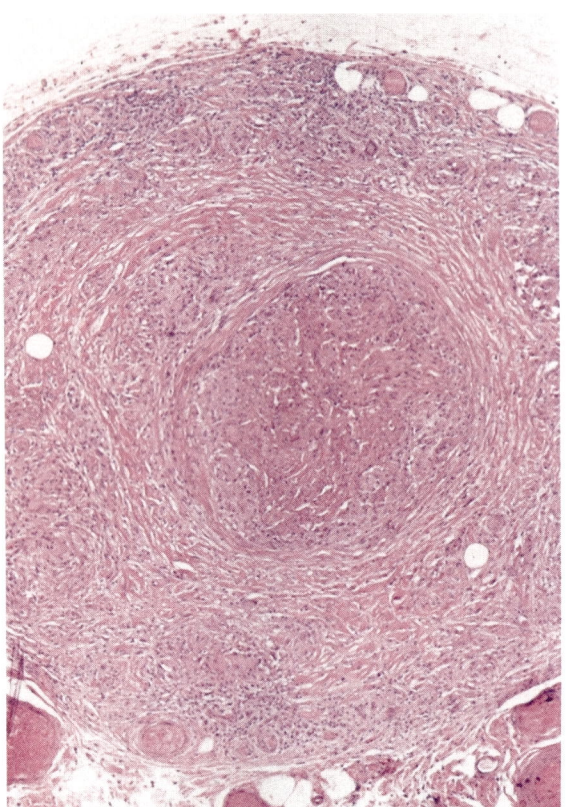 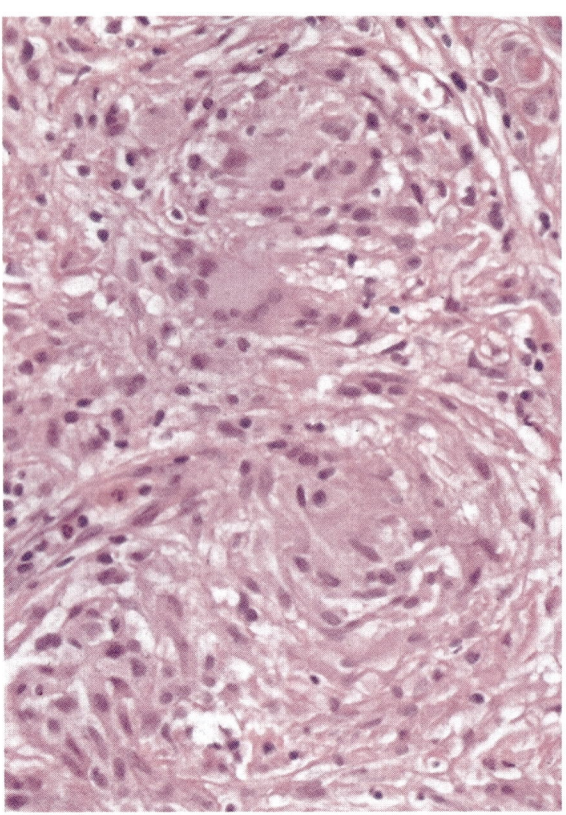

Figure 4-5
SARCOIDOSIS
This section of the sural nerve shows involvement of epineurium, perineurium, and endoneurium (left) by noncaseating granulomas (right). (Courtesy of Dr. C. Giannini, Treviso, Italy and Dr. P. J. Dyck, Rochester, Minnesota.)

as by other, albeit less reliable methods, including: 1) the Kveim test which yields a significant proportion of both false-positive and false-negative results; 2) measurement of serum levels of angiotensin-converting enzyme (ACE), which is often positive when the diagnosis is apparent; and 3) cerebrospinal fluid examination, which may demonstrate an elevated protein level, a slight increase in lymphocytes, and sometimes a decrease in glucose level.

Gross and Microscopic Findings. Peripheral neuropathy in sarcoidosis has been exhaustively studied (17). Affected nerves appear firm and thickened but do not resemble tumors. Although not diagnostic, the histologic finding of sarcoidal-type granuloma at any site is of clinical value. Typically, the noncaseating granulomas of sarcoidosis are sharply demarcated and consist, in varying proportion, of epithelioid histiocytes and multinucleate giant cells in association with only a

small number of lymphocytes. Schaumann bodies can occasionally be seen within giant cells. Although frank necrosis is lacking, fibrinoid material may be evident at the center of some granulomas. Sarcoidal granulomas often exhibit interstitial reticulin staining. Marked fibrosis is a common feature of chronic lesions. By definition, sarcoidal granulomas are devoid of microorganisms on special stain and are culture negative.

Neuropathy may result from granulomatous inflammation, but the mechanism of nerve injury in sarcoidal neuropathy is controversial. Diffuse involvement of perineurium, epineurium, and endoneurium by sarcoidal granulomas (fig. 4-5) is thought to mediate nerve fiber damage resulting in multiple mononeuropathy, radiculopathy, and progressive polyneuropathy. Both nerve fiber compression, as well as ischemia due to accompanying lymphocytic angiitis, have been suggested as possible pathogenetic mechanisms.

The pathologic basis of the acute sarcoidal polyradiculoneuropathy resembling Guillain-Barré syndrome is unclear.

Differential Diagnosis. The principle differential diagnoses are *fungal* and *mycobacterial infections.* The likelihood of infection is high in the face of necrotizing granulomas. Special stains, including silver preparations for fungi and acid fast or fluorescent stains for mycobacteria are useful, but a negative reaction is no assurance that a lesion is noninfectious. Correlation with clinical data, skin tests, and culture results is mandatory. Other processes in the differential diagnosis are *necrotizing vasculitis* and *lymphoma.*

Treatment and Prognosis. The outcome in sarcoidal neuropathy is favorable. Recoveries were documented even prior to the introduction of steroid therapy. The latter has a beneficial effect upon cranial as well as spinal nerve disease. In general, the prognosis of patients with peripheral nervous system sarcoidosis is more favorable than for those with central nervous system involvement.

LEPROUS NEUROPATHY

General Comments. Leprosy, the most common and treatable cause of peripheral neuropathy worldwide, is a chronic disease resulting from *Mycobacterium leprae* infection. It affects any part of the body, but shows a particular tendency to involve superficially situated nerves, as well as skin, eyes, respiratory tract, and testes. Bacterial invasion of peripheral nerve is noted in all cases. Although the disease is most common in the tropics and subtropics, it also occurs in more temperate zones. Leprosy has been reported in association with human immunodeficiency virus (HIV) infection (22), although not to the extent that atypical mycobacterial infection occurs in this setting. The mechanism of spread is uncertain, but a respiratory route and direct inoculation into skin appear most likely. Untreated patients are the major source of infection, but in North America infected armadillos also represent a potential reservoir. Only a minority of the population is susceptible to infection and children are more readily affected than adults.

M. leprae, the only bacterium that regularly invades peripheral nerve, is morphologically indistinguishable from *M. tuberculosis.* It consists of an acid-fast rod measuring 1 to 8 μm in length and up to 0.5 μm in diameter. Although the organism has not been cultured in vitro, the mouse foot pad (26) and the armadillo (24) serve as experimental models of infection. The optimal growth temperature of *M. leprae* is low (27° to 30°C).

Clinical Features. Patients with leprosy mainly present with peripheral neuropathy. Sensory loss often precedes other evidence of disease and manifests sequentially as loss of temperature, touch, pain, and pressure sensations. Affected nerves are more often the small, intracutaneous or subcutaneous nerves than the major peripheral nerve trunks. As a rule, frank nerve enlargement is not clinically discernible.

Depending upon the capacity of the patient to respond to the infection, three major clinicopathologic forms of leprosy are generally recognized: tuberculoid, lepromatous, and borderline varieties, each of which features peripheral nerve involvement. Most patients fall into the borderline category, although it is preferable both conceptually and in practical terms, to consider leprosy as a complete spectrum of host response to the pathogen rather than as a disease having various forms.

It is the nature of the cellular immune response that determines whether an exposed individual develops leprosy, as well as its subtype (20). In normal individuals the organisms are taken up by macrophages which become activated by their interaction with T lymphocytes. The result is destruction of the bacillus. An abnormality of T-cell function probably plays a major role in the pathogenesis of leprosy, but the exact mechanisms are not understood. A minor excess in activity results in localized lesions (tuberculoid leprosy), whereas more a marked abnormality results in a major defect of cell-mediated immunity and the development of generalized disease (lepromatous leprosy). Patients with defects of intermediate severity develop a borderline form. Measurement of the cellular immune response is the basis of the lepromin skin test, which is positive in tuberculoid and negative in lepromatous leprosy.

Gross and Microscopic Findings. Presenting as localized disease, *tuberculoid leprosy* is characterized by asymmetric cutaneous lesions occurring over the extensor surfaces of the extremities, the face, or the buttocks. Microscopically, the lesions consist of epithelioid granulomas, only rarely associated with caseation, and a peripheral

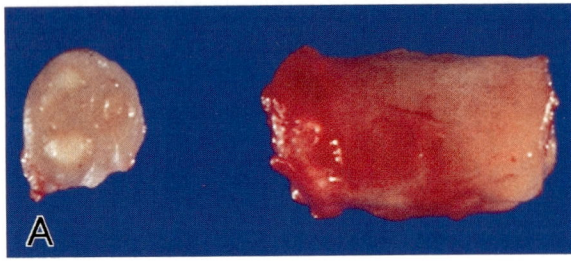

Figure 4-6
TUBERCULOID LEPROSY, NEUROPATHY

This form of the disease may markedly enlarge peripheral nerves (A). It features extensive noncaseating granulomatous inflammation (B) associated with nerve fibers and myelin (C). Necrosis of large nerves in advanced cases results in "cold abscess" formation that may grossly mimic tumor (D). (D, courtesy of Dr. P. Brand, Carville, Louisiana.)

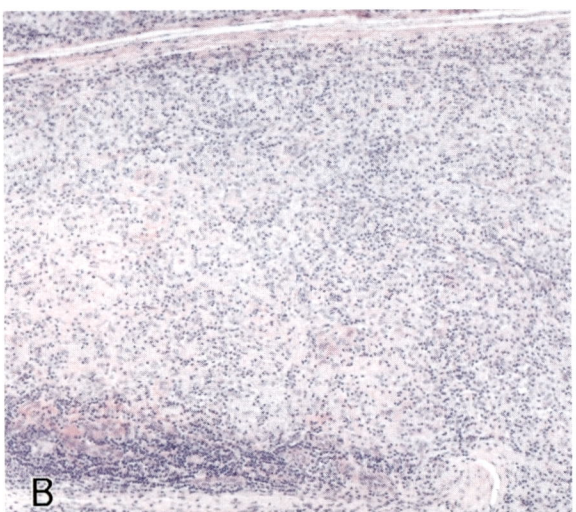

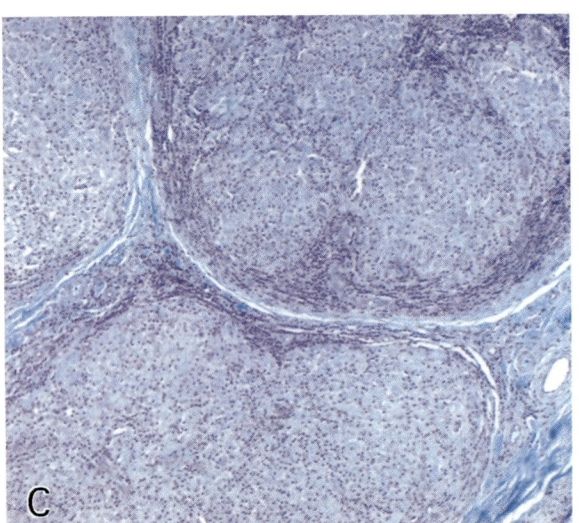

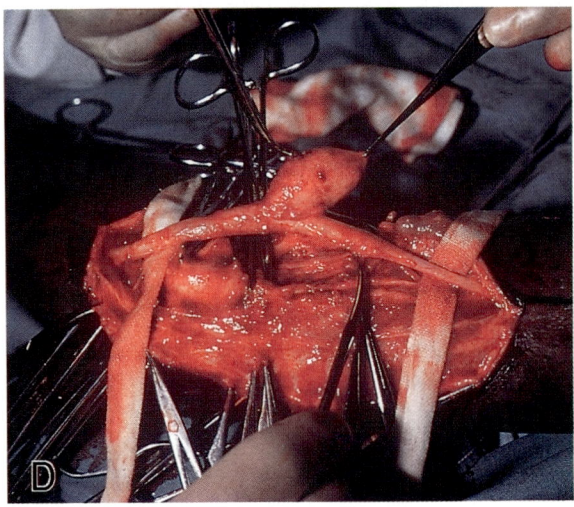

infiltrate of lymphocytes. Epithelioid histiocytes are numerous. The inflammatory process is concentrated about dermal appendages and to a great degree involves cutaneous and subcutaneous nerves (fig. 4-6A). Destruction of nerve fibers and loss of myelin is extensive. Although the fibers are invaded and destroyed, even a careful search under oil immersion reveals only rare Fite stain–positive organisms within epithelioid histiocytes (fig. 4-6B,C) and Langhans-type giant cells.

The spread of tuberculoid leprosy to surrounding tissues is by direct extension, but the manner in which nerve trunks beneath cutaneous lesions become involved is unclear. Transaxonal bacillary spread has not been proven to occur. Affected nerves are palpably enlarged (fig. 4-6A). Of major sensorimotor nerves, those most

frequently affected include the ulnar, median, peroneal, and facial; of sensory nerves it is the cutaneous radial, digital, posterior auricular, and sural. The inflammatory response to bacilli consists primarily of noncaseating granulomatous inflammation (fig. 4-6B,C). In cases with intense response to bacilli, necrosis may result in the formation of a so-called cold abscess (fig. 4-6D) (25). Associated dystrophic calcification may occur and be radiographically apparent. Cold abscesses heal with time, resulting in widespread fibrosis of all nerve compartments. Microscopically, the changes resemble those occurring in smaller nerves. The infiltrate consists of epithelioid histiocytes and giant cells and, although concentrated within the epineurium and perineurium, may also extend to involve the endoneurium. Bacilli

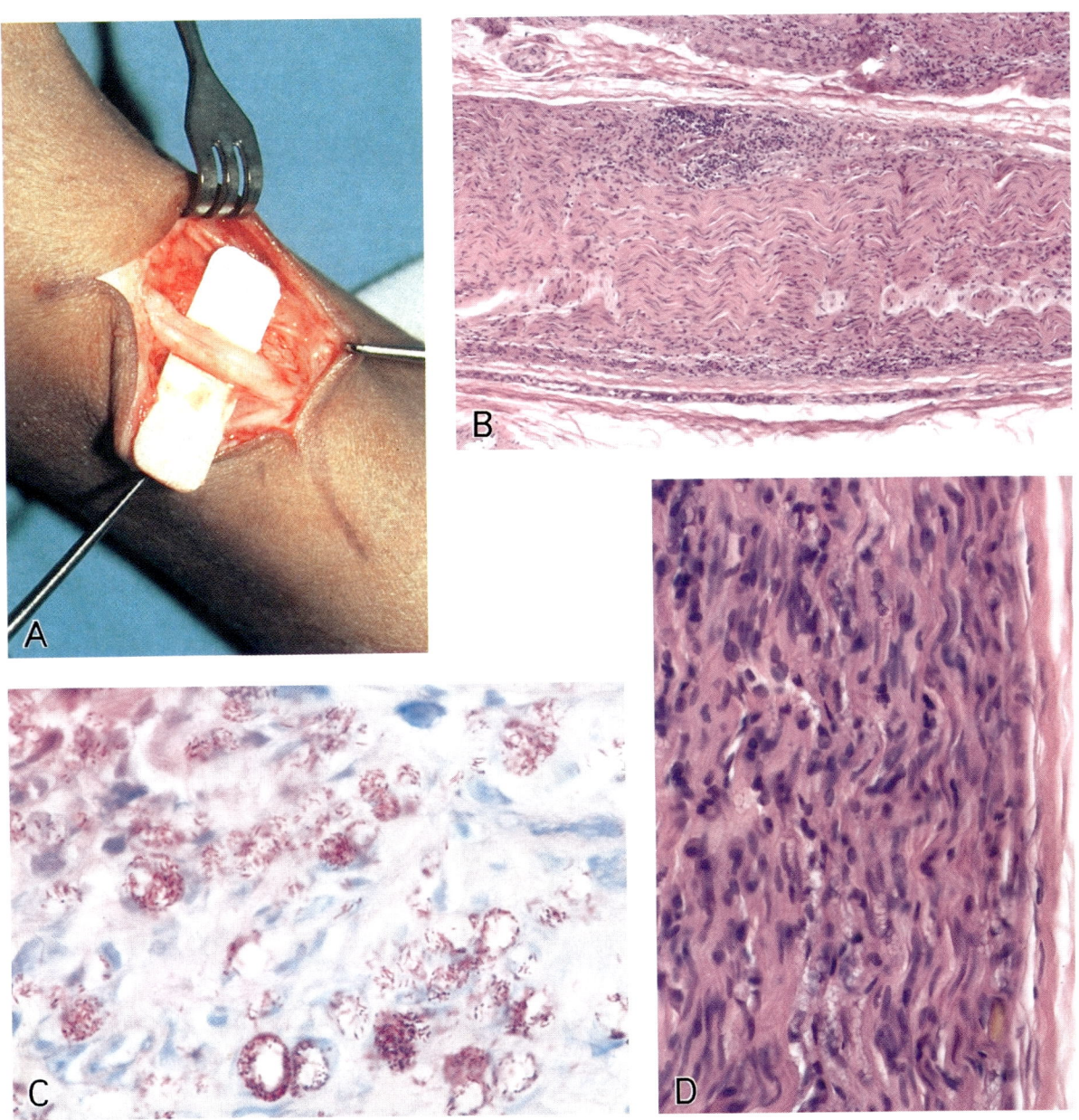

Figure 4-7
LEPROMATOUS LEPROSY, NEUROPATHY
    This form of leprosy only occasionally produces nerve enlargement, in this case, of a segment of the superficial radial nerve of an adult patient with a 5-year history of the disease (A). Nerve involvement in yet another case features only mild chronic inflammation, primarily histiocytic infiltration of perineurium and peripheral endoneurium (B). Such cells contain masses of Fite stain–positive mycobacteria (C). Bacilli-containing vacuoles within Schwann and perhaps endothelial cells are best seen in longitudinal sections of the nerve (D).

may not be demonstrable. Fascicular abnormalities are variable; some are destroyed and others are relatively spared.

    In contrast to the tuberculoid variant, *lepromatous leprosy* is characterized by a florid prolifera-

tion of bacteria and by their hematogenous dissemination. As in tuberculoid leprosy, superficial tissues are affected. In skin the process is concentrated upon blood vessels, nerves, and adnexa. Gross infiltration of the skin of the face results in leonine facies, a feature of advanced disease. The upper respiratory tract, eyes, testes, and lymph nodes, particularly inguinal and epitrochlear nodes, may also be affected. A cutaneous biopsy in lepromatous leprosy shows an infiltrate of foamy histiocytes (Virchow cells) containing masses of bacilli, as well as scattered plasma cells. Unlike tuberculoid leprosy, the lepromatous form shows little in the way of an inflammatory reaction and no significant tissue destruction.

Although nerve trunk involvement can occur in longstanding disease (fig. 4-7A), nerve enlargement is generally not as prominent a feature as in tuberculoid leprosy. Nonetheless, we have seen an example of nerve-centered lepromatous infection presenting as a palpable mass in the neck. It was regarded as a possible neoplasm of peripheral nerve by the referring pathologist. The correct diagnosis was achieved only after the demonstration of acid-fast organisms. Affected nerves are architecturally preserved (fig. 4-7B), but bacteria-rich histiocytes involve the perineurium (fig. 4-7B),

splitting it in an "onion skin" fashion. Fascicular involvement may be uneven. In addition to epineural and perineurial involvement, vacuoles containing abundant bacilli may be seen within endoneurium (fig. 4-7C), particularly at its interface with the perineurial sheath. Longitudinal sections of the nerve show the bacilli-containing vacuoles seen in Schwann cells aligned along nerve fibers (fig. 4-7D). Endothelial cells within endoneurium may also contain bacilli. Wallerian degeneration and segmental demyelination may be seen (21). In longstanding cases, the endoneurium may undergo considerable fibrosis, but organisms may still be demonstrable.

Differential Diagnosis. A complete discussion is beyond the scope of this work. The reader is referred to the excellent review by Sabin et al. (23). The diagnosis is predicated upon the demonstration of acid-fast or Fite stain–positive microorganisms in the appropriate clinical setting.

Treatment and Prognosis. In most instances, specific antimicrobial therapy is curative.

REFERENCES

Inflammatory Pseudotumor of Nerve

1. Beer TW, Carr NJ, Weller RO. Inflammatory pseudotumor of peripheral nerve [Letter]. Am J Surg Pathol 1998;22:1035–6.
2. Chan JK. Inflammatory pseudotumor: a family of lesions of diverse nature and etiologies. Am J Surg Pathol 1995;19:859–72.
3. Davis RE, Warnke RA, Dorfman RF. Inflammatory pseudotumor of lymph nodes. Additional observations and evidence for an inflammatory etiology. Am J Surg Pathol 1991;15:744–56.
4. Diaz-llopis M, Menezo JL. Idiopathic orbital pseudotumor and low-dose cyclosporine. Am J Ophtholmol 1989;107:547–8.
5. Fanous MM, Margo CE, Hamed LM. Chronic idiopathic inflammation of the retropharyngeal space presenting with sequential abducens palsies. J Clin Neuro-Ophthalmol 1992;12:154–7.
6. Figarella-Branger D, Gambarelli D, Perez-Castillo M, Garbe L, Grisoli F. Primary intracerebral plasma cell granuloma: a light, immunocytochemical, and ultrastructural study of one case. Neurosurgery 1990;27:142–7.
7. Keen M, Conley J, McBride T, Mutter G, Silver J. Pseudotumor of the pterygomaxillary space presenting as anesthesia of the mandibular nerve. Laryngoscope 1986;96:560–3.
8. Matsubara O, Tan-Liu NS, Kenney RM, Mark EJ. Inflammatory pseudotumor of the lung: progression from organizing pneumonia to fibrous histiocytoma or to plasma cell granuloma in 32 cases. Hum Pathol 1988;19:807–14.
9. Weiland TL, Scheithauer BW, Rock MG, Sargent JM. Inflammatory pseudotumor of nerve. Am J Surg Pathol 1996;20:1212–8.
10. Wiseman JB, Arriaga MA, Houston GD, Boyd EM. Facial paralysis and inflammatory pseudotumor of the facial nerve in a child. Otolaryngol Head Neck Surg 1995;113:826–8.
11. Wold LE, Weiland LH. Tumefactive fibro-inflammatory lesions of the head and neck. Am J Surg Pathol 1983;7:477–82.
12. Yanagihara N, Segoe M, Gyo K, Ueda N. Inflammatory pseudotumor of the facial nerve as a cause of recurrent facial palsy: case report. Am J Otol 1991;12:199–202.

Sarcoidosis

13. Campbell JN, Black P, Ostrow PT. Sarcoid of the cauda equina. Case report. J Neurosurg 1977;47:109–12.
14. Cesaro P, Defer G, Barbizet J, Degos JD. Sarcoïdose du système nerveux central et périphérique. Ann Med Interne (Paris) 1984;135:144–8.
15. Delaney P. Neurologic manifestations of sarcoidosis: review of the literature with a report of 23 cases. Ann Intern Med 1977;87:336–45.
16. Kömpf D, Neundörfer B, Kager-Gutchalian C, et al. Mononeuritis multiplex bei Boeckscher-Sarkoidose. Nervenarzt 1976;47:687–9.
17. Matthews WB. Sarcoid neuropathy. In: Dyck PJ, Thomas PK, eds. Peripheral neuropathy. 3rd ed. Philadelphia: W.B. Saunders Co., 1993:1418–23.
18. Mayock RL, Bertrand P, Morrison CE, Scott JH. Manifestations of sarcoidosis. Analysis of 145 patients with a review of nine series selected from the literature. Am J Med 1965;35:67–89.
19. Silverstein A, Feuer MM, Siltzbach LE. Neurologic sarcoidosis: study of 18 cases. Arch Neurol 1965;12:1–11.

Leprous Neuropathy

20. Adams LB, Krahenbuhl JL. Granulomas induced by Mycobacterium leprae. Methods (Duluth) 1996;9:220–32.
21. Gibbels E, Henke U, Klingmuller G, Haupt WF. Myelinated and unmyelinated fibers in sural nerve biopsy of a case with lepromatous leprosy—a quantitative approach. Int J Lepr Other Mycobact Dis 1987;55:333–7.
22. Ponnighaus JM, Mwamjsi LJ, Fine PE, et al. Is HIV infection a risk factor for leprosy? Int J Lepr 1991;59(2):221–8.
23. Sabin TD, Swift TR, Jacobson RR. Leprosy. In: Dyck PJ, Thomas PK, eds. Peripheral neuropathy. 3rd ed. Philadelphia: W.B. Saunders Co., 1993:1354–79.
24. Scollard DM, Lathrop GW, Truman RW. Infection of distal peripheral nerves by M. leprae in infected armadillos; an experimental model of nerve involvement in leprosy. Int J Lepr 1996;64(2):146–51.
25. Sehgal VN. Nerve abscesses in leprosy in Northern India. Lepr Rev 1966;37:109–12.
26. Shepard CC. Experimental chemotherapy in leprosy, then and now. Int J Lepr Other Mycobact Dis 1973;41:307–19.

5

HYPERPLASTIC LESIONS

PALISADED ENCAPSULATED NEUROMA

Definition. This is a usually cutaneous true neuroma, nodular or occasionally plexiform in appearance, consisting of Schwann cells and numerous axons within a delicate perineurium-derived capsule. It is also called *solitary circumscribed neuroma.*

General Comments. Since its first description by Reed et al. (10), several additional series (2, 3,6–8) have established palisaded encapsulated neuroma (PEN) as a clinically and morphologically distinct form of true neuroma. Although underdiagnosed and often unrecognized, it is a relatively common lesion. Originally considered a primary hyperplasia of nerve fibers or a hamartoma consisting of axons and their complement of Schwann cells, recent publications suggest an analogy to traumatic neuroma (3,7), a notion weakened by the absence of scarring in adjacent dermis. In any case, PEN can be viewed as one of several forms of true neuroma, a category that includes traumatic, pacinian, and mucosal neuromas.

Clinical Features. PENs are longstanding lesions. Most (90 percent) affect the face, particularly the nose, cheek, forehead, and lips. Many lie in proximity to mucocutaneous junctions and affect the oral mucosa (5,9). Although occurring from adolescence to old age, the peak age incidence is in the 5th to 7th decades, with a slight female predominance. Occasional examples involve skin of the extremities. The lesions are typically solitary, nonpigmented, painless papules or nodules which, though not ballottable or hard, are firm. The overlying skin is usually smooth and intact, and lacks hair. Hyperpigmentation is absent. Clinically, PENs resemble melanocytic nevi, basal cell carcinoma, or adnexal tumors. None have been associated with neurofibromatosis or mucosal neuromatosis (6). Although there are no known predisposing factors, such as trauma, PENs are associated with acne more often than is expected (1,7).

Microscopic Findings. At low power, PENs appear circumscribed, smooth contoured, and round or pear-shaped; the largest or bulbous component is often superficial (fungating pattern) (fig. 5-1). A significant minority are multinodular (fig. 5-2) or even plexiform (3). Most measure around 3 mm (range, 1 to 15 mm) and are located in the skin, usually the reticular dermis. Subcutaneous tissue is rarely involved. In approximately 20 percent of cases a nerve of origin is microscopically apparent; serial sectioning increases the likelihood of finding the associated nerve at either the base or apex of the lesion (fig. 5-1B). Despite the use of the descriptive terms palisaded and encapsulated, PENs are often not entirely encapsulated and, as a rule, do not show significant palisading. Most are only partially encapsulated: the delicate, compacted perineurial layer and connective tissue surrounding them is often lacking in superficial portions of the lesion where vertical alignment of the microfascicles may be seen (fig. 5-2, top). PENs situated entirely within the reticular dermis may appear totally encapsulated. A cracking artifact, presumably related to fixation, frequently separates the lesions from surrounding dermis (fig. 5-1A), and individual fascicles (fig. 5-1B,C).

At higher power, the bulk of the process consists of spindled Schwann cells, often aligned and fasciculated, coursing in various directions or forming occasional nodules (figs. 5-1B, 5-2, bottom, 5-3). The bundles or microfascicles of Schwann cells surround small numbers of often aligned, silver-positive axons variously distributed throughout the lesion (fig. 5-4C). Axons are present in greatest concentration within distinctly fascicular areas. In a physiologic manner, the Schwann cells are orderly aligned about axons which are often concentrated at the base or apex of the lesion, areas in which contiguity with a small nerve is most often seen. The Schwann cells are normal in appearance, having a sinuous configuration with elongate tapering nuclei (fig. 5-4A). No atypia or mitotic activity is evident. Stains for myelin are usually negative. Only a minority of lesions (3) show focal fibrosis, chronic inflammation, or stromal mucopolysaccharide accumulation. Mast cells are infrequent. Overlying skin occasionally shows mild hyperkeratosis but no hyperpigmentation.

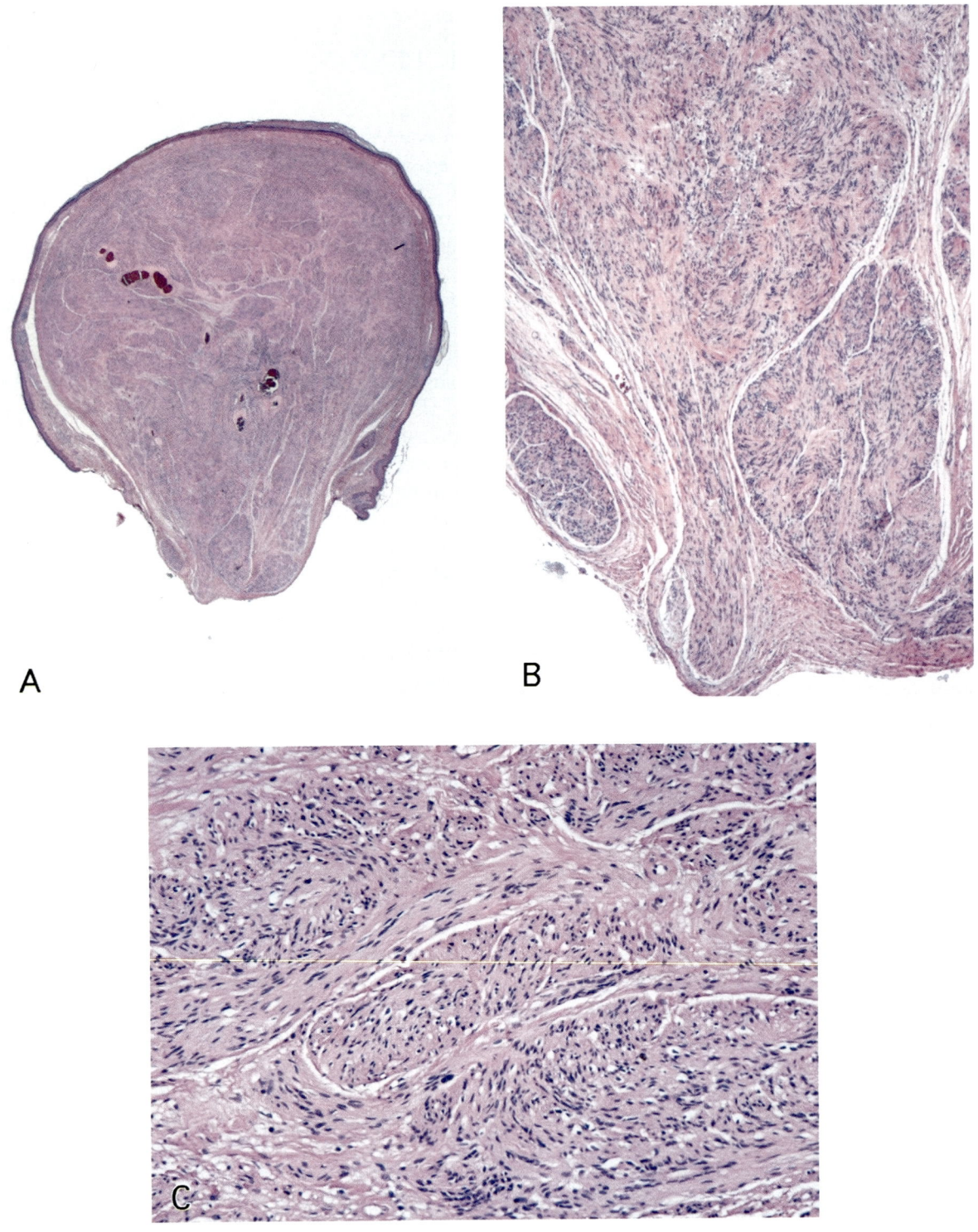

Figure 5-1
PALISADED ENCAPSULATED NEUROMA

A: This whole-mount section of a somewhat pedunculated example shows the pear-shaped lesion beneath intact skin.

B: The entering nerve is readily apparent on the inferior aspect of the lesion. Note artifactual "cracking" between the lesion and its interface with surrounding dermal tissues.

C: The microfascicular growth pattern is readily apparent.

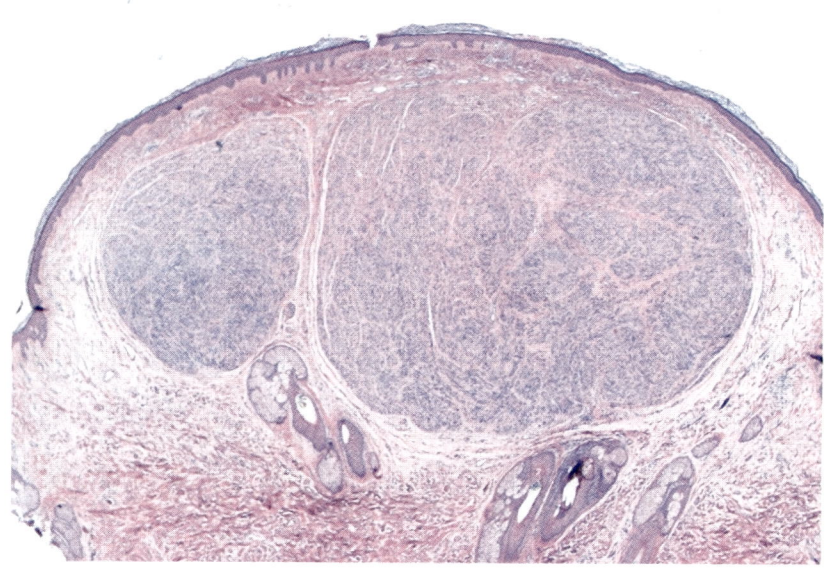

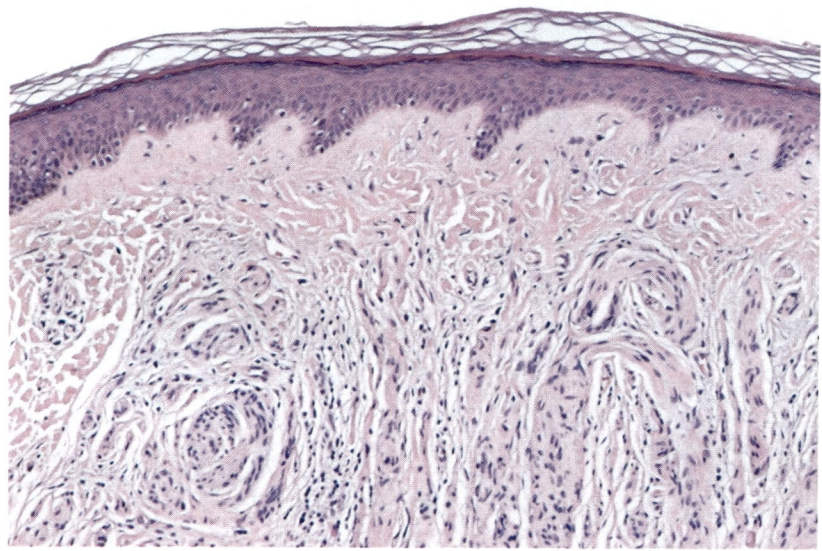

Figure 5-2
PALISADED
ENCAPSULATED NEUROMA
Top: This multinodular lesion is
dome-shaped. Despite the descriptive
term "encapsulated," only a thin layer
of perineurium and compressed connective tissue surrounds the process.
Bottom: Some lack of circumscription is apparent on the superficial
aspect.

Immunohistochemical Findings. Immunostains help distinguish PEN from other, similar
appearing cutaneous lesions. The Schwann cell
component of PEN shows strong, uniform S-100
protein reactivity (fig. 5-4B). Staining for myelin
basic protein and Leu-7 have also been observed,
as has reactivity for type 4 collagen (4). Neurofilament protein–reactive axons are demonstrated in
varying number throughout the lesion (fig. 5-4D).
Epithelial membrane antigen (EMA) stains occasionally highlight perineurial cells within the
thin capsule but not within the lesion.

Ultrastructural Findings. PENs consist of
well-differentiated Schwann cells often com-
pletely encircling axons and surrounded by basement membrane. Myelin sheath formation is
minimal or focal at best (7).
Differential Diagnosis. Despite their frequency of occurrence, PENs are often misdiag-
nosed. Most are considered nerve sheath tumors
of indeterminate type. Alternative diagnoses include schwannoma, neurofibroma, mucosal neuroma, traumatic neuroma, and angioleiomyoma
(vascular leiomyoma).

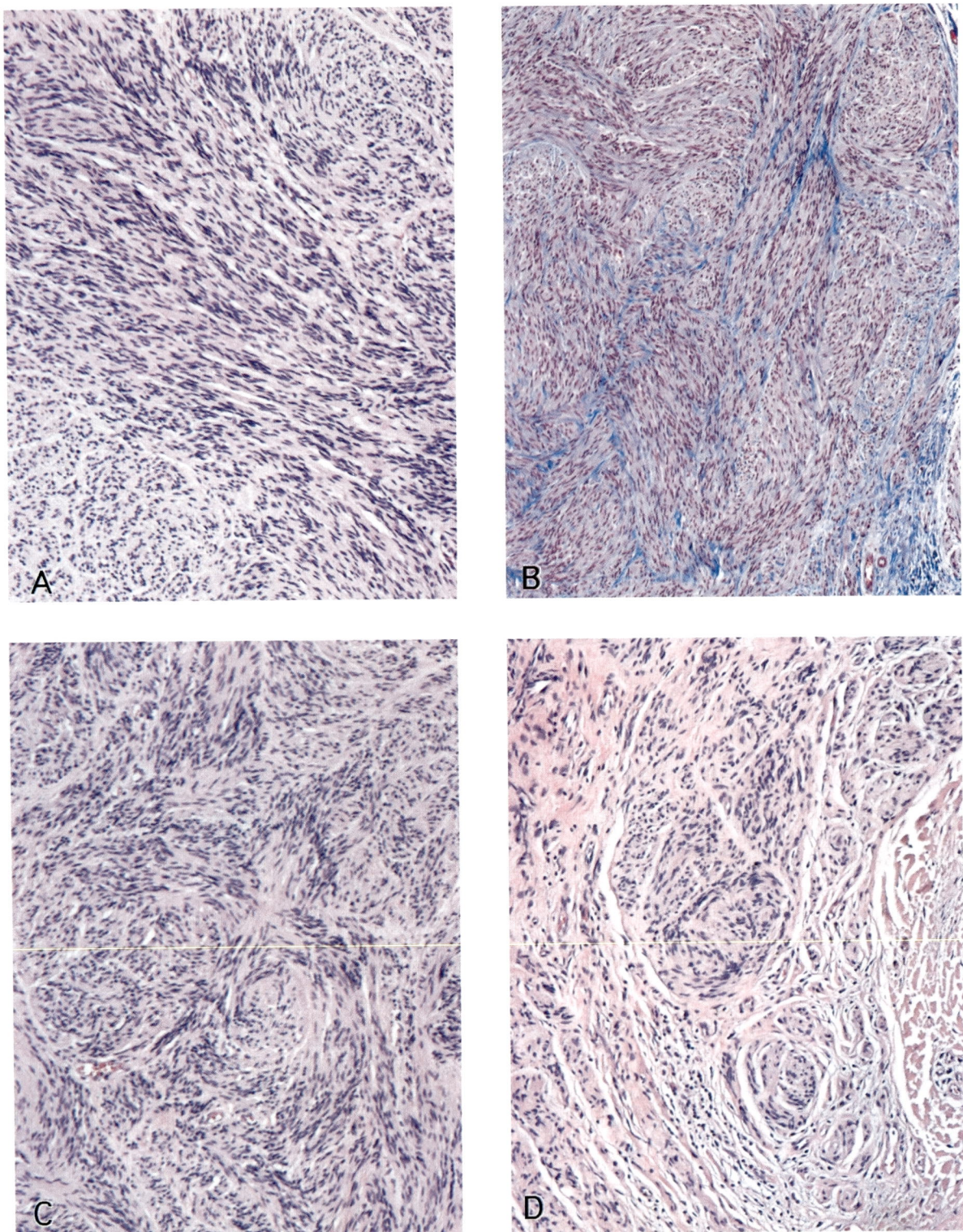

Figure 5-3
PALISADED ENCAPSULATED NEUROMA
Typically the constituent cells show alignment (A), vague fasciculation, here accentuated on trichrome stain (B), or random sweeping (C). Whorl formation is an inconspicuous feature (D), and palisading is only rarely observed.

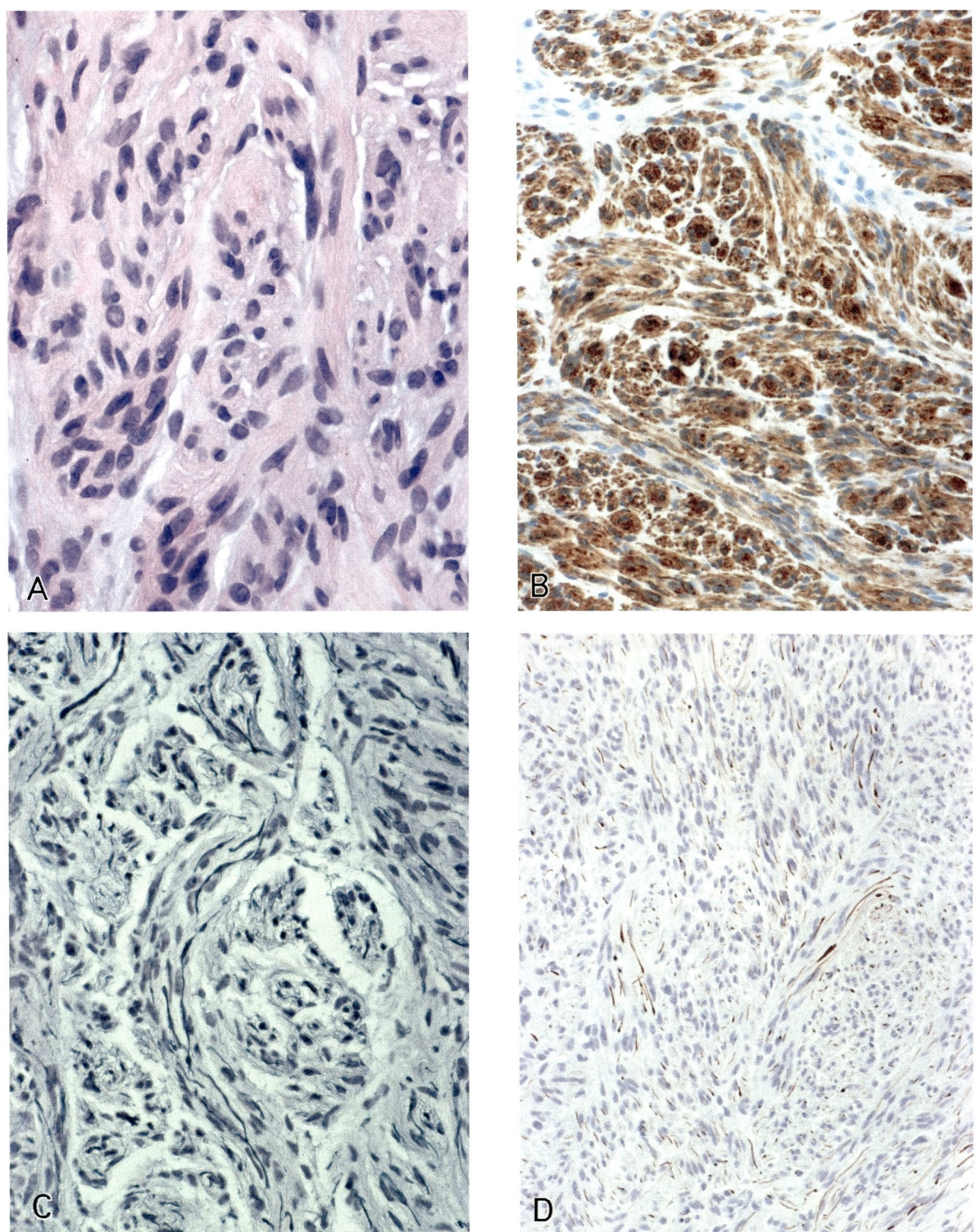

Figure 5-4
PALISADED ENCAPSULATED NEUROMA
The fascicles consist of typical, cytologically benign Schwann cells (A) which show generalized immunoreactivity for S-100 protein (B). Axons vary in number. Although inapparent with H&E stain, they are readily apparent with silver impregnation (C, Bodian) and immunostains for neurofilament protein (D).

At times, it is difficult to distinguish PEN from *schwannoma*. Unlike PENs, schwannomas usually affect subcutaneous tissue and uncommonly occur in the dermis. Nonetheless, like PEN, cutaneous and mucosal schwannomas lack a thick, fibrous capsule (see fig. 7-7). In contrast to PEN, schwannomas show Antoni A and B patterns and generally lack axons. Hyalinized, thick-walled vessels similar to those of schwannomas may be seen in plexiform PEN (3).

Unlike the compact architecture and coarse fasciculation of PENs, *neurofibromas* are more loosely textured, have a myxoid stroma, and show a delicate fibrillary pattern of collagen deposition. Since most of the cells in PEN are normal Schwann cells, nuclear size is larger and more homogeneous than in neurofibromas. No association of PEN with neurofibromatosis has been reported.

Although PENs only infrequently involve mucosa, those that do may prompt consideration of *mucosal neuromatosis*. The latter lesions are often multiple and exhibit a plexiform pattern of growth. Compared to PEN, axons in mucosal neuromas are numerous and a well-formed perineurium is readily identified around each nerve. A significant proportion of patients with mucosal neuromatosis show stigmata of multiple endocrine neoplasia (MEN) type IIb, an inherited condition which includes medullary carcinoma of the thyroid and pheochromocytoma (see below). No such association has been described with PEN.

Traumatic neuromas (4) are generally unencapsulated and are often associated with an obvious nerve. Compared with PEN, the microfascicles of fully developed traumatic neuromas are better formed, each being ensheathed by an EMA-immunopositive layer of perineurial cells. In PEN, such cells are limited primarily to the capsular zone. In addition, traumatic neuromas contain more axons and myelin products, and exhibit greater degrees of stromal fibrosis and acidic mucin deposition. Chronic inflammation or foreign body reaction, an occasional feature in traumatic neuroma, is not seen in PEN.

Lastly, *angioleiomyoma* (vascular leiomyoma) enters into the differential diagnosis in that they are circumscribed cellular dermal proliferations. In contrast to PEN, they lack intralesional perifascicular clefting, are more vascular, and are devoid of axons. Unlike Schwann cells, the smooth muscle cells of angioleiomyoma lack a sinuous configuration, show more defined cytoplasmic margins, contain stainable cytoplasmic fibrils, and possess nuclei with blunt rather than tapered ends. Immunostaining shows reactivity for smooth muscle antigens but generally not for S-100 protein. If present in angioleiomyoma, S-100 protein reactivity is usually weak. Unlike in PEN, hemosiderin deposition and extravasation of red blood cells are common in angioleiomyoma.

Prognosis. PENs are benign. Simple excision is curative since recurrence is exceptional (6). None have undergone malignant change or metastasized.

MUCOSAL NEUROMA, MUCOSAL NEUROMATOSIS, AND INTESTINAL GANGLIONEUROMATOSIS OF MEN IIB

Definition. These lesions, occurring in the setting of multiple endocrine neoplasia (MEN) type IIb, result from hypertrophy of autonomic nerves and ganglia, with the formation of either discrete masses or extensive plexus enlargement. Synonyms include *multiple mucosal neuroma* and *intestinal ganglioneuromatosis of the alimentary tract*.

General Comments. Inasmuch as mucosal neuromas and intestinal ganglioneuromatosis are early markers of MEN IIb, it is important that pathologists be familiar with their clinical and pathologic features. Individuals with this syndrome are at risk of dying at an early age of thyroid medullary carcinoma, pheochromocytoma, or even of direct complications of intestinal ganglioneuromatosis (17,23,35). Like MEN IIa, subtype IIb is a multisystem disorder occurring either sporadically or inherited in an autosomal dominant manner. Affected individuals frequently develop multicentric thyroid medullary carcinoma, parathyroid hyperplasia, and bilateral pheochromocytoma (36). The distinction of MEN IIb from MEN IIa is based upon the additional presence in the former of mucosal neuromas, intestinal ganglioneuromatosis, and musculoskeletal abnormalities (25–27,44,49). In addition, MEN IIb generally features a less pronounced degree of parathyroid hyperplasia (17). Present in childhood and generally antedating clinical manifestations of thyroid and adrenal neoplasms are true neuromas often involving the tongue, lips, eyelids, and eyes (conjunctiva, cornea); ganglioneuromatosis of the esophagus and intestines; or both. Less often, neuromas affect the buccal mucosa, gingiva, palate, nasal mucosa, larynx, or bronchi. Ganglioneuromatosis may also involve salivary glands, pancreas, gallbladder, or urinary bladder (17). Rarely, neuromas histologically similar to those in the oral cavity are found in skin (17). Musculoskeletal abnormalities in MEN IIb resemble those of Marfan's syndrome (fig. 5-5A), and include excessive length of the limbs, loose-jointedness, scoliosis, anterior chest deformity, and a high arched palate (17,26,27). Muscular underdevelopment and hypotonia are also frequent (17).

Clinical Features. There is a slight female predominance (56 percent) among patients with MEN IIb (17), as well as among those presenting with mucosal neuromas or intestinal ganglioneuromatosis. Lesions invariably become clinically apparent during the first three decades of life. The most common sites of involvement are the lips, tongue, and eyelids. Affected lips are diffusely enlarged, patulous or occasionally everted, and have a multinodular or bumpy appearance (fig. 5-5A) (17,18). When involved, the tongue is typically studded by numerous hemispherical nodules at the tip, anterior one third, and occasionally along the lateral aspects. The nodules usually range from pinhead size to a few millimeters in diameter (fig. 5-5B) (17,18). Eyelids are similarly thickened by a diffuse or nodular process and may be everted (fig. 5-5C). Common but less obvious lesions include broadening of the base of the nose, diffuse gingival hypertrophy, palatal nodules, and such ocular changes as conjunctival nodules and thickened corneal nerves (11,14,26,28,42). The latter are best seen on slit-lamp examination (fig. 5-5D).

Intestinal ganglioneuromatosis is common in patients with MEN IIb, and often provides the earliest clinical clue that a patient has the syndrome (15–17). Other prominent features include constipation and diarrhea, generalized colonic diverticulosis, megacolon (fig. 5-6), and disturbance of esophageal motility (17,20). A diagnosis of MEN IIb is occasionally made upon finding ganglioneuromatosis in an appendix removed either incidentally (fig. 5-7) or for symptoms of appendicitis.

Pathologic Findings. Mucosal neuromas, whether localized or diffuse, consist of markedly enlarged nerves within the submucosa of the lips, oral cavity, and tongue, as well as in conjunctiva. Polypoid, dome-shaped, or diffuse, their basic elements are the same (figs. 5-8, 5-9). The numerous, tortuous, highly branched and loosely arrayed nerve bundles vary in size and shape. Less frequently, nerve bundles are compact and fascicular in arrangement (36). The perineurium of affected nerves is usually thickened and a mucoid matrix (fig. 5-8B) may be present between nerve fiber bundles. Reactive fibrosis is not a feature of mucosal neuroma. In contrast to the mass of affected nerves encountered at oral sites, linear thickening of discrete nerves is more common in the cornea. Most occur in the limbus (fig. 5-5D); the conjunctiva and iris are less often affected (46). Proliferation of endoneurial cells has been reported to occur in mucosal neuromas (17), but at the ultrastructural level the ratio of Schwann cells to axons appears to be normal (41,46). As a rule, ganglion cells are not present in mucosal neuromas, but they have been noted in neuromas of lingual and ciliary nerves (18,31,40), as well as at the root of the iris and in the uveal meshwork (41,46).

The principle histologic feature of intestinal ganglioneuromatosis in patients with MEN IIb is band-like and nodular enlargement of both the submucosal and myenteric nerve plexuses (figs. 5-10A,B, 5-11) (21). This process consists of an increase in all nerve elements, including ganglion cells, their processes, and accompanying Schwann cells (fig. 5-10). Ganglion cells are commonly identified in affected plexuses and are arranged singly or in clusters; their content of Nissl substance is variable (fig. 5-11A,B). Whether there is actual hyperplasia of ganglion cells has not been determined by comparative studies. The abnormality is less pronounced in the submucosa (fig. 5-10B) than in the muscularis propria (myenteric plexus) (figs. 5-10A, 5-11), a site in which enlarged nerve plexuses form an almost uninterrupted band between the longitudinal and circular muscle coats. In addition, hypertrophic neural tissue often lies dispersed within the muscularis propria and may even be seen in subserosal fat. Whereas proliferative neural tissue, with or without ganglion cells, may be seen within the lamina propria in patients with MEN IIb (fig. 5-10C), mucosal involvement is usually focal and is invariably associated with enlargement of the myenteric plexus. For practical purposes,

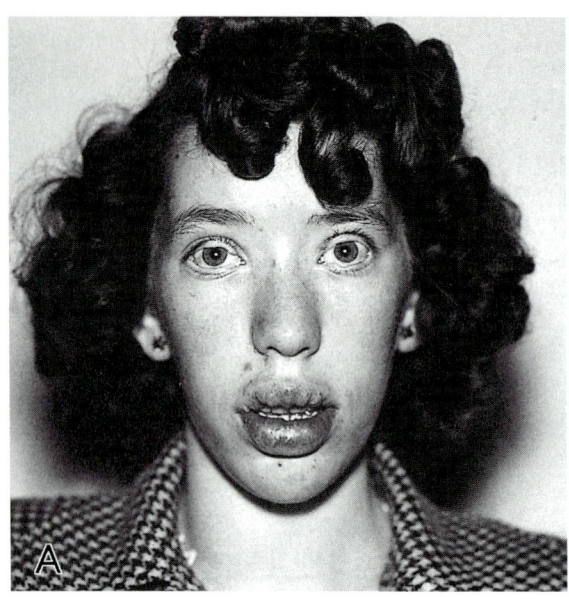

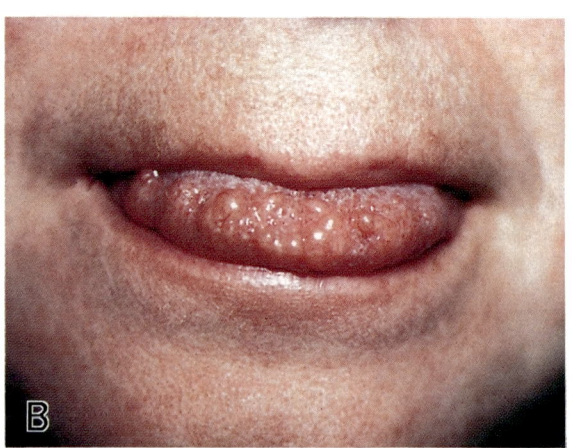

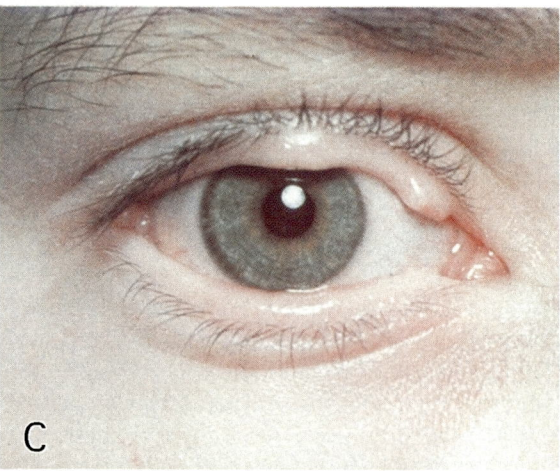

Figure 5-5
MEN IIB

In addition to a long, narrow face, patients often have prominent bumpy lips (A), as well as nodularity of the anterolateral tongue (B) and eyelid margin (C) due to the presence of submucosal neuromas. On slit lamp examination enlarged corneal nerves are evident as delicate threads (D). Although greatly enlarged, the microanatomy of these affected nerves is essentially normal. (A and B, courtesy of Dr. J. A. Carney, Rochester, Minnesota.)

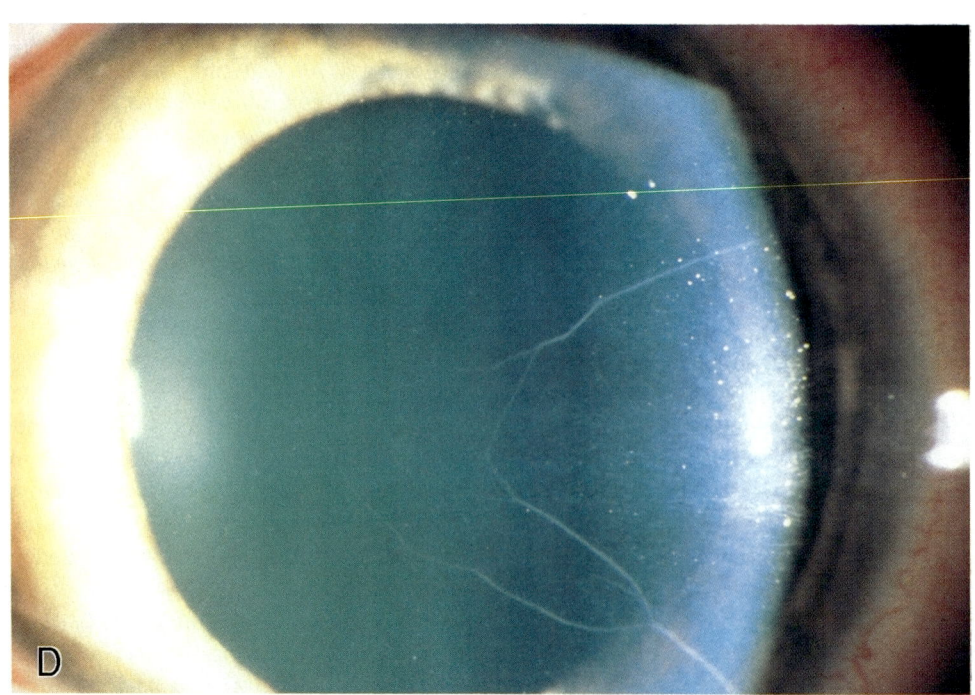

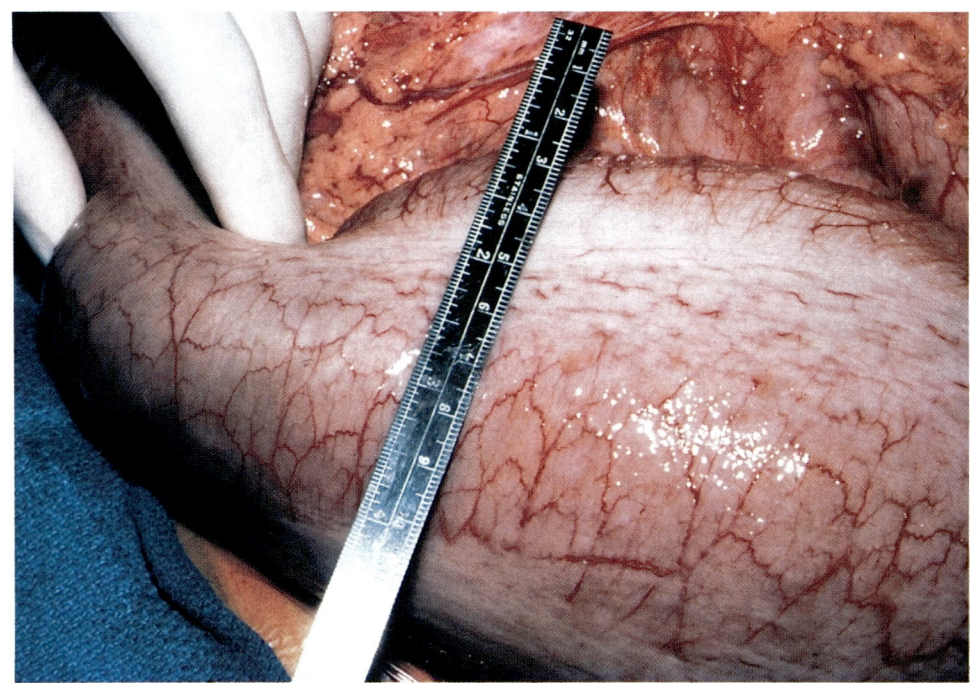

Figure 5-6
GANGLIONEUROMATOSIS OF THE COLON IN MEN IIB
Megacolon commonly results. Note dilation of the affected segment.

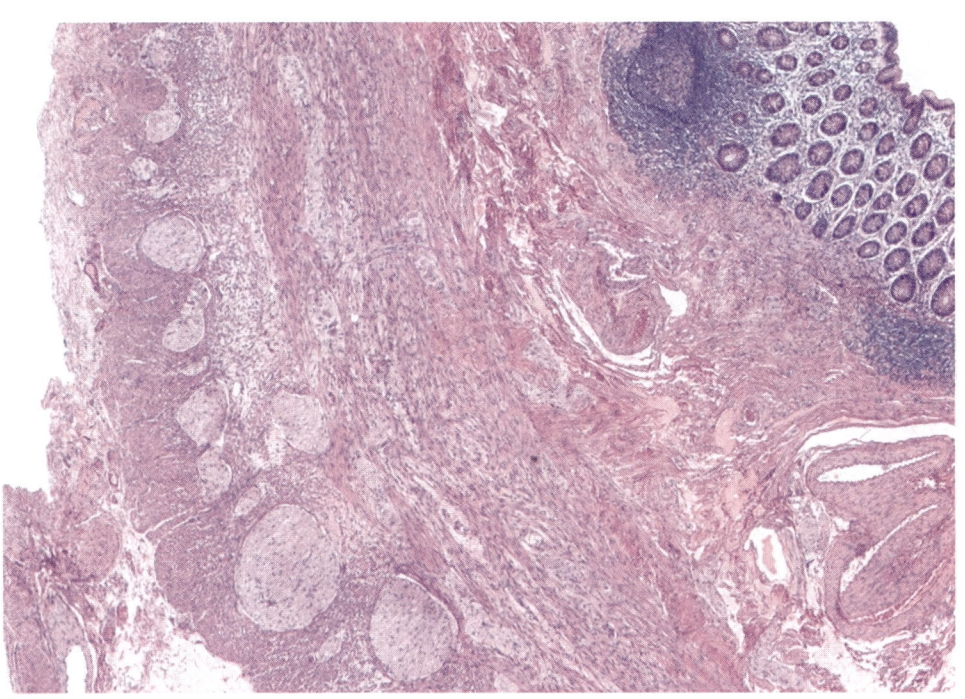

Figure 5-7
GANGLIONEUROMATOSIS OF THE APPENDIX IN MEN IIB
On occasion, the diagnosis may be suspected at incidental appendectomy. The changes are identical to those in the colon (see figs. 5-10, 5-11).

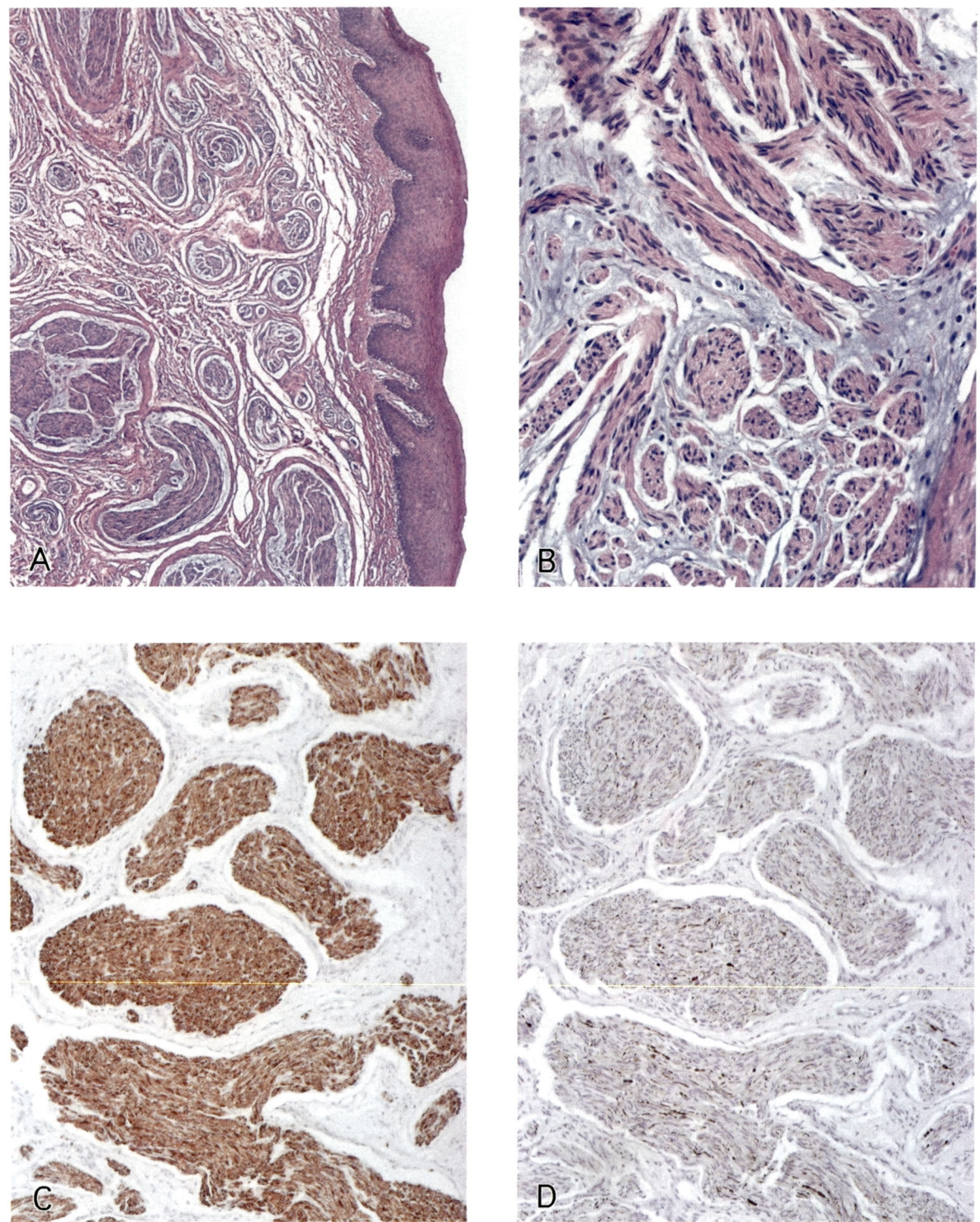

Figure 5-8

MUCOSAL NEUROMATOSIS OF THE LIPS IN MEN IIB

A: A biopsy demonstrates hypertrophic submucosal nerves unassociated with ganglion cells.

B: Note the increase of endoneurial mucin, a feature best seen at higher magnification.

C,D: The relatively normal microanatomy of the nerves is illustrated with immunostains for S-100 protein (C) and neurofilament protein (D).

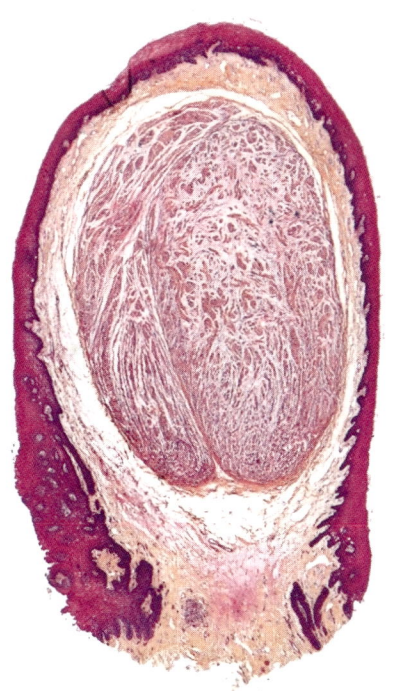

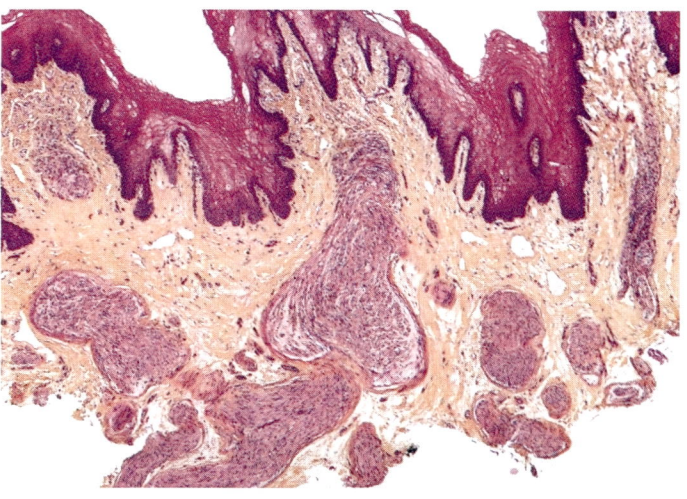

Figure 5-9
MUCOSAL NEUROMATOSIS OF THE TONGUE IN MEN IIB
The process varies from polypoid (left) to plexiform (above).

Figure 5-10
GANGLIONEUROMATOSIS OF
THE COLON IN MEN IIB
Note massive, nearly continuous, band-like hypertrophy of Auerbach's myenteric plexus (A), hypertrophy of the submucosal plexus (B), and lesser involvement of the lamina propria (C).

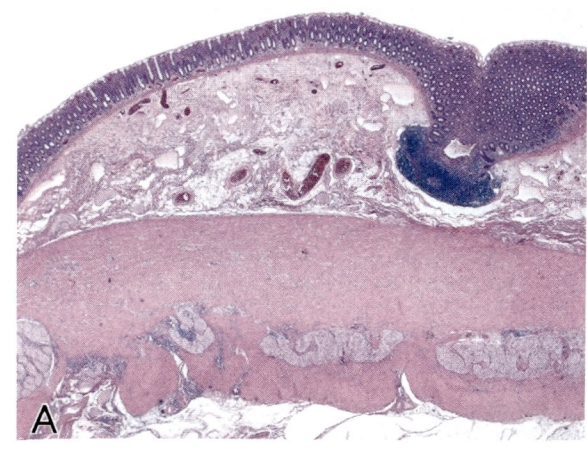

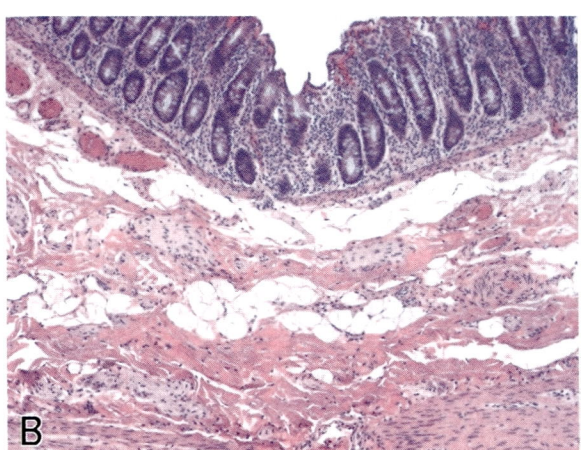

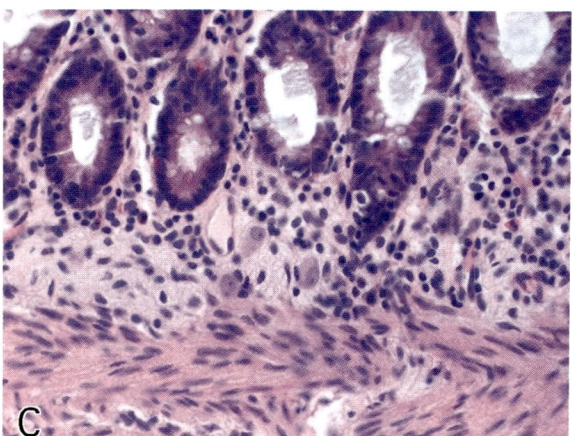

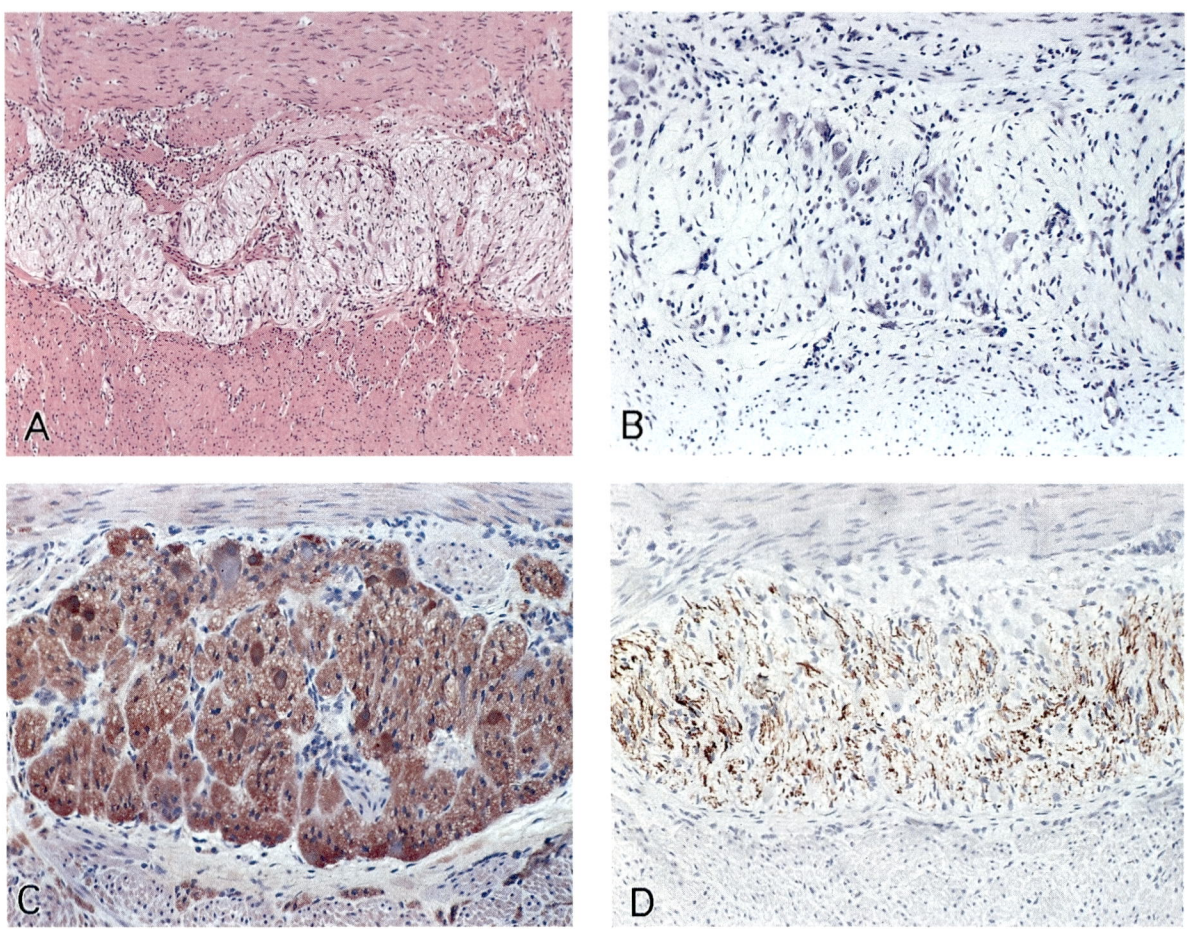

Figure 5-11
GANGLIONEUROMATOSIS OF THE COLON IN MEN IIB
The myenteric ganglia are markedly enlarged (A) but their cellular elements, Schwann cell-ensheathed axons and ganglion cells, are essentially normal on Nissl preparations (B), and neuron-specific enolase (C) and neurofilament protein (D) immunostains.

ganglioneuromatous involvement of all layers of the intestine is seen only in patients with MEN IIb; similar changes in neurofibromatosis type 1 (NF1) are rare (see fig. 5-15).

Immunohistochemical Findings. As expected, the cells of mucosal neuromas stain like normal nerve cells. Schwann cells and axons strongly stain for S-100 protein and neurofilament protein, respectively (fig. 5-8C,D). In addition, the ganglion cells of ganglioneuromas are reactive for neuron specific enolase (fig. 5-11C), neurofilament protein (fig. 5-11D), and synaptophysin.

Differential Diagnosis. Histologically, mucosal neuromas of MEN IIb may resemble either traumatic neuroma or palisaded encapsulated neuroma (PEN), both of which have been reported to occur in oral mucosa (19). The lesion may also resemble schwannoma. Cross sections of *traumatic neuroma* generally reveal a jumble of closely packed nerve fiber bundles. These vary in size and shape, show scant or only focal perineurial ensheathment, and lie in a background of reactive fibrosis with or without associated chronic inflammation. A readily recognized nerve is often seen to enter and occasionally to exit the mass. In contrast, the mucosal neuromas of MEN IIb represent a more orderly increase in distinct, well-formed nerves in an otherwise unremarkable submucosa. In contrast to mucosal neuromas, *schwannomas* usually present as discrete lesions, and feature Antoni A and B tissue as well as palisading of tumor cells. Even when plexiform, schwannomas show a relative absence of axons. Although mucosal PEN, particularly multinodular examples, may be difficult to distinguish from the mucosal neuromas of MEN IIb, the compact, ill-defined microfascicles of the former are very cellular, consist almost entirely of Schwann cells, and contain fewer axons than are present in mucosal neuromas. Further clues to their distinction include the presentation of mucosal PEN as a solitary lesion occurring in an older age group (middle age versus childhood and adolescence) as well as the occasional appearance of palisaded Schwann cells. A diagnosis of mucosal neuromatosis is obviously aided by the identification of other manifestations of the MEN IIb syndrome, either in the patient or in a family member.

Also to be considered is focal or diffuse intestinal ganglioneuromatosis associated with disorders other than MEN IIb. These include *Cowden's disease* (29,47), *juvenile polyposis* (22,33,37,48), *colonic adenoma* and *adenocarcinoma* (45,48), and *Hirschsprung's disease* (12,38,43). Isolated intestinal ganglioneuromatosis has also been reported (13,24,30,32,34,39). Unlike the intestinal ganglioneuromatosis of MEN IIb, the above-noted examples are usually focal and, with the exception of occasional extension into the submucosa, do not involve deeper layers of the intestinal wall. Far more difficult to distinguish from intestinal ganglioneuromatosis of MEN IIb are similar lesions rarely occurring in *NF1*.

NEUROMA, GANGLIONEUROMA/ GANGLIONEUROMATOSIS, AND NEURONAL INTESTINAL DYSPLASIA OF THE ALIMENTARY TRACT UNASSOCIATED WITH MEN TYPE IIB

These lesions consist of hyperplasia of nerve fibers or hypertrophy of autonomic plexuses, either localized and tumefactive or diffuse, but unassociated with MEN IIb. The disorders and lesions included here fall under the categories of neuroma, likely a reactive condition, ganglioneuroma/gangliomatosis, and neuronal intestinal dysplasia.

Neuromas

The appendiceal neuroma, a commonly observed reactive lesion also termed mucosal neurogenic appendicopathy, reportedly affects 10 to 27 percent of excised vermiform appendices (59, 67,82). The lesion was originally studied by Masson in the 1920s (64,65), but a number of series have subsequently been reported (50,54,59,67, 68,82,84). In most instances the lesion is an incidental finding in appendices excised for other reasons (82). Only rare examples cause luminal obstruction and are responsible for symptoms simulating acute appendicitis (60,64,68).

In terms of gross pathology, appendiceal neuromas are usually indistinguishable from fibrous obliteration of the appendiceal tip. On cut section, they are gray and often glistening (82). Histologically, appendiceal neuromas somewhat resemble traumatic neuroma, a lesion to which they may be related. They feature variable replacement of the appendiceal wall and luminal obliteration by a proliferation of loosely arranged, spindle-shaped cells with delicate eosinophilic processes (fig. 5-12A,B). Immunoreactive for S-100 protein (fig. 5-12C), these cells represent Schwann cells investing nerve fibers. They are not readily seen with hematoxylin and eosin (H&E) stain; instead they are demonstrated with Bodian or Bielschowski preparations and immunostain for neurofilament protein. Unlike the ganglioneuromatous lesions noted above, appendiceal neuromas lack a ganglion cell component.

Three growth patterns have been described (67): intramucosal, subserosal, and axial. Intramucosal examples expand the lamina propria, spreading apart crypts and depressing the muscularis mucosae. Axial neuromas are the most common and account for nearly half of all examples (67). Longitudinally oriented, such lesions involve the tip of the obliterated appendix, are encased by fibromuscular and adipose tissue, and only proximally contact the mucosa. Their boundary with adjacent lamina propria is often indistinct. Appendiceal neuromas are frequently associated with an increase of argentaffin-positive neuroendocrine cells in the lamina propria (fig. 5-12D) and may be found within the neuromatous tissue. Regressive changes are seen in approximately 25 percent of cases and include atrophy of neurites, absence or loss of argentaffin cells, chronic

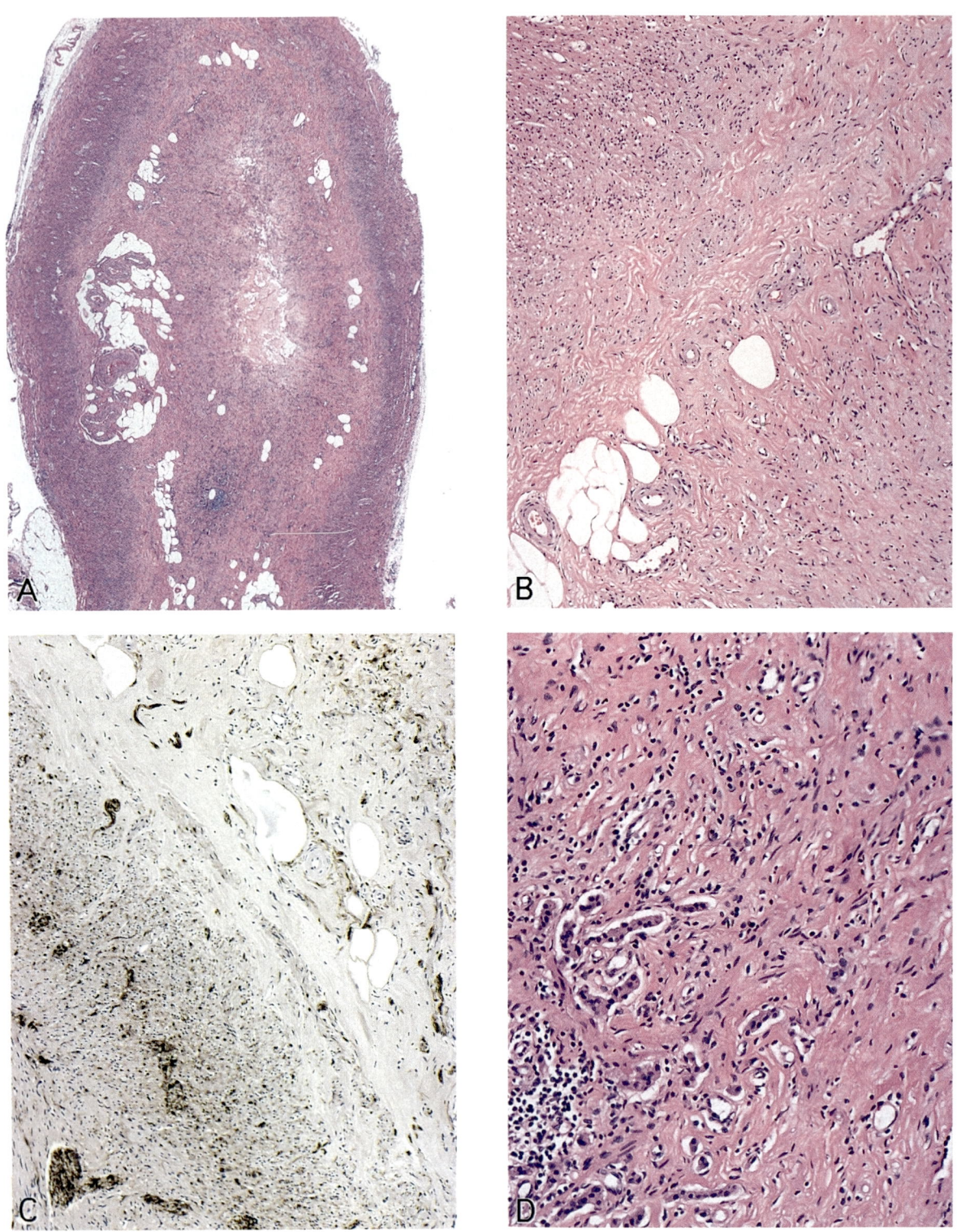

Figure 5-12
APPENDICEAL NEUROMA
The obliterated tip of the appendiceal lumen (A) is replaced by a tangle of hypertrophic nerve fibers which also involve the submucosa (B). Some single and others grouped, their Schwann sheaths immunoreact for S-100 protein (C). Clusters of neuroendocrine cells are a common finding within such neuromas (D).

inflammation, fibrosis, and occasionally stromal myxoid change (67).

We have seen and others have reported neuromas of the intestinal tract unassociated with other neoplasms (85). Among these are biliary tract and duodenal neuromas. Examples typically occur in the wall of the gallbladder, the common bile duct, and in the second portion of the duodenum (fig. 5-13A,B). They arise from submucosal or myenteric plexuses, and may be multinodular. Devoid of ganglion cells, their architecture somewhat resembles that of traumatic neuroma (fig. 5-13B,C) (76). One example was reported as a neurofibroma (86). This point of confusion can be avoided by the performance of silver impregnation stains or immunostains for the demonstration of axons. The differential diagnosis with gangliocytic paraganglioma of the duodenum (61,79) generally poses no problem.

Ganglioneuroma/Ganglioneuromatosis

Solitary Polypoid Intestinal Ganglioneuroma. Focal ganglioneuroma is most often an incidental colonoscopic finding unassociated with an underlying condition (fig. 5-14) (80). Most are small, sessile, or pedunculated polyps that grossly resemble juvenile polyps, adenomas, or hyperplastic polyps, and measure less than 2 cm. The microscopic pattern (80) of the ganglioneuromatous tissue varies: there may be a patchy distribution within the lamina propria; a nodular, neurofibroma-like distribution in mucosa and submucosa; or a combined pattern. Ganglion cells vary in number (fig. 5-14B,C). Shekitka and Sobin (80) showed no association with multiple tumors, NF1, or MEN IIb.

Ganglioneuromatosis. This condition, consisting of hypertrophy of the diffuse autonomic plexus of the alimentary tract, may occur in several settings aside from MEN IIb (see Mucosal Neuroma, Mucosal Neuromatosis, and Intestinal Ganglioneuromatosis of MEN IIb). There are reports of intestinal ganglioneuromatosis in patients with NF1 (56,74,77,80). Such lesions are rare (fig. 5-15) and may affect both the submucosal and myenteric plexuses or only the former (56). Most often, the changes are limited to the mucosa. The confusing term "ganglioneurofibromatosis" has also crept into use to describe a sprinkling of ganglion cells within the mucosa in patients with

NF1. We, as well as others (74), do not consider this an entity and discourage the use of the term. In our opinion, most reported examples of transmural hypertrophy of the autonomic plexus in patients with NF1 more closely resemble involvement by plexiform neurofibroma (53,58,83). Subtle morphologic features distinguish intestinal ganglioneuromatosis of MEN IIb from such lesions. Whereas the enlarged plexuses and discrete nodules noted in neurofibroma may exhibit a myxomatous matrix, such stromal change is not a feature of MEN IIb-associated intestinal ganglioneuromatosis. Furthermore, the altered nerves are arranged both horizontally and vertically, whereas in the ganglioneuromatosis of MEN IIb and rarely of NF1, the enlarged hypertrophic plexuses are arranged only in a horizontal manner.

Mucosal ganglioneuromatosis may also be part of a systemic disorder termed *Cowden's disease* (63), an autosomal dominant disorder characterized by ectodermal, mesodermal, and endodermal abnormalities, including hypoplastic mandible and prominent forehead (52); verrucous-like cutaneous papules occurring in an acral distribution; facial trichilemmomas arising predominantly about the mouth, nose, eyes, and ears (52, 62,70); squamous papules of the oral mucosa (70); multifocal esophageal acanthosis (62); gastric lymphoid and hyperplastic polyps (71); small bowel polyposis (71); benign polyps of the colon (71); carcinoma of the thyroid (57); and a high incidence of mammary carcinoma in females (75). An association has also been noted between Cowden's disease and dysplastic gangliocytoma of the cerebellum (Lhermitte-Duclos disease) (69).

Hyperplasia of neural tissue of the intestinal mucosa, sometimes accompanied by ganglion cells, has also been seen in association with *juvenile polyposis* (55,66,72,87) and *colonic adenoma* and *adenocarcinoma* (81,87). In patients with such lesions, as well as in the setting of Cowden's disease, mucosal ganglioneuromatosis is invariably an incidental finding and does not contribute to presenting symptoms. The mucosal ganglioneuromatosis occurring in association with the above conditions consists of mucosal thickening due to abundance of neural processes, their parent ganglion cells, and accompanying Schwann cells. When associated with benign polyps, the ganglioneuromatous proliferation may involve either the polyps or surrounding normal mucosa (87). In one

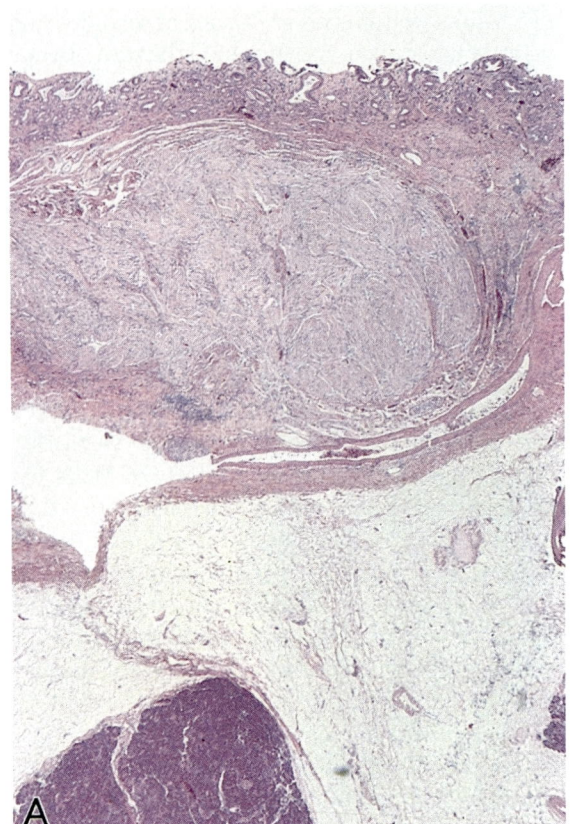

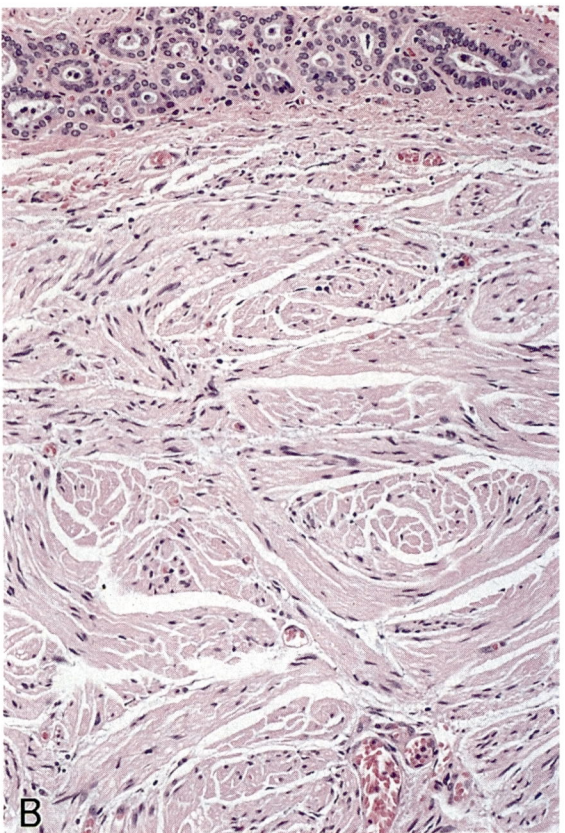

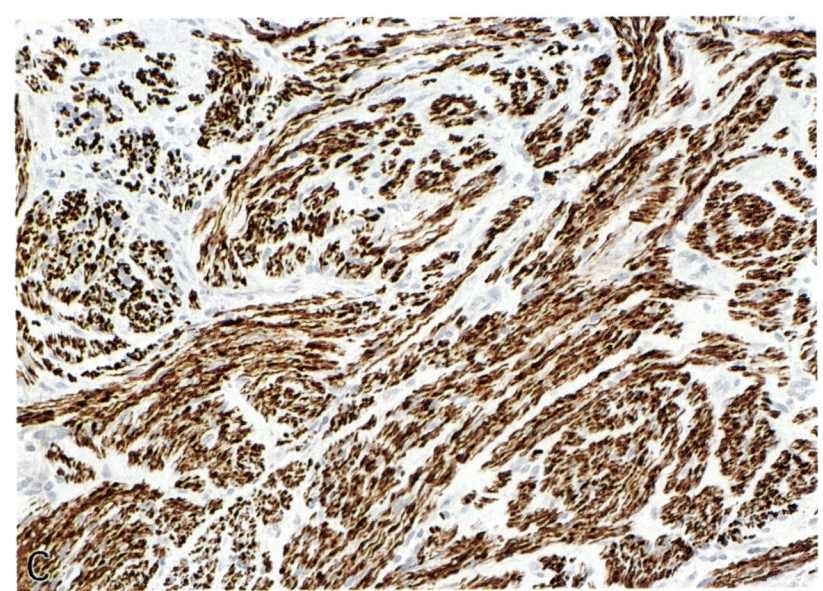

Figure 5-13
DUODENAL NEUROMA

This submucosal lesion (A) consists of spindle-shaped Schwann cells (B) associated with nerve fibers. Individual or disposed in fascicles, the Schwann sheaths and axons are immunoreactive for both neurofilament protein (C) and S-100 protein.

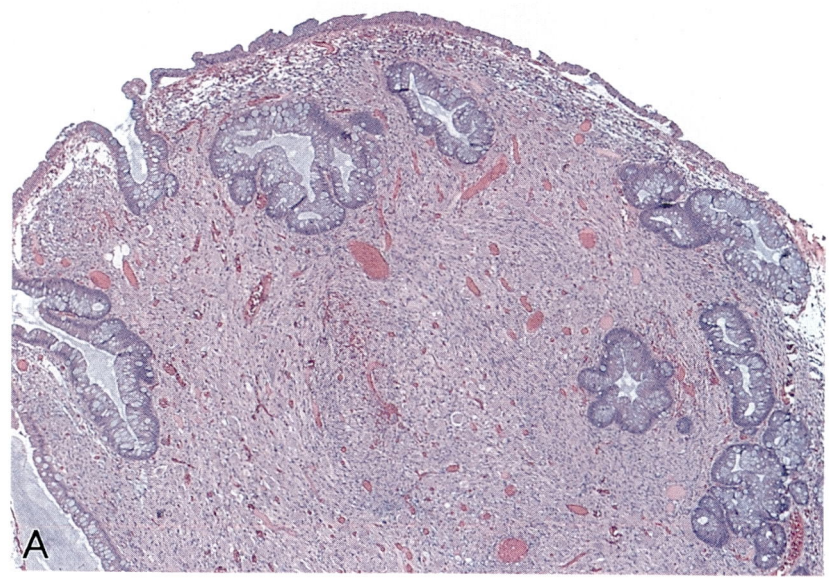

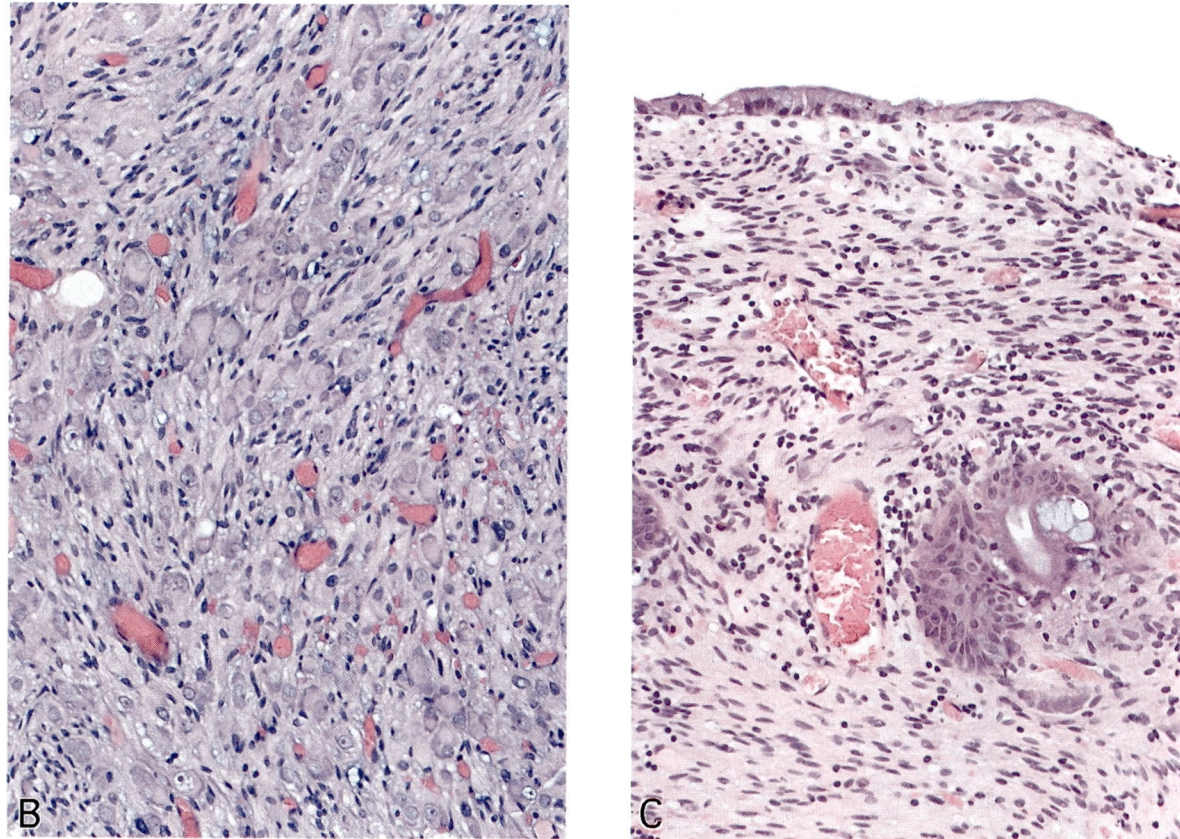

Figure 5-14
SOLITARY POLYPOID GANGLIONEUROMA

As isolated lesions such as this colonic example in a 50-year-old male (A), polypoid ganglioneuromas are of no clinical significance. Superficial in location, they expand the lamina propria and submucosa and consist of numerous mature ganglion cells and nerve fibers. The former may be numerous (B) or, as in another example, sparse (C). (Courtesy of Dr. L. J. Burgart, Rochester, Minnesota.)

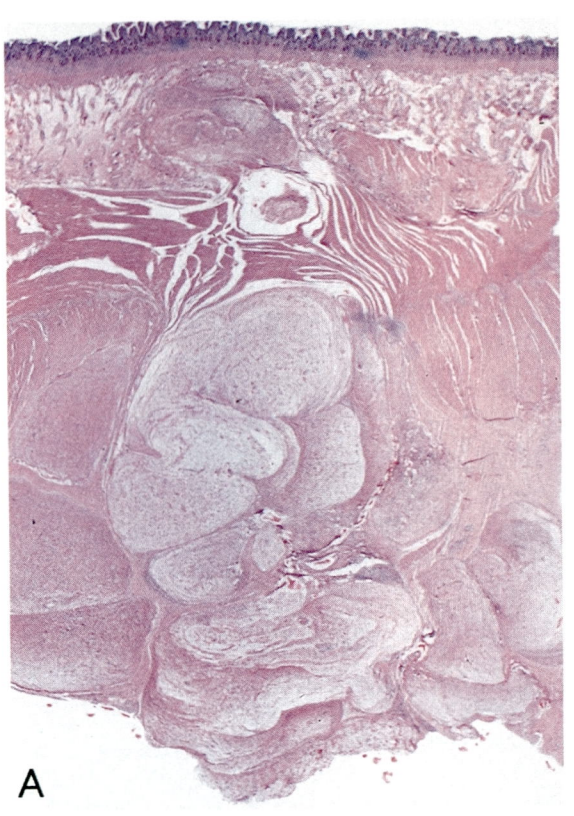

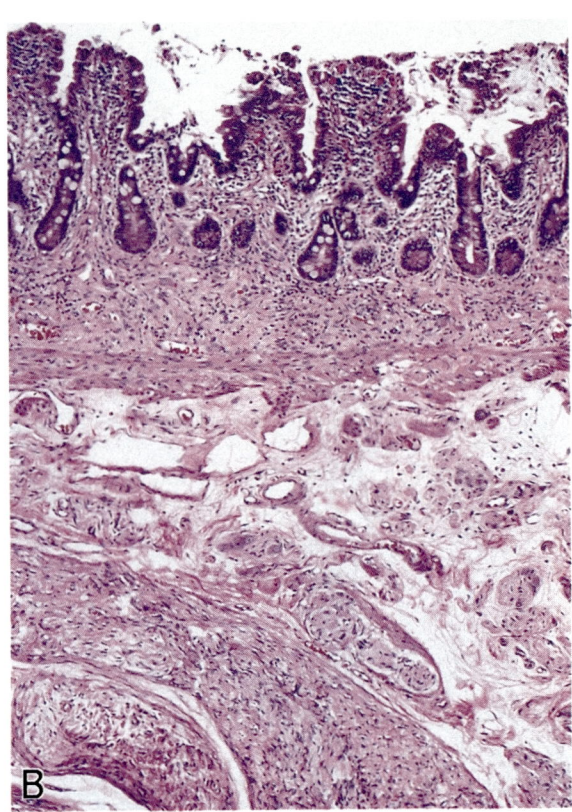

Figure 5-15
GANGLIONEUROMATOSIS IN NF1

In addition to plexiform neurofibroma affecting both the submucosa and serosa (A), ganglioneuromatous involvement of the submucosa (B) and mucosa (C) is also seen. (Courtesy of Dr. L. Sobin, Washington, DC, and K.M. Shekitka, Annapolis, Maryland.) (Also see figure 13-13.)

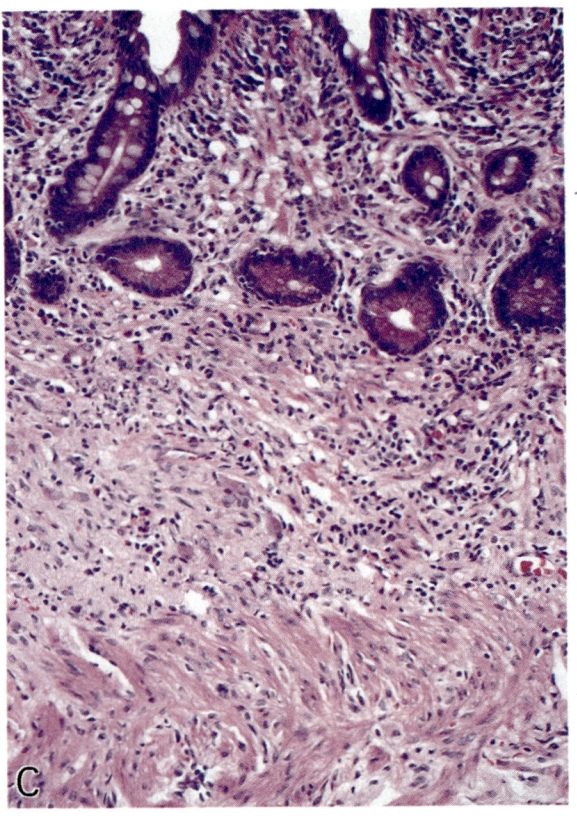

case of colonic adenocarcinoma, the ganglio-neuromatosis was diffuse, involving not only the tumor-affected cecum, but the vermiform appendix and terminal ileum as well (81).

Neuronal Intestinal Dysplasia

Usually a disorder of newborns and associated with Hirschsprung's disease (51,73,78), neuronal intestinal dysplasia (NID) is characterized by localized or diffuse hypertrophy of the submucosal and myenteric plexuses, often in the distal large bowel. Hypertrophic neural tissue occasionally extends into the lamina propria. The diffuse form may extend to involve more proximal large bowel, the vermiform appendix, small bowel, or even the stomach (51). NID may present as an isolated disorder or, as in 20 to 75 percent of cases, in association with distal bowel aganglionosis (Hirschsprung's disease). In a minority of instances, the patients exhibit major malformations (51).

Affected newborns and young children have symptoms resembling those of *Hirschsprung's disease*. Clinically, the disorder is divided into three groups: A (15 percent), B (70 percent), and C (15 percent). Group C cases exhibit the combined features of groups A and B (51). Individuals in group A experience an early onset of severe symptoms including constipation, diarrhea, and those of "ulcerative colitis." The acute, stormy course of group A disease is due to hypoplasia of the sympathetic innervation of the gut. Patients in group B commonly present with constipation, and the disease is less severe and more protracted. Fatality due to NID of any type is infrequent (51).

A familial disorder of small intestinal neuronal dysplasia associated with multiple gastrointestinal autonomic nerve tumors (GANT) has recently been described (70a).

LOCALIZED HYPERTROPHIC NEUROPATHY

Definition. Localized hypertrophy of a peripheral nerve is caused by onion bulb-like hyperplasia of Schwann cells, leading to fascicular enlargement.

General Comments. The term localized hypertrophic neuropathy (LHN) has long been used to denote two distinct lesions: a rare, nonhereditary, localized Schwann cell proliferation characterized by onion bulb formation and a more common intraneural tumor of perineurial cells engaged in pseudo-onion bulb formation, now designated intraneural perineurioma. Unlike some authors (89), we do not consider LHN to be a part of a lesion spectrum that includes perineurioma.

The nature of LHN has not been determined, but most consider it a reactive rather than a neoplastic process. It involves isolated nerves and should not be considered a variant of the hereditary hypertrophic sensorimotor neuropathy, eg. Dejerine-Sottas or Charcot-Marie-Tooth disease. Onion bulb formation, the hallmark of Schwann cell hypertrophy, follows repeated episodes of demyelination and remyelination, and can also be seen in chronic inflammatory demyelinating neuropathy (92), as well as other polyneuropathies.

Clinical Features. To date only four examples of LHN have been described (88–90,93). All have occurred in adults. Although one patient had several café au lait spots, no cases have been reported in association with NF1. Since in one instance the process did involve two nerves (93), the designation localized hypertrophic "mononeuropathy" should be avoided. Cranial (88,89) or spinal nerves (90,93) may be affected. Both reported cranial nerve examples involved the trigeminal nerve. One spinal nerve case, a tibial nerve lesion, was associated with chronic inflammation (90) and the other, a cauda equina example, involved two nerve roots and was associated with a sacral meningocele (93).

Gross Findings. The four cases reported to date have involved nerves of differing size as well as cranial nerve ganglia. Grossly, these structures are enlarged and usually yellow to gray. Affected nerves appear fusiform with markedly enlarged fascicles; maximal lesion length and diameter were 15 cm (90) and 2 cm (93), respectively. Adherence to normal surrounding roots was noted in the cauda equina lesion (93).

Microscopic Findings. LHN is characterized by nerve fascicle expansion (fig. 5-16A) due to the formation of onion bulbs, each consisting of whorls of uniform, cytologically normal Schwann cells encircling a variably myelinated axon (fig. 5-16B). The onion bulbs contain considerable collagen (fig. 5-16C) and typically lie within a watery, Alcian blue–positive matrix (fig. 5-16D). Stains for myelin show it to be scant (fig. 5-17, left) but axons are readily demonstrated on silver preparations (fig. 5-17, right).

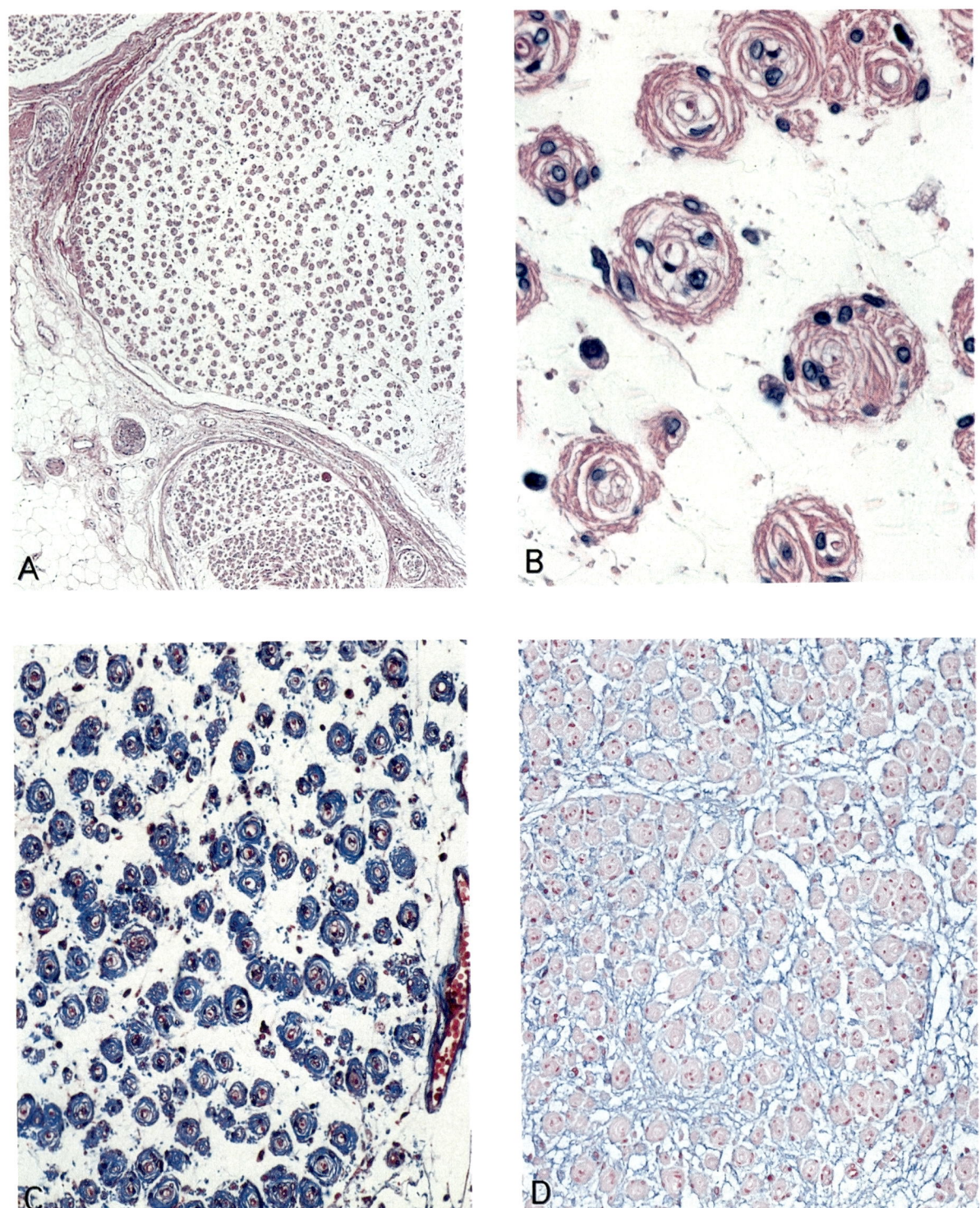

Figure 5-16
LOCALIZED HYPERTROPHIC NEUROPATHY
A: A portion of two affected fascicles show the onion bulbs to be widely separated.
B: Onion bulbs consist of lamellae of Schwann cells surrounding a nerve fiber.
C: Considerable collagen accompanies the Schwann cells (trichrome).
D: The endoneurium contains Alcian blue–positive mucin. (Courtesy of Dr. D. Horoupian, Palo Alto, California.)

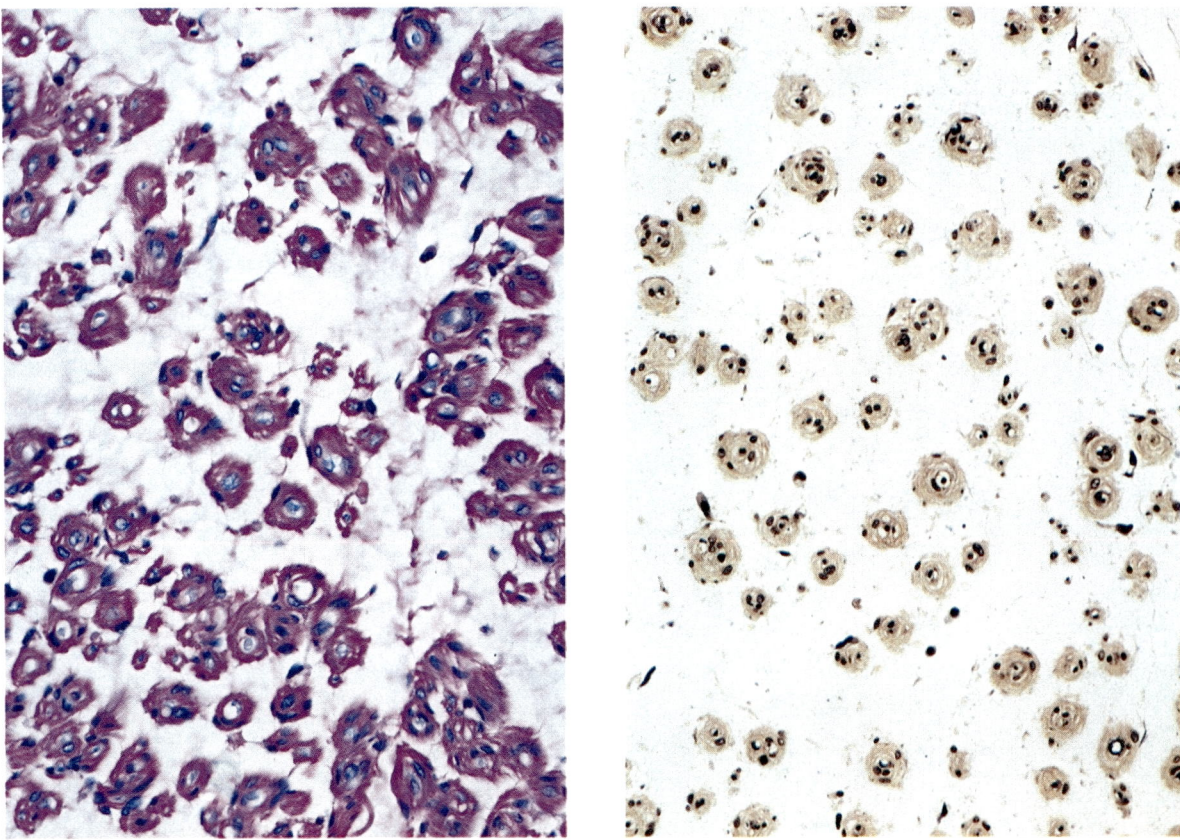

Figure 5-17
LOCALIZED HYPERTROPHIC NEUROPATHY
Routine histochemical stains show myelin to be scant or lacking (left, Luxol-fast blue), but axons are readily visible on silver preparation (right, Bielschowsky). (Courtesy of Dr. D. Horoupian, Palo Alto, CA.)

Immunohistochemical Findings. In keeping with their composition of multilayered Schwann cells, onion bulbs are strongly S-100 protein immunoreactive (fig. 5-18A). Each surrounds a central, neurofilament protein–positive axon (fig. 5-18B). Epithelial membrane antigen (EMA) reactivity is limited to perineurium (fig. 5-18C).

Ultrastructural Findings. Individually, the onion bulbs are composed of multiple layers of Schwann cells encircling a variably myelinated axon. The reduplicated Schwann cells have a continuous basement membrane and loosely apposed cytoplasmic processes, and lack the numerous intercellular junctions and micropinocytotic vesicles of perineurial cells.

Differential Diagnosis. The principle differential diagnosis of LHN is *intraneural perineurioma,* a lesion long included in the spectrum of LHN but now recognized to be a neoplasm rather than a reactive process (91). Perineuriomas affect major nerves, involve perineurium and endoneurium, and consist of proliferating, multilayered perineurial cells surrounding one or more axons and their Schwann sheaths. The result is pseudo-onion bulb formation. Encirclement of vessels may also be seen. Given their composition of predominantly perineurial cells, perineuriomas differ from LHN by being EMA immunoreactive. S-100 protein stains demonstrate only preexisting normal, centrally located Schwann sheaths. The ultrastructural features of the multilayered cells are those of well-differentiated perineurial cells, rather than of Schwann cells. A detailed description of the ultrastructural of intraneural perineurioma is presented in chapter 9.

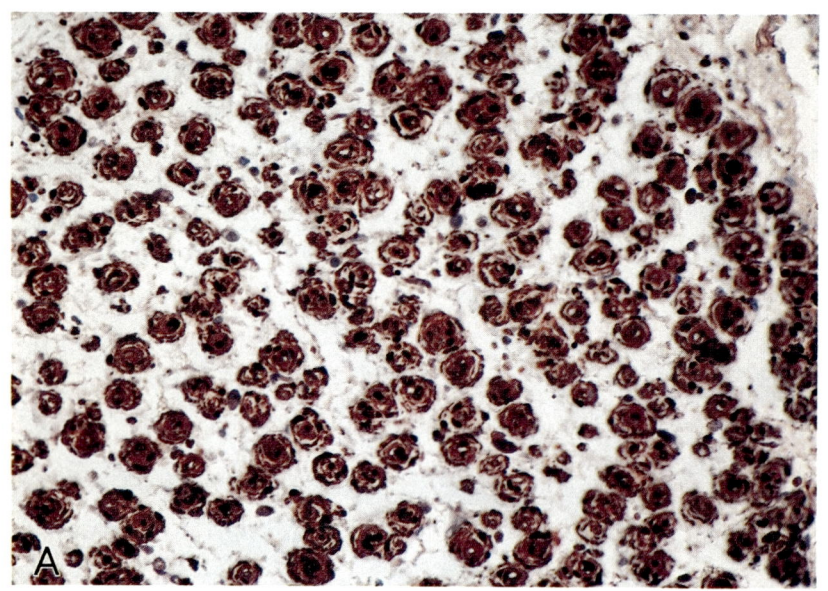

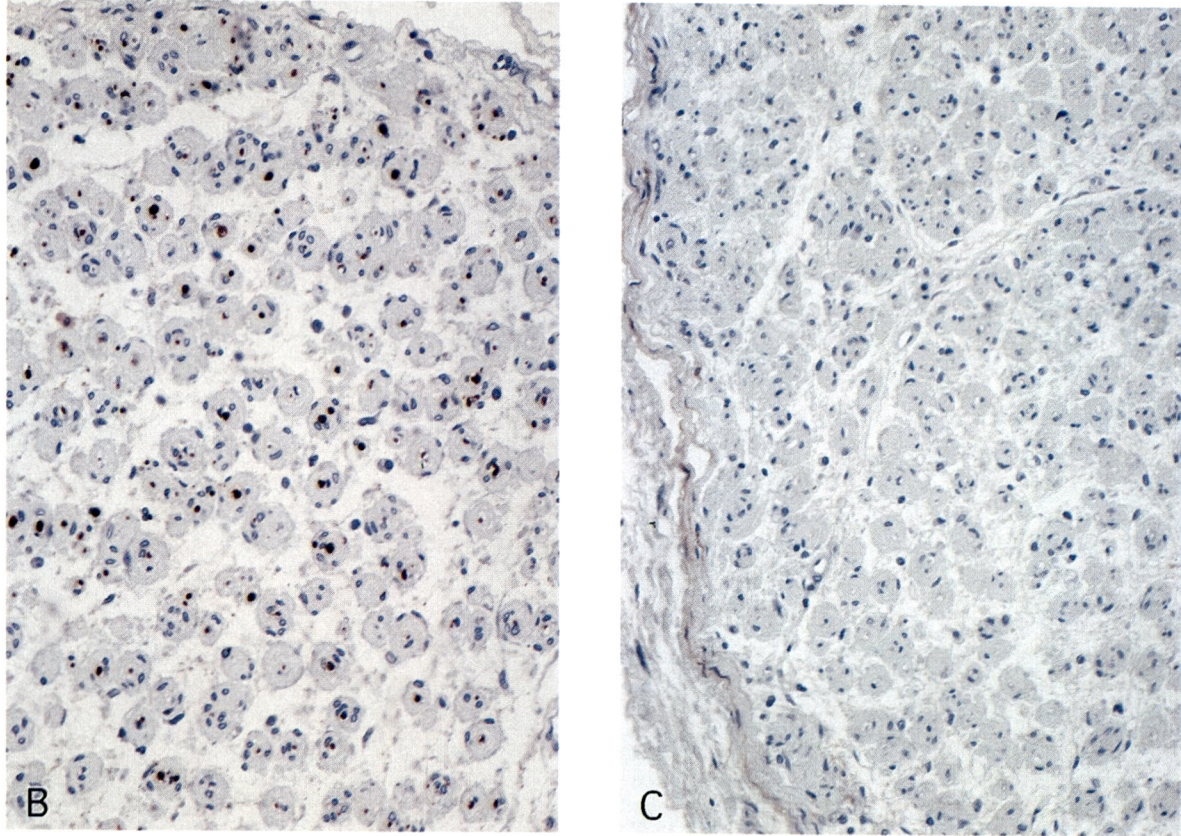

Figure 5-18
LOCALIZED HYPERTROPHIC NEUROPATHY
A: The Schwann cell nature of the cells comprising onion bulbs is evidenced by strong S-100 protein immunoreactivity.
B: Note central axons on neurofilament protein immunostain.
C: Staining for EMA is limited to normal perineurium.

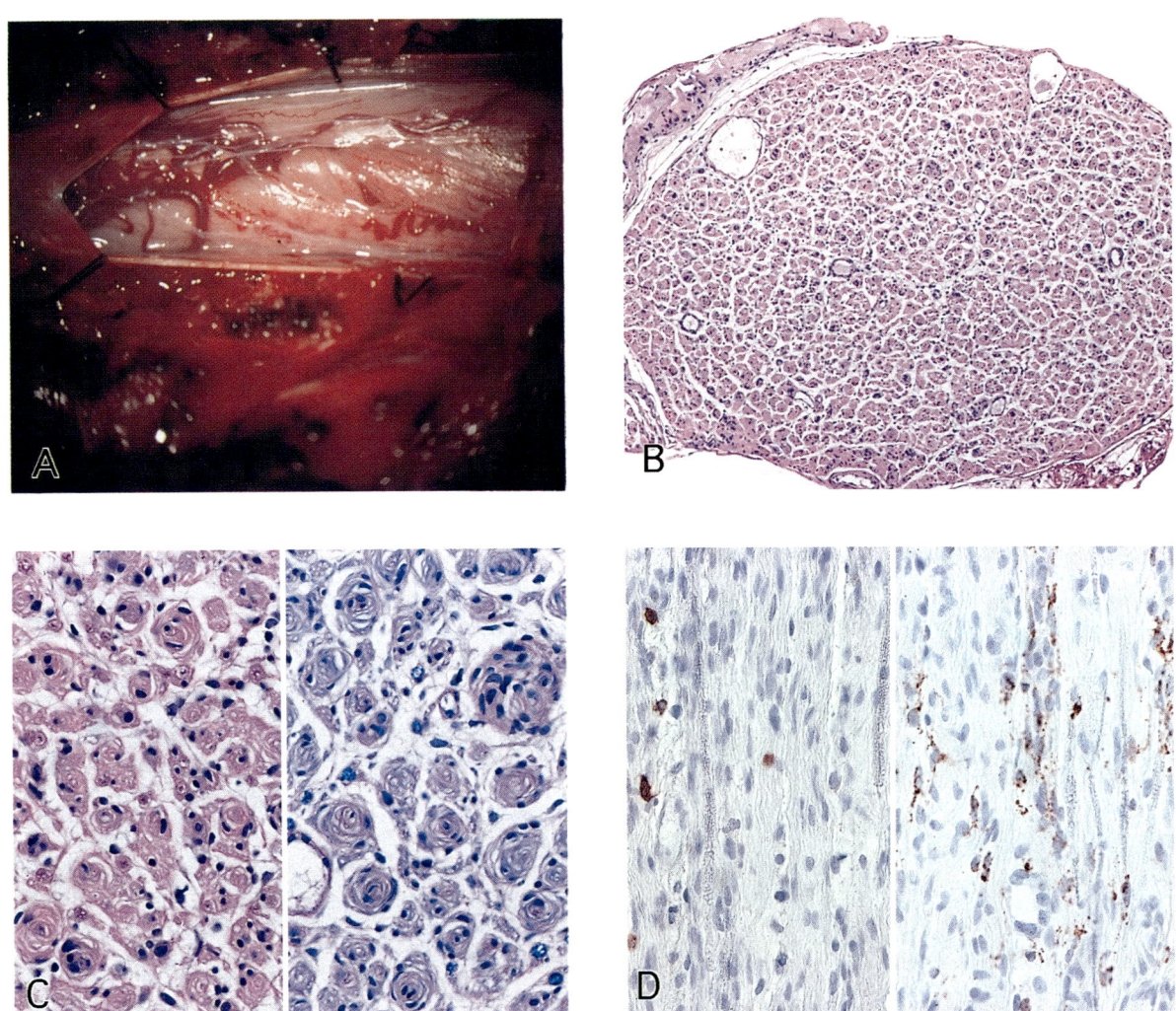

Figure 5-19
CHRONIC INFLAMMATORY DEMYELINATING POLYNEUROPATHY (CIDP)
This sporadic, often relapsing autoimmune condition varies in extent. This impressive example involved cranial and spinal nerve roots, including the cauda equina (A). The roots are markedly enlarged (A,B) and show prominent onion bulb formation (C, left). Many fibers are affected, having lost their myelin (C, right; Luxol fast-blue) and being surrounded by hypertrophic Schwann cells. Inflammatory cells are few but include lymphocytes (D, left; CD45) and histiocytes (D, right; CD68).

More generalized disorders characterized by onion bulb formation, such as hereditary sensorimotor neuropathies (Charcot-Marie-Tooth disease, Dejerine-Sottos disease) and chronic inflammatory demyelinating polyneuropathy (CDIP) (fig. 5-19) are easily distinguished from LHN on clinicopathologic grounds.

Treatment and Prognosis. LHN is an indolent process. Only one example was tumefactive (89), a trigeminal lesion that occupied the left cavernous sinus. The treatment is similar to that of intraneural perineurioma, biopsy confirmation of the diagnosis followed by observation.

REFERENCES

Palisaded Encapsulated Neuroma

1. Argenyi ZB. Immunohistochemical characterization of palisaded encapsulated neuroma. J Cutan Pathol 1990;17:329–35.
2. Argenyi ZB. Newly recognized neural neoplasms relevant to the dermatopathologist. Dermatol Clin 1992; 10(1):219–34.
3. Argenyi ZB, Cooper PH, Santa Cruz D. Plexiform and other unusual variants of palisaded encapsulated neuroma. J Cutan Pathol 1993;20:34–9.
4. Argenyi ZB, Santa Cruz D, Bromley C. Comparative light-microscopic and immunohistochemical study of traumatic and palisaded encapsulated neuromas of the skin. Am J Dermatopathol 1992;14:504–10.
5. Chauvin PJ, Wysocki GP, Daley TD, Pringle GA. Palisaded encapsulated neuroma of oral mucosa. Oral Surg Oral Med Oral Pathol 1992;73:71–4.
6. Dakin MC, Leppard B, Theaker JM. The palisaded, encapsulated neuroma (solitary circumscribed neuroma). Histopathology 1992;20:405–10.
7. Dover JS, From L, Lewis A. Palisaded encapsulated neuromas. A clinicopathologic study. Arch Dermatol 1989;125:386–9.
8. Fletcher CD. Solitary circumscribed neuroma of the skin (so-called palisaded, encapsulated neuroma). A clinicopathologic and immunohistochemical study. Am J Surg Pathol 1989;13:574–80.
9. Magnusson B. Palisaded encapsulated neuroma (solitary circumscribed neuroma) of the oral mucosa. Oral Surg Oral Med Oral Pathol Oral Radiol Endod 1996;82:302–4.
10. Reed RJ, Fine RM, Meltzer HD. Palisaded, encapsulated neuromas of the skin. Arch Dermatol 1972;106:865–70.

Mucosal Neuroma, Mucosal Neuromatosis, and Intestinal Ganglioneuromatosis of MEN IIb

11. Braley AE. Medullated corneal nerves and plexiform neuromas associated with pheochromocytoma. Trans Am Ophthal Soc 1954;52:189–97.
12. Briner J, Oswald HW, Hirsig J, et al. Neuronal intestinal dysplasia—clinical and histochemical findings and its association with Hirschsprung's disease. Z Kinderchir 1986;41:282–6.
13. Brody A, Hoover HC. Polypoid ganglioneurofibromatosis of the colon. Br J Radiol 1971;47:494–5.
14. Calmettes L, Bazex A, Deodati F, Dupre A, Bec P. Manifestations oculo-palpebrales des neuromes myeliniques muqueux. Arch Ophthalmol 1959;19:257–69.
15. Carney JA, Go VL, Sizemore GW, Hayles AB. Alimentary-tract ganglioneuromatosis: a major component of the syndrome of multiple endocrine neoplasia, type 2b. N Engl J Med 1976;295:1287–91.
16. Carney JA, Hayles AB. Alimentary tract manifestations of multiple endocrine neoplasia type 2b. Mayo Clin Proc 1977;52:543–8.
17. Carney JA, Sizemore GW, Hayles AB. Multiple endocrine neoplasia, type 2b. Pathobiol Annu 1978;8:105–53.
18. Carney JA, Sizemore GW, Lovestedt SA. Mucosal ganglioneuromatosis, medullary thyroid carcinoma and pheochromocytoma: multiple endocrine neoplasia, type 2b. Oral Surg 1976;41:739–52.
19. Chauvin PJ, Wysocki GP, Daley TD, Pringle GA. Palisaded encapsulated neuroma of oral mucosa. Oral Surg Oral Med Oral Pathol 1992;73:71–4.
20. Cope R, Schleinitz PF. Multiple endocrine neoplasia, type 2b, as a cause of megacolon. Am J Gastroenterol 1983;78:802–5.
21. d'Amore ES, Manivel JC, Pettinato G, Niehans GA, Snover DC. Intestinal ganglioneuromatosis: mucosal and transmural types. A clinicopathologic and immunohistochemical study of six cases. Hum Pathol 1991;22:276–86.
22. Donnelly WH, Sieber WK, Yunis EJ. Polypoid ganglioneurofibromatosis of the large bowel. Arch Pathol Lab Med 1969;87:537–41.
23. Frank K, Raue F, Gottswinter J, Heinrich V, Meybier H, Ziegler R. Importance of early diagnosis and follow-up in multiple endocrine neoplasia (MEN IIb). Eur J Pediatr 1984;143:112–6.
24. Gleason IO, Beauchemin J, Busks A. Polypoid ganglioneuromatosis of the large bowel. Arch Neurol 1962;6:242–7.
25. Gorlin RJ, Mirkin BL. Multiple mucosal neuromas, pheochromocytoma, medullary carcinoma of the thyroid and marfanoid body build with muscle wasting. Syndrome of hyperplasia and neoplasia of neural crest derivatives—a unitarian concept. Z Kinderheilkd 1972;113:313–25.
26. Gorlin RJ, Sedano HO, Vickers FA, Cervenka J. Multiple mucosal neuromas, pheochromocytoma and medullary carcinoma of thyroid—a syndrome. Cancer 1968;22:293–9.
27. Khairi MR, Dexter RN, Burzynski NJ, Johnston CC Jr. Mucosal neuroma, pheochromocytoma and medullary thyroid carcinoma: multiple endocrine neoplasia type 3. Medicine 1975;54:89–112.
28. Koke MP, Braley AE. Bilateral plexiform neuromata of the conjunctiva and medullated corneal nerves. Report of a case. Am J Ophthal 1940;23:179–82.
29. Lashner BA, Riddell RH, Winans CS. Ganglioneuromatosis of the colon and extensive glycogenic acanthosis in Cowden's disease. Dig Dis Sci 1986;31:213–6.
30. Legros A, Leconte D, Huguet C. Pseudo-obstruction de l'intestin grele par ganglioneuromatose. Gastroenterol Clin Biol 1980;4:333–7.
21. Levy M, Habib R, Lyon G, Schweisguth O, Lemerle J, Royer P. Neuromatose et epithelioma a stroma amyloide de la thyroide chez l'enfant. Arch Franc Pediatr 1970;27:561–83.
32. Masson P, Branch A. Gigantisme et ganglioneuromatose de l'appendice. Rev Canad Biol 1945;4:219–63.
33. Mendelsohn G, Diamond MP. Familial ganglioneuromatous polyposis of the large bowel: report of a family with associated juvenile polyposis. Am J Surg Pathol 1984;8:515–20.
34. Nezelof C, Guy-Grand D, Thomine E. Les megacolons avec hyperplasie des plexus myenteriques. Une entite anatomo-clinique, a propos de 3 cas. Presse Med 1970;78:1501–6.

35. Norton JA, Froome LC, Farrell RE, Wells SR Jr. Multiple endocrine neoplasia type IIb: the most aggressive form of medullary thyroid carcinoma. Surg Clin North Am 1979;59:109–18.

36. O'Riordain DS, O'Brien T, Crotty TB, Gharib H, Grant CS, van Heerden JA. Multiple endocrine neoplasia type 2B: more than an endocrine disorder. Surgery 1995;118:936–42.

37. Pham BN, Villanueva RP. Ganglioneuromatous proliferation associated with juvenile polyposis coli. Arch Pathol Lab Med 1989;113:91–4.

38. Puri P, Lake BD, Nixon HH, Mishalany H, Claireaux AE. Neuronal colonic dysplasia: an unusual association of Hirschsprung's disease. J Pediatr Surg 1977;12:681–5.

39. Rescorla FJ, Vane DW, Fitzgerald JF, et al. Vasoactive intestinal peptide-secreting ganglioneuromatosis affecting the entire colon and rectum. J Pediatr Surg 1988;23:635–7.

40. Reza MJ, Young RT, van Herle AJ, et al. Multiple endocrine adenomatosis type IIb (Sipple's syndrome) in twins. West J Med 1975;123:441–6.

41. Riley FC Jr, Robertson DM. Ocular histopathology in multiple endocrine neoplasia type 2b. Am J Ophthalmol 1981;91:57–64.

42. Robertson DM, Gordon H. Thickened corneal nerves as a manifestation of multiple endocrine neoplasia. Trans Am Acad Ophthalmol Otolaryngol 1975;79:OP772–87.

43. Scharli AF, Meier-Ruge W. Localized and disseminated forms of neuronal intestinal dysplasia mimicking Hirschsprung's disease. J Pediatr Surg 1981;16:164–70.

44. Schimke RN, Hartmann WH, Prout TE, Rimoin DL. The syndrome of bilateral pheochromocytoma, medullary thyroid carcinoma and multiple neuromas. A possible regulatory defect in the differentiation of chromaffin tissue. N Engl J Med 1968;279:1–7.

45. Snover DC, Weigent CE, Sumner HW. Diffuse mucosal ganglioneuromatosis of the colon associated with adenocarcinoma. Am J Clin Pathol 1981;75:225–9.

46. Spector B, Klintworth GK, Wells SA Jr. Histologic study of the ocular lesions in multiple endocrine neoplasias syndrome type IIb. Am J Ophthalmol 1981;91:204–15.

47. Weary PE, Gorlin RJ, Gentry WC. Multiple hamartoma syndrome (Cowden's disease). Arch Dermatol 1972;106:682–90.

48. Weidner N, Flanders DJ, Mitros FA. Mucosal ganglioneuromatosis associated with multiple colonic polyps. Am J Surg Pathol 1984;8:779–86.

49. Williams ED, Pollock DJ. Multiple mucosal neuromata with endocrine tumors: a syndrome allied to von Recklinghausen's disease. J Pathol Bacteriol 1966;91:71–80.

Neuroma, Neuromatosis, and Ganglioneuromatosis of the Alimentary Tract Unassociated with MEN Type IIb

50. Aubock L, Ratzenhofer M. Extraepithelial enterochromaffin cell-nerve-fiber complexes in the normal human appendix, and in neurogenic appendicopathy. J Pathol 1982;136:217–26.

51. Briner J, Oswald HW, Hirsig J, et al. Neuronal intestinal dysplasia—clinical and histochemical findings and its association with Hirschsprung's disease. Z Kinderchir 1986;41:282–6.

52. Burnett JW, Goldner R, Calton GJ. Cowden disease. Report of two additional cases. Brit J Dermatol 1975;93:329–36.

53. Castleman B, Scully RE, McNeely BU. Case record of the Massachusetts General Hospital (Case 24–1974). N Engl J Med 1974;290:1426–31.

54. Collins DC. 71,000 human appendix specimens: a final report summarizing 40 years of study. Am J Proctol 1963;14:365–81.

55. Donnelly WH, Sieber WK, Yunis EJ. Polypoid ganglioneurofibromatosis of the large bowel. Arch Pathol Lab Med 1969;87:537–41.

56. Fuller CE, Williams GT. Gastrointestinal manifestations of type 1 neurofibromatosis (von Recklinghausen's disease). Histopathology 1991;19:1–11.

57. Harach HR, Williams GT, Williams ED. Familial adenomatous polyposis associated thyroid carcinoma: a distinct type of follicular cell neoplasm. Histopathology 1994;25:549–61.

58. Hochberg FH, Dasilva AB, Galdabini J, Richardson EP. Gastrointestinal involvement in von Recklinghausen's neurofibromatosis. Neurology 1974;24:1144–51.

59. Hofler H, Kasper M, Heitz PU. The neuroendocrine system of normal human appendix, ileum, colon, and in neurogenic appendicopathy. Virchows Arch [A] 1983;399:127–40.

60. Isaacson NH, Blades B. Neuroappendicopathy: review of the literature and report of 52 cases. Arch Surg 1951;4:455–67.

61. Kepes JJ, Zacharias DL. Gangliocytic paragangliomas of the duodenum. Report of two cases with light and electron microscopic examination. Cancer 1971;27:61–70.

62. Lashner BA, Riddell RH, Winans CS. Ganglioneuromatosis of the colon and extensive glycogenic acanthosis in Cowden's disease. Dig Dis Sci 1986;31:213–6.

63. Lloyd KM, Dennis M. Cowden's disease. A possible new symptom complex with multiple system involvement. Ann Intern Med 1963;58:136–42.

64. Masson P. Carcinoids (argentaffin-cell tumors) and nerve hyperplasia of the appendicular mucosa. Am J Pathol 1928;4:181-211.

65. Masson P. Neural proliferations in the vermiform appendix. In: Penfield W, ed. Cytology of the nervous system. Vol. III, 1932:1095–130.

66. Mendelsohn G, Diamond MP. Familial ganglioneuromatous polyposis of the large bowel. Report of a family with associated juvenile polyposis. Am J Surg Pathol 1984;8:515–20.

67. Michalany J, Galindo W. Classification of neuromas of the appendix. Beitr Pathol 1973;150:213–28.

68. Millikin PD. Extraepithelial enterochromaffin cells and Schwann cells in the human appendix. Arch Pathol Lab Med 1983;107:189–94.

69. Nelson J, Mena H, Ross KF, Martz KL. Lhermitte-Duclos disease (LDD): clinicopathologic features and association with Cowden's disease (CD). Lab Invest 1994;70:139A.

70. Nuss DD, Aeling JL, Clemons DE, Weber WN. Multiple hamartoma syndrome (Cowden's disease). Arch Dermatol 1978;114:743–6.

70a. O'Brien P, Kapusta L, Dardick I, Axler J, Gnidec A. Multiple familial gastrointestinal autonomic nerve tumors and small intestinal neuronal dysplasia. Am J Surg Pathol 1999;23:198–204.

71. Ortonne JP, Lambert R, Daudet J. Involvement of the digestive tract in Cowden's disease. Int J Dermatol 1980;19:570–6.

72. Pham BN, Villanueva RP. Ganglioneuromatous proliferation associated with juvenile polyposis coli. Arch Pathol Lab Med 1989;113:91–4.

73. Puri P, Lake BD, Nixon HH, et al. Neuronal colonic dysplasia: an unusual association of Hirschsprung's disease. J Pediatr Surg 1977;12:681–5.

74. Raszkowski HJ, Hufner RF. Neurofibromatosis of the colon: a unique manifestation of von Recklinghausen's disease. Cancer 1971;27:134–42.

75. Rendler S. Cowden's disease. Curr Concepts Skin Dis 1981;2:7–11.

76. Rush BF Jr, Stefaniwsky AB, Sasso A, Dumitrescu I, Wexler D. Neuroma of the common bile duct. J Surg Oncol 1988;39:17–21.

77. Saul RA, Sturner RA, Burger PC. Hyperplasia of the myenteric plexus. Its association with early infantile megacolon and neurofibromatosis. Am J Dis Child 1982;136:852–4.

78. Scharli AF, Meier-Ruge W. Localized and disseminated forms of neuronal intestinal dysplasia mimicking Hirschsprung's disease. J Pediatr Surg 1981;16:164–70.

79. Scheithauer BW, Nora FE, Lechago J, et al. Duodenal gangliocytic paraganglioma. Clinicopathologic and immunocytochemical study of 11 cases. Am J Clin Pathol 1986;86:559–65.

80. Shekitka KM, Sobin LH. Ganglioneuromas of the gastrointestinal tract. Relation to von Recklinghausen disease and other multiple tumor syndromes. Am J Surg Pathol 1994;18:250–7.

81. Snover DC, Weigent CE, Sumner HW. Diffuse mucosal ganglioneuromatosis of the colon associated with adenocarcinoma. Am J Clin Pathol 1981;75:225–9.

82. Stanley MW, Cherwitz D, Hagen K, Snover DC. Neuromas of the appendix. A light-microscopic, immunohistochemical and electron-microscopic study of 20 cases. Am J Surg Pathol 1986;10:801–15.

83. Staple TW, McAlister WH, Anderson MS. Plexiform neurofibromatosis of the colon simulating Hirschsprung's disease. Am J Rad 1964;91:840–5.

84. Stephenson J, Snoddy WT. Appendiceal lesions: observations of 4,000 appendectomies. Arch Surg 1961;83:661–6.

85. Sugahara K, Yamamoto M, Iizuka H, Yoshioka M, Miura K. Spontaneous neuroma of the bile duct: a case report. Am J Gastroenterology 1985;80:807–9.

86. Walsh MM, Drew M, Bleiweiss IJ. Neurofibroma of the common bile duct. A case report and review of the literature. Int J Surg Pathol 1997;4:245–8.

87. Weidner N, Flanders DJ, Mitros FA. Mucosal ganglioneuromatosis associated with multiple colonic polyps. Am J Surg Pathol 1984;8:779–86.

Localized Hypertrophic Neuropathy

88. Baskin DS, Townsend JJ, Wilson CB. Isolated hypertrophic interstitial neuropathy of the trigeminal nerve associated with trigeminal neuralgia. J Neurosurg 1981;55:987–90.

89. Chang Y, Horoupian DS, Jordan J, Steinberg G. Localized hypertrophic mononeuropathy of the trigeminal nerve. Arch Pathol Lab Med 1993;117:170–6.

90. Chow SM. Role of macrophages in onion-bulb formation in localized hypertrophic mononeuritis (LHN). Clin Neuropathol 1991;10:112–21.

91. Emory TS, Scheithauer BW, Hirose T, Wood M, Onofrio BM, Jenkins RB. Intraneural perineurioma. A clonal neoplasm associated with abnormalities of chromosome 22. Am J Clin Pathol 1995;103:696–704.

92. Suarez GA, Giannini C, Bosch EP, et al. Immune brachial plexus neuropathy: suggestive evidence for an inflammatory immune pathogenesis. Neurology 1996;46:559–61.

93. Yassini PR, Sauter K, Schochet SS, Kaufman HH, Bloomfield SM. A localized hypertrophic mononeuropathy involving spinal roots and associated with sacral meningocele. J Neurosurg 1993;79:774–8.

6

HAMARTOMA AND CHORISTOMA

LIPOFIBROMATOUS HAMARTOMA OF NERVE

Definition. This is a benign overgrowth of epineurial adipose and fibrous tissue, with or without associated macrodactyly, most often affecting the distal upper extremity. Synonyms include *fibrolipomatous hamartoma, lipofibroma,* and *fibrolipomatosis.*

General Comments. Lipofibromatous hamartoma is an uncommon lesion: only about 50 cases have been reported (1,4,7,8,10,13). The process occurs sporadically and has no association with neurofibromatosis. Females are twice as often affected as males. At presentation, the majority of patients are adolescents or young adults; occasional examples occur in the neonatal period or in late adulthood (1). Distal peripheral nerves are most often affected; cranial nerve involvement is rare (3). Lipofibromatous hamartomas affect the upper extremities three times more frequently than the lower limbs. Proximal lesions are few, and include a lesion of the radial nerve at the elbow (5) and one involving the whole of the brachial plexus (11). The median nerve is far more often affected than the ulnar or radial nerve. Digital enlargement due to an increase of perineural soft tissue and skin commonly results (fig. 6-1). When accompanied by "true macrodactyly," enlargement of bone as well as soft tissue (fig. 6-2), the lesion has been referred to as *macrodystrophia lipomatosa.* The fact that lipofibromatous hamartomas of the lower extremities are rarely associated with true macrodactyly suggests that a genetically determined abnormality in end-organ tissue responsiveness to trophic factors may underlie the morphologic distinction (13). Lipofibromatous hamartomas are rarely bilateral (1). Although there is no relationship with neurofibromatosis, one patient with hamartomatous involvement of two digits in one hand was reported to also have Klippel-Trenaunay-Webber syndrome (bony hypertrophy of extremities and a concomitant vascular anomaly) (1). Aside from the clinically obvious mass, patients with lipofibromatous hamartoma tend to develop sensorimotor defi-

cits. Involvement of the median nerve at the wrist may manifest as carpal tunnel syndrome.

Gross Findings. Lipofibromatous hamartomas consist of a lobulated, yellow, sausage-shaped expansion of peripheral nerve by adipose tissue (fig. 6-3). In some instances, hypertrophy of surrounding skin and soft tissue is associated with bone enlargement (macrodystrophia lipomatosa) (fig. 6-2). When totally resected, relatively normal-appearing proximal and distal nerves are often identified (fig. 6-3, right).

Microscopic Findings. In cross section, the epineurium of the affected nerve and often of its branches is expanded by adipose tissue (fig. 6-4A). It is in the proximal and distal portions of the lesion that the relative proportion of fibrous tissue to fat may be increased. Additional fibro-adipose overgrowth is often evident outside the vague, delicate confines of the epineurium. Since small branches of a nerve may also be affected, the diagnosis may in some cases be confidently made on a very limited biopsy. In addition to adipose tissue, the most conspicuous component of the lesion, the affected nerve may show other alternations, particularly perineurial septation of nerve fascicles and microfascicle formation (fig. 6-4B) (5,14). Onion bulb-like hypertrophic change due to an increase in perineurial cells may also be seen and should not be misinterpreted as intraneural perineurioma, a lesion discussed in chapter 9 (fig. 6-4E). Chronic alterations also include collagen deposition and marked axonal loss (fig. 6-4).

Ultrastructural Findings. The hypertrophic change that may be seen in entrapped nerves has been shown to consist of multilayering of perineurial cells (14). Minimal changes are observed in myelinated and unmyelinated nerve fibers and their accompanying Schwann cells.

Differential Diagnosis. A number of adipose lesions, either intrinsic or extrinsic, may affect nerve (fig. 6-5) (7,14). Soft tissue *lipoma* and lipoma of nerve sheath may compress nerve fascicles to produce neurologic symptoms. Their distinction from lipofibromatous hamartoma may be made at surgery. Composed entirely of adipose

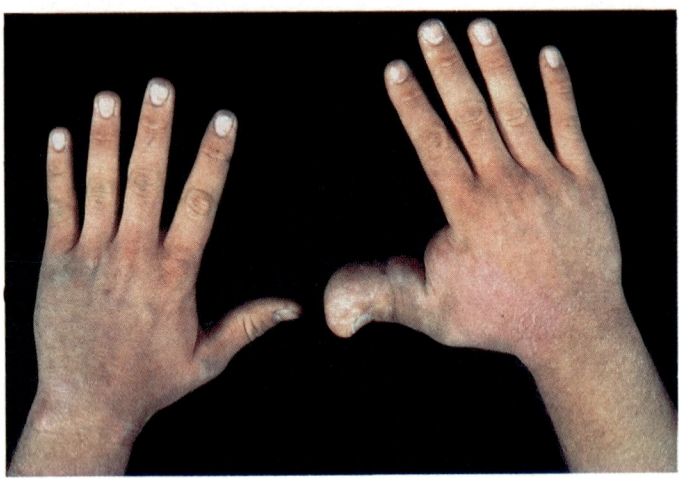

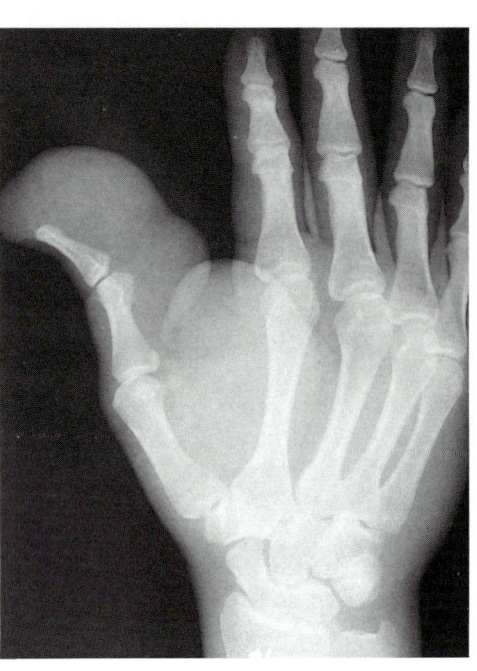

Figure 6-1
LIPOFIBROMATOUS HAMARTOMA

In this case, massive involvement of the thumb and thenar eminence (above) was radiographically unassociated with a skeletal abnormality (right). (Figures 6-3, right and 6-4, right are from the same case.)

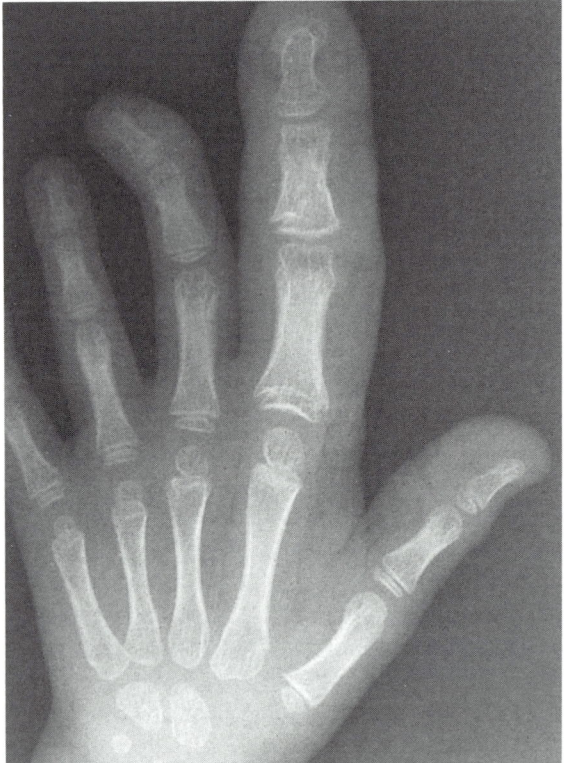

Figure 6-2
LIPOFIBROMATOUS HAMARTOMA

This example, affecting the index finger, was associated with true macrodactyly and conforms to the "macrodystrophia lipomatosa" variant.

tissue, lipomas are delicately encapsulated, and lack an intimate association with nerve branches and fascicles or, for that matter, with macrodactyly. Lipoma of soft tissue secondarily affecting nerve and epineurial lipomas are discussed in greater detail in the section Miscellaneous Tumor of Nerve.

The relation of lipofibromatous hamartoma to "lipoma" of cranial and cauda equina nerve roots is unclear. In that such lesions occasionally contain other tissue elements, including muscle, they are discussed under the differential diagnosis of neuromuscular choristoma (see below).

Treatment and Prognosis. The therapeutic approach to lipofibromatous hamartoma must take into account both the integrity of the affected nerve and the frequently associated macrodactyly. Since older patients often have a more profound neurologic deficit than do young ones, approaches to therapy vary with patient age. Some, noting a degree of preservation of sensation despite nerve excision, recommend simple excision of the entire lesion (2,9). Microsurgical intraneural dissection of hamartomatous tissue also has its proponents (6,14), but the procedure may meet with only limited success (1). One recent study (1) suggests that simple excision of epineurial tissue, leaving the intact nerve in situ, preserves nerve function. Others have suggested no or only minimal surgical intervention (12). As a rule,

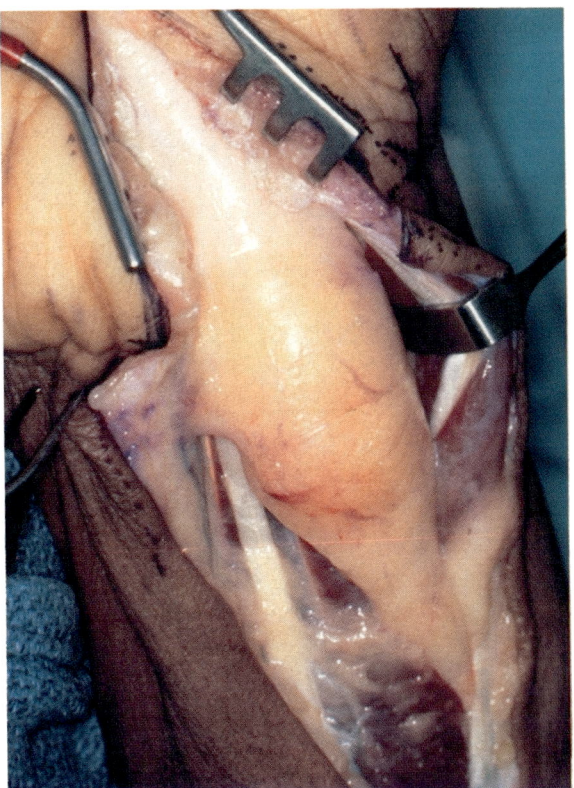
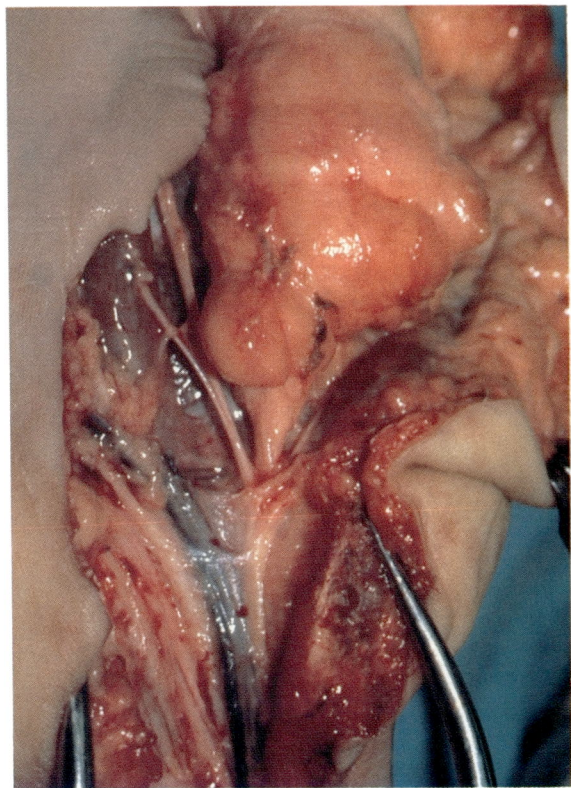

Figure 6-3
LIPOFIBROMATOUS HAMARTOMA

Left: Operative view of a lipofibromatous hamartoma of the median nerve after release of the transverse carpal ligament. The lesion occurred in a 63-year-old female with a 6-month history of weakness, numbness, and clumsiness of the right hand. Note the enormously swollen median nerve containing adipose tissue in the distal forearm and wrist. (Fig. 2 from Guthikonda M, Rengachary SS, Balko MG, van Loveren H. Lipofibromatous hamartoma of the median nerve: case report with magnetic resonance imaging correlation. Neurosurgery 1994;35:127–32.)

Right: Yet another more massive example shows more abrupt transition to normal nerve.

resection is curative, but recurrence of symptoms, such as carpal tunnel syndrome, or of a discernible mass is rarely reported (1).

NEUROMUSCULAR CHORISTOMA

Definition. This non-neoplastic mass is composed of mature skeletal muscle and peripheral nerves in which myocytes are intimately associated with nerve fibers. It is also known as *neuromuscular hamartoma*.

General Comments. The nature of neuromuscular choristoma is as yet unsettled. When viewed in the context of limb components, the once popular designation neuromuscular hamartoma may seem reasonable. On the other hand, since skeletal muscle is not a normal component of nerve, the term choristoma is more appropriate when the lesion is viewed as one intrinsic to nerve. The hamartoma concept is also hard to reconcile with the occurrence of similar lesions in the central nervous system (23,40) (see below).

The original suggestion of Orlandi (33), that the process is malformative in nature and results from the entrapment of muscle into the substance of developing nerve, is indirectly supported by the report of a lipoma-associated example in the lumbar dural sac (23). Lipomas at this site are considered malformations and often, in addition to nerve, contain other mesenchymal elements including skeletal muscle. An alternative suggestion that neuromuscular choristomas represent hamartomas of muscle spindles is inviting (29), but the often strap-shaped myocytes with subplasmalemmal nuclei that comprise neuromuscular choristoma resemble normal, ordinary

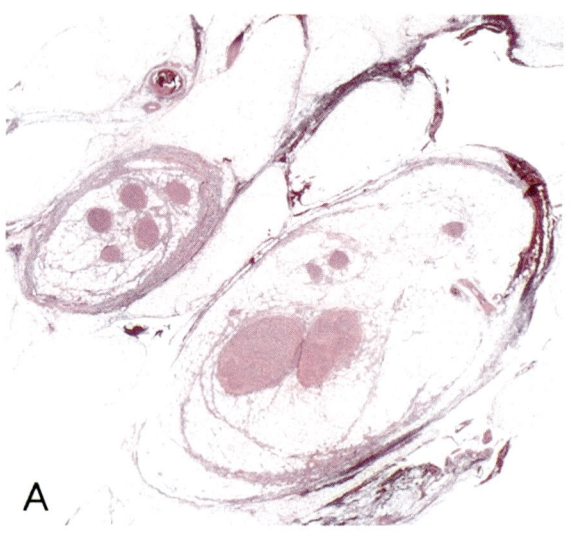

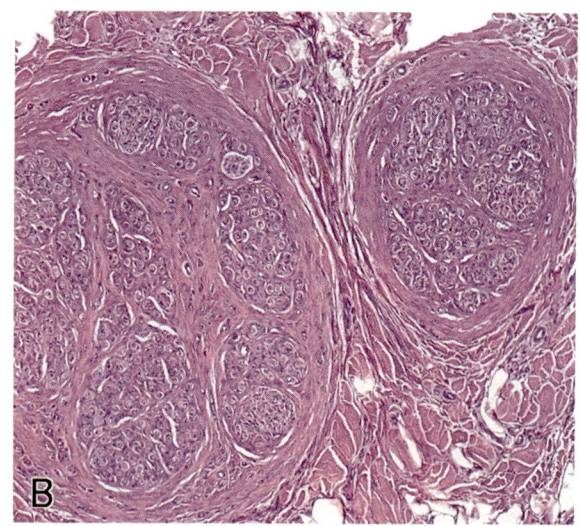

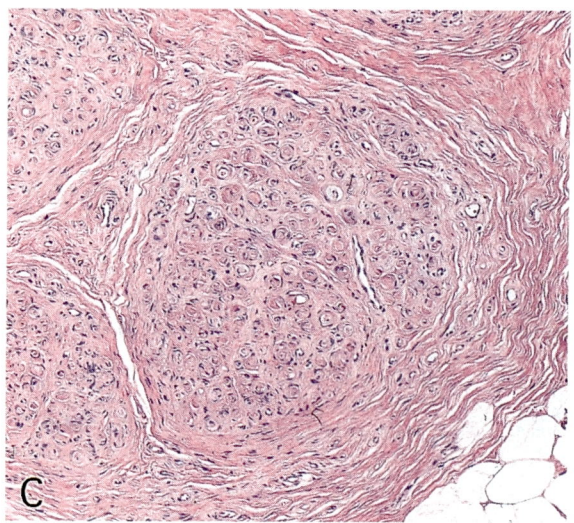

Figure 6-4
LIPOFIBROMATOUS HAMARTOMA
Note expansion of the epineurium of two nerve branches by adipose tissue (A). Another example shows secondary, chronic changes in the nerve including microfasciculation (B). Longstanding involvement is also associated with pseudo-onion bulb formation (B,C), collagen deposition (D), and severe axonal loss (E, Bielschowski stain). (C-E: Courtesy of Dr. D. Horoupian, Stanford, CA.)

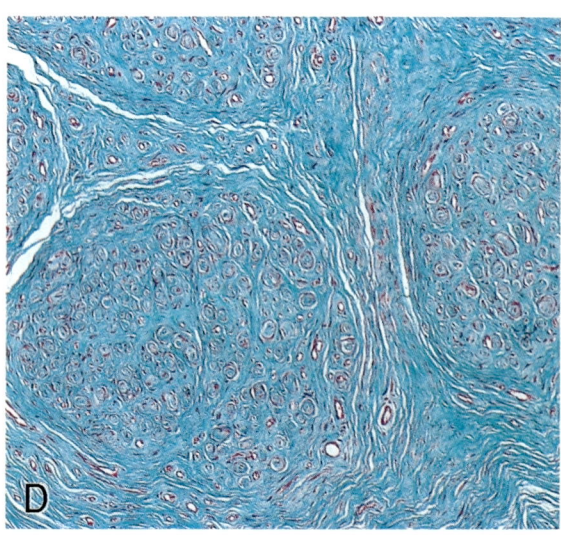

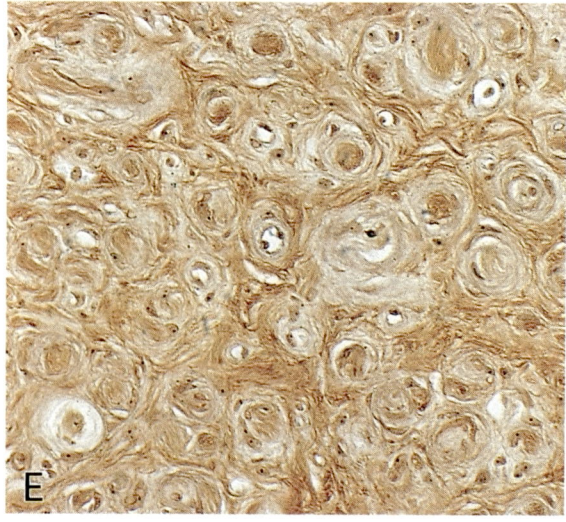

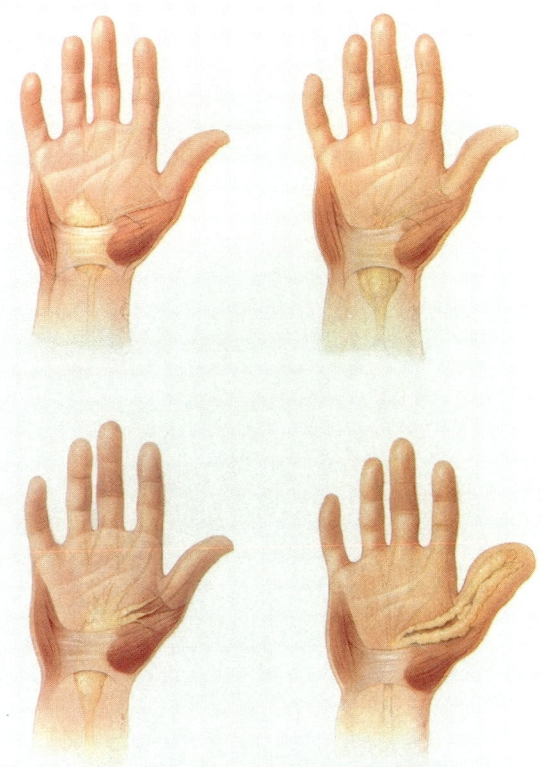

Figure 6-5
ADIPOSE LESIONS AFFECTING NERVE

Four major forms of lipomatous lesions occur in the forearm and hand. Soft tissue lipoma compresses the median nerve, with no intrinsic abnormality of the nerve (upper left). Intraneural lipoma of the median nerve, a discrete and benign neoplasm, arises from adipose tissue within the epineurium and splays the median nerve fascicles (upper right). A cleavage plane permits separation of the fascicles from the lipoma. Lipofibromatous hamartoma with diffuse inter- and perifascicular infiltration by fibrofatty tissue, without a defined plane of cleavage between the lesion and nerve fascicles (lower left). Lipofibromatous hamartoma, macrodystrophia lipomatosa variant, with marked enlargement of a digit due to fatty infiltration of the epineurium and its surroundings, as well as hypertrophy of skin, subcutaneous tissue, and bone (lower right). (Fig. 4 from Guthikonda M, Rengachary SS, Balko MG, van Loveren H. Lipofibromatous hamartoma of the median nerve: case report with magnetic resonance imaging correlation. Neurosurgery 1994;35:127–32.)

striated muscle cells rather than the bag and chain fibers of muscle spindles. Furthermore, although a capsule composed of perineurial-like cells surrounds normal muscle spindles, choristomas lack a perineurial ensheathment (31). Lastly, Masson's (30) suggestion that neuroectoderm is capable of mesenchymal differentiation, hence the term "ectomesenchyme," may be relevant to the genesis of this lesion. Normal examples of such differentiation in the human include the development of iris muscles from the eye cup (32); the formation of cranial bones, soft tissue, and a portion of the leptomeninges from neuroectoderm (37); and the occurrence of skeletal muscle "heterotopias" within the leptomeninges (15) or within normal nerve in the larynx (39). The same mechanism has been used to explain the occurrence of skeletal muscle in a spinal nerve of a frog (16). The ectomesenchyme concept has also been invoked to explain the occurrence of skeletal muscle components in benign (19) and malignant nerve sheath tumors (25,38). Which of these mechanisms, if any, underlies the development of neuromuscular choristoma remains unresolved.

Clinical Features. Neuromuscular choristoma is a rare lesion. Since its first description as an incidental autopsy finding in an adult (33), 14 bona fide clinical cases have been reported (18,20, 21,23,24,26,28,29,31,36,40). The majority present in early childhood, some being congenital, or in adolescence. No sex predilection has been noted. Most patients with neuromuscular choristomas present with neurologic signs, but in some cases symptoms are simply a reflection of the mass effects. Lesion location and size determine clinical manifestations, which include sensorimotor deficits and muscle atrophy. Whereas neuromuscular choristomas typically affect major nerve trunks, exceptional lesions affect smaller nerves, such as of the chest wall (21) or cranial nerves (40). Only a minority are multiple (21,33). Accompanying malformations have been reported, including skeletal abnormalities (33) and an intimately associated spinal intradural lipoma (23). No association with heritable disorders has been noted.

Gross Findings. Neuromuscular choristomas form nodular, firm, gray-brown masses. More often single than multiple, they lie within or are loosely attached to a major nerve which is usually seen to enter and exit the demarcated or encapsulated mass. Nerve branches meander among entangled muscle bundles. On cut surface, the neuromuscular nodules are often separated by fibrous bands of varying thickness.

Microscopic Findings. Neuromuscular choristomas consist of a disordered proliferation of skeletal muscle and peripheral nerve tissue. The skeletal muscle fibers are well differentiated, vary in size, and are haphazardly distributed among variably myelinated nerves (fig. 6-6). Careful

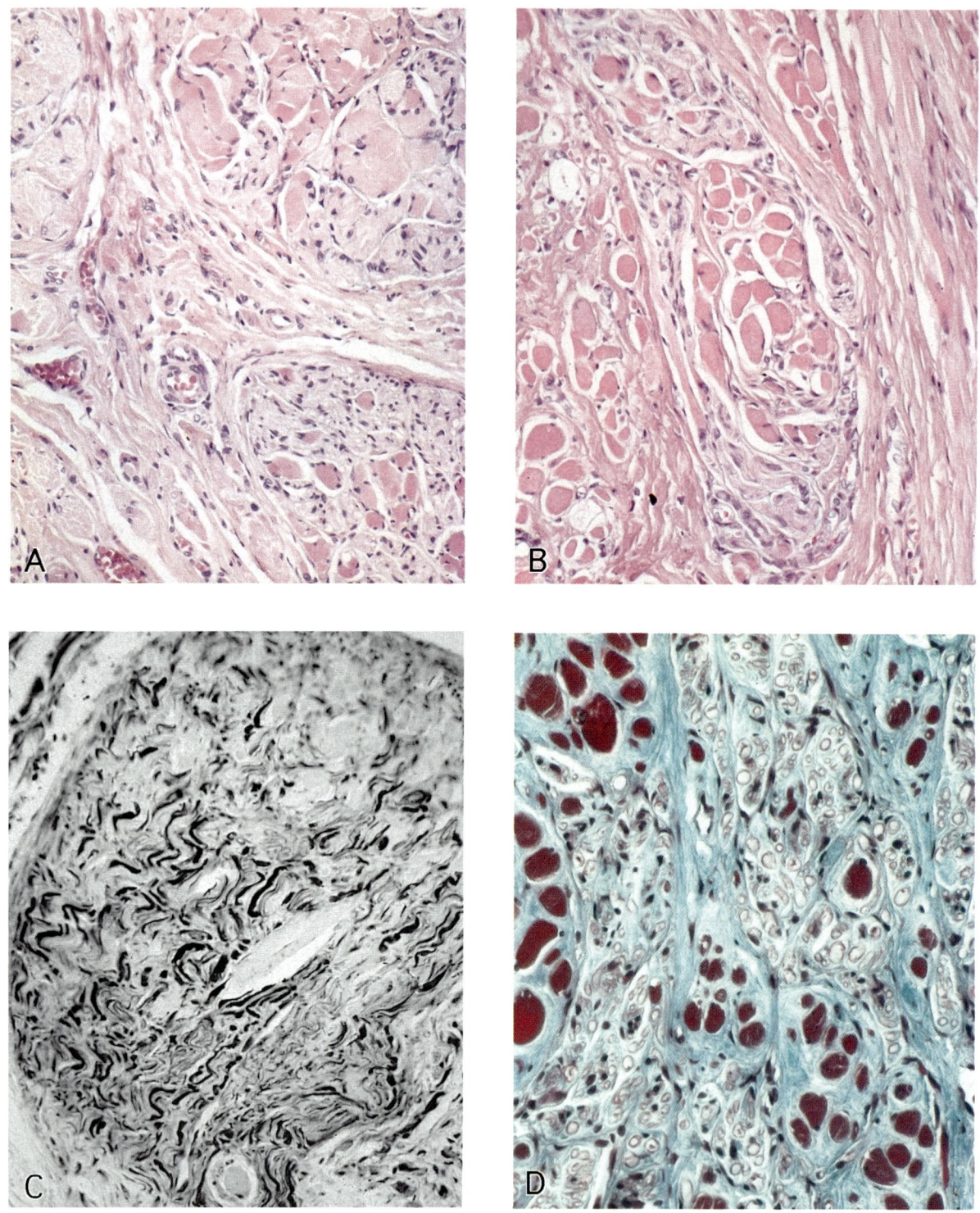

Figure 6-6
NEUROMUSCULAR CHORISTOMA

A low-power view of one published example (17) shows separation of smoothly contoured nodules of skeletal muscle by varying sized bundles (A). The intimate relationship between muscle fibers and nerve tissue (A, upper right; B) is also evident on Bodian stain for axons which clearly shows skeletal muscle fibers lying among nerve fibers (C). In yet another published example (D), a trichrome stain shows connective tissue septa outlining neuromuscular bundles (7).

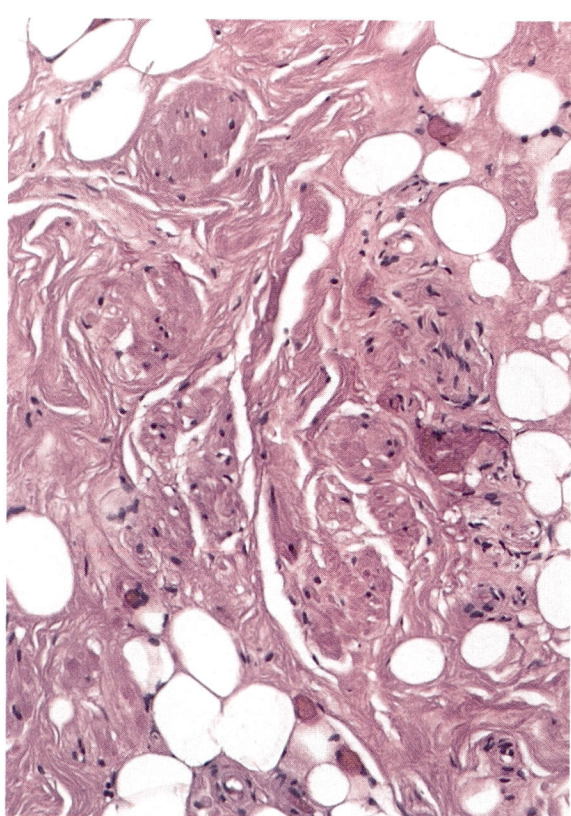 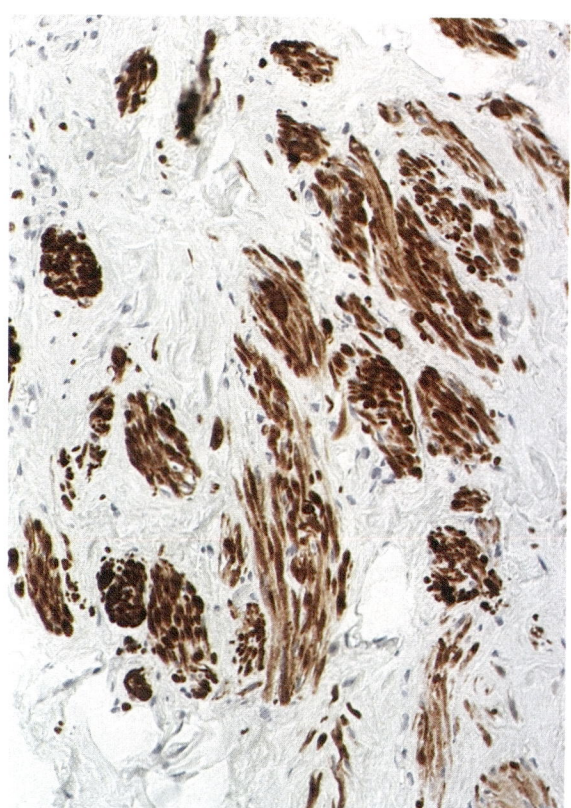

Figure 6-7
LIPOMA OF EIGHTH CRANIAL NERVE

Lipomas of the central nervous system, such as affect the cerebellopontine angle and cauda equina region, may feature skeletal muscle components. This example (left) involving the eighth nerve entrapped nerve fascicles and contains bundles of myocytes. The latter are well seen on immunostain for desmin (right).

scrutiny typically shows the myocytes to reside not only between fascicles but among nerve fibers (fig. 6-6). Despite their disarray, the muscle fibers resemble normal skeletal muscle cells, being strap-shaped and multinucleate with subplasmalemmal nuclei and cross striations. One unusual example featured both skeletal and smooth muscle (36). The relative proportion of nerve and muscle varies, but myocytes usually predominate, particularly at the center of the nodules. Nerve fibers are readily apparent with silver impregnation stains for axons, such as Bielschowsky or Bodian preparations (fig. 6-6C), whereas myelin may or may not be present. Stroma takes the form of connective tissue septa separating nodules of neuromuscular tissue (fig. 6-6D). Cytologic atypia is lacking, as are mitoses.

Immunohistochemical Findings. Not surprisingly, the neural component of neuromuscular hamartoma shows neurofilament protein staining of axons whereas S-100 protein reactivity is seen in accompanying Schwann cells. The presence or absence of a perineurial cell element has not been adequately studied by EMA stain (31). The muscular component of the tumor is reactive for all markers of striated muscle including desmin, HHF-35, sarcomeric actin, myogenin, and myoglobin.

Ultrastructural Findings. To date, only a single brief ultrastructural description of an unusual, smooth muscle–containing neuromuscular choristoma has been published (36).

Differential Diagnosis. The term "benign Triton tumor" has been inappropriately applied to neuromuscular choristoma (18,29), a non-neoplastic lesion. Nonetheless, peripheral nerve sheath tumors with myogenic differentiation do enter into the differential, as does rhabdomyoma.

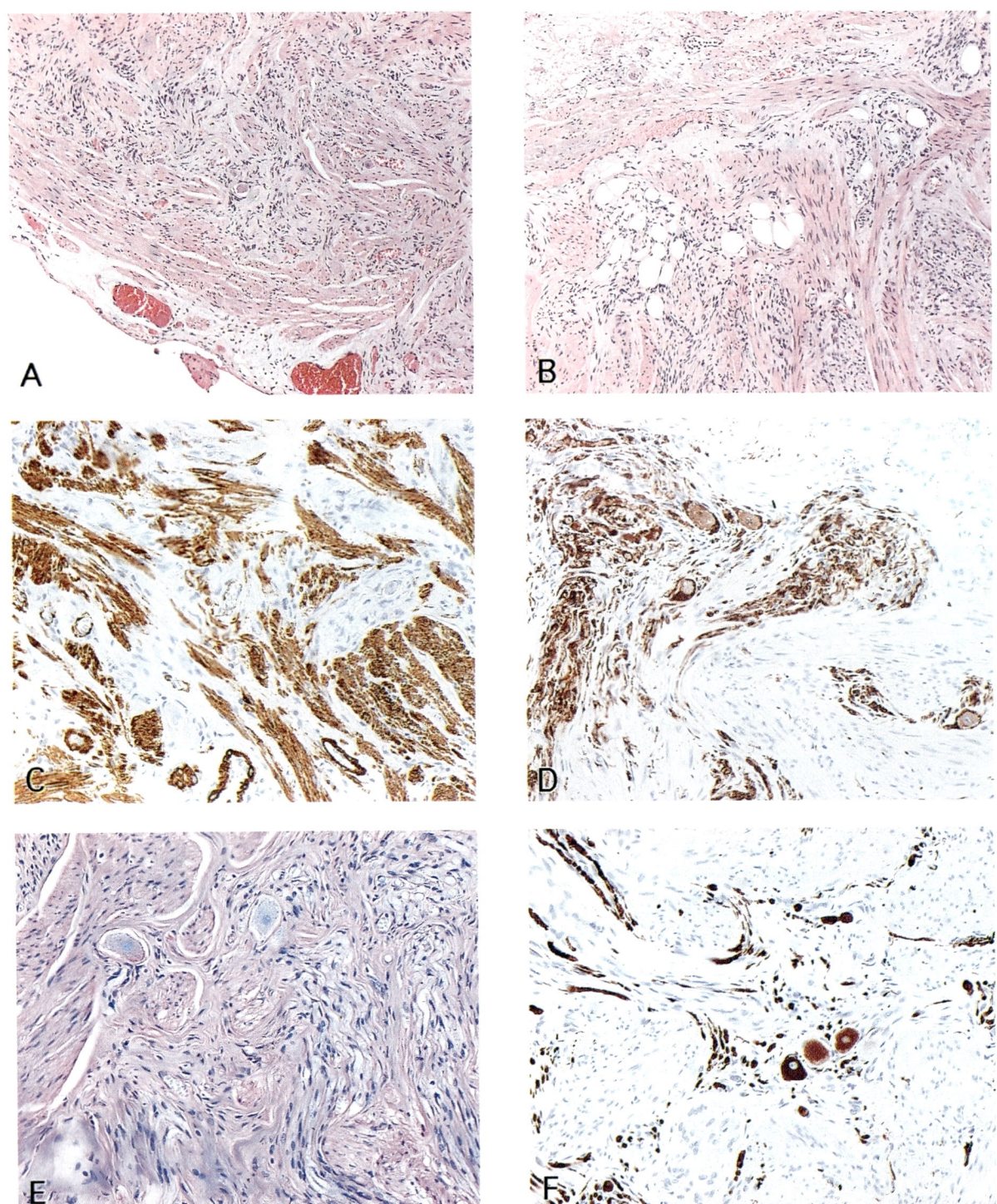

Figure 6-8

NEUROMUSCULAR CHORISTOMA OF 8TH NERVE AND GANGLION

The circumscribed, delicately encapsulated lesion consists primarily of smooth muscle intimately associated with Schwann cells and axon bundles as well as ganglion cells (A). A very minor adipose element was also noted (B). The components of the lesion are highlighted on stains for smooth muscle actin (C), S-100 protein (D), Luxol-fast blue for myelin (E), and neurofilament protein (F). Given the presence of a minor adipose component, the relation of this lesion to lipoma of eighth nerve is unclear. (Courtesy of Dr. Renate Kalnins, Heidelberg, Victoria, Australia.)

Neuromuscular choristomas differ from *neurofibroma with a rhabdomyomatous component,* the only form of benign Triton tumor reported to date (19). Unlike neurofibromas, choristomas are not patternless and lack a loose textured, mucinous stroma. Instead, choristomas grossly and at low power microscopy exhibit nodularity and contain abundant nerve fibers accompanying groups of mature skeletal muscle fibers. Choristomas differ markedly from *malignant Triton tumor,* a lesion often associated with neurofibromatosis type 1 (NF1), in that the striated muscle elements of choristomas are truly abundant, cytologically benign, and unassociated with a neoplastic proliferation of nerve sheath cells.

The high concentration of muscle cells at the center of choristoma nodules may also simulate *rhabdomyoma.* An example is the case of Zwick et al. (40) in which a sparing removal of the choristoma from within the trigeminal nerve revealed primarily skeletal muscle and only occasional nerve fibers. It could be argued that it, like the case of Gersdorff et al. (26), simply represents rhabdomyoma, but the variable association with nerve argues otherwise, as does the occurrence of similar lesions consisting in small part of adipose tissue (35).

The occurrence of muscle-containing lipomatous lesions enveloping or disrupting cranial nerve roots and ganglia (17) causes confusion of neuromuscular choristoma with so-called *"cranial nerve lipoma"* (see fig. 10-6) (22,27,34). Many such lesions contain skeletal muscle (fig. 6-7), but we have observed one 8th nerve tumor composed primarily of smooth muscle with only scant adipose tissue (fig. 6-8).

As reported in three cases (20,31,31), a deep-seated *fibromatosis* (desmoid tumor) may overshadow or postoperatively follow upon the neuromuscular choristoma. Thus thorough sampling is important in order to establish a correct diagnosis.

Treatment and Prognosis. Neuromuscular choristomas are benign. Although resection is curative, biopsy or incomplete excision is occasionally accompanied by spontaneous regression (28). Treatment should, therefore, be conservative and focused upon preservation of nerve function.

In three instances, two nondiagnostic biopsies (20,21) and one gross total resection (31), the procedure was followed by the development of postoperative fibromatosis. In each case, recurrence of the fibromatosis necessitated an amputation which resulted in cure.

REFERENCES

Lipofibromatous Hamartoma of Nerve

1. Amadio PC, Reiman HM, Dobyns JH. Lipofibromatous hamartoma of nerve. J Hand Surg 1988;13A:67–75.
2. Bergman FO, Blom SE, Stenström SJ. Radical excision of a fibro-fatty proliferation of the median nerve, with no neurological loss of symptoms. Plast Reconstr Surg 1970;46:375–80.
3. Berti E, Roncaroli F. Fibrolipomatous hamartoma of a cranial nerve. Histopathology 1994;24:391–2.
4. Frykman GK, Wood VE. Peripheral nerve hamartoma with macrodactyly in the hand: report of three cases and review of the literature. J Hand Surg 1978;3:307–12.
5. Gouldesbrough DR, Kinny SJ. Lipofibromatous hamartoma of the ulnar nerve at the elbow: brief report. J Bone Joint Surg 1989;71:331–2.
6. Greene TL, Louis DS. Compartment syndrome of the arm—a complication of the pneumatic tourniquet. A case report. J Bone Joint Surg 1983;65A:270–3.
7. Guthikonda M, Rengachary SS, Balko MG, van Loveren H. Lipofibromatous hamartoma of the median nerve: case report with magnetic resonance imaging correlation. Neurosurgery 1994;35:127–32.
8. Johnson RJ, Bonfiglio M. Lipofibromatous hamartoma of the median nerve. J Bone Joint Surg 1969;51A:984–90.
9. Paletta FX, Senay LC Jr. Lipofibromatous hamartoma of median nerve and ulnar nerve: surgical treatment. Plast Reconstr Surg 1981;68:915–21.
10. Patel ME, Silver JW, Lipton DE, Pearlman HS. Lipofibroma of the median nerve in the palm and digits of the hand. J Bone Joint Surg 1979;61A:393–7.
11. Price AJ, Compson JP, Calonje E. Fibrolipomatous hamartoma of nerve arising in the brachial plexus. J Hand Surg 1995;1:16–8.
12. Rowland SA. Case report: ten year follow-up of lipofibroma of the median nerve in the palm. J Hand Surg 1977;22:316–7.
13. Silverman TA, Enzinger FM. Fibrolipomatous hamartoma of nerve. A clinicopathologic analysis of 26 cases. Am J Surg Pathol 1985;9:7–14.
14. Terzis JK, Daniel RK, Williams HB, Spencer PS. Benign fatty tumors of the peripheral nerves. Ann Plast Surg 1978;1:193–216.

Neuromuscular Choristoma

15. Ambler MW. Striated muscle cells in the leptomeninges in cerebral dysplasia. Acta Neuropathol 1977;40:269–71.

16. Anzil AP, Wernig A. Muscle cells in a nerve trunk of a frog muscle. Cell Tissue Res 1981;219:433–6.

17. Apostiledes PJ, Spetzler RF, Johnson PC. Ectomesenchymal hamartoma (benign "ectomesenchymoma") of the VIIIth nerve: case report. Neurosurgery 1995;37:1204–7.

18. Awasthi D, Kline DG, Bechman EN. Neuromuscular hamartoma (benign "Triton" tumor) of the brachial plexus. J Neurosurg 1991;75:795–7.

19. Azzopardi JG, Eusebi V, Tison V, Betts BM. Neurofibroma with rhabdomyomatous differentiation: benign "Triton" tumor of the vagina. Histopathology 1983;7:561–72.

20. Boman F, Palan C, Floquet A, Floquet J, Lascombes P. Neuromuscular hamartoma. Ann Pathol 1991;11:36–41.

21. Bonneau R, Brochu P. Neuromuscular choristoma. A clinicopathologic study of two cases. Am J Surg Pathol 1983;7:521–8.

22. Burger PC, Scheithauer BW. Tumors of the central nervous system. Atlas of Tumor Pathology. 3rd Series, Fascicle 10. Armed Forces Institute of Pathology, 1994:301–2.

23. Chapon F, Hubert P, Mandard JC, Rivrain Y, Lechevalier B. Spinal lipoma associated with a neuromuscular hamartoma. Report of one case. Ann Pathol 1991;11:345–8.

24. Chen KT. Neuromuscular hamartoma. J Surg Oncol 1984;26:158–60.

25. Ducatman BS, Scheithauer BW. Malignant peripheral nerve sheath tumors with divergent differentiation. Cancer 1984;54:1049–57.

26. Gersdorff MC, Decat M, Duprez T. Neuromuscular hamartoma of the internal auditory canal. Eur Arch Otorhinolaryngol 1996;253:440–2.

27. Kato T, Sawamure Y, Abe H. Trigeminal neuralgia caused by a cerebellopontine-angle lipoma: case report. Surg Neurol 1995;44:33–5.

28. Louhimo I, Rapola J. Intraneural muscular hamartoma: a report of two cases in small children. J Pediatr Surg 1972;7:696–9.

29. Markel SF, Enzinger FM. Neuromuscular hamartoma—a benign "Triton" tumor composed of mature neural and striated muscle elements. Cancer 1982;49:140–4.

30. Masson P. Tumeurs humaines. Paris: Librairie Maloine, 1956:973–5.

31. Mitchell A, Scheithauer BW, Ostertag H, Sepehrnia A, Sav A. Neuromuscular choristoma. Am J Clin Pathol 1995;103:460–5.

32. Moore KL. The developing human: clinically oriented embryology. Philadelphia: WB Saunders Co., 1973:339.

33. Orlandi E. A case of rhabdomyoma of the sciatic nerve. Arch Scienze Med 1895;19:113–37.

34. Singh SP, Cottingham SL, Slone W, Boesel CP, Welling DB, Yates AJ. Lipomas of the internal auditory canal. Arch Pathol Lab Med 1996;120:681–3.

35. Vandewalle G, Brucher JM, Michotte A. Intracranial facial rhabdomyoma. Case report. J Neurosurg 1995;83:919–22.

36. Van Dorpe JV, Sciot R, De Vos R, Uyttebroeck A, Stas M, Van Damme B. Neuromuscular choristoma (hamartoma) with smooth and striated muscle component: case report with immunohistochemical and ultrastructural analysis. Am J Surg Pathol 1997;9:1090–5.

37. Weston JA. The migration and differentiation of neural crest cells. In: Abercrombie M, Brachet J, King TJ, eds. Advances in morphogenesis. Vol 8. New York: Academic Press, 1970:41–114.

38. Woodruff JM, Chernik NL, Smith MC, et al. Peripheral nerve tumors with rhabdomyosarcomatous differentiation (malignant "Triton" tumors). Cancer 1973;32:426–39.

39. Zak FG, Lawson W. An anatomic curiosity: intraneural striated muscle fibers in the human larynx. J Laryngol Otol 1975;89:199–201.

40. Zwick DL, Livingston K, Clapp L, Kosnik E, Yates A. Intracranial trigeminal nerve rhabdomyoma/choristoma in a child: a case report and discussion of possible histogenesis. Hum Pathol 1989;20:390–2.

❖❖❖

7

SCHWANNOMA

The classification of peripheral nerve sheath tumors (PNSTs), of which schwannoma and neurofibroma are the most frequent, is based upon which normal nerve sheath cell(s) the neoplastic cells resemble. Currently, the most precise determination of a tumor's cell type is established by its immunohistochemical profile, ultrastructural features, or both. A tumor composed of cells with distinctly schwannian characteristics is designated schwannoma. Neurofibroma, the other major form of benign PNST, is less well characterized in terms of its cellular makeup. Numerous clinicopathologic differences exist between schwannoma and neurofibroma (Table 7-1).

There are four major forms of schwannoma: conventional, cellular, plexiform, and melanotic. To varying extents, these differ in clinical and pathologic terms.

CONVENTIONAL SCHWANNOMA

Definition. This benign, usually encapsulated, nonmelanotic nerve sheath tumor is composed entirely of cells with the immunophenotype and ultrastructural features of Schwann cells. Synonyms include *neurilemoma* and *neurinoma*.

General Comments. For several reasons the schwannoma is the prototypic PNST. In ultrastructural and immunohistochemical terms it is the best defined of such tumors, with cells having the features of differentiated Schwann cells. In the overall spectrum of PNSTs, schwannomas have a limited capacity to undergo divergent, usually limited mesenchymal differentiation. An appreciation of the morphologic variability and clinical behavior of schwannoma and its variants is basic to an understanding of other PNSTs.

Table 7-1

CLINICOPATHOLOGIC DISTINCTION OF SCHWANNOMA AND NEUROFIBROMA

Schwannoma	Neurofibroma*
Non-NF1-associated/occasional NF2-associated	NF1-associated/non-NF2-associated
Frequently affects extremities	Frequently involves the trunk
Usually solitary	Frequently solitary
Nerve often identified	Nerve infrequently identified
Eccentric to nerve	Incorporates nerve
Globular	Globular, fusiform, or diffuse
Encapsulated	Delicately surrounded by perineurium and epineurium (solitary and plexiform neurofibroma); no capsule (diffuse neurofibroma)
Nonmucoid, soft to firm	Mucoid and firm
Tan to yellow, opaque	Gray-tan, opalescent
Occasionally cystic	Noncystic
High cellularity	Low to moderate cellularity
Biphasic Antoni A and B patterns	Uniphasic pattern with gradual changes in cellularity
Scant or no stromal mucin	Mucin-rich matrix
Axons often absent	Axons often present
Palisading and Verocay bodies	Wagner-Meissner or rarely Pacinian-like corpuscles; no palisading
Composed of Schwann cells	Composed of Schwann cells, perineurial-like cells, fibroblasts, and transitional cells
Mast cells infrequent	Mast cells frequent
Malignant transformation extremely rare	Malignant transformation rare (2 percent of patients with NF1)

*Exclusive of plexiform neurofibroma.

It was Verocay (93) who first successfully popularized the notion that nerve sheath tumors are neuroectodermal rather than mesenchymal in nature. The terms neurinoma (94) and neurilemoma (meaning nerve sheath tumor) are legacies of the period when there was uncertainty as to the cellular makeup of this tumor. Stout (88) coined the term neurilemoma, basing it on the Greek word "eilema," a closely applied sheath or covering (87). A mistaken belief by some that the base word was "lemma," a loosely applied sheath or bark, led to a frequently used, alternative spelling for this tumor (neurilemmoma). Given the cellular composition of this tumor, the term schwannoma is now preferred (43).

Predisposing Factors. The etiology of schwannomas is poorly understood, but is thought in part to be related to alteration or loss of the neurofibromatosis type 2 (NF2) gene product of chromosome 22 (also designated Merlin), a presumed tumor suppressor gene (76).

Neurofibromatosis, Type 2. Most schwannomas are unassociated with a syndrome. Although rare examples are associated with NF1, by far the strongest association is with NF2. Tumors occurring in the latter setting usually affect cranial or spinal nerve roots. More peripherally situated nerve and dermal lesions are infrequent. The occasional schwannoma occurring in the setting of NF1 is typically solitary. In contrast, a high proportion of NF2-associated schwannomas are multiple (48), particularly those affecting vestibular or spinal nerves roots; so-called acoustic tumors actually arise from the vestibular nerve. Whether sporadic or occurring in the setting of NF2, a majority of schwannomas show aberrations of chromosome 22 (49,79). This takes the form of partial or complete monosomy of the chromosome (5,6,15) and NF2 gene (22q12) mutations (56,74). Examples in which there was a loss of one allele and inactivation of the second have also been reported (6). In a study of 30 vestibular schwannomas, Sainz et al. (76) identified 18 mutations of the NF2 protein, most of which were predicted to result in a truncated NF2 protein; 7 cases demonstrated loss or mutation of both NF2 alleles. An immunohistochemical study in all tumors using NF2 protein antibody revealed absence of staining in schwannoma cells, suggesting that loss of NF2 protein function is a necessary step in schwannoma formation.

Schwannomatosis. The precise nature of the association of multiple schwannomas with NF2 is becoming clearer. In early reports of patients with multiple schwannomas, the tumors often involved both the peripheral and central nervous systems, and included bilateral vestibular schwannomas (80). Nonetheless, meningiomas and glial tumors were far less common in these cases than in NF2. Despite the occasional occurrence of symptoms referable to 8th nerve dysfunction and/or other findings associated with NF2, Shishiba et al. (80) proposed the term "neurilemomatosis" to denote this situation and suggested the disorder was a distinct entity. In contrast, subsequent publications describing similar cases (70–72), suggested that schwannomatosis (neurilemomatosis) is simply a variant of NF2 (71). Although NF2 is an autosomal dominant disorder with full penetrance, very few familial cases of schwannomatosis have been reported.

Recent publications use a more restricted definition of schwannomatosis as multiple, histologically proven schwannomas without the vestibular tumors diagnostic of NF2 (58,64a,72a). In one series (58), the tumors were entirely subcutaneous, 90 percent being typical encapsulated schwannomas and 10 percent plexiform tumors. In a more recent, updated series (72a), the tumors occurred at a variety of sites including the neck, trunk, and extremities. Visceral lesions were infrequent. All patients were adults; no sex predilection was apparent. The tumors were typical schwannomas, one being plexiform. To date, no examples have undergone malignant transformation. Molecular genetic studies of these cases suggest that they represent a third form of neurofibromatosis, one in which patients are prone to somatic alterations of the NF2 gene rather than having germline mutations (18,58).

Postirradiation Schwannoma. Aside from genetic factors predisposing to the development of schwannomas, irradiation has also been implicated (75,81,92). Over 150 cases of radiation-induced intracranial and peripheral schwannomas have been reported, their mean latency period being approximately 20 years (75). Only a small minority were multiple.

Schwannoma Variants. The clinical and morphologic spectrum of schwannomas is broad. With the exception of very rare malignant examples, schwannomas are benign. Their morphologic similarity, both within and outside the setting of neurofibromatosis, permits their consideration as an entity, with only minor variations. Thus, conventional schwannoma forms the substance of much of this chapter

The *cellular schwannoma* deserves separate mention in as much as it mimics MPNST (119–121) and, if subtotally excised, shows a higher likelihood of recurrence than does conventional schwannoma (102). Cellular schwannomas are discussed in detail below.

Whereas most schwannomas are globular, uninodular masses, a small minority, usually dermal tumors, show a multinodular or plexiform growth pattern (see below). Unlike plexiform neurofibroma, such tumors are unassociated with neurofibromatosis (32,46,75,99). *Plexiform schwannomas* are separately discussed below.

A special form of inherited schwannoma, the *psammomatous melanotic* variant, occurs in the setting of Carney's complex (9). This rare disorder is discussed in detail in a later part of this chapter.

Clinical Features. Schwannomas occur in individuals of all ages, but show a peak incidence between the third and sixth decades. No sex predilection is evident, although females are twice as often affected by central nervous system schwannomas, while radiation-induced examples most often occur in males (75).

The most common sites of occurrence of peripheral nerve schwannomas are the head and neck region and the flexor surfaces of the extremities. Of tumors involving sizable nerves, sensory cranial and spinal nerve roots are particularly affected; motor roots (11,77) and sympathetic nerves are uncommonly involved. Outside the setting of NF2, most schwannomas are solitary. As a rule, they grow slowly over a period of years. Their size varies from microscopic (fig. 7-1A,B), through barely palpable tumors (fig. 7-1C), to larger lesions which on physical examination are mobile (figs. 7-2, 7-3A,B). As is true of nerve sheath tumors in general, schwannomas resist movement along the longitudinal axis of their parent nerve. They rarely present as primary bone tumors (22).

Patients with schwannomas are often asymptomatic but may present with pain, particularly in the setting of schwannomatosis. Cutaneous schwannomas are typically small, grossly unasso-

ciated with a nerve, and rare. Mediastinal, retroperitoneal, and sacral examples are well known for their large size (figs. 7-3C, 7-4) and usually come to attention due simply to mass effects. Paraspinous tumors usually present with sensory disturbance, whereas those with a significant intraspinal component may compress the spinal cord to produce motor signs (figs. 7-4A, 7-5B,C).

Radiographic Findings. On routine X ray, schwannomas generally appear as sharply circumscribed masses (figs. 7-3C, 7-5A). Computerized tomography (CT) scans show circumscribed, low attenuation masses (fig. 7-5C) which demonstrate uniform or heterogeneous contrast enhancement. Magnetic resonance imaging (MRI) shows a high T2 signal, as well as heterogeneous contrast enhancement (fig. 7-6). A recent correlative MRI and histopathologic study found that imaging characteristics are related not only to relative proportions of Antoni A and B tissue, but to superimposed degenerative changes (7a). Both CT and MRI show that large tumors often have cystic changes (fig. 7-4B,C). If in the vicinity of bone (fig. 7-5A) or arising within bony confines such as the spinal canal (fig. 7-5B,C) or the sacral canal (fig. 7-4B,C), the tumor causes compressive remodeling and occasional destruction of bone. Respective examples include intraspinal schwannomas which often straddle and expand a spinal foramen to assume a dumbbell shape (figs. 7-4A, 7-5B,C), and so-called giant sacral schwannoma (fig. 7-4B,C) (1). In contrast, active, irregular invasion of bone is a feature of malignancy seen in association with malignant PNST (see fig. 11-8).

Geographic Considerations. Schwannomas can be conveniently subdivided according to location into intracranial, intraspinal, peripheral, and visceral tumors.

Intracranial schwannomas arise from nerve roots distal to their transition zone, a region in which central portions of a nerve root become peripheral nerve, and are associated with a change of myelination by oligodendrocytes to Schwann cells (8). Sensory nerves are far more often involved than are motor nerves. When arising in the 8th nerve, the vestibular portion of that nerve is most often affected. Such lesions typically expand the internal auditory meatus, but only rarely destroy bone focally. Particularly large examples frequently compress the brain stem and cerebellum, as well as a peduncle. Similarly,

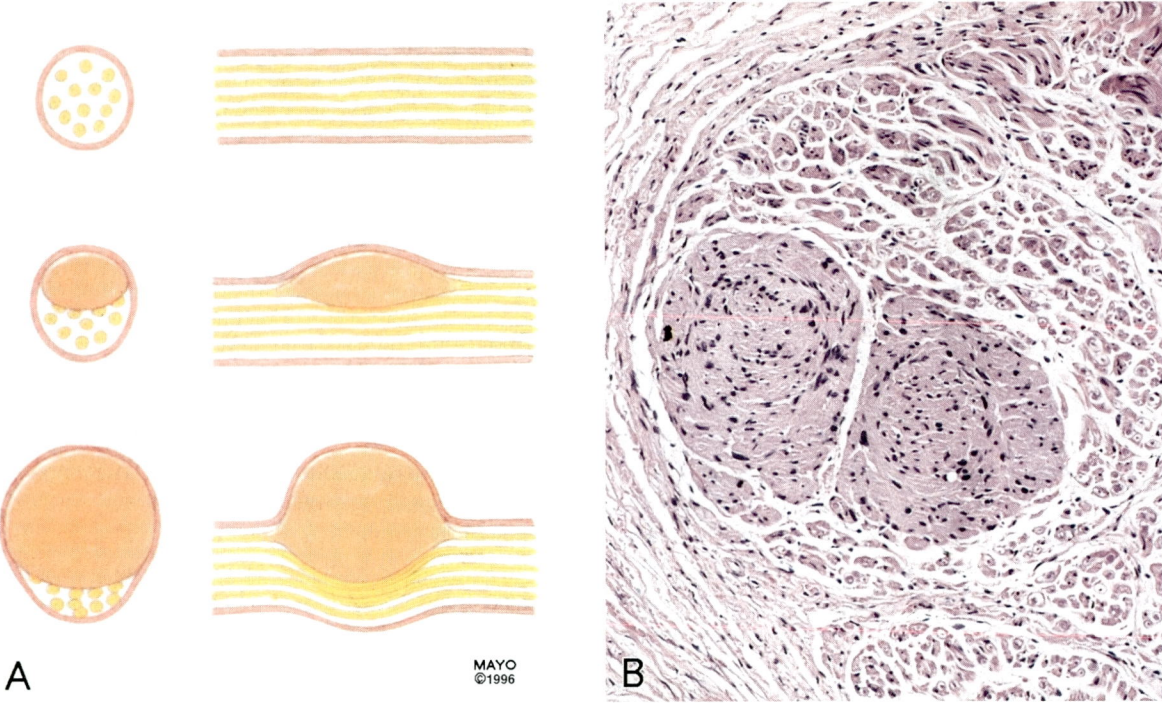

Figure 7-1
SCHWANNOMA

This illustration shows the essential features of schwannoma, a solid lesion here shown arising within a nerve consisting of a single fascicle (A). The tumor peripherally displaces nerve fibers to produce a globoid eccentric mass. In their early intrafascicular growth phase, minute schwannomas displace nerve fibers (B) and lack a capsule. Somewhat larger tumors only minimally enlarge the parent nerve (C) and become separated from surrounding fascicles by a capsule derived from the perineurium and epineurium. (C: Fig. 3.423 from Okazaki H, Scheithauer BW. Atlas of neuropathology, 1988. With permission from the Mayo Foundation.)

large schwannomas arising from the trigeminal nerve often extend into the middle cranial fossa. Involvement of motor or other cranial nerves, such as the 9th and 10th, is more likely to occur in the setting of neurofibromatosis. Multiple schwannomas are uncommon; many are seen in NF2 (see figs. 13-24, 13-25). Bilateral vestibular schwannomas are diagnostic of NF2 (fig. 7-24) and often occur in association with gliomas and meningiomas; gross and microscopic multinodularity is a common feature of such schwannomas. On rare occasion, an intracranial schwannoma may arise within the sella (36) or the cavernous sinus (47).

Decidedly uncommon are parenchymal schwannomas arising in the substance of the brain or within the ventricular system (10,86). Such lesions presumably arise from nerves innervating the meninges or from Schwann cell ectopias. Parenchymal schwannomas occur primarily in males. Since both conventional and cellular schwannomas arise at intracranial sites, the finding of increased cellularity and occasional mitoses should not prompt a diagnosis of malignancy.

Intraspinal schwannomas far more often arise from sensory than from motor nerve roots. Whether intradural, extradural, or both, intraspinal

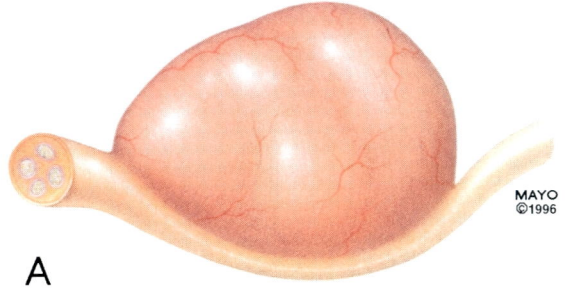

A

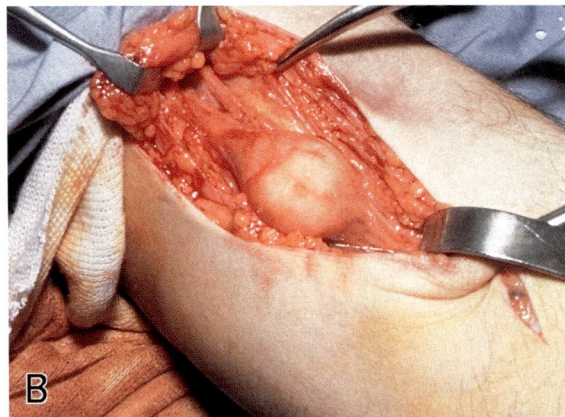

B

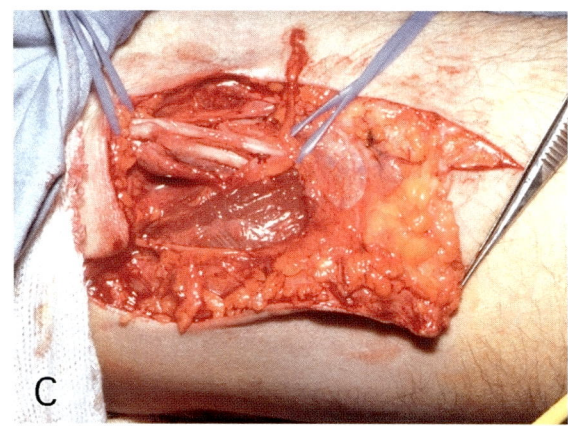

C

Figure 7-2
SCHWANNOMA
Due to their encapsulation and eccentric growth (A), sizable schwannomas lend themselves to gross total resection (B) with sparing of the parent nerve (C).

schwannomas occur at any level. Sporadic tumors are most often lumbar in location, whereas those occurring in NF2 show a predilection for cervicothoracic roots (42). Most solitary examples are sporadic. When multiple, consideration should be given to NF2 (42). Spinal schwannomas with intradural and extradural components ("dumbbell tumors") usually arise in the cervicothoracic region (figs. 7-4A, 7-5B,C). Cauda equina lesions are often sausage-shaped, lie distal to the conus medullaris, and displace surrounding nerve roots (fig. 7-8F,G). Schwannomas arising within the spinal cord are rare (73).

Peripheral schwannomas affect nerves of all sizes and frequently present on the flexor surfaces of the extremities (fig. 7-2B,C) at the level of the elbow, wrist, or knee, or arise in nerve roots in the posterior mediastinum, retroperitoneum, or sacrum (figs. 7-3C, 7-4B,C). Of nerve root examples, at least half partly extend into an intervertebral foramen. Unlike neurofibromas, peripheral or soft tissue schwannomas infrequently affect superficial nerves of the trunk. Unusual sites of peripheral nerve involvement

include the tongue, palate, and larynx. As previously noted, intraosseous schwannomas are rare (22). Most affect either the mandible, where they arise in the dental foramen (85) or, less frequently, a vertebral body (69).

Visceral schwannomas are rare. Those we have seen were unassociated with neurofibromatosis. Most reported examples have arisen in the gastrointestinal tract, nearly all in the stomach (fig. 7-7A) (16,60,78). The majority are incidental findings, although on occasion patients present with pain or hemorrhage due to mucosal ulceration. Visceral schwannomas may be pigmented (see Melanotic Schwannoma). Schwannomas only rarely occur in other organs, such as the heart (28), lung (83), or kidney (fig. 7-7B,C). Visceral tumors, although demarcated, often lack a well-formed capsule (fig. 7-7).

Gross Findings. Most schwannomas are nodular and smooth surfaced, and measure less than 10 cm in diameter. The majority affect small nerves. The fibrocollagenous capsule evident in most tumors, whether thick, thin, or focally discontinuous, is derived from perineurium and

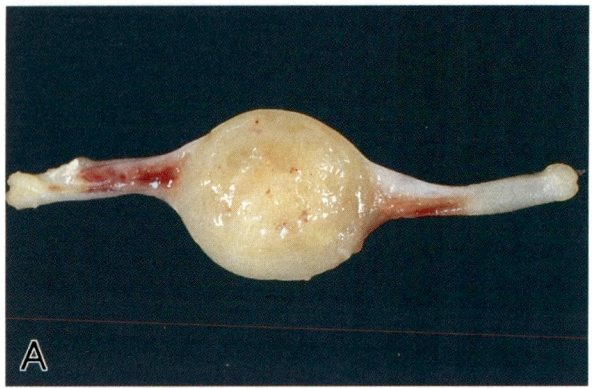

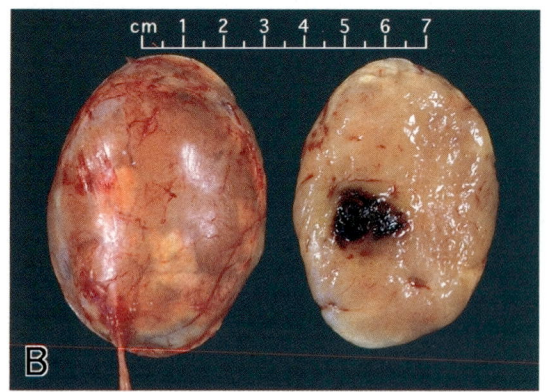

Figure 7-3
SCHWANNOMA
The majority of schwannomas are grossly recognizable. Most are solid, globular masses, with the parent nerve embedded within their fibrous capsule (A,B). Large tumors such as those that arise in the mediastinum (C), retroperitoneum, pelvis, or sacrum dwarf the parent nerve. (C: Fig. 3.426 from Okazaki H, Scheithauer BW. Atlas of neuropathology. New York: JB Lippincott, 1988:186.)

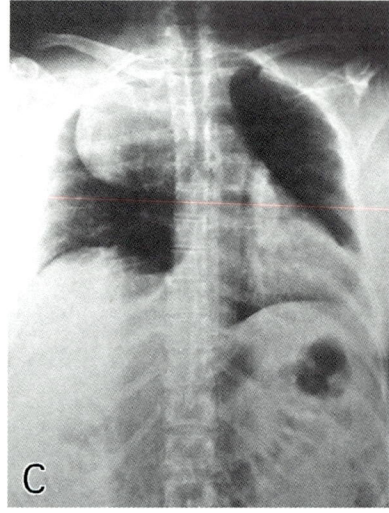

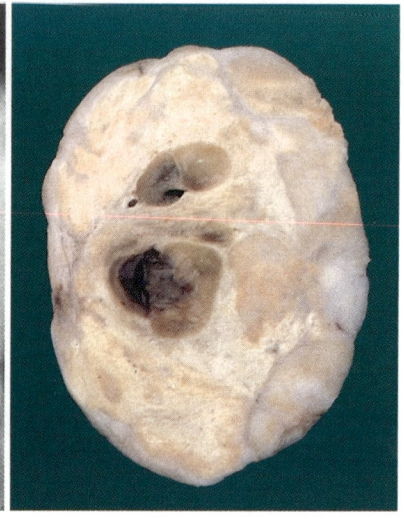

epineurial tissue. Schwannomas of the central nervous system and those arising in viscera or at mucosal sites, such as the nose and nasopharynx (44), often lack a capsule (fig. 7-7). Although early, small lesions are clearly intraneural (fig. 7-1) and may produce focal nerve enlargement, almost all schwannomas are globular and lie eccentric to the parent nerve, thus causing it to be splayed over the tumor or to be incorporated into its capsule (figs. 7-2A, 7-3A,B). Understandably, the parent nerve is more often evident in tumors that arise in large nerves (17). The largest schwannomas are usually found in the mediastinum (fig. 7-3C), retroperitoneum, or pelvis (fig. 7-4B,C). The gross appearance of schwannoma is quite variable (figs. 7-8–7-10). Occasional cutaneous or extracutaneous examples may appear plexiform (fig. 7-8C) or multinodular (fig. 7-8D). Multinodularity is particularly common

in bilateral, NF2-associated 8th nerve tumors. Less common are widely separated tumors on a single nerve (fig. 7-8E). The same is true of thin walled, entirely cystic schwannomas (fig. 7-8G).

The cut surface of conventional schwannomas is often smooth or somewhat lobulated, and tan (fig. 7-9A) or patchy yellow (fig. 7-9B) due to lipid accumulation (figs. 7-3B,C, 7-9B–D). Ill-defined, poorly formed fibrous septa may appear to separate tumor lobules in large examples (figs. 7-3C, 7-5B, 7-9D). Sizable tumors frequently show degenerative features, including marked lipidization (fig. 7-9D,E), cystic change (figs. 7-8G, 7-9D,E, 7-10B), hemorrhage (fig. 7-10A,B), and calcification (fig. 7-9F). Hemorrhage may occasionally be extensive and followed by cystic change (fig. 7-10B) (37). We have seen large, symptomatic schwannomas of the retroperitoneum, pelvis, and lower extremity presenting

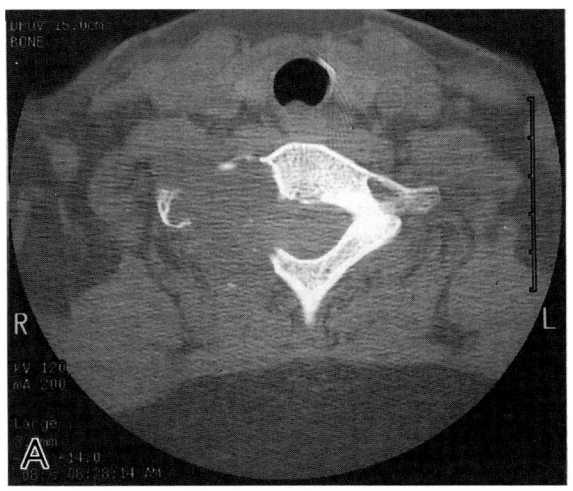

Figure 7-4
SCHWANNOMA OF NERVE ROOT,
BONE DESTRUCTION

This axial CT study of a "dumbbell tumor" shows both bone remodeling and destruction, as well as massive paraspinous extension (A). A giant sacral schwannoma, here seen on sagittal T1- and T2-weighted images (B,C), expands the sacral canal, displaces and in part destroys the sacrum, and emerges in the presacral space via intervertebral foramina. Note the central cystic change (bright signal on T2 image) (C).

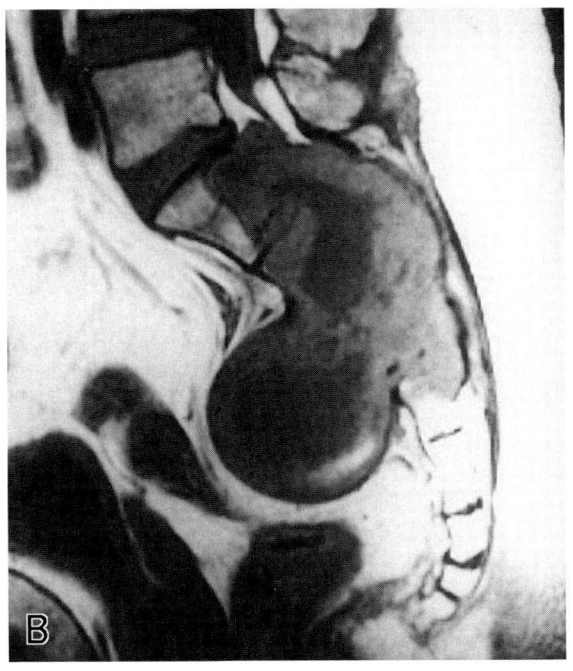

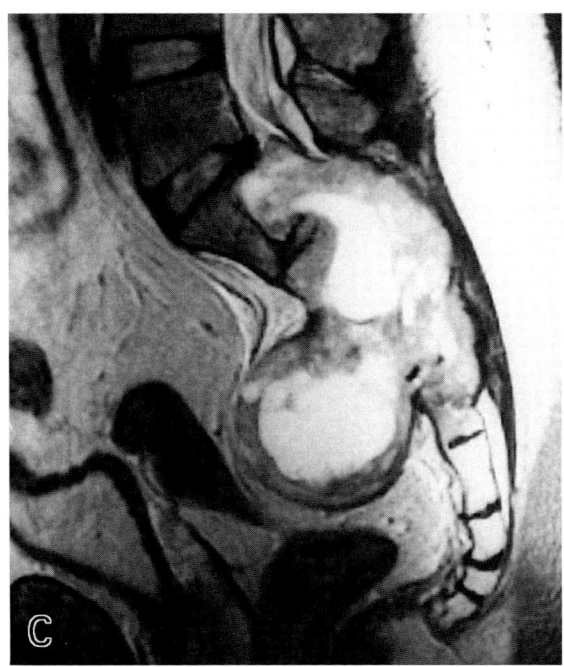

as cystic, thin-walled, hemorrhagic masses. In one such case the presence of a few, minute fragments of Antoni A tissue was the only clue to the diagnosis. These tumors, when subject to needle aspiration, pose a diagnostic challenge (fig. 7-10C,D). The effects of schwannoma upon nearby or surrounding bone has been discussed (figs. 7-4, 7-5).

Microscopic Findings. A common feature of adequately sampled schwannoma is a well-formed fibrous capsule (fig. 7-11A,B). Properly oriented sections show it to contain the displaced parent nerve (fig. 7-11C). In intradural tumors a capsule may be lacking (fig. 7-11D). Occasional schwannomas incorporate a nearby ganglion, a dorsal root ganglion in spinal examples and Scarpa's ganglion in vestibular tumors (63).

Conventional schwannomas consist entirely of Schwann cells arranged in two characteristic patterns, referred to as Antoni A and B (fig. 7-12). The proportion of each pattern varies. The interface between them may be either gradual or abrupt, and is highlighted by differences in histochemical staining, collagen being most abundant

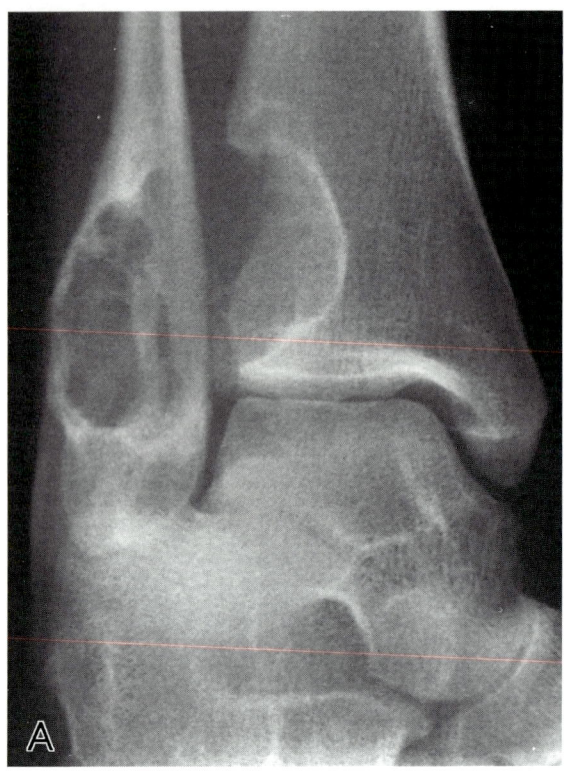

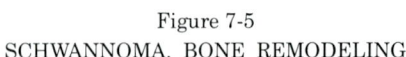

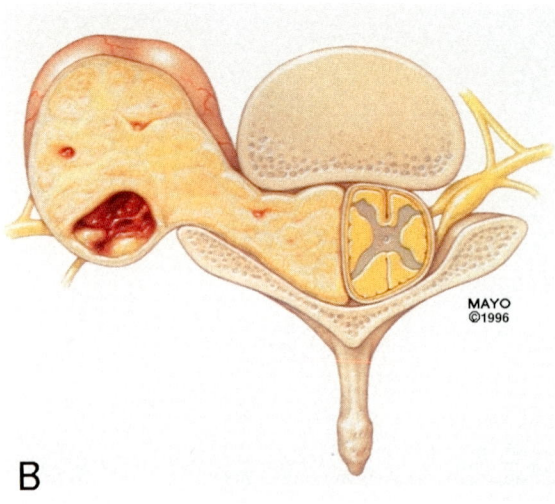

Figure 7-5
SCHWANNOMA, BONE REMODELING

Smooth contoured bone impression is illustrated by a schwannoma arising between the distal tibia and fibula (A). Due to intraspinal and paraspinal growth, spinal examples may assume a "dumbbell" configuration (B). Note spinal cord displacement and focal cystic degeneration of the tumor. An axial CT study of such a lesion (C) shows unilateral expansion of a spinal foramen and extension of the tumor into the paraspinous space. The spinal cord is compressed.

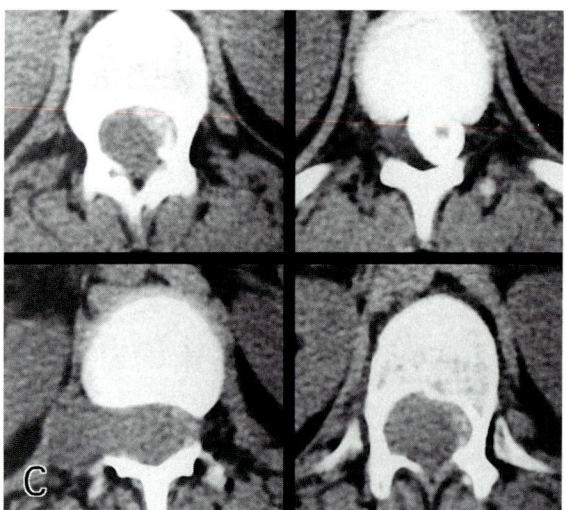

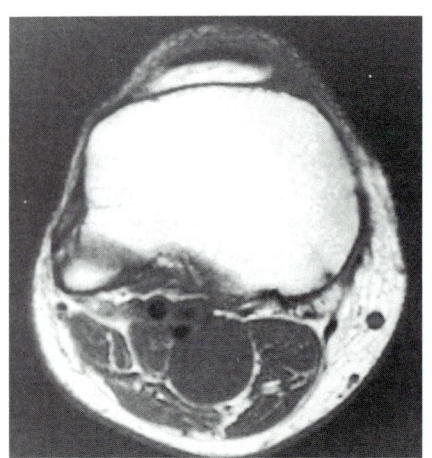

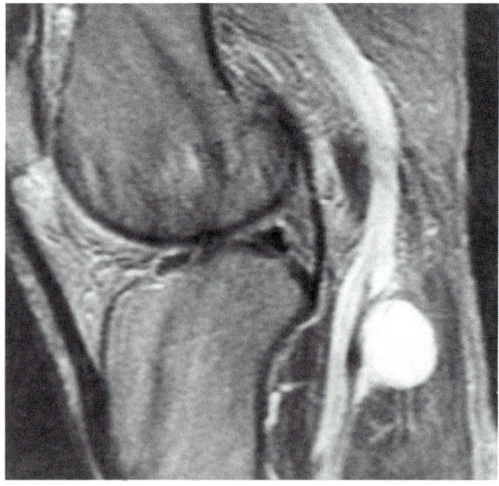

Figure 7-6
SCHWANNOMA, NEUROIMAGING

Left: An axial T1-weighted image shows the spherical tumor as a low signal (bottom) beneath the bright tibial plateau.

Right: On the sagittal T2 study, the uniform bright signal clearly demonstrates the solid tumor attached to its parent nerve.

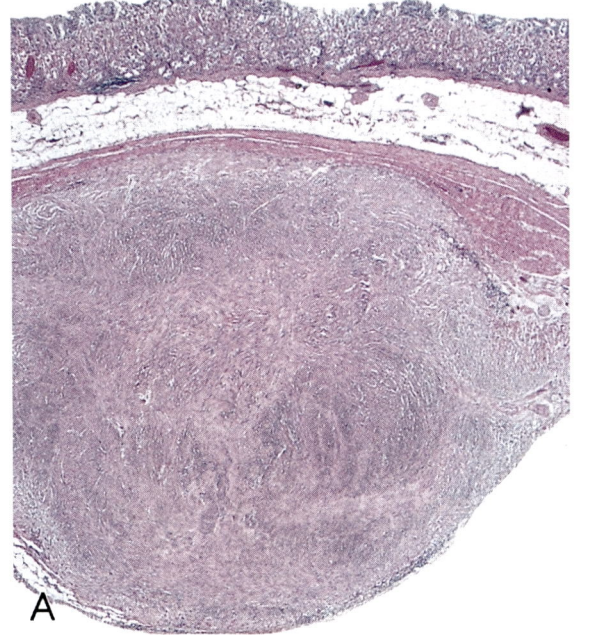

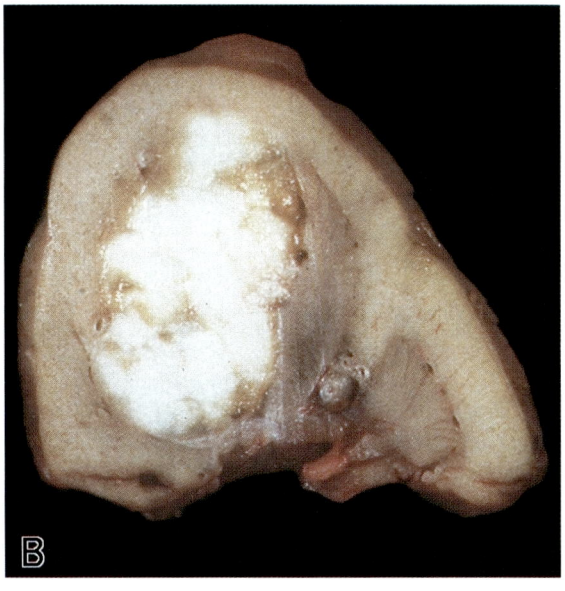

Figure 7-7
VISCERAL–MUCOSAL SCHWANNOMA
Visceral tumors are infrequent in occurrence and affect mainly the gastrointestinal tract, usually the stomach (A). Other organs, such as the kidney, are rarely affected (B,C). Mucosal involvement, as of the nose or paranasal sinuses, is also uncommon (D). In each instance, note the lack of a well-formed capsule. Limited infiltration of surrounding tissue should not be interpreted as evidence of malignancy.

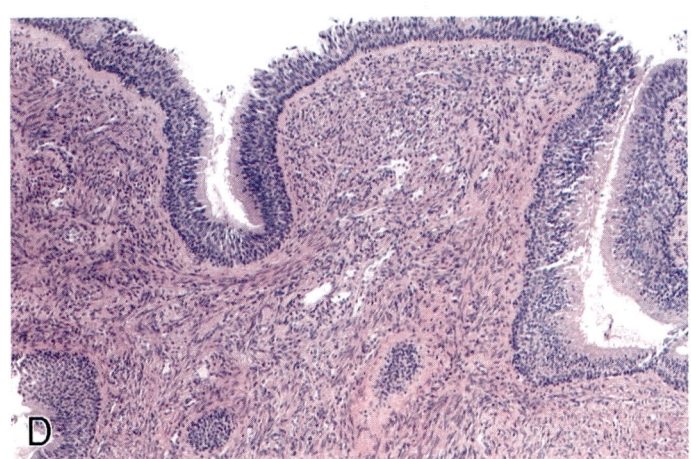

in Antoni A and mucopolysaccharide in Antoni B tissue (fig. 7-13).

The Antoni A pattern predominates in tumors of the spinal canal and in cellular schwannomas (see below). It consists of compacted, elongate cells with tapered, spindle-shaped nuclei, variable chro-

masia, ample pink cytoplasm, and no discernible cell membrane (fig. 7-12A,B). The nuclei are several times larger than those of most neurofibromas. On histologic sections and smears, intranuclear cytoplasmic pseudoinclusions may be seen, but nucleoli are inconspicuous (fig. 7-14).

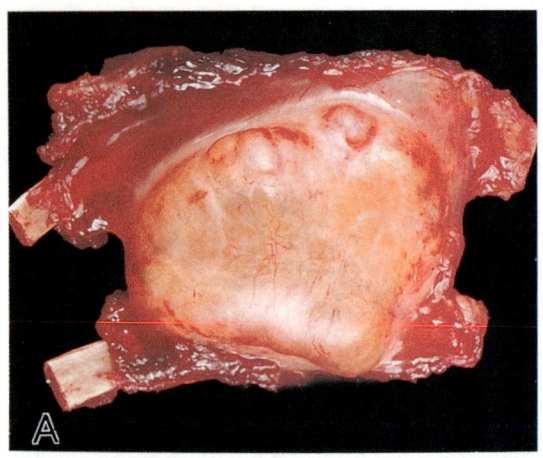

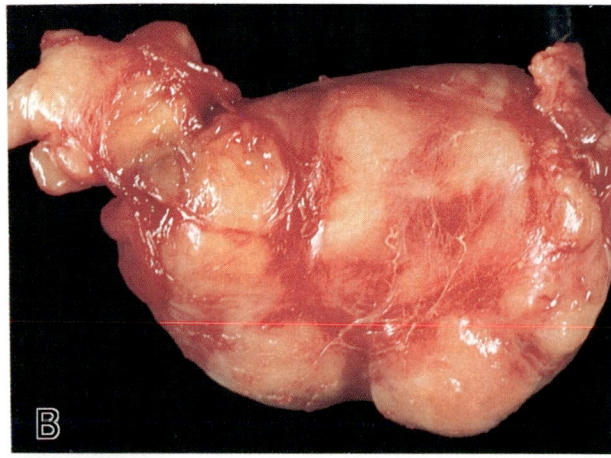

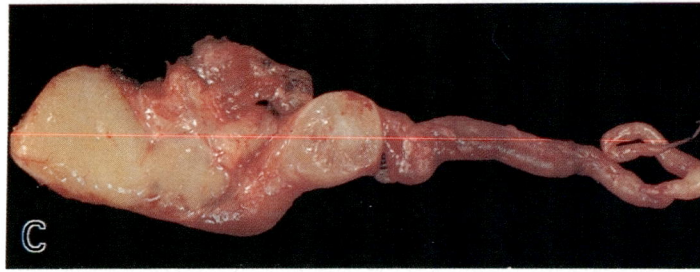

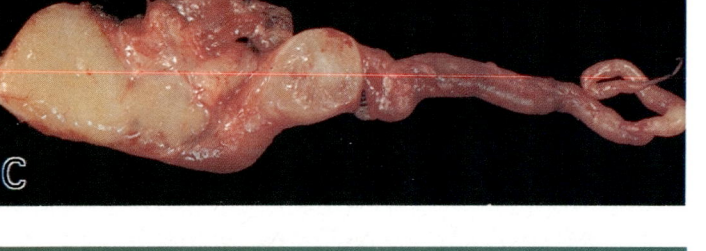

Figure 7-8
SCHWANNOMA

Tumor configuration may vary. Some schwannomas, such as this intercostal nerve example, are misshapen by surrounding osseous structures (A). Lobulation is also an unusual feature (B). Occasional tumors exhibit sinuous plexiform growth (C). Multiple tumors may be closely apposed (D), or separate as in this intradural lumbar lesion (E). Due to their axial orientation, tumors arising in the lumbar intradural space are often sausage-shaped (F). Almost entirely cystic lesions, such as this transilluminated, lumbar intradural example, are unusual (G).

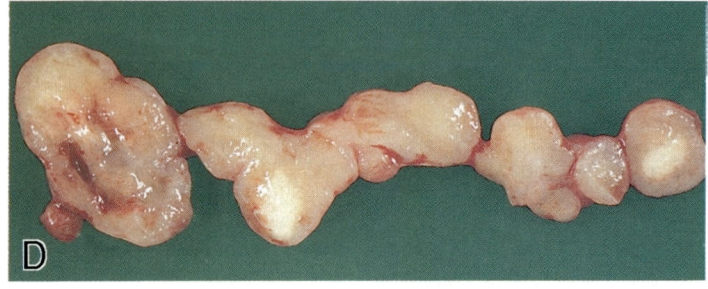

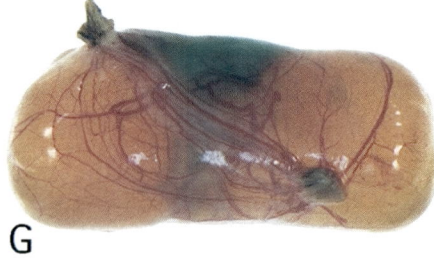

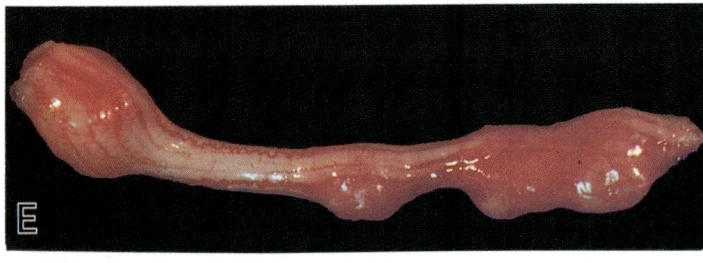

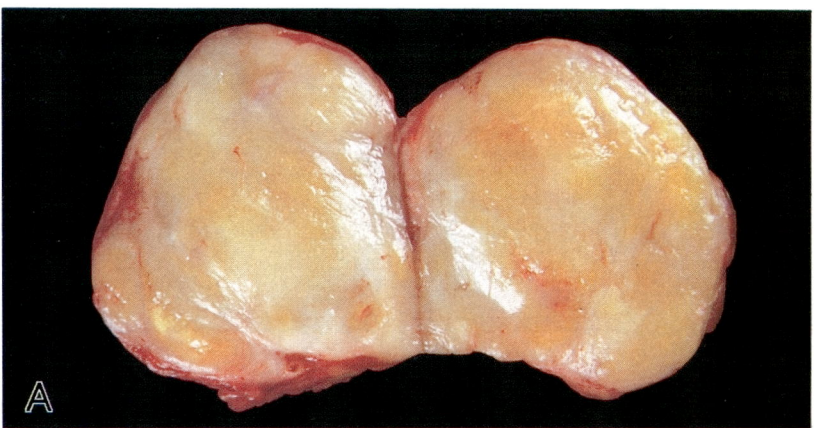

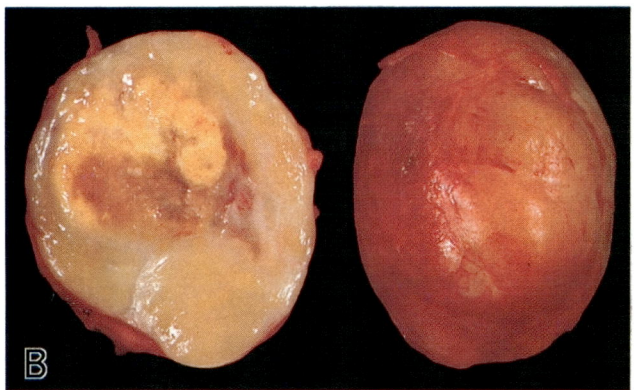

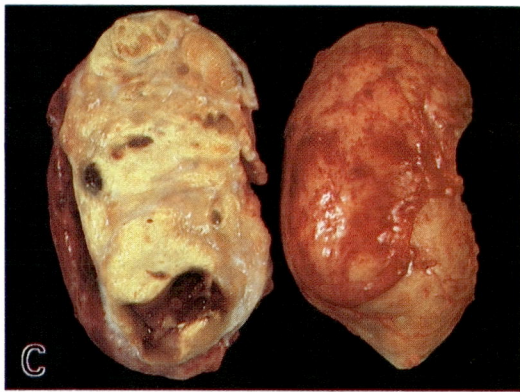

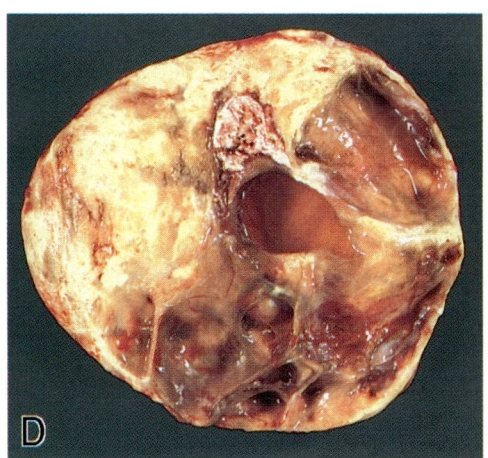

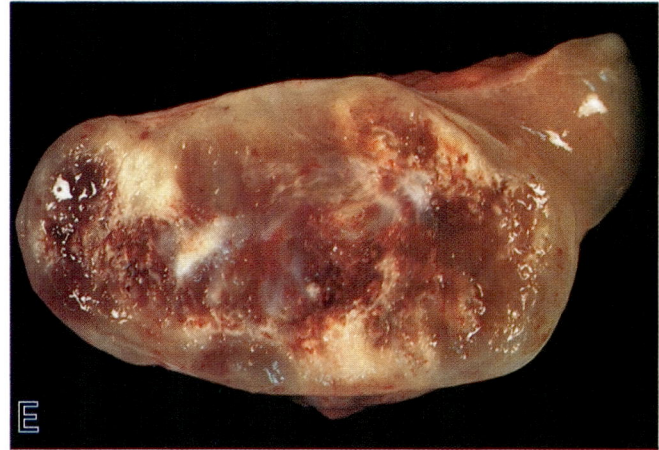

Figure 7-9
SCHWANNOMA

On cut section, typical schwannomas are solid and homogeneously tan. Lipid deposition, a common degenerative feature that produces yellow coloration (A), may be focally accentuated (B) or extensive (C). The same is true of cystic degeneration (D,E). Calcification when seen is usually focal.

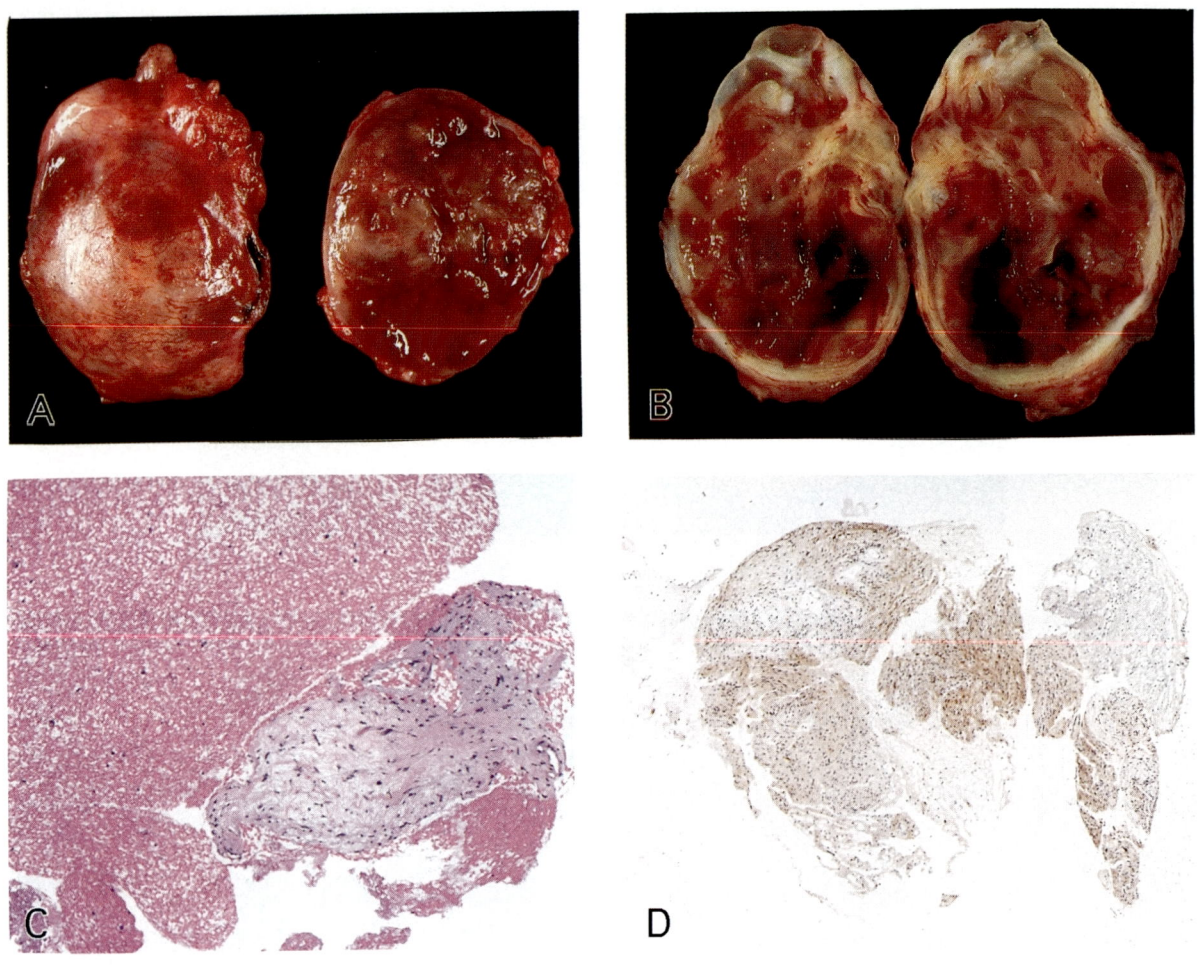

Figure 7-10
SCHWANNOMA

Hemorrhage is a common finding and may be focal (see fig. 7-5B) or extensive (A) with resultant cystic degeneration (B). On occasion a schwannoma enlarged by hemorrhage may clinically mimic a metastatic neoplasm (C), as in this woman with a history of mammary carcinoma who underwent needle aspiration biopsy of a mass in the adrenal region. Only rare fragments of a schwannoma were identified; an immunostain for S-100 protein (D) confirmed the diagnosis.

The cells in Antoni A tissue are aligned and compactly disposed in broad bundles (fig. 7-12A), interlacing fascicles (fig. 7-15A), or occasionally in whorls (fig. 7-16E). These histologic features are highly characteristic, often allowing a diagnosis of schwannoma on small tissue fragments in the case of large cystic or hemorrhagic schwannomas or in needle aspiration specimens (fig. 7-10C,D). Nuclear clusters of one form or another are also common, the most frequent being a palisaded arrangement in which well-regimented, often double rows of nuclei lie separated by aligned eosinophilic cell processes. Often distinct from their surroundings, these Verocay bodies (figs. 7-15B,C, 7-16A) have long been recognized as a cardinal feature of schwannoma (94). Verocay bodies vary in frequency. Although uncommon in 8th nerve schwannomas, they are frequent in intraspinal examples. Truly, Verocay body–rich tumors are rare (figs. 7-15D, 7-16A). In occasional Antoni A areas, Verocay bodies superficially resemble Homer Wright rosettes (fig. 7-16B) (31,38) or the neoplastic Schwann cells are arranged in tight clusters (fig. 7-16C); such cell arrangements (fig. 7-14) should not prompt an erroneous diagnosis of malignancy. Rare schwannomas exhibit pseudopapillary or other odd patterns (fig. 7-16D,F).

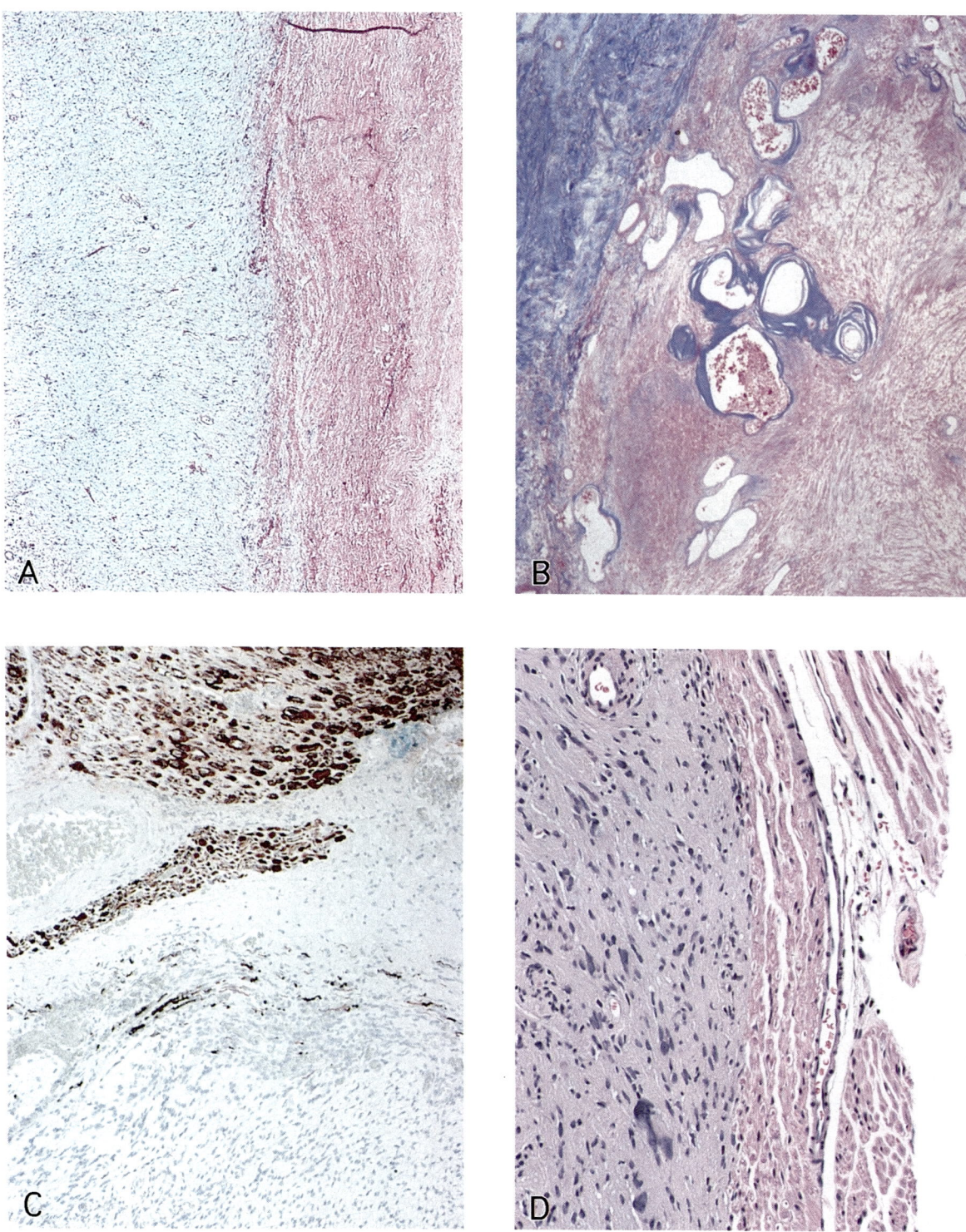

Figure 7-11
SCHWANNOMAS

Schwannomas of peripheral nerve typically possess a thick hyaline capsule (A), a feature highlighted with trichrome stains (B), as are the hyalinized vessels (B). It is within the capsule that remnants of the parent nerve may be found (C, neurofilament protein immunostain) (see also fig. 7-25F). Intradural tumors such as this cauda equina lesion and schwannomas arising within the brain or spinal cord often lack a thick capsule (D) (see also fig. 7-7).

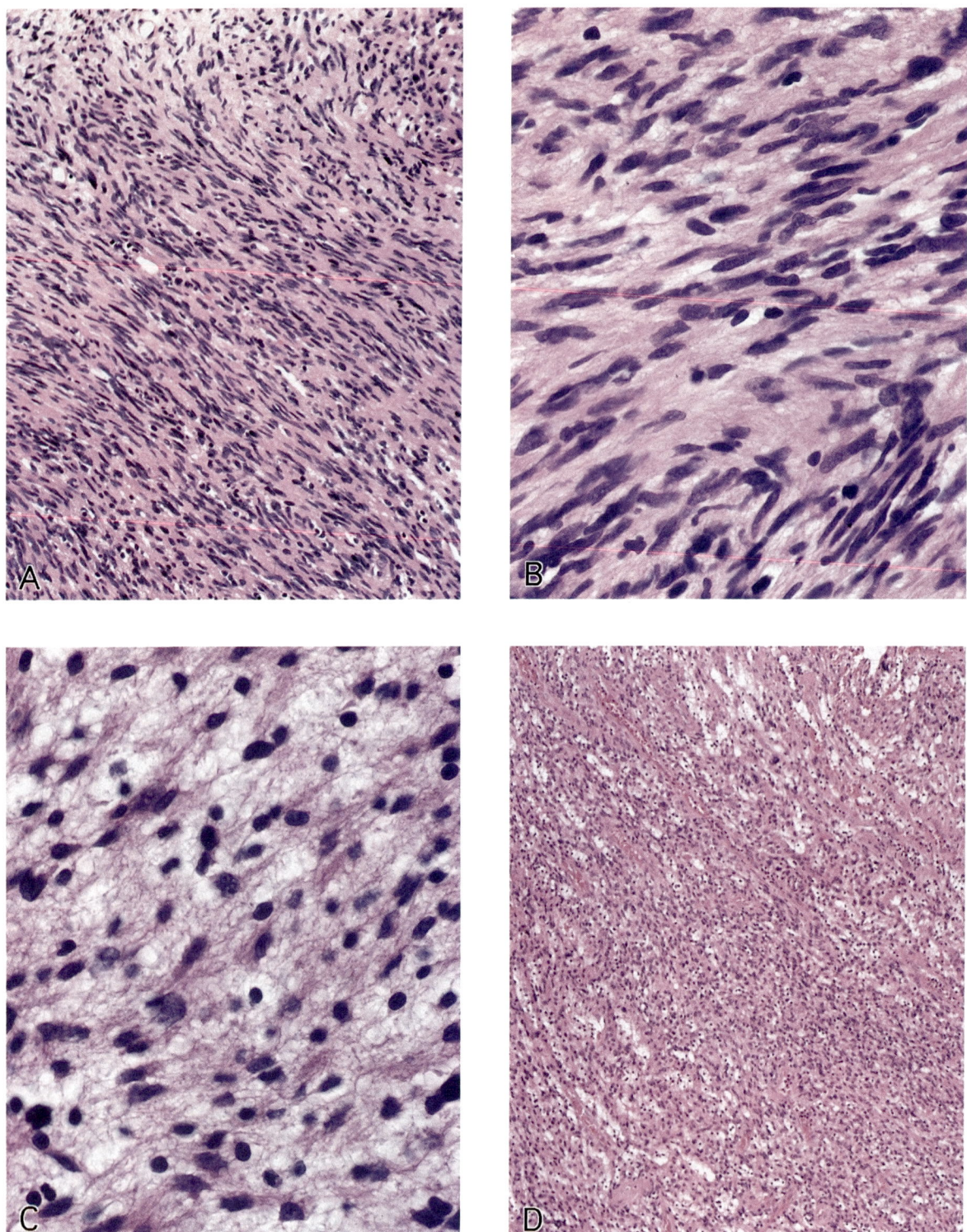

Figure 7-12
SCHWANNOMA

Of the two principal histologic patterns, the compact Antoni A pattern featuring aligned spindle cells with elongate nuclei is that most obviously schwannian in nature (A,B). In contrast, the Antoni B pattern (C) consists of loose textured cells with round nuclei and delicate cobweb-like processes. On occasion, Antoni B tissue may appear focally cellular (D).

The Antoni B pattern consists of a loose-textured, cobweb-like meshwork of cells with multipolar processes (fig. 7-12C,D). Their round to oval, occasionally hyperchromatic nuclei may feature cytoplasmic nuclear pseudoinclusions. The loose texture of Antoni B tissue may give way to microcyst formation. Also a common feature is the presence of hemosiderin about vessels (fig. 7-17A). The vessels are typically hyalinized and thick-walled (fig. 7-17A,B), but thin-walled, ectatic vessels may also be seen (fig. 7-17C). On occasion, abnormal vessels may be so conspicuous as to resemble a vascular malformation (53). Thrombosis and recanalization of vessels is common and may be related to patches of non-palisading necrosis (fig. 7-17D). Infiltrates of foamy cells are often seen in schwannomas (fig. 7-18A), particularly in 8th cranial nerve tumors. It has been suggested that such delicately periodic acid–Schiff (PAS)- and oil red O-positive, lipid-laden cells (fig. 7-18B) represent phagocytic Schwann cells (26). Whereas lipofuscin is commonly seen in normal and neoplastic Schwann cells (fig. 7-18C,D), melanin is rare and is limited to melanotic variants of this tumor (see below). Iron deposition, apparently related to vascular abnormalities, may be conspicuous (fig. 7-18E). Stromal mucin formation can be substantial (fig. 7-18F), but is less a feature of schwannoma than of neurofibroma. Occasional examples are sufficiently mucin rich as to appear myxoid (fig. 7-19) and be confused with other myxoid soft tissue tumors.

The biologic relationship between Antoni A and B tissues remains unclear. Tissue culture studies showing substantial differences in their metabolic state suggest that the Antoni B element has a broader range of metabolic activity (62).

Although plump, epithelial-appearing cells are occasionally seen in otherwise conventional or plexiform schwannomas (fig. 7-48), only rare schwannomas are composed largely of plump epithelioid cells (fig. 7-20). Loosely termed *"epithelioid schwannomas,"* such tumors remain to be fully characterized. Of reported cases, most are subcutaneous and presumably behave as ordinary schwannomas (54a).

Special stains provide diagnostically useful information regarding the microanatomy of schwannomas (fig. 7-13). In longstanding tumors, trichrome stains often reveal considerable collagen deposition in both the Antoni A and B components (fig. 7-13A). As compared to the abundance of mucopolysaccharide-rich matrix in neurofibromas, Alcian blue stains for mucin are usually only mildly reactive in schwannomas (fig. 7-13C). Reticulin stains in a dense pericellular pattern in Antoni A components (fig. 7-13B) highlighting not only intercellular collagen bundles, but the pericellular distribution of basement membrane so typical of Schwann cells. As previously noted, it is unusual for fibers of the parent nerve to be distributed within the substance of all but the subcapsular portions of a schwannoma (fig. 7-11C). Since both the Bielschowsky and Bodian silver impregnation methods may nonspecifically stain reticulin fibers, residual nerve fibers are more reliably identified by immunohistochemical stains for neurofilament protein. Mast cells are readily seen in schwannoma, particularly in the Antoni B component.

Although uncommon, *metaplasia* to cartilaginous, osseous, and even adipose tissue may be observed in schwannomas (40,51,65). It is doubtful whether schwannomas ever show true epithelial (glandular or squamous) differentiation. Most purported examples (3,7,21,33,100) were located in skin, a site in which the "epithelial elements" could be explained as trapped cutaneous adnexae. Woodruff and Christensen (98) found no evidence of a myoepithelial cell layer in glandular peripheral nerve sheath tumors arising at noncutaneous sites. Instead, the glands in so-called cutaneous glandular schwannomas were seen to be invested by a layer of myoepithelial cells (fig. 7-21), a feature of the coiled secretory portions of sweat glands (29). Also commonly mistaken for glands in schwannoma are small, single or multiple spaces lined by eosinophilic, S-100 protein–immunoreactive Schwann cells superficially resembling epithelium (fig. 7-23) (30). Tumors with such degenerative pseudoglandular spaces should not be termed glandular schwannomas and do not represent a schwannoma variant (13).

As previously noted, infarct-like necrosis unassociated with palisading may be seen in schwannomas, particularly in large examples (fig. 7-17D). The finding is of no prognostic significance. The same is true of mitotic figures. Cellular lesions composed entirely of Antoni A tissue sometimes feature 4 or more mitoses per

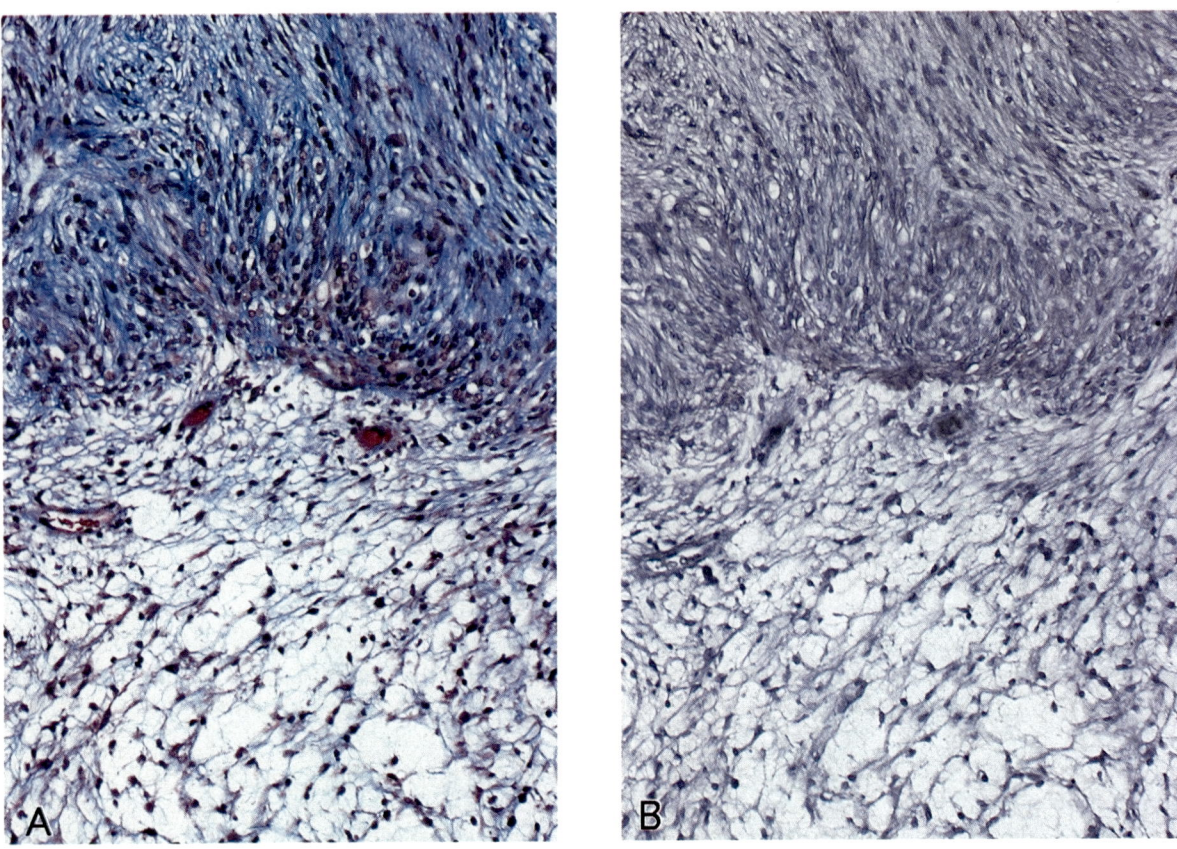

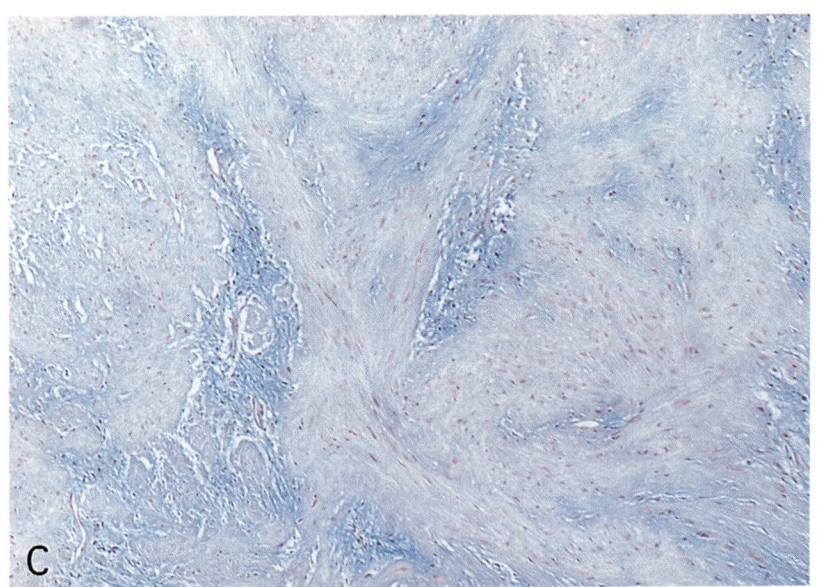

Figure 7-13
SCHWANNOMA
Antoni A and B tissues feature variable degrees of collagen deposition (A, Masson's trichrome; B, reticulin) and mucin accumulation (C, Alcian blue).

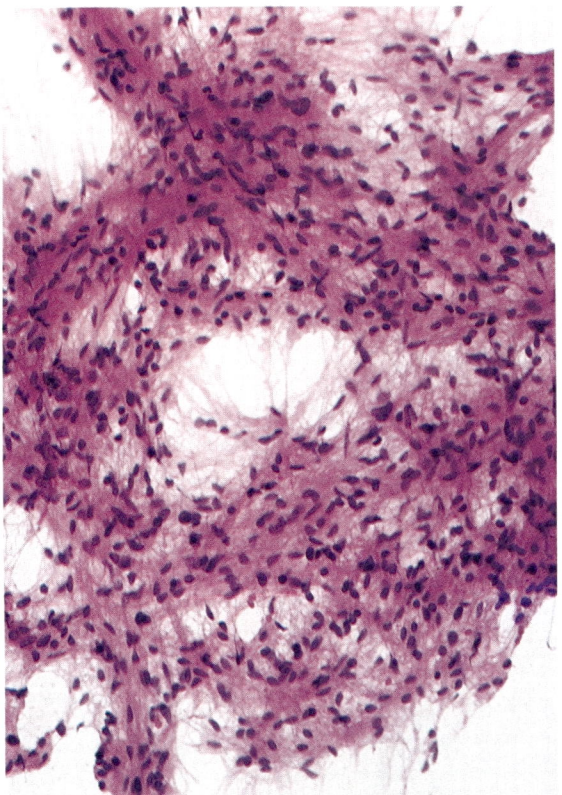 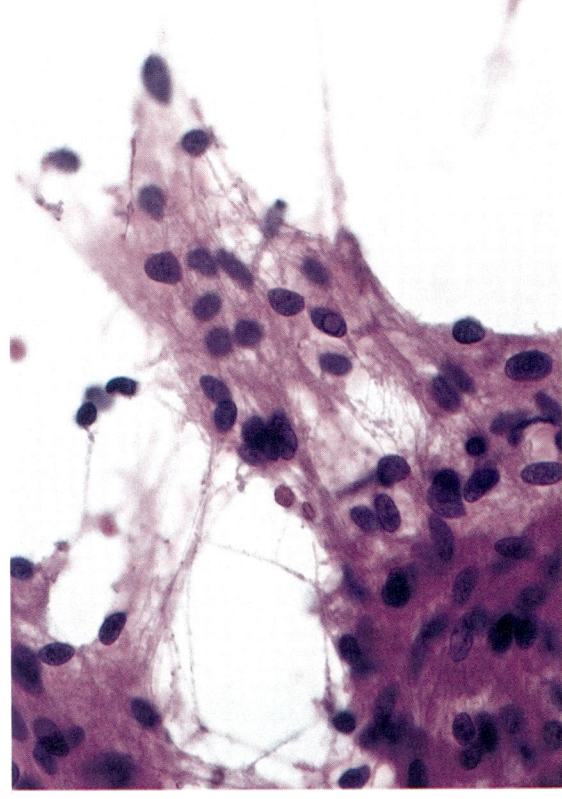

Figure 7-14
SCHWANNOMA, CYTOLOGY

Left: The constituent cells possess elongate to plump nuclei with stippled chromatin, inconspicuous nucleoli, and delicate wispy cell processes of varying length.

Right: Nuclear cytoplasmic pseudoinclusions may also be seen.

10 high-power fields; such tumors should be designated cellular schwannoma, not malignant peripheral nerve sheath tumor (MPNST).

Longstanding schwannomas often show extensive stromal and vascular degenerative changes, including organization of remote hemorrhage, widespread hyalinization (fig. 7-24), and calcification (fig. 7-9F). Such tumors may also show advanced degenerative nuclear changes characterized by marked pleomorphism, hyperchromasia, and cytoplasmic pseudoinclusion formation (fig. 7-24D). Once termed *"ancient schwannomas"* (2), tumors with these findings are in no way clinically distinctive. We recognize such lesions, but do not consider them a specific variant of schwannoma. Chronic inflammation may also be seen (fig. 7-22, left). Lymphoplasmacellular infiltrates are seen in approximately 5 percent of schwannomas and occasionally accompany other degenerative changes. Noncaseating microgran-

ulomas of unknown etiology and significance are rarely seen in otherwise typical schwannomas (fig. 7-22, right).

Schwannomas of NF2. Unusual histologic features may be exhibited by NF2-associated schwannomas. These include: multifocality within a nerve, a tendency to nodularity and whorl formation (fig. 7-16E), and peripheral ingrowth of surrounding exuberant arachnoidal tissue. On rare occasion the latter progresses to the formation of a mixed schwannoma-meningioma (34,84).

Immunohistochemical Findings. The immunophenotype of schwannomas is highly distinctive. Staining for S-100 protein is very useful in identifying schwannomas; all optimally fixed tumors are uniformly immunopositive for this antigen (50,54,97). We attribute rare lack of reactivity to artifacts of tissue fixation or processing. Staining for S-100 protein is often stronger in Antoni A tissue than in the less cellular Antoni B

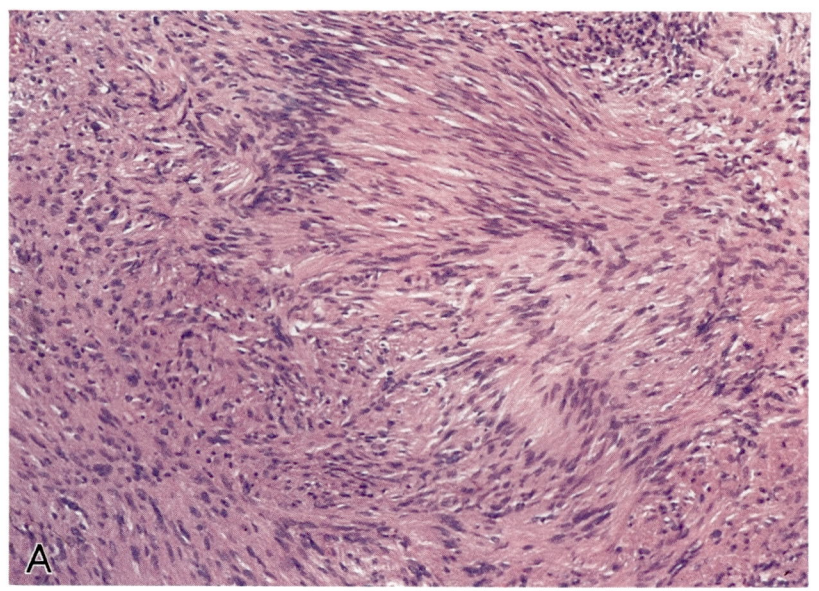

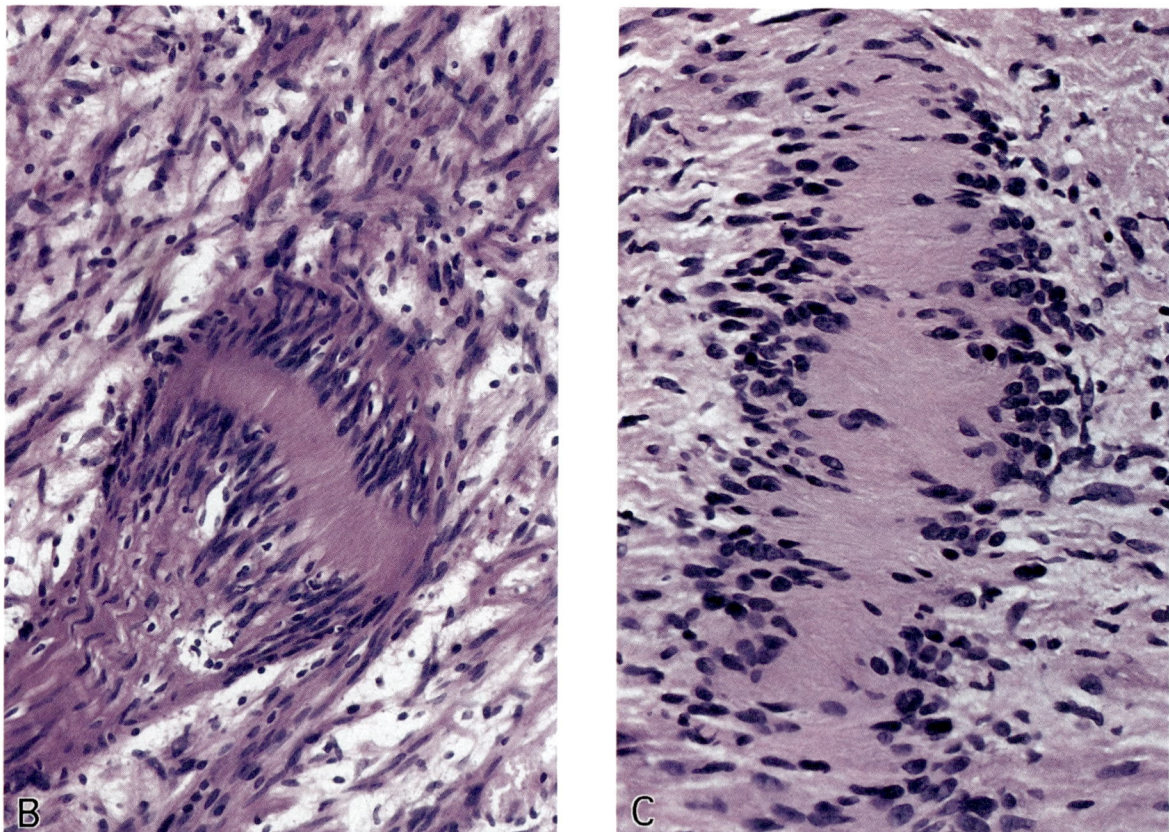

Figure 7-15
SCHWANNOMA, VEROCAY BODIES
A distinctive feature of schwannomas is the tendency to cellular regimentation which varies from indistinct (A) to the formation of tight, occasionally discrete aggregates termed Verocay bodies (B,C).

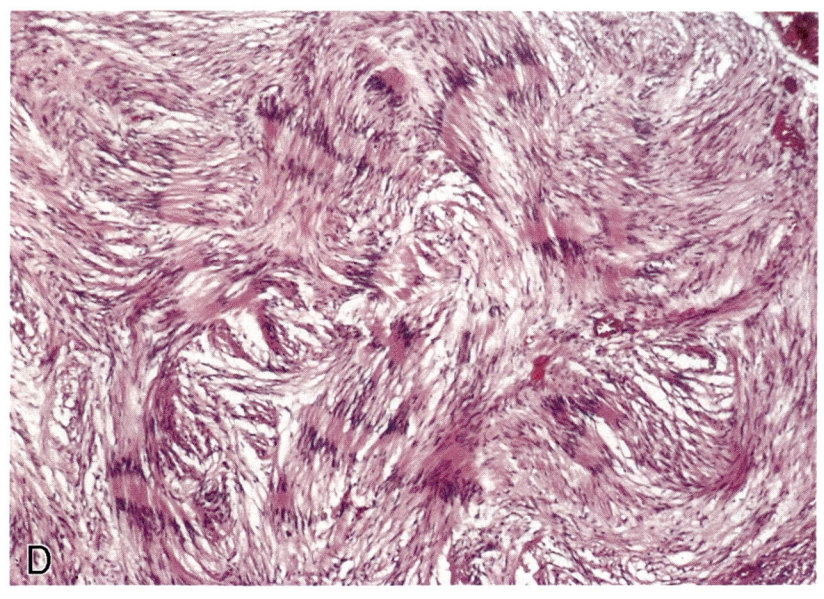

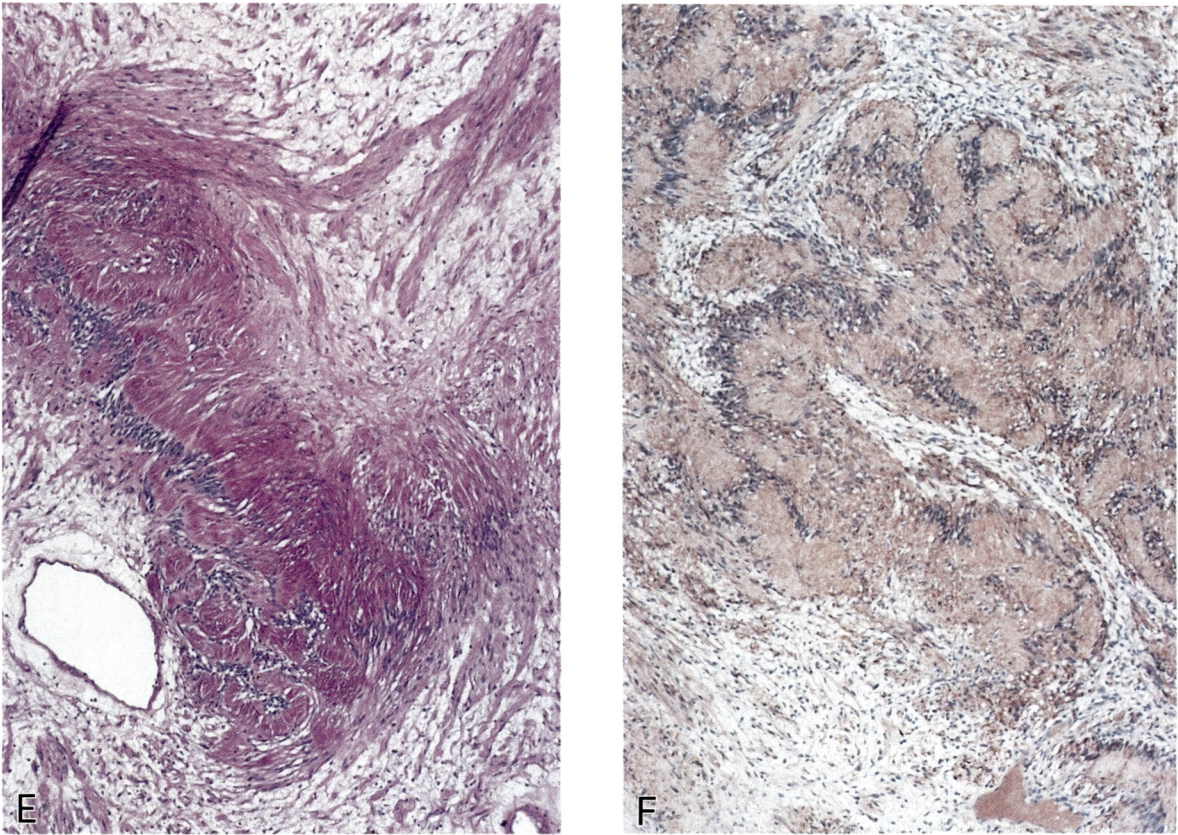

Figure 7-15 (Continued)

Verocay bodies may be numerous in intraspinal schwannomas (D). Strong PAS staining (E) and S-100 protein immunore-activity (F) in Verocay bodies result from compaction of basement membranes and cell processes.

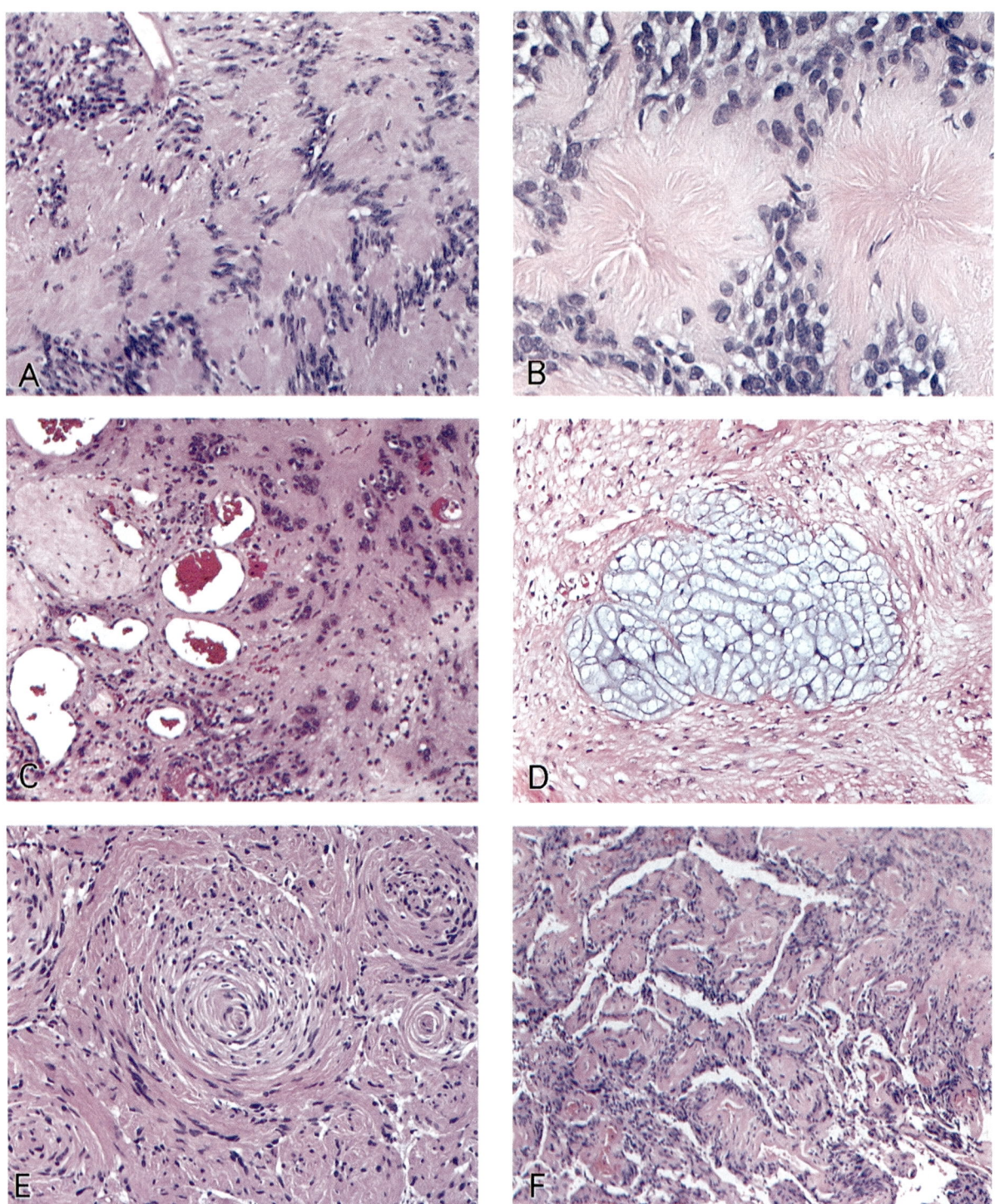

Figure 7-16
SCHWANNOMA, UNUSUAL PATTERNS

Coalescence of miniature Verocay bodies occasionally results in irregular nuclear crowding (A). When nuclei are plump and cell processes radiate toward a center, the result is an exaggerated Homer Wright rosette-like pattern (B). Tight clusters of epithelioid cells are an uncommon finding (C), as is a loose, geometric cell arrangement resembling vegetable matter (D). Whorl formation is more often seen in NF2-associated schwannomas (E). Papillary degeneration is rarely seen (F). (D, courtesy of Dr. A. Tsutsumi, Osaka, Japan.)

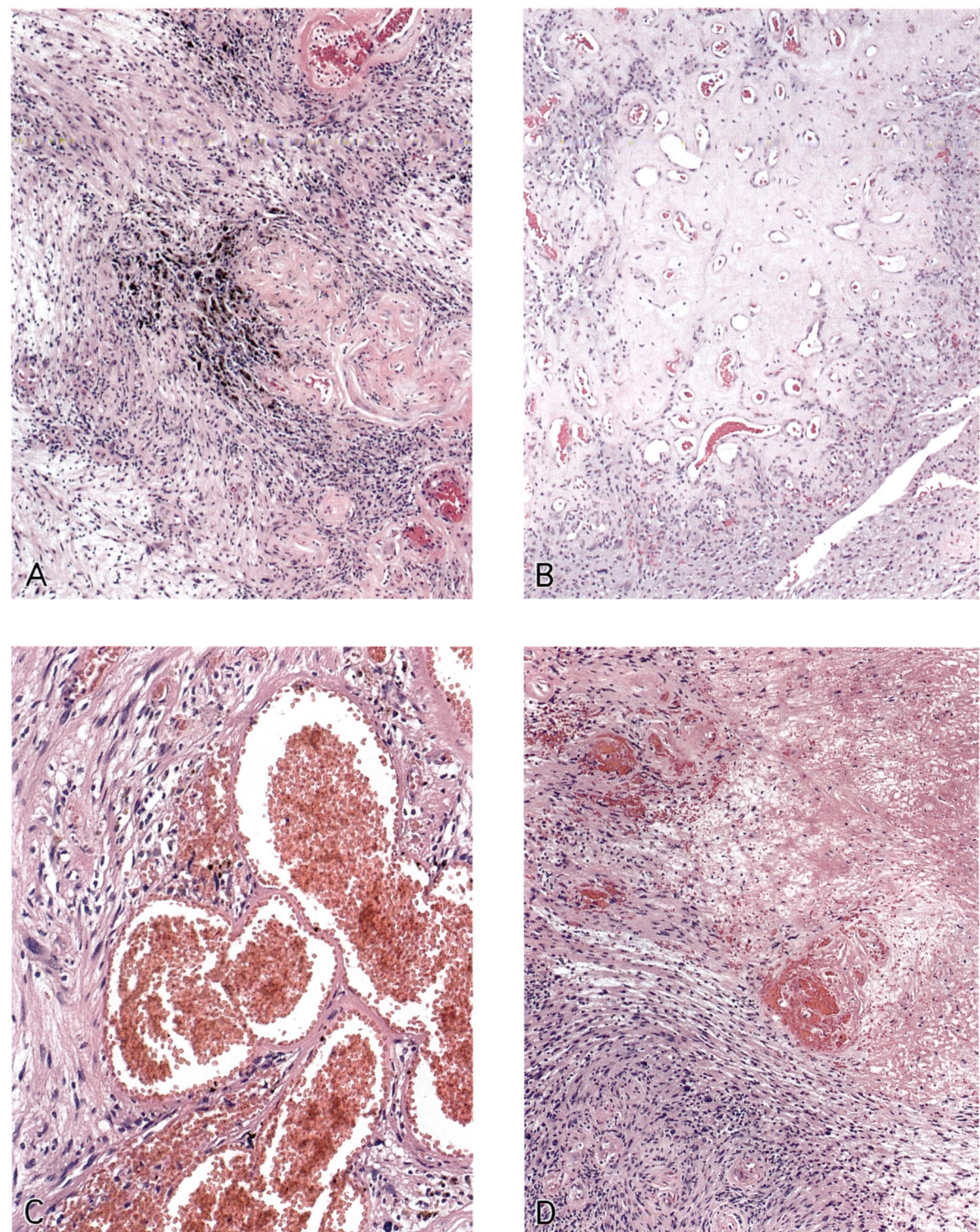

Figure 7-17
SCHWANNOMA, DEGENERATIVE CHANGES

Perivascular hemosiderin deposits are commonly seen surrounding hyalinized vessels (A). Such hyalinization may be prominent (B). Thin-walled, ectatic vessels are also a frequent finding (C). Such altered vessels tend to undergo thrombosis and microhemorrhage. The latter accounts for iron deposition (see fig. 7-18E) and probably underlies the occasional finding of nonpalisading necrosis (D).

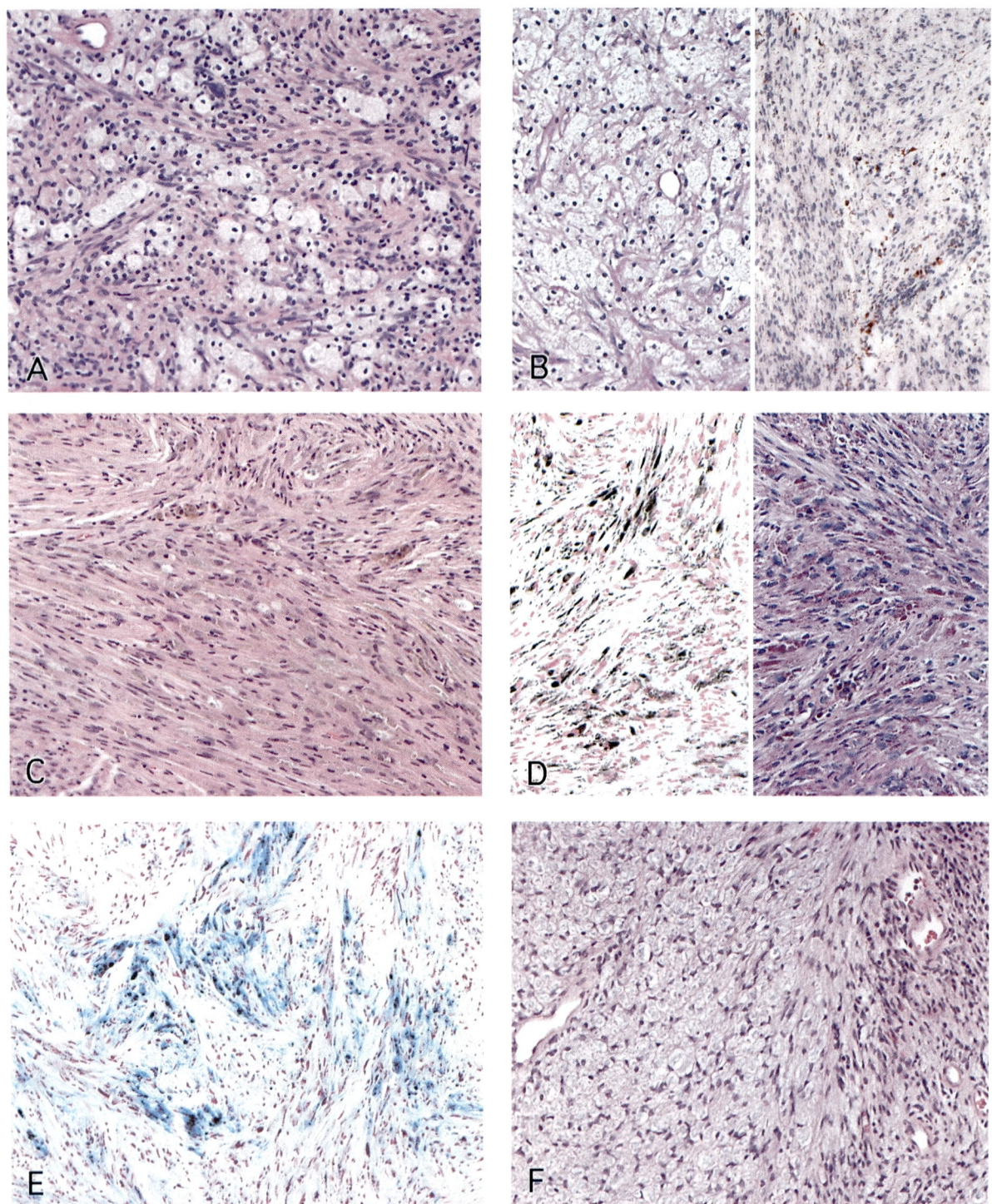

Figure 7-18
SCHWANNOMA, DEGENERATIVE CHANGES

Foam cells with xanthic changes (A) are clearly seen on PAS stain (B, left) and are accentuated with oil red O preparations (B, right). Lipofuscin accumulation is a less frequent finding (C); such tumors should not be confused with melanotic schwannoma. Although this pigment is argentaffin reactive (D, left; Fontana stain) it is also PAS positive (D, right). Iron deposition is commonly seen in longstanding tumors with advanced vascular degeneration (E; Prussian blue). On occasion, otherwise typical schwannomas show extensive stromal mucin accumulation wherein the cells actually surround small puddles of mucin (F).

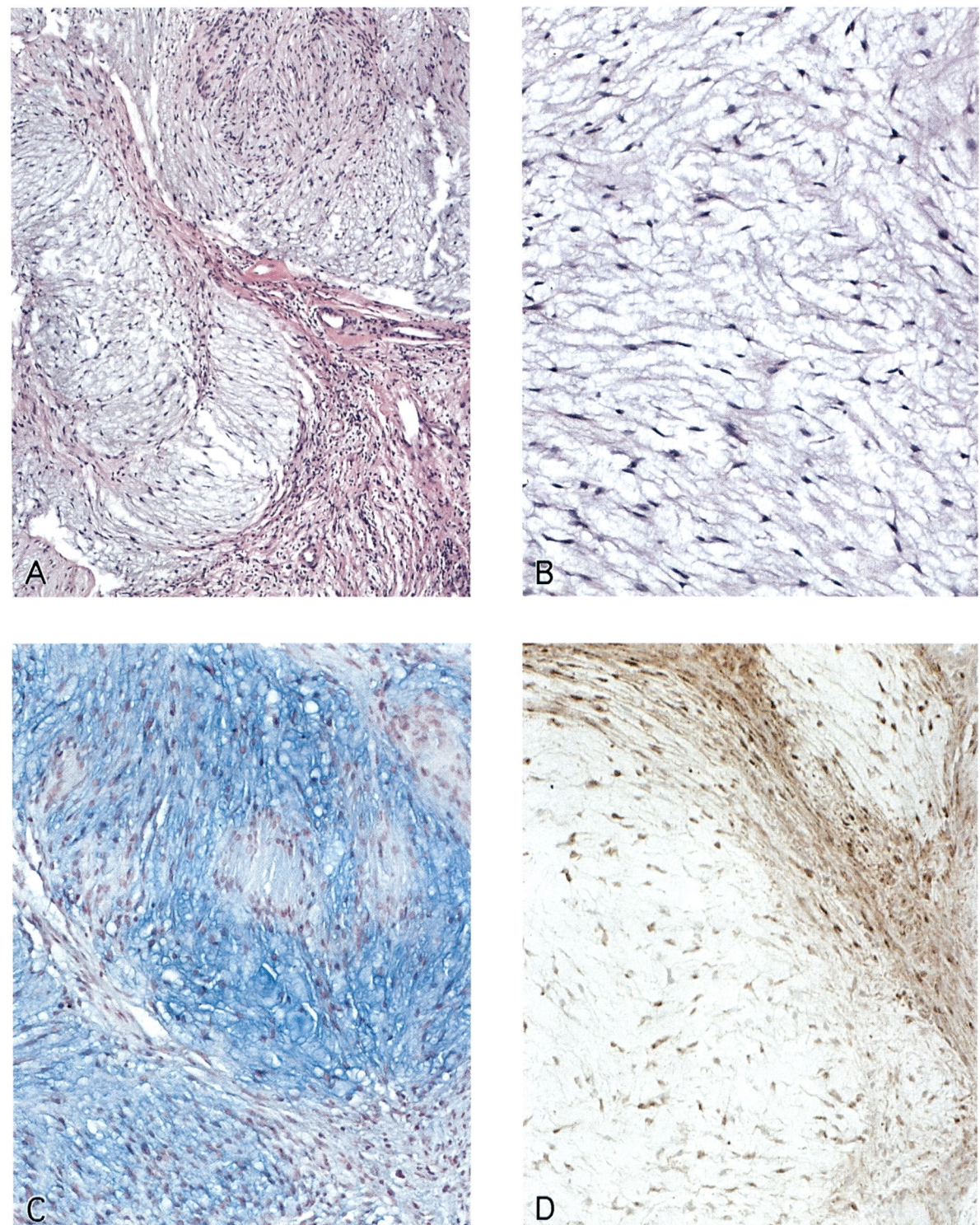

Figure 7-19
SCHWANNOMA PARTLY SIMULATING MYXOMA

On occasion, myxoid change in schwannoma is so extensive (A,B) as to mimic nerve sheath myxoma or even conventional myxoma of soft tissue. Such mucin-rich schwannomas are strongly Alcian blue positive (C) and uniformly S-100 protein immunoreactive (D).

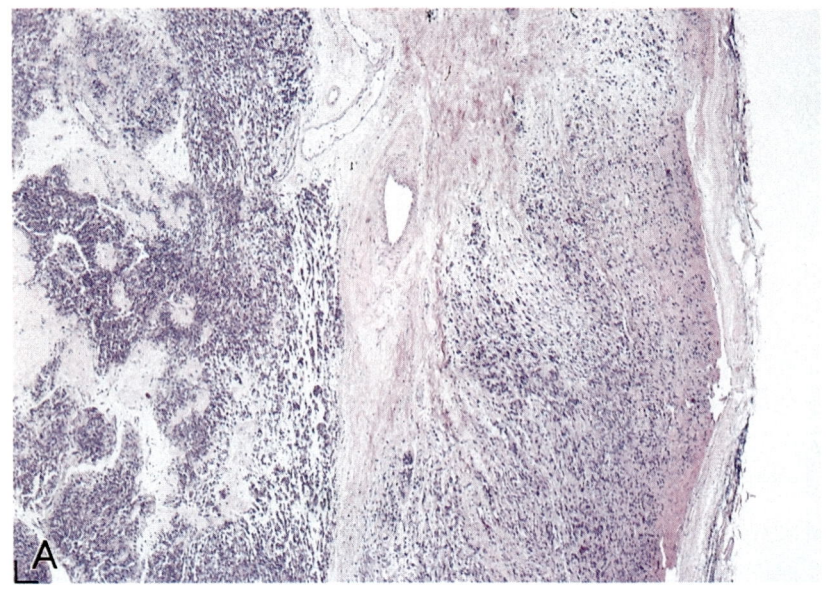

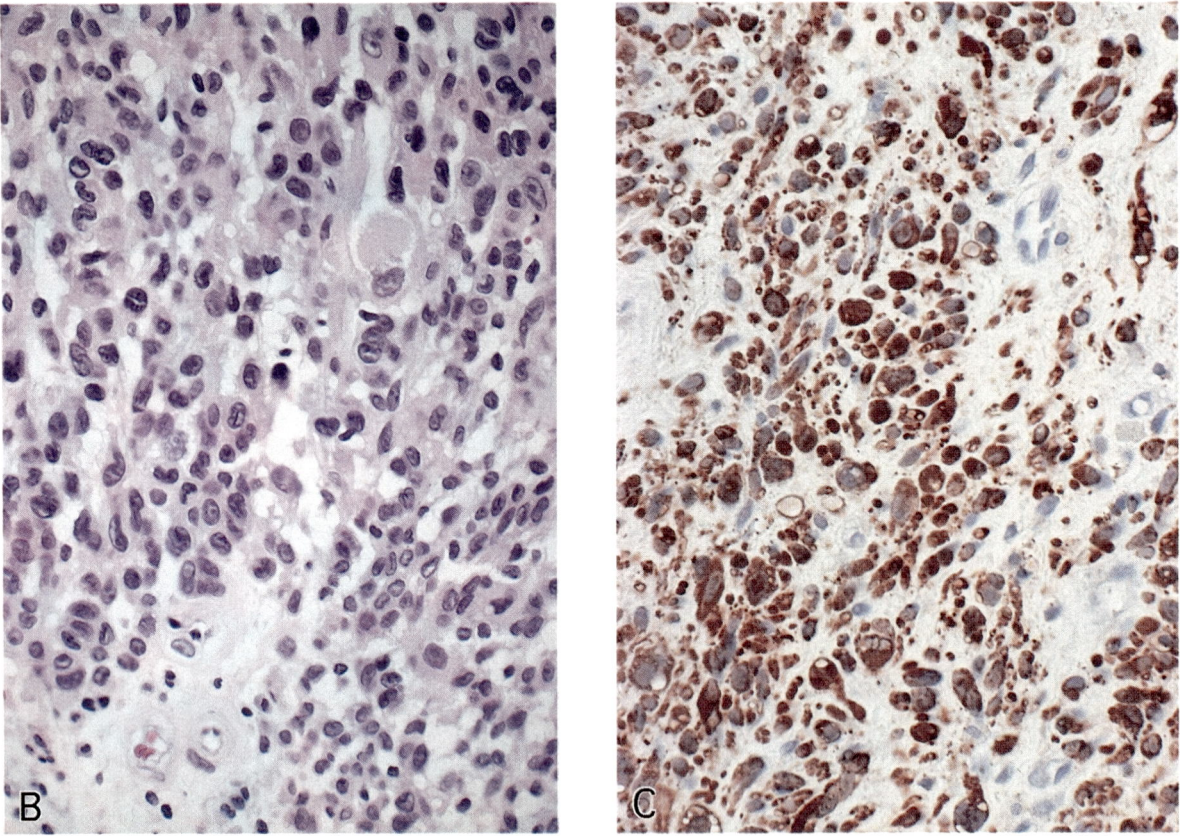

Figure 7-20
EPITHELIOID SCHWANNOMA

These tumors are rare, may exhibit a somewhat lobular pattern (A), and consist of often clustered cells with ample eosinophilic cytoplasm (B). They are strongly S-100 protein immunoreactive (C).

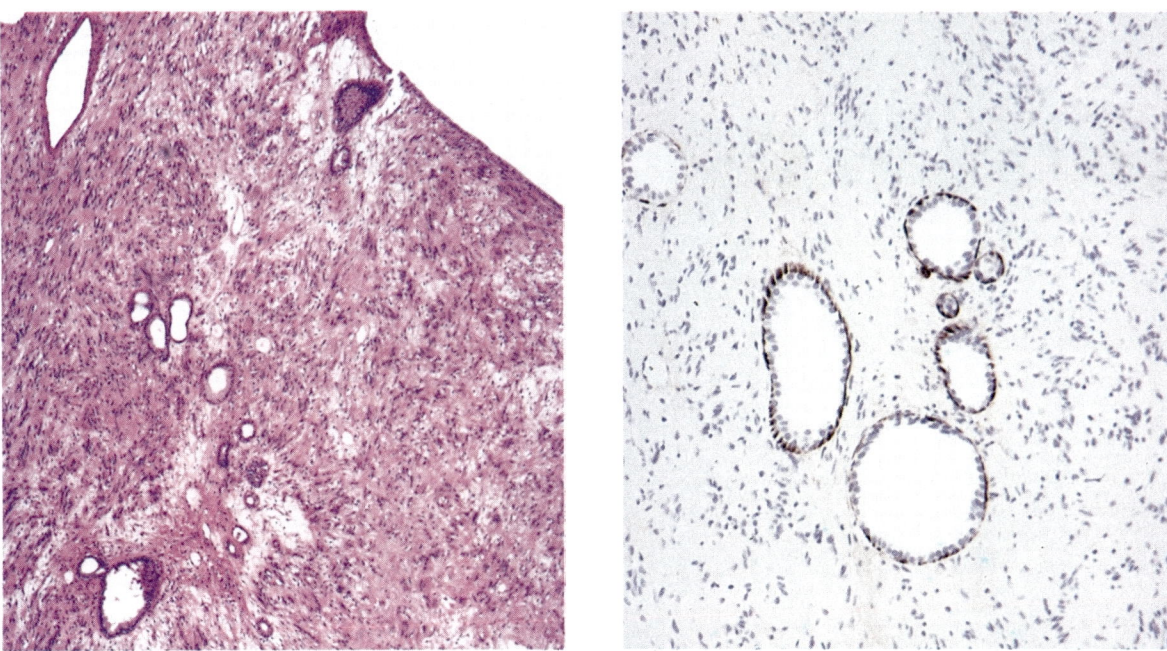

Figure 7-21
CUTANEOUS SCHWANNOMA WITH ENTRAPPED SWEAT GLAND

Left: This conventional schwannoma involving skin and subcutaneous tissue of the left arm entraps sweat gland tissue which mimics glandular differentiation.

Right: An immunostain for muscle common actin shows these "glands" to be surrounded by myoepithelial cells, a finding indicating their sweat gland derivation rather than a diagnosis of glandular schwannoma.

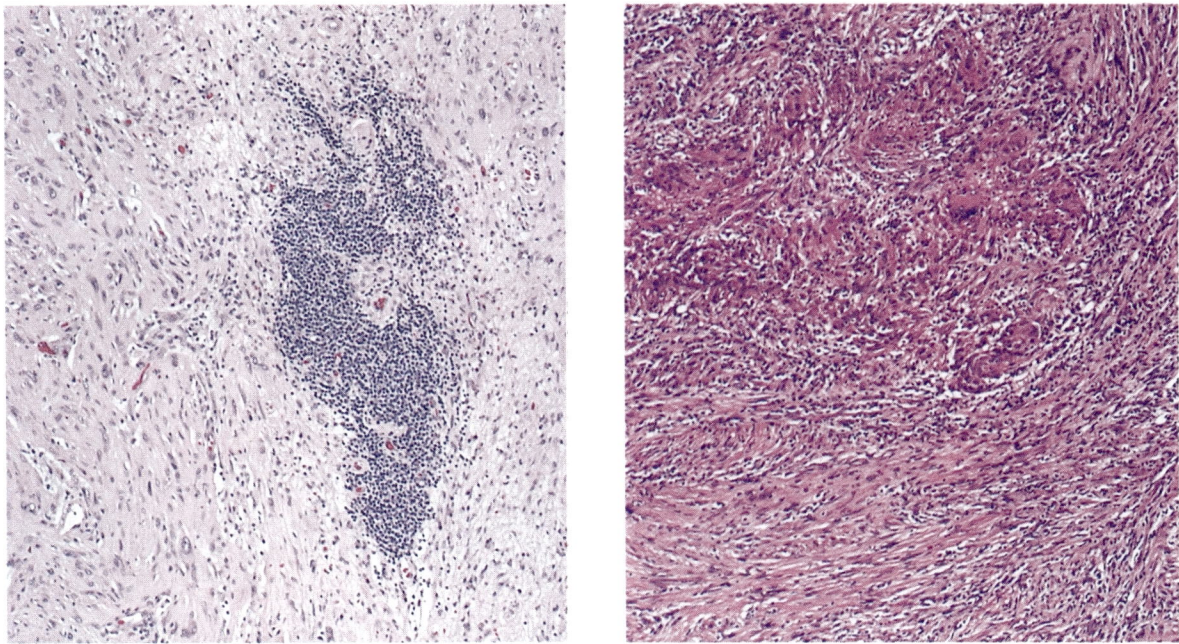

Figure 7-22
SCHWANNOMA

Left: Chronic inflammation is common, particularly as large tumor infiltrates, and consists primarily of lymphoid cells.
Right: Noncaseating granulomas are a rare finding in schwannomas and are of unknown significance.

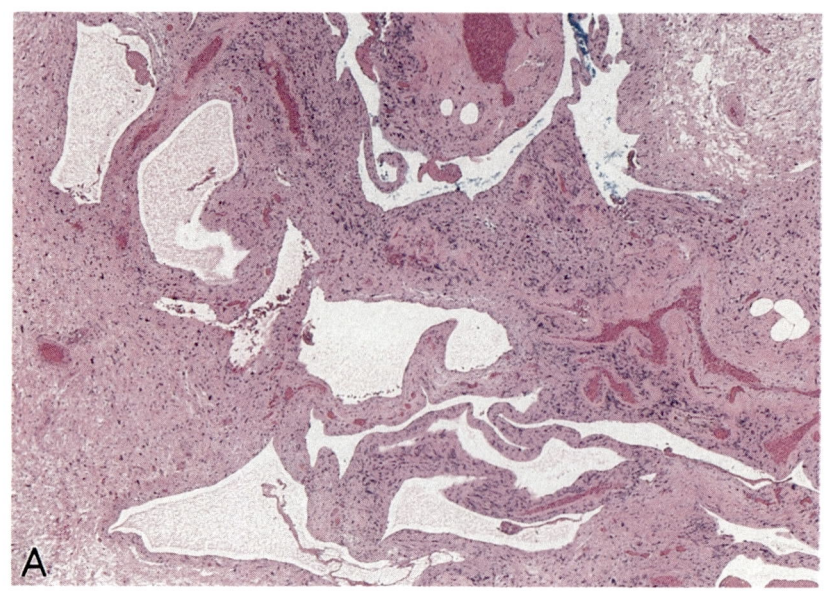

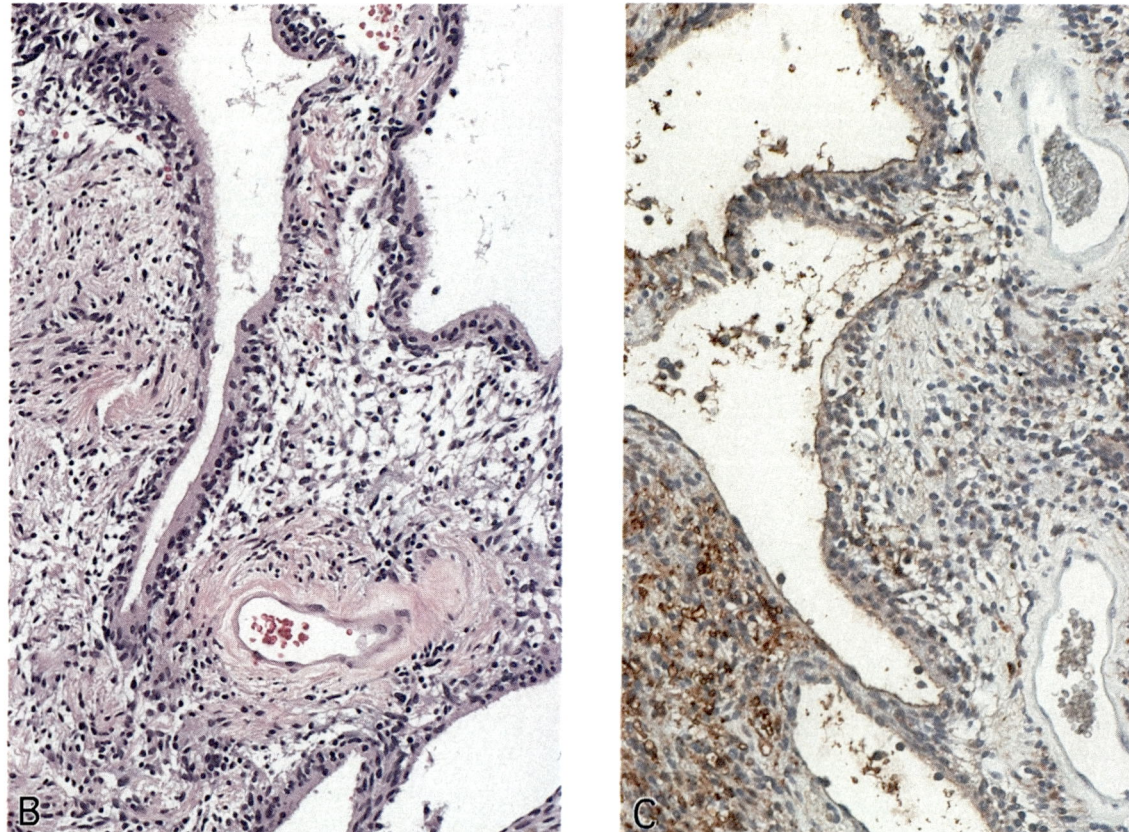

Figure 7-23
SCHWANNOMA, PSEUDOGLANDS

The occasional formation of microcysts (A) with a pseudoepithelial lining of Schwann cells (B) is considered a degenerative change. The lining cells are S-100 protein immunoreactive (C) and lack immunoreactivity for epithelial markers.

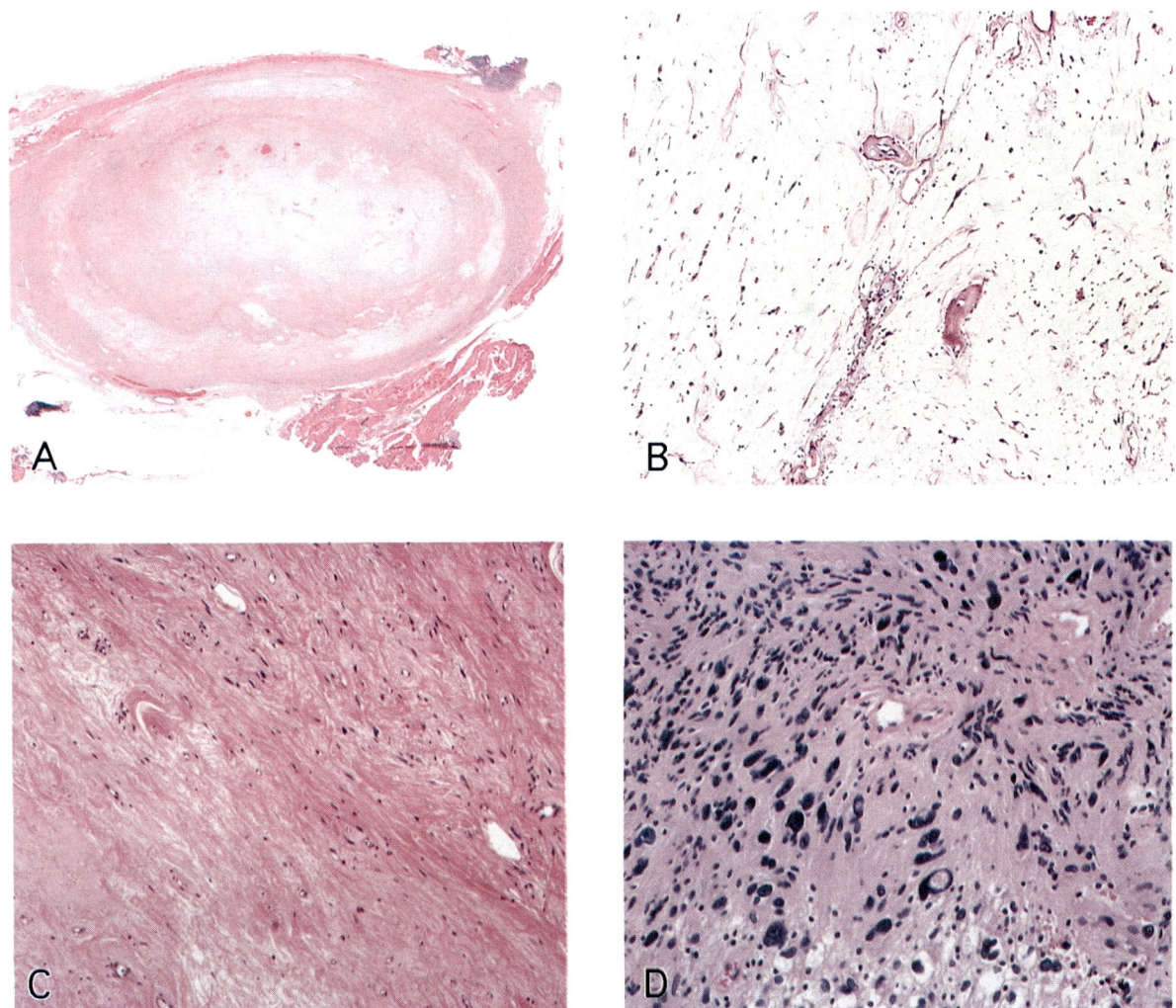

Figure 7-24
"ANCIENT SCHWANNOMA"
Schwannomas of long standing often show degenerative changes including central tissue loss (A,B), necrosis unassociated with nuclear palisading (see fig. 17-17D), widespread hyalinization (C), focal calcification (see fig. 7-9F), and degenerative nuclear atypia (D). (A,B: Courtesy of Dr. D. Horoupian, Stanford, CA.)

areas (fig. 7-25A). A similar pattern of staining, although less frequent and uniform, is seen with Leu-7 (fig. 7-25B) (50). Myelin basic protein (MBP) staining has been reported by some authors (67), but most have reported no reactivity for this antigen (14,50). Negative results are not surprising, since MBP has not been biochemically demonstrated in schwannomas (68). Immunoreactivity for glial fibrillary acidic protein (GFAP) may be seen in a significant number of schwannomas (fig. 7-25C) (35,41,50,61). The frequency and degree of staining varies with the source of the antibody used. The reaction is

thought to detect a GFAP-like substance distinct from that found in glial cells of the central nervous system. Such reactivity is of practical diagnostic significance, since benign nerve sheath tumors are more often GFAP reactive than are malignant ones, which are either nonreactive (41,54) or only sparsely reactive (see fig. 11-19F) (35). Unlike neurofibroma, wherein CD34-positive cells may be seen throughout, schwannomas show reactivity only in Antoni B tissue, usually nearby the capsule (13a). Despite the demonstration of CD68 staining in schwannoma (fig. 7-25D) (54c), we have not seen widespread granular cell

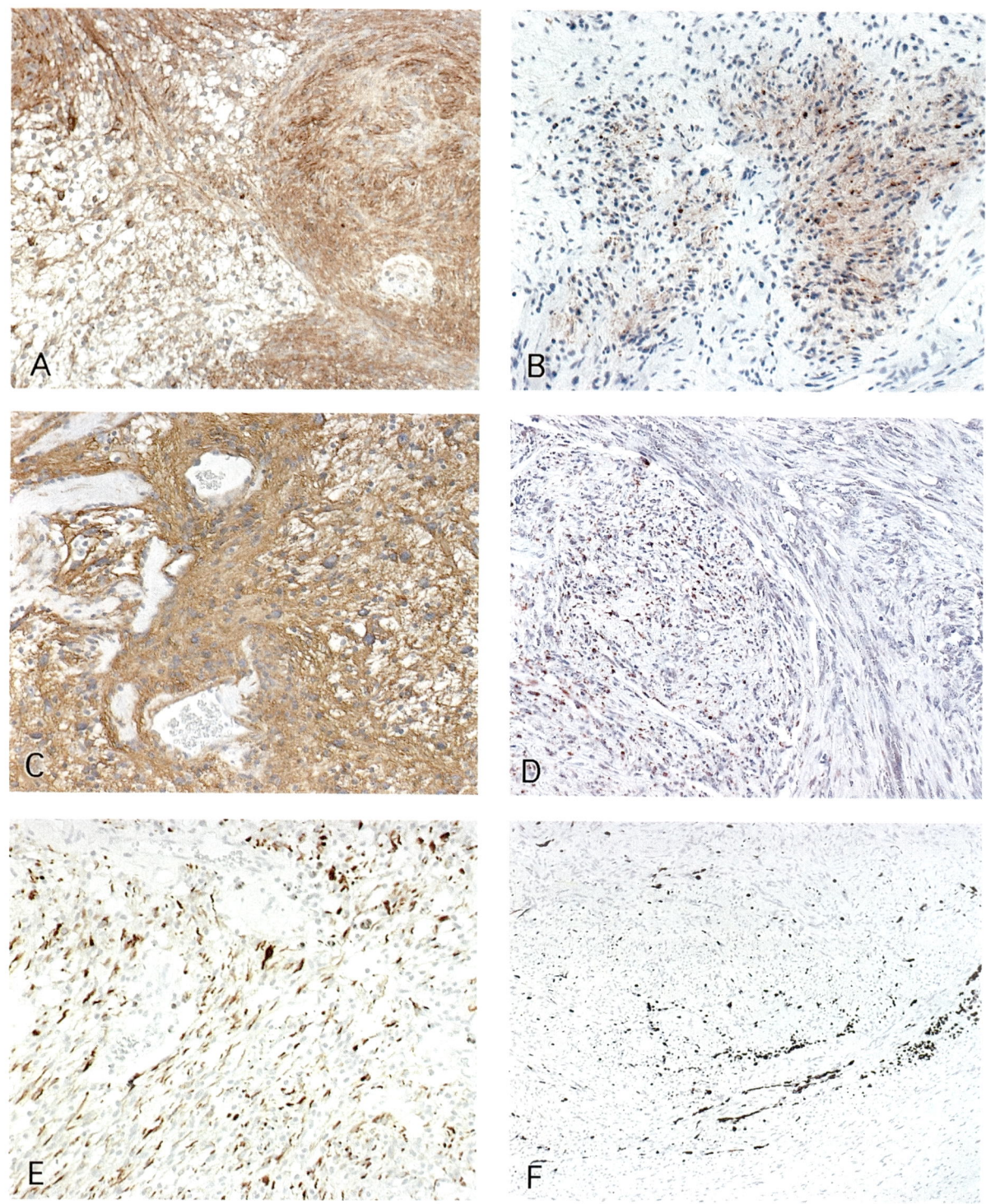

Figure 7-25
SCHWANNOMA

The immunoprofile of schwannoma includes uniform staining of Antoni A and B tissues for vimentin as well as for S-100 protein (A). Stains for Leu-7 are variably positive (B). Reactivity for glial fibrillary acidic protein is commonly seen, but is usually patchy (C). Although granular cell change is rare in schwannomas, patchy CD68 staining is a common finding (D). Collagen 4 reactivity corresponds to pericellular basement membranes (E). Neurofilament protein-positive axons, if present within the substance of schwannomas, are usually limited to the subcapsular region (F).

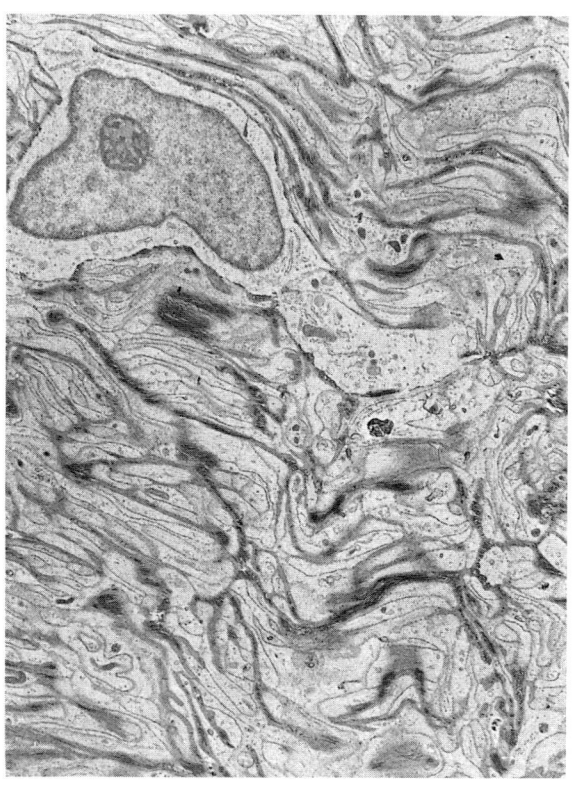

Figure 7-26
SCHWANNOMA

Antoni type A tissue consisting of prominent arrays of Schwann cell processes that are coated on their free surfaces by basement membrane substance (X5,800).

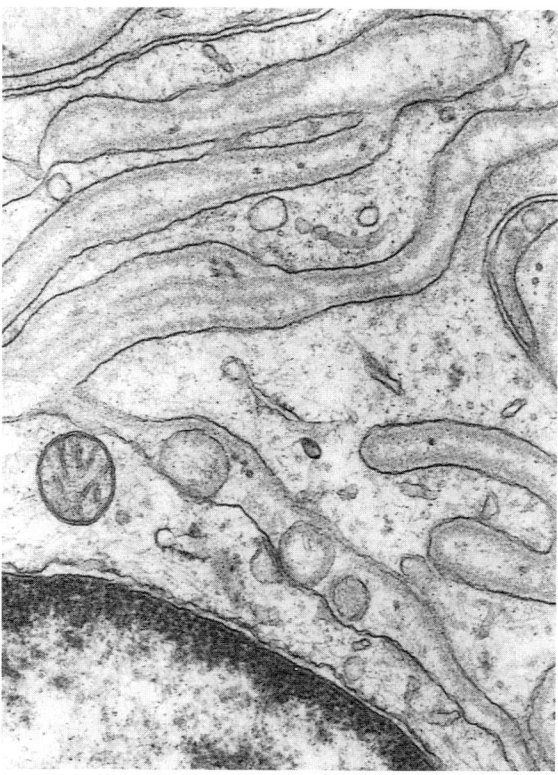

Figure 7-27
SCHWANNOMA

Detail of a complex Schwann cell process. Note the occasionally reduplicated lamina densa of the basement membrane in the intercellular spaces (X32,400).

change in this tumor. Basement membrane staining for collagen 4 (fig. 7-25E) and laminin shows a pattern corresponding to that of reticulin (59). Both are particularly strong in Antoni A tissue and among the aligned, compact cells and processes that comprise areas of palisading and Verocay bodies. The types of collagen represented vary somewhat: Antoni A regions are collagen 4 immunoreactive, whereas Antoni B areas reportedly stain for collagen types 1, 3, and 4 (64). Stains for neurofilament protein are useful in assessing the relationship of a schwannoma to its parent nerve, the fibers of which reside in the capsule (fig. 7-11C) and are scant or only occasionally encountered in subcapsular portions of the lesion (fig. 7-25F). As previously noted, immunostaining for neurofilament protein is more sensitive in demonstrating nerve fibers than are silver impregnation methods. Lastly, whereas staining for vimentin is of little

diagnostic utility, a positive reaction serves as evidence of immunoviability. Reactivity is strong in schwannomas, as well as in other nerve sheath tumors (39).

Ultrastructural Findings. Although electron microscopy usually is not required for the routine diagnosis of schwannoma, a working knowledge of the ultrastructural features of this lesion is important in the differential diagnosis. Antoni A tissue is composed of neoplastic Schwann cells having prominent, long, thin cytoplasmic processes often complexly entangled (fig. 7-26) and joined by widely scattered rudimentary cell junctions (12,19,20,23–25,55,83,95,99). The tumor cell nuclei are elongate with generally smooth contours, finely dispersed chromatin, and one or two small nucleoli (fig. 7-26). Perinuclear cytoplasm contains a small Golgi apparatus, scattered mitochondria, short profiles of rough endoplasmic reticulum, ribosomes and polysomes, various

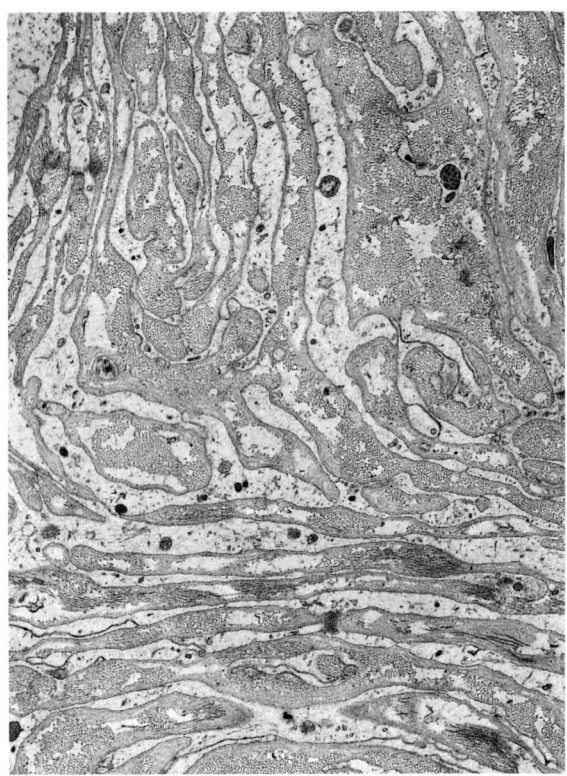

Figure 7-28
SCHWANNOMA
The central portion of a Verocay body consists of a relatively straight Schwann cell process with a prominent intervening collagen/basement membrane substance stroma (X8,400).

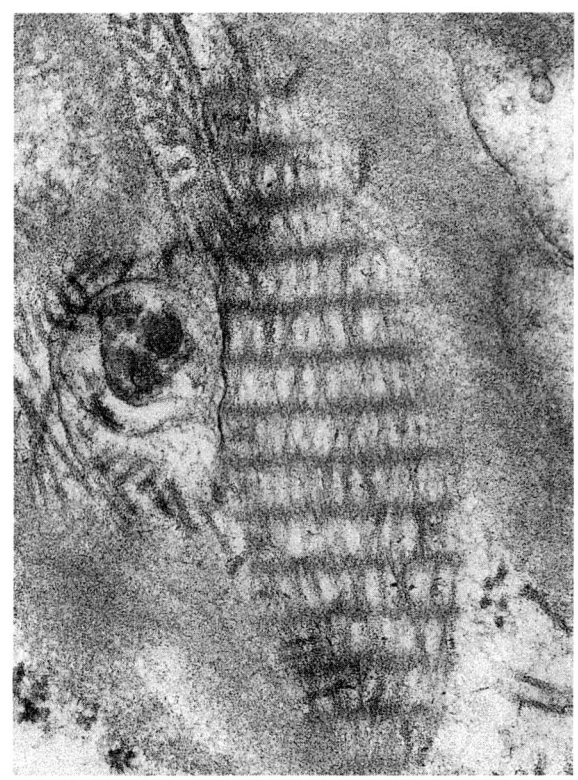

Figure 7-29
SCHWANNOMA
A portion of intercellular stroma contains a Luse body, typical collagen fibrils, and basement membrane substance (X52,500).

types of primary and secondary lysosomes, and occasional small lipid droplets (fig. 7-27). The prominent, undulating, intertwining cell processes generally contain few organelles, other than scattered arrays of intermediate filaments and microtubules, as well as small vesicles (fig. 7-27). The central anucleate portions of the Verocay bodies are composed of long, parallel cytoplasmic processes separated in varying proportion by basement membrane substance and collagen fibrils (fig. 7-28). The main constituents of the generally sparse stroma include reduplicated basement membrane, scattered small bundles of thin collagen fibrils (figs. 7-26, 7-27), and variable numbers of long-spaced (130-nm periodicity) collagen fibrils often referred to as Luse bodies (fig. 7-29).

In contrast, Antoni type B tissue is less cellular and consists of neoplastic Schwann cells dispersed within flocculent material of low electron density, basement membrane substance, and scat-

tered collagen fibrils (fig. 7-30). Schwann cell nuclei in Antoni B areas often are somewhat more pleomorphic and may contain more clumped chromatin than do those in Antoni A tissue. In addition, the frequent finding of secondary lysosomes and myelin figures may be a reflection of cell degeneration (fig. 7-31) (82). The blood vessels of schwannoma characteristically exhibit a thickened basement membrane (23,52, 82) and are fenestrated (45).

Differential Diagnosis. A number of lesions enter into the differential diagnosis of conventional schwannoma. Principal among these are cellular schwannoma (see later in this chapter), neurofibroma, and MPNST. Ganglioneuroma, leiomyoma, and palisaded myofibroblastoma must also be considered.

Distinguishing schwannoma from *neurofibroma* usually poses no problem (Table 7-1). Confusion may occur, however, since the loose

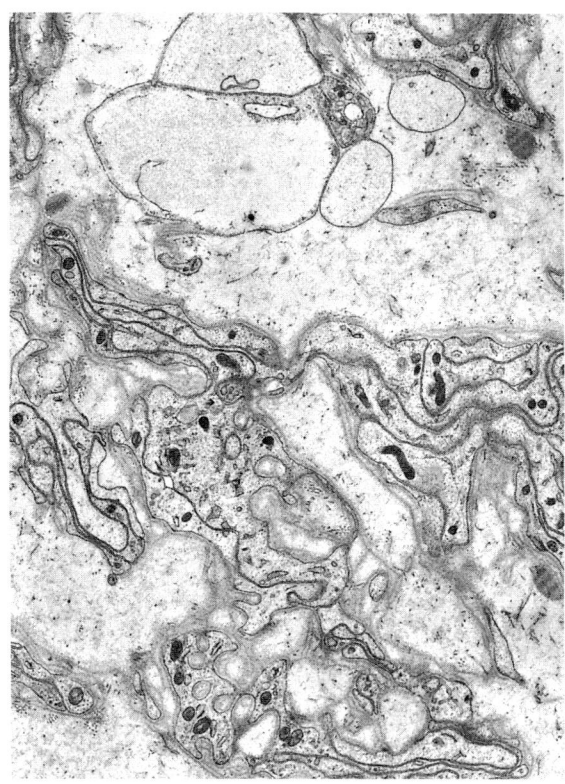

Figure 7-30
SCHWANNOMA, ANTONI TYPE B TISSUE
Schwann cell processes in a prominent stroma contain sparse basement membrane substance and collagen fibrils. Dilated Schwann cell processes are present (X9,900).

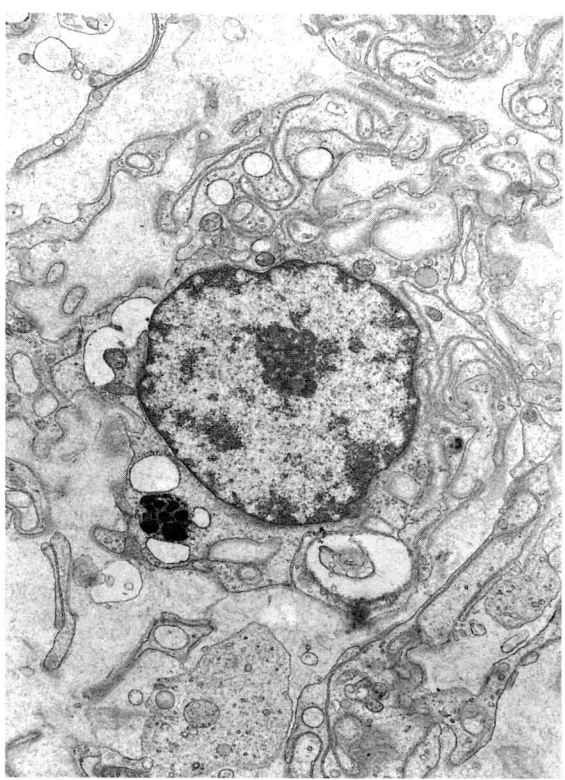

Figure 7-31
SCHWANNOMA, ANTONI TYPE B TISSUE
Note the cluster of lysosomes in the perinuclear cytoplasm as well as the dilated rough endoplasmic reticulum (RER) cisternae (X7,200).

textured Antoni B tissue of schwannoma may closely mimic neurofibroma (fig. 7-32A–C). Attention to overall architectural and immunocytochemical features usually resolves the issue. Neurofibromas may be surrounded by a variably thickened perineurium and epineurium but lack the thick, collagenous capsule of schwannoma. Furthermore, many neurofibromas, particularly plexiform examples, diffusely infiltrate surrounding soft tissue. Neurofibromas usually lack the Antoni A and B patterns so typical of schwannoma, but occasional examples, particularly plexiform or lumbosacral intradural neurofibromas, may contain nodules of Schwann cells resembling mini-schwannomas (see fig. 8-28). Unlike most schwannomas, neurofibromas often possess a mucinous matrix and contain scattered myelinated and unmyelinated axons. Immunoreactivity for S-100 protein is seen in only a portion of the cells comprising neurofibroma, whereas reactiv-

ity is uniform throughout schwannoma (fig. 7-32D). Neurofibromas also show cellular heterogeneity at the ultrastructural level; in contrast to the homogeneous composition of schwannomas, they contain not only Schwann cells, but fibroblasts and perineurial-like cells.

Schwannomas rich in mucopolysaccharide matrix may mimic *dermal nerve sheath myxoma* (fig. 7-21). Nerve sheath myxomas are not encapsulated and do not exhibit Antoni A and B patterns or Verocay bodies (see fig. 9-20). Immunohistochemistry is of little use since both lesions are composed of Schwann cells. Nonetheless, reactivity for S-100 protein is variable and occasionally absent in nerve sheath myxomas (see fig. 9-30).

Although, unlike most schwannomas, *MPNSTs* are invasive of surrounding tissues, infiltration may be grossly or even microscopically inapparent. The fibrous tissue-rich pseudocapsule of such MPNSTs is composed of infiltrated soft tissue

135

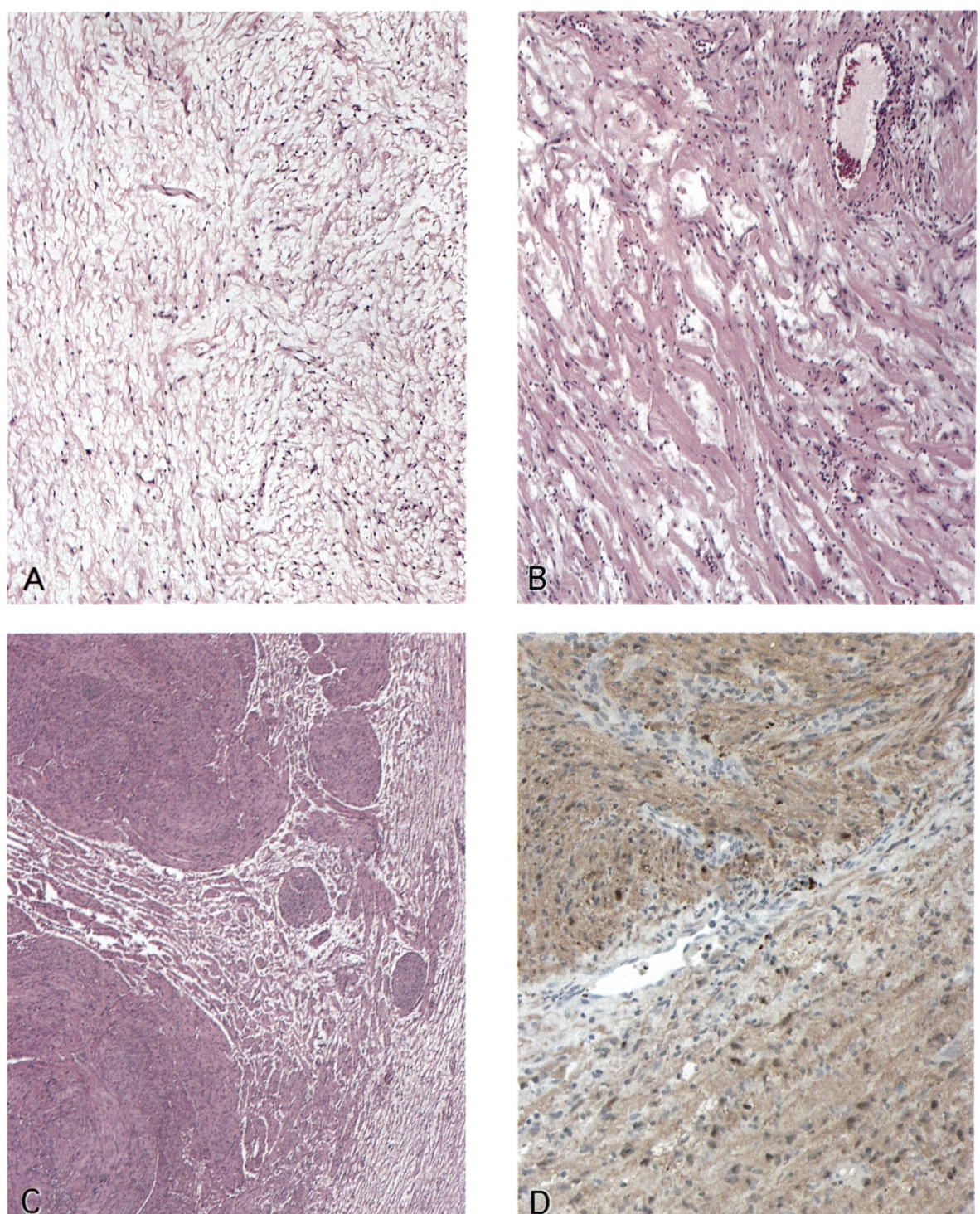

Figure 7-32
SCHWANNOMA SIMULATING NEUROFIBROMA

Loose textured components (A), particularly in spinal intradural tumors, may mimic neurofibroma. The same is true of tumors in which collagen accumulation mimics the "shredded carrots" pattern of neurofibroma (B). More often, neurofibroma-like tissue lies interposed between nodules of obvious schwannoma (C). In addition to sampling, a strong and uniform S-100 protein staining (D) and lack of nerve fibers support the diagnosis of schwannoma.

and should not be mistaken for the true capsule of schwannoma. The finding of skeletal muscle, densely adherent at the gross level or microscopically incorporated into the fibrous periphery of an MPNST, is indicative of invasion and malignancy. As previously noted, visceral schwannomas and those occurring at mucosal sites, such as in the nose or paranasal sinuses (44), often lack a capsule (fig. 7-7). Limited infiltration in such instances should not be overinterpreted as evidence of malignancy. The same is true of schwannomas associated with osseous destruction, e.g., "giant sacral" schwannoma. Their effects upon bone are due to compression, not to permeative growth; the latter is a feature of MPNST (19,22). Hyalinized vasculature accompanied by histiocytes and hemosiderin deposition are characteristic features of schwannoma, and are usually lacking in MPNST. As a rule, all but a minority of low-grade MPNSTs are more cellular than schwannomas. MPNSTs lack distinctive Antoni A and B patterns as well as Verocay bodies. The degenerative nuclear atypia in schwannoma, which includes bizarre hyperchromatic cells and intranuclear cytoplasmic inclusions, is readily distinguished from the more typically uniform, malignant cytologic features of MPNST, which includes marked cell crowding and hyperplasia. Unlike schwannoma, necrosis in MPNST is far more likely to be accompanied by surrounding palisaded tumor cells. Lastly, the presence of heterologous mesenchymal differentiation, a feature of approximately 10 percent of MPNSTs, does not occur in schwannoma. On occasion, however, schwannomas may show osseous metaplasia. Immunohistochemistry also aids in the distinction of schwannoma from MPNST in that the latter generally shows only patchy or scant S-100 protein and Leu-7 staining. Reactivity for GFAP, a common feature of schwannomas and other benign PNSTs (61), is rare in MPNST (35,41).

The differential diagnosis with *leiomyoma* arises primarily in tumors of skin, deep soft tissue, and the retroperitoneum and gastrointestinal tract. Leiomyomas are unassociated with nerve and generally lack the thick hyaline capsule and hyalinized vasculature of schwannoma. Although smooth muscle tumors do not feature well-formed Antoni A and B components, nuclear palisading may be seen. Indeed, the palisaded areas of some leiomyomas, notably uterine examples, may closely simulate Verocay bodies,

but sometimes differ by being disposed in a wave-like pattern. Nuclear shape may be of assistance in that the nuclei of smooth muscle tumors, especially leiomyomas, are often blunt-ended rather than tapered. Smooth muscle cells also have a more densely eosinophilic cytoplasm and, unlike neoplastic Schwann cells, often distinct cell borders. Trichrome and phosphotungstic acid hematoxylin (PTAH) stains often show red and blue longitudinal fibrils, respectively, within the cytoplasm of smooth muscle cells. The longitudinal fibrils are also sometimes seen on hematoxylin and eosin (H&E) stained material. Immunohistochemistry readily settles the issue: smooth muscle tumors, with some exceptions (90,91), lack S-100 protein staining and Leu-7 reactivity is not observed; instead they are reactive for myogenic markers such as smooth muscle actin and sometimes desmin. The ultrastructure of smooth muscle tumors is highly distinctive. Their cells usually are bounded by a basement membrane and often contain parallel arrays of abundant cytoplasmic microfilaments (actin) with interspersed fusiform dense bodies, subplasmalemmal attachment plaques, and pinocytotic vesicles.

The distinction of schwannoma from *ganglioneuroma* only becomes an issue if the schwannoma, usually paraspinous examples, overruns a dorsal root ganglion. The anatomic distribution and uniform cytology generally distinguish normal ganglion cells of residual dorsal root ganglia from the haphazardly arrayed, often cytologically abnormal ganglion cells that typify ganglioneuroma. Since ganglion cells in ganglioneuroma are surrounded by varying numbers of satellite Schwann cells, the simple presence of the latter does not distinguish ganglioneuroma from either schwannoma or neurofibroma involving a ganglion. The spindle cell component of ganglioneuroma is usually less cellular than that of schwannoma and more closely resembles neurofibroma. Ganglioneuromas are rich in unmyelinated axons, structures generally lacking in schwannoma and readily identified on immunostains for neurofilament protein. Myelinated axons are a prominent feature in normal and overrun dorsal root ganglia.

By its content of palisaded cells and Verocay-like bodies, the *palisaded myofibroblastoma* can mimic schwannoma (96). Palisaded myofibroblastomas typically involve lymph nodes, usually of the inguinal region; unequivocal lymph node involvement by schwannoma has yet to be described. Palisaded myofibroblastomas do not express S-100 protein but may show smooth muscle actin staining. What appear at first glance to be Verocay-like bodies are in actuality patches of amianthoid collagen fibers (89,96). Any fibroblastic or myofibroblastic process that may be mistaken for schwannoma can readily be distinguished by a lack of immunoreactivity for S-100 protein.

Treatment and Prognosis. The optimal treatment of schwannomas is gross total resection with sparing of the parent nerve, when one is identified (fig. 7-2B,C). Although conventional schwannomas are benign, incompletely excised examples are capable of slow recurrence.

So-called "giant sacral schwannomas" are especially prone to local recurrence (1); as a result, the parent nerve may have to be sacrificed. As a rule, however, the overall favorable outcome of schwannoma permits a conservative approach, such as "gutting" or enucleation in which it is necessary to spare nerve function.

A recent clinicopathologic study found that patients symptomatic schwannomas occurring in association with NF2 not only present with more severe neurologic deficits, but experience little postoperative improvement and a higher rate of tumor recurrence (54b). There is no evidence supporting the notion that schwannomas undergo accelerated growth during pregnancy (4). Lastly, malignant transformation of schwannoma is an exceedingly rare event (see chapter 11).

CELLULAR SCHWANNOMA

Definition. This schwannoma is characterized by high cellularity, a largely Antoni A pattern, and absence of well-formed Verocay bodies.

General Comments. Since its original characterization by Woodruff et al. (121), several studies have, despite initial doubt (106,116), confirmed that cellular schwannomas are benign and do not represent well-differentiated MPNST. While they may recur nonaggressively, they lack metastatic potential (103,104,108,113,119,121). The recognition of cellular schwannoma permits nerve-sparing surgery and obviates both radical surgery and adjuvant radiation or chemotherapy. Its slow clinical progression, lack of a significant association with neurofibromatosis, and

failure to metastasize all distinguish this tumor from conventional MPNST.

Clinical Features. With rare exception (103, 119), cellular schwannomas are solitary lesions. In the Mayo Clinic experience, they represent approximately 5 percent of benign PNST (103). Females are twice as often affected as males. Although they occur over a wide age range, with a maximal incidence in the fourth decade (119), nearly 5 percent present in childhood and adolescence (103). A similar small proportion, 2 to 4 percent, arise in the setting of NF1 (103,108, 119). Cellular schwannomas grow slowly, some enlarging imperceptibly over a period of as many as 20 years. Most present as painless, palpable masses, but a minority produce neurologic symptoms including pain, paresthesia, or weakness. Occasional examples are incidentally encountered on physical examination or at radiography. Cellular schwannomas show a tendency to involve either the paravertebral region of the mediastinum, pelvis, or retroperitoneum, or the intraspinal space (103). Of tumors related to the spinal space, approximately one third have a dumbbell configuration, and a similar number show bone erosion. In one large series, nearly 10 percent were intracranial, some affecting cranial nerves 5 and 8 (103). Other favored sites include the head and neck as well as the extremities (119). Tumors involving the limbs rarely occur distal to the wrists and ankles (119). Dermal lesions are similarly rare (103). Resectability is in large part dependent upon tumor location. As is further discussed below, recurrences are few and are slow to present; no metastases have been described, nor has transformation to MPNST.

Gross Findings. Like conventional schwannomas, cellular schwannomas are well circumscribed and encapsulated. Approximately one third arise from a recognizable nerve (119); these are globular, lie eccentric to the parent nerve, and lack the fusiform configuration often seen with nerve-associated MPNSTs (fig. 7-33A). On occasion, they are multinodular (fig. 7-33B) or even assume a plexiform configuration (see fig. 7-50). Cellular schwannomas range in size from 1 to 20 cm (mean, 5 cm). Typically rubbery and tan with gray-white or yellow areas (fig. 7-33), only a small minority grossly show areas of cystic degeneration. Foci of hemorrhage are common but, unlike in MPNST, gross necrosis is generally not

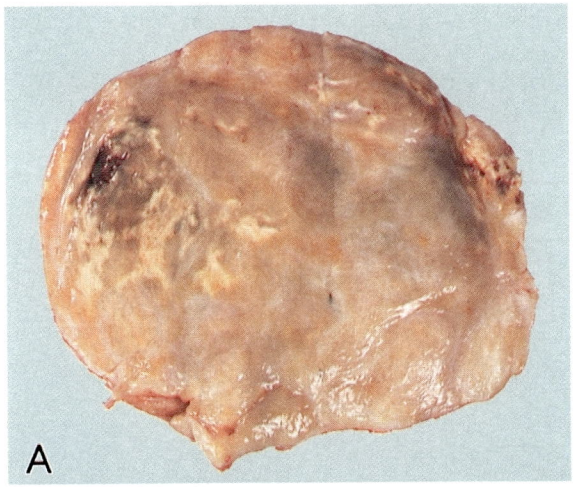

Figure 7-33
CELLULAR SCHWANNOMA
Unlike conventional schwannoma, the cellular variant is often more fleshy (A). Nonetheless, in terms of its gross encapsulation and the eccentric position of nerve-associated examples, it clearly represents a variant of schwannoma. Gross multinodularity (B) is an uncommon feature. Conventional schwannomas occasionally feature a cellular component (C). This example, consisting only in large part of pale cellular schwannoma tissue, underscores the close relationship between conventional and cellular tumors.

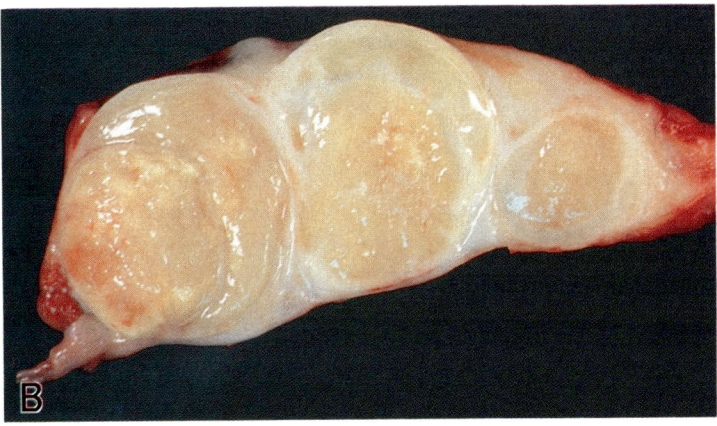

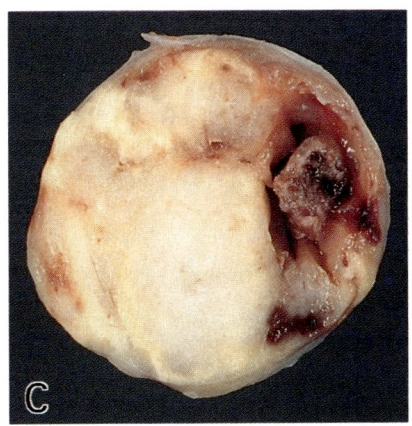

a feature. Most exhibit a smooth margin, even in areas of bone erosion. Radiographic or operative evidence of the latter is most frequently seen in tumors of the lumbosacral region (119). An irregular surface is decidedly unusual, as is partial lack of a capsule (119) or focal infiltration of nearby tissue (fig. 7-34, right).

Microscopic Findings. Microscopically, cellular schwannomas exhibit many features of conventional schwannoma, including their characteristic cytology (fig. 7-35), the presence of a well-formed capsule (fig. 7-36A), hyalinization of tumor vasculature (fig. 7-36B), and collections of lipid-laden histiocytes (fig. 7-36C). Architecturally, they differ from conventional schwannoma by their higher cellularity (fig. 7-35); more uniform pattern; frequent capsular, subcapsular, and perivascular lymphocytic infiltrates (fig. 7-36D); and the less frequent occurrence of hemosiderin depos-

its. All examples are dominated by Antoni A tissue (fig. 7-35) (119). The Antoni B pattern, although focally present in nearly two thirds of cases in one series (103), generally occupies no more than 10 percent of the tumor area and is often subcapsular in location (119). Cellularity varies, among and within tumors (fig. 7-37). Gross cysts are unusual, but nearly one fourth exhibit microcyst formation (103). Microfoci of necrosis are rare, and are usually solitary findings. Such foci commonly consist of circumscribed areas of pale-staining tissue devoid of nuclear detail. Unlike the geographic necrosis of MPNST, foci of necrosis in cellular schwannoma are not sharply demarcated and almost always lack pseudopalisading (fig. 7-34, left). In some instances, the presence of necrosis may be related to prior trauma (119). On close inspection, hematoxylin and eosin–stained sections show the

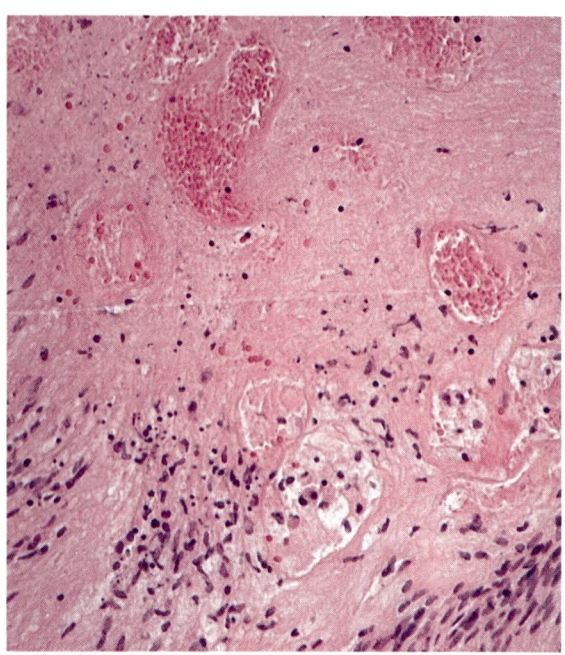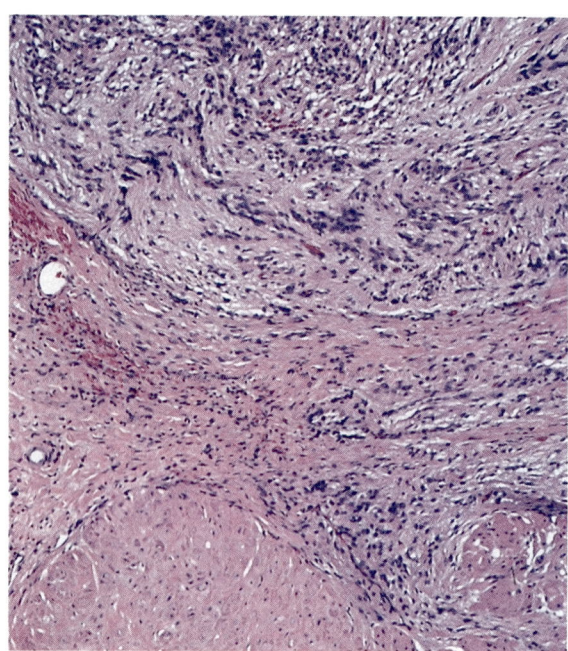

Figure 7-34
CELLULAR SCHWANNOMA
Focal nonpalisading necrosis (left) and occasional limited infiltration of nearby structures, the urinary bladder in this case (right), are not indicative of malignancy and are seen in a minority of cases.

presence of residual nerve within the capsule in approximately 15 percent of cases (103).

The predominant Antoni A component of cellular schwannomas consists of sheets of occasionally interlacing spindle cells. These have thin tapered nuclei with frequent but not invariable hyperchromasia. The cytoplasm is eosinophilic and afibrillar, and cell borders are indistinct (fig. 7-39). Some nuclear pleomorphism may be present but usually does not approach that noted in "ancient" schwannomas (fig. 7-39B,C). In a minority of cases, vague storiform and ill-defined fascicular or whorling patterns may be evident (fig. 7-40). Nuclear palisading has been noted in 10 to 15 percent of cases (fig. 7-38A)(103,119), but well-formed Verocay bodies are lacking (119). Aggregation of nuclei into tight clusters is also occasionally seen (fig. 7-38B). Otherwise typical schwannomas, when seen with such clustering, do not qualify as "cellular" (114). Foci of loose textured myxoid stroma superficially resembling that of neurofibroma are noted in approximately 10 percent of cases (fig. 7-38C)(103,119). Mitotic figures are present in up to 70 percent of tumors and generally range from 1 to 4 per 10 high-power fields. In one large series (103), half of the tumors exhibited an average of 1 mitotic figure per 10 high-power fields. Although examples with as many as 8 mitoses per 10 high-power fields have been reported (fig. 7-35, left)(119), we have occasionally encountered even greater proliferative indices (fig. 7-39D). Thus, we do not agree with those who believe brisk mitotic activity is indicative of malignancy in these tumors.

Immunohistochemical Findings. As with conventional schwannomas, cellular schwannomas almost always show strong, uniform S-100 protein immunoreactivity (fig. 7-41A)(103,104, 108,119,121). In contrast, Leu-7 stains in only one third to half the cases and is irregular and patchy (fig. 7-41B). Myelin basic protein reactivity was observed commonly in one series (119). GFAP staining is evident in nearly half of tumors (103) and may be strong (fig. 7-41C). As in ordinary schwannomas, the presence of basement membrane is reflected in pericellular laminin or collagen 4 reactivity (fig. 7-41D). Unlike perineurioma, the neoplastic cells of cellular schwannoma do not stain for epithelial membrane antigen

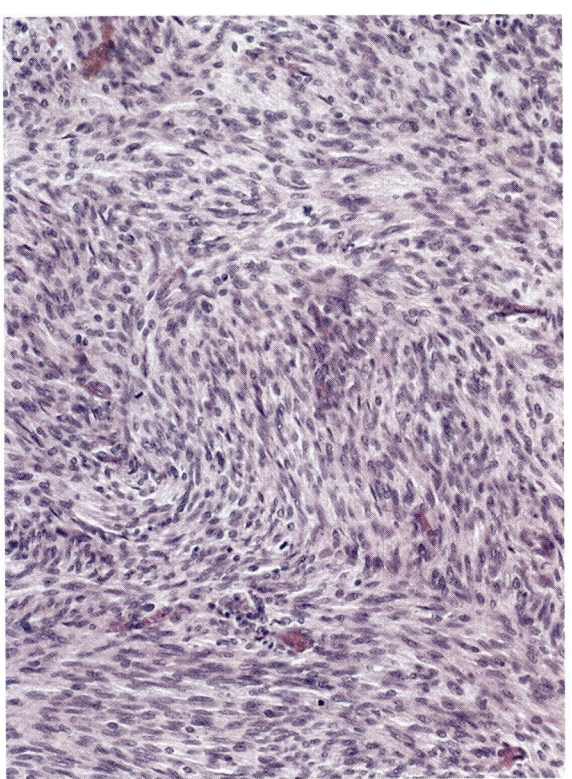
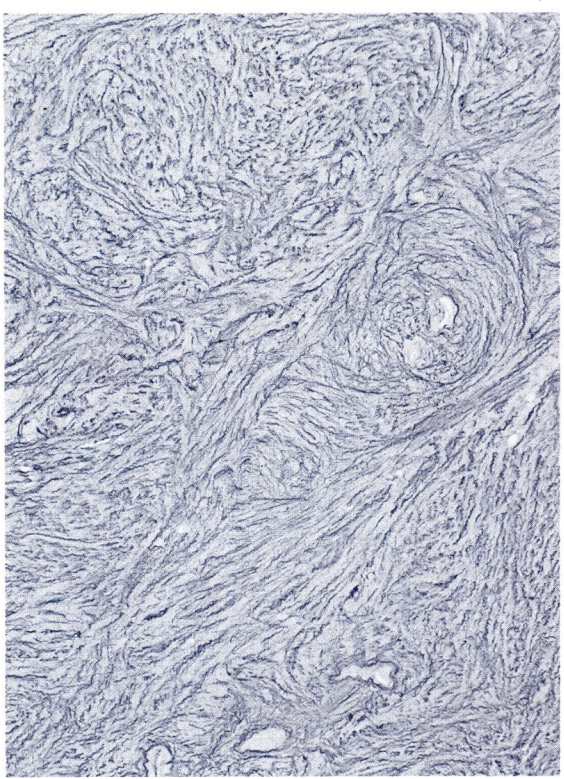

Figure 7-35
CELLULAR SCHWANNOMA
The essential histologic feature is cellular Antoni A tissue (left). Due to the presence of pericellular basement membrane, cells are individually surrounded by reticulin (right).

(EMA). The scant capsular EMA reactivity noted in half of cellular schwannomas simply reflects the presence of residual normal perineurial cells (119). Although the bulk of the parent nerve usually lies within the capsule of conventional schwannomas, individual neurofilament-positive axons are occasionally seen within peripheral portions of cellular schwannomas, particularly in the subcapsular region (fig. 7-41E) (103,104).

Immunostaining for proliferation markers, including proliferating cell nuclear antigen (PCNA) and MIB-1 (Ki-67 antigen), has been studied in a large series of cellular schwannoma (103). Nuclear labeling for both proliferation markers varied widely; median values were 6 percent and 8 percent, respectively (fig. 7-41F). One recent series compared PCNA and MIB-1 staining in benign PNSTs, including conventional and cellular schwannomas, to that in MPNST (112). Whereas nearly all MPNSTs showed MIB-1 labeling indices in the range of 5

to 65 percent, neither conventional nor cellular schwannoma had indices in excess of 1 percent. Overlap of PCNA indices between MPNST and schwannoma was considerable, and the most reliable cutoff value was 75 percent.

Ultrastructural Findings. Electron microscopy plays a role in the diagnosis of cellular schwannoma and in its distinction from light microscopically similar tumors (see below). Although it has been suggested that cellular schwannomas may be less fully differentiated than conventional schwannomas (105), we view them as well-differentiated neoplasms showing the full spectrum of Schwann cell features (103,104,108, 119,121). Most conspicuous are elongate, interlacing processes covered with a continuous, occasionally duplicated basement membrane and joined by poorly developed intercellular junctions. As previously noted, nuclei are more abundant and often more atypical than those of conventional schwannoma (fig. 7-42). This is manifested

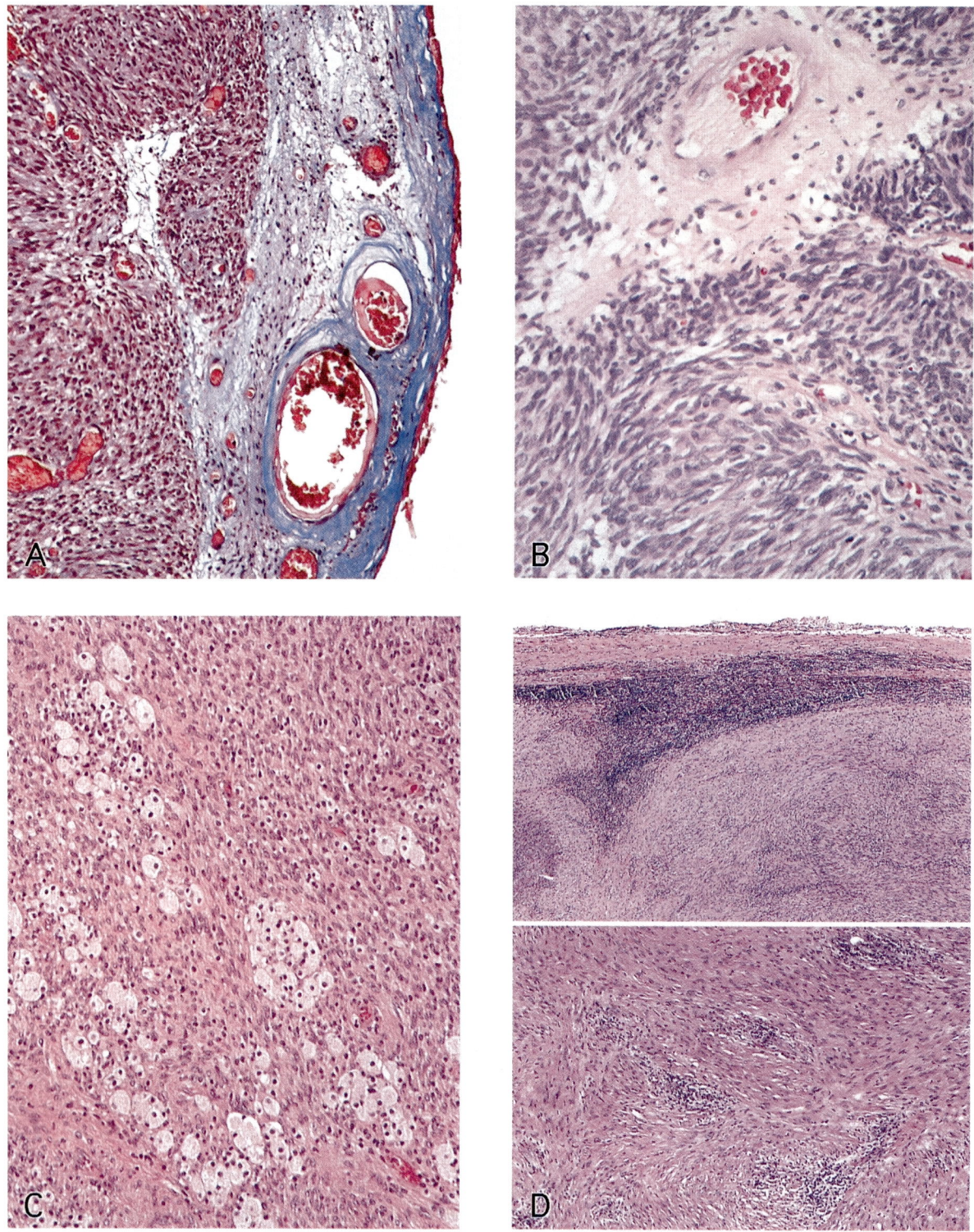

Figure 7-36
CELLULAR SCHWANNOMA

Encapsulation is a characteristic feature (A), here highlighted on trichrome stain. Also diagnostically helpful is the finding of vascular hyalinization (B) and patchy histiocyte accumulation (C). Patchy capsular (D, top) and perivascular (D, bottom) chronic inflammation is also a common finding.

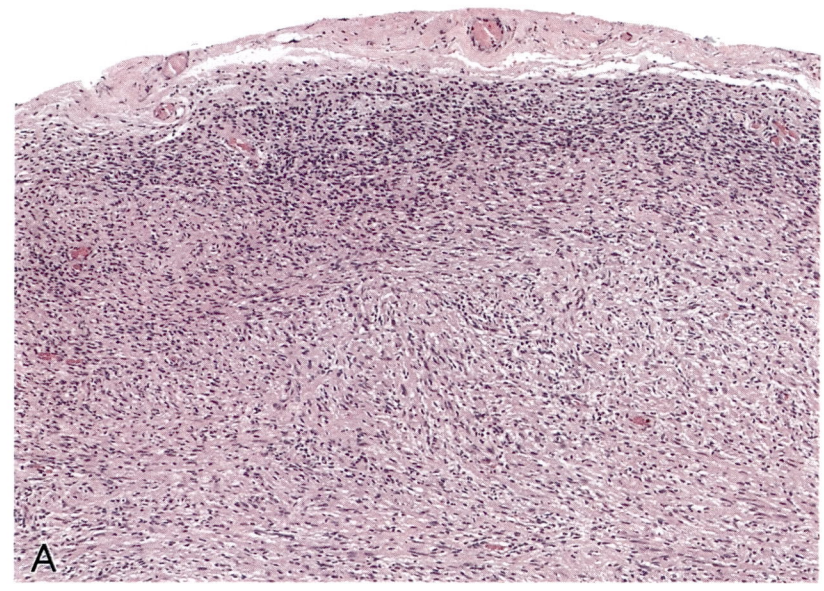

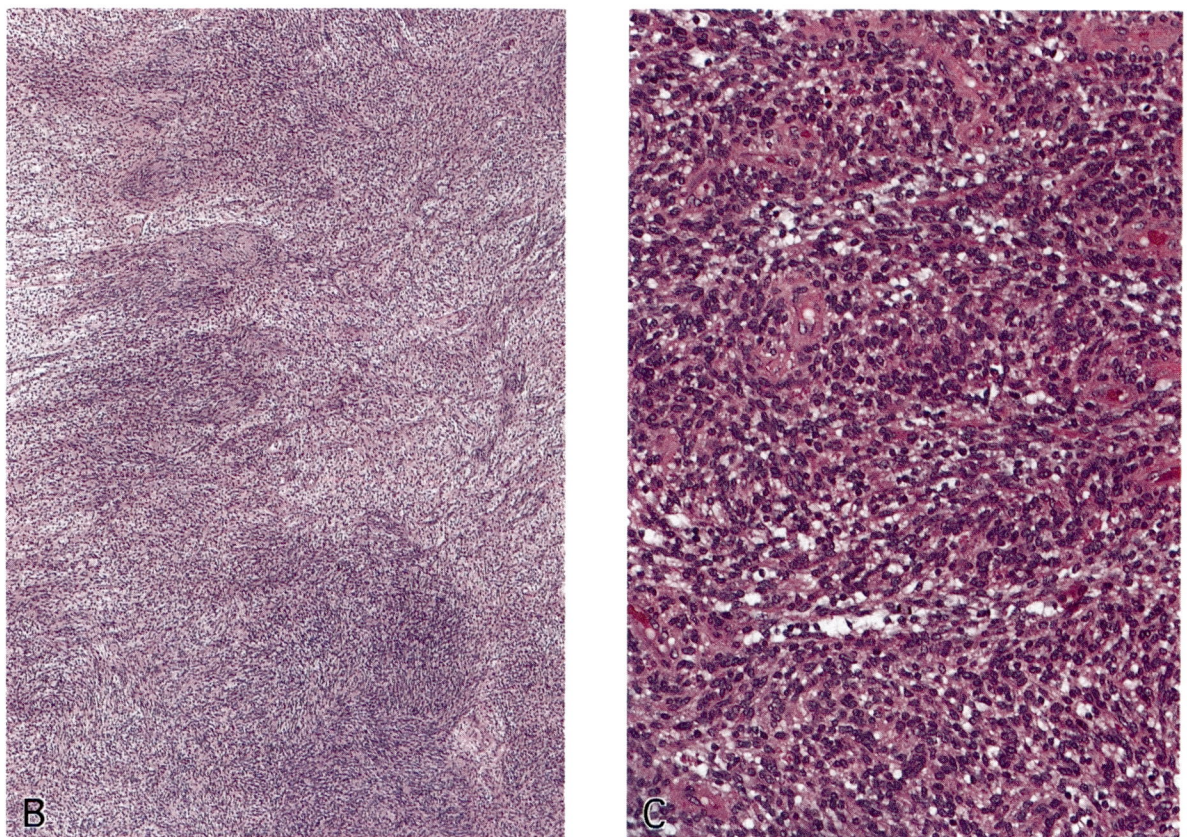

Figure 7-37
CELLULAR SCHWANNOMA

Hypercellularity may be uniform (A) or patchy (B). Fields in which cells are transversely sectioned may appear particularly cellular (C).

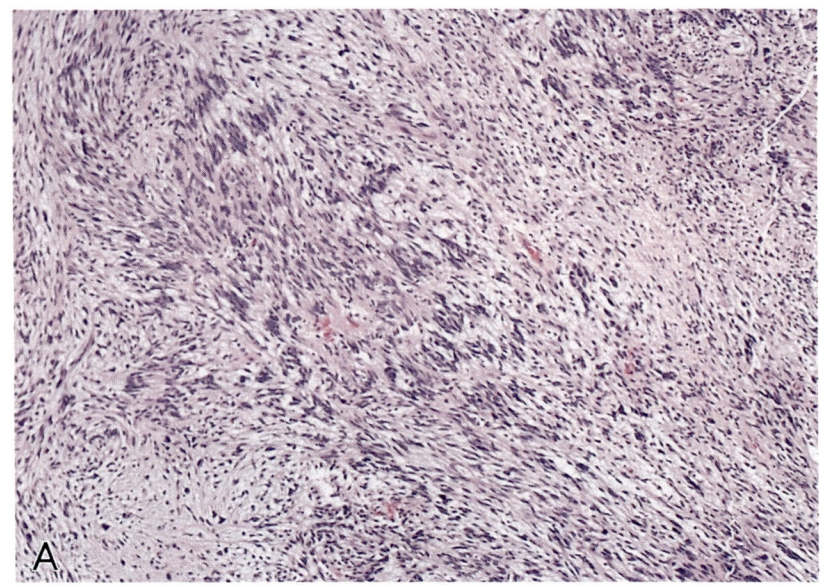

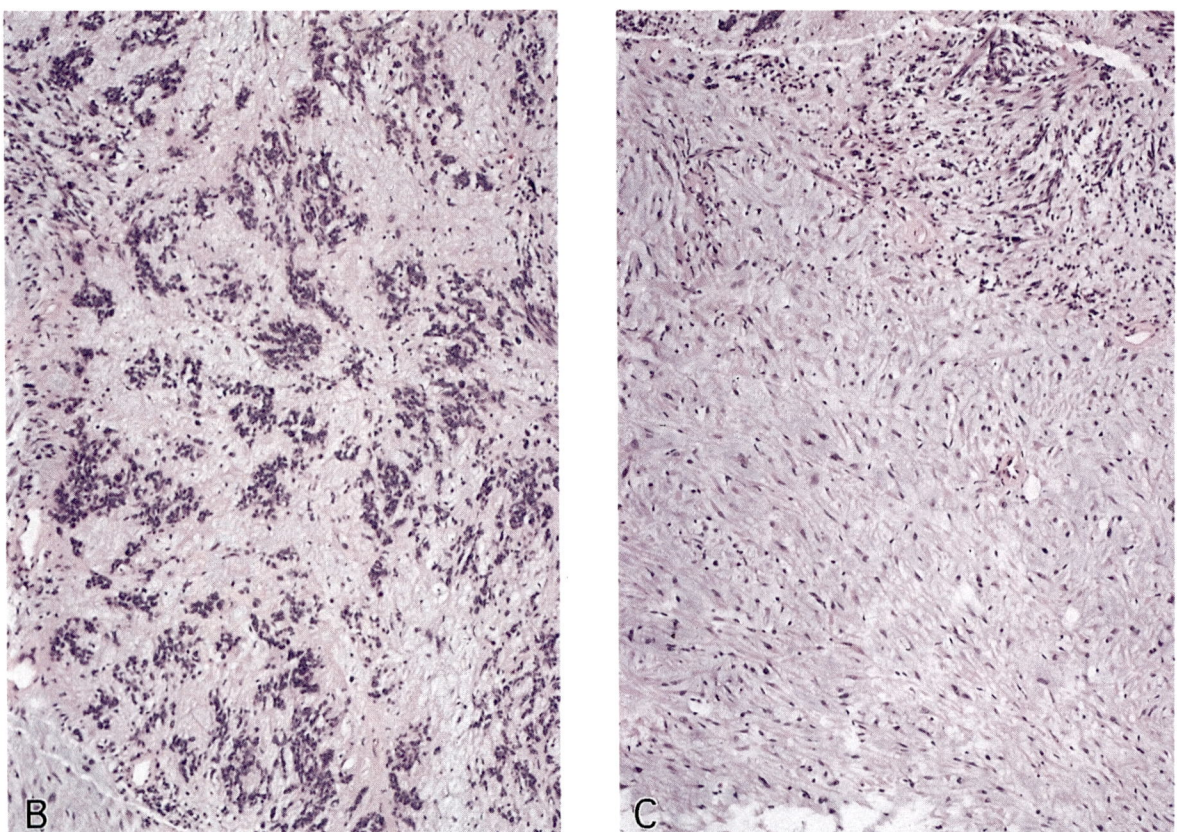

Figure 7-38
CELLULAR SCHWANNOMA
Unusual features of cellular schwannoma include regimentation of nuclei in a Verocay body–like manner (A), clustering of nuclei (B), and focal stromal myxoid change (C).

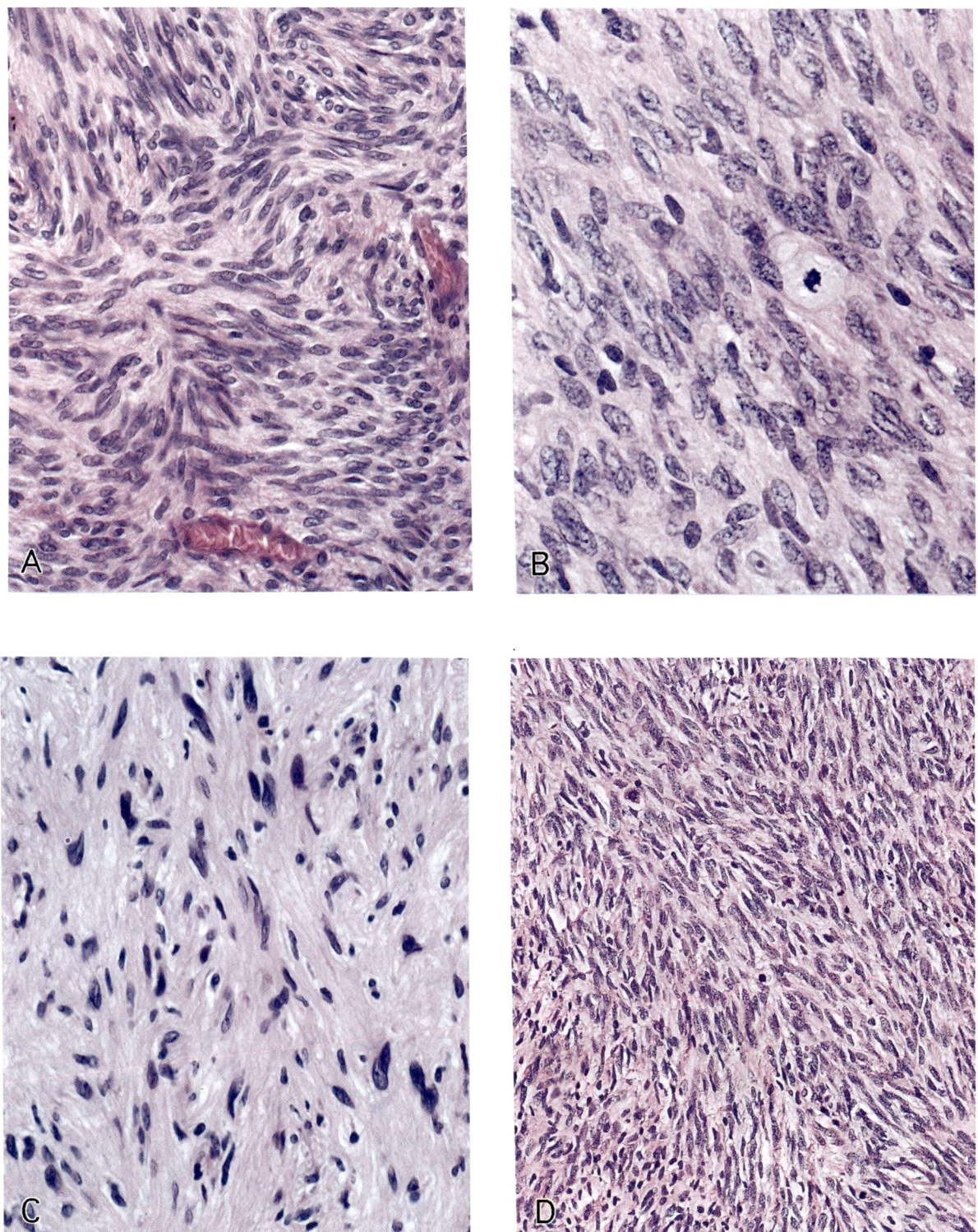

Figure 7-39
CELLULAR SCHWANNOMA

Nuclear uniformity is the rule (A), but some pleomorphism and nucleolar prominence may be seen (B). Smudgy degenerative nuclear atypia (C) is less common than in conventional schwannomas. Although mitoses vary in frequency, from scant to occasional in most cases, they may be conspicuous (D).

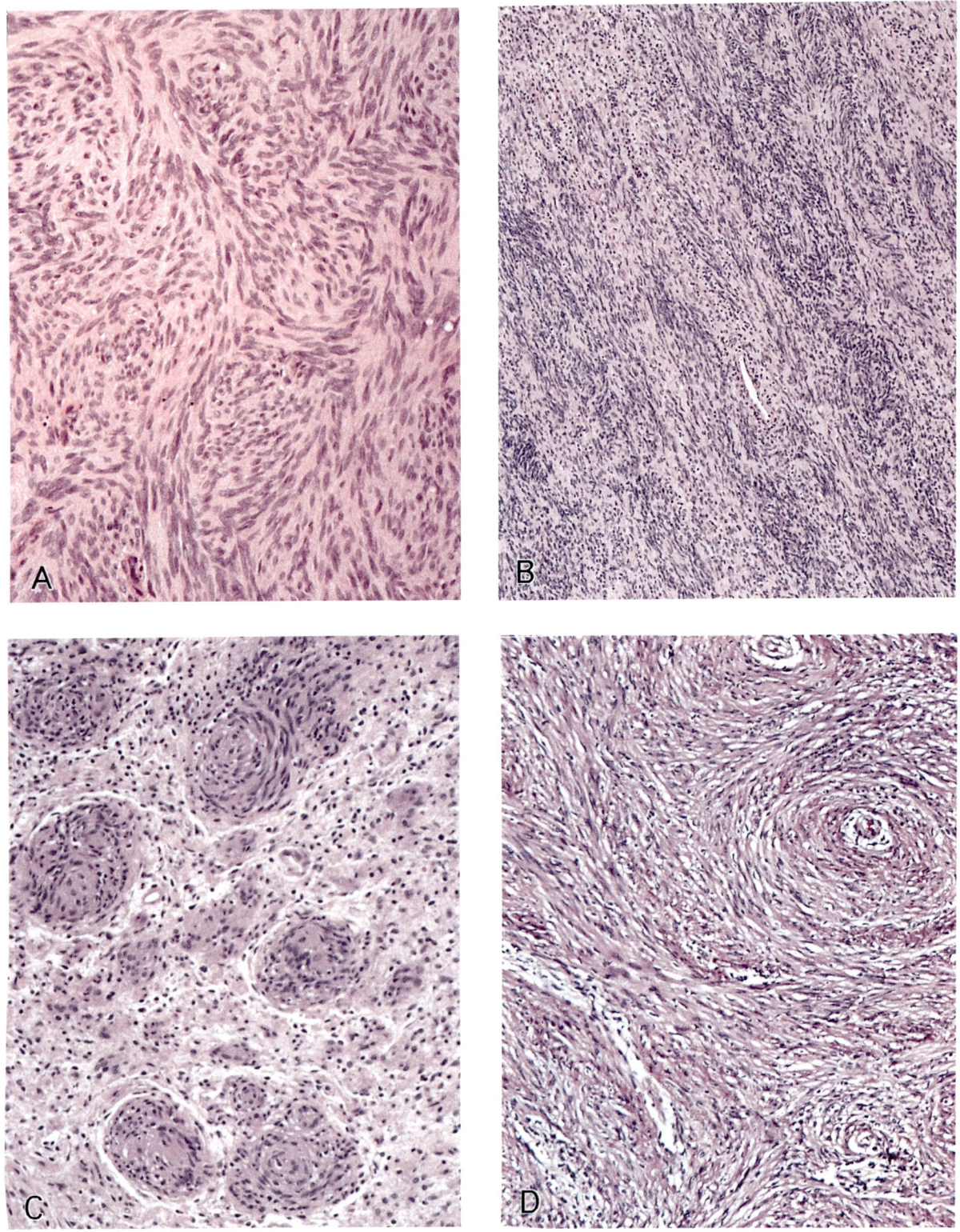

Figure 7-40
CELLULAR SCHWANNOMA
Although Antoni A tissue comprises most if not all of these tumors, the histologic pattern varies and includes curving fascicles (A), straight fascicles (B), and compact or loose cellular whorls (C,D).

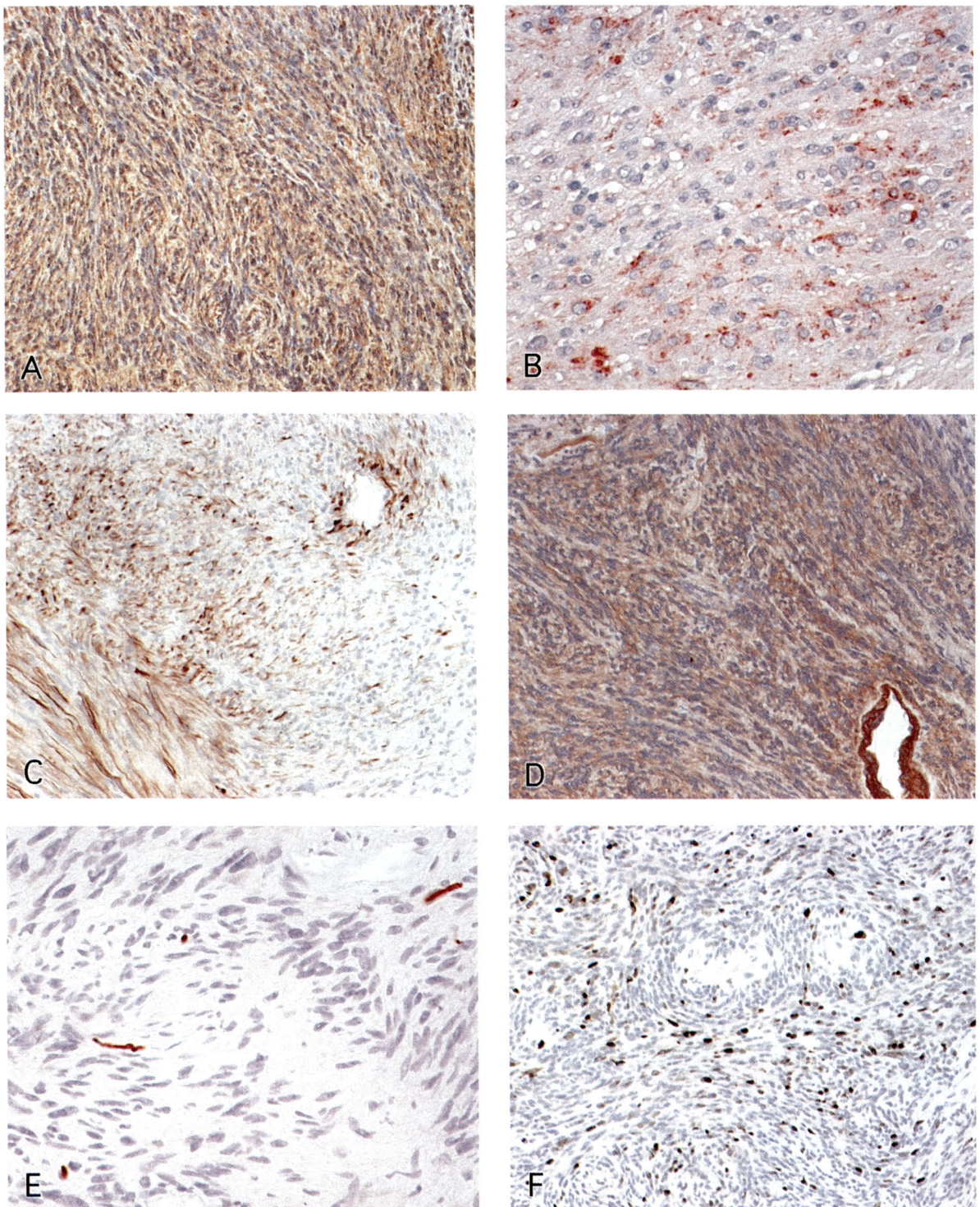

Figure 7-41
CELLULAR SCHWANNOMA

Like conventional schwannoma, the cellular variant is characterized by uniform immunoreactivity for S-100 protein (A), patchy Leu-7 staining (B), frequent staining for glial fibrillary acidic protein (C), and uniform pericellular reactivity for laminin or collagen 4 (D). While residual neurofilament-positive axons, when encountered, are usually seen in the capsule, they may occasionally be found within subcapsular portions of the tumor (E). Stains for the proliferation marker MIB-1 often show moderate labeling indices (F).

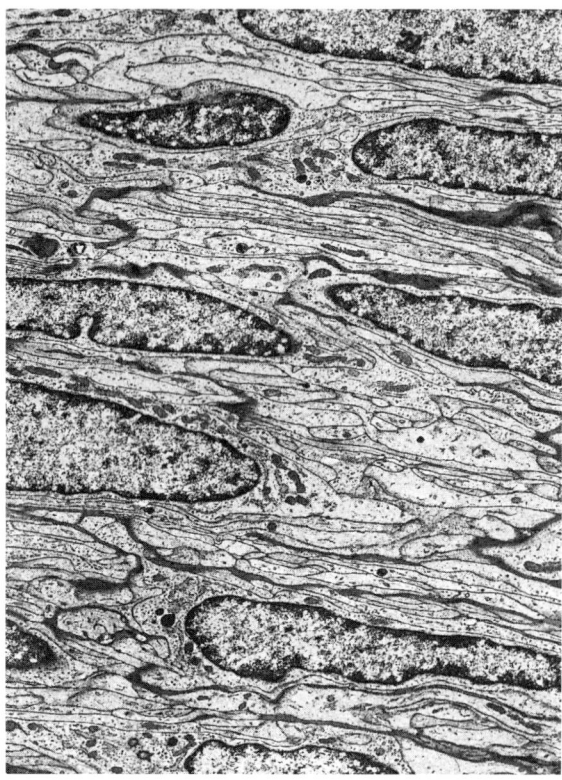

Figure 7-42
CELLULAR SCHWANNOMA
Nuclei are more abundant in cellular than in conventional schwannomas (X6,800).

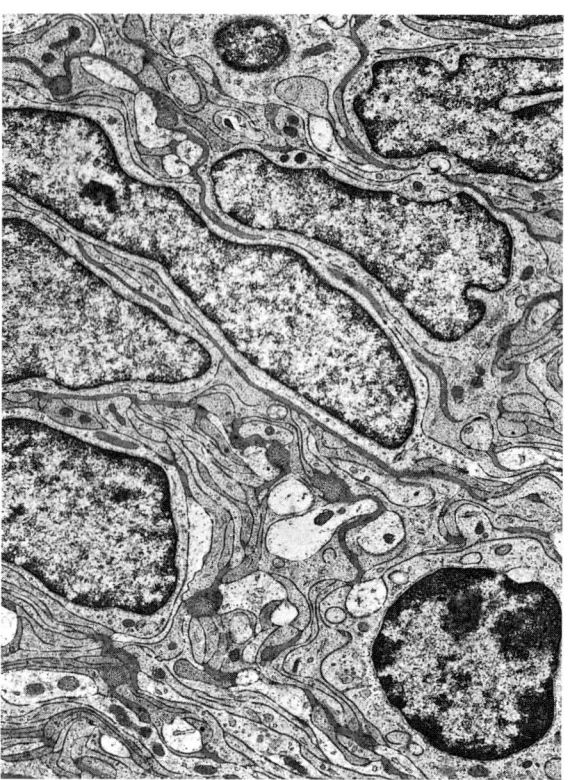

Figure 7-43
CELLULAR SCHWANNOMA
Note nuclear pleomorphism, marginated chromatin, and tortuous arrays of Schwann cell processes (X10,600).

by irregular contours, increased heterochromatin, and larger nucleoli (fig. 7-43). Abortive mesaxon formation, often around bundles of stromal collagen, is less commonly seen than in conventional schwannoma. Cytoplasm is moderate in quantity and contains scattered nonspecific organelles, small numbers of intermediate filaments, and occasional microtubules. If sampling includes an Antoni B component, scattered lysosomes and cytoplasmic lipid droplets may be seen. The intercellular matrix varies in quantity, particularly in terms of its collagen content. Long-spacing collagen is less commonly observed in cellular schwannomas (15 percent) than in conventional tumors (103,119).

DNA Flow Cytometry. A recent study of the DNA flow cytometric characteristics of cellular schwannoma (103) found two thirds to be diploid and the remainder equally divided among tetraploid and aneuploid examples. S-phase determinations ranged from 1 to 26 percent (mean, 6.6 percent);

values for diploid, tetraploid, and aneuploid tumors were 5.5, 5.5, and 11.5 percent, respectively. No differences in S-phase determinations were noted among nonrecurring and recurring tumors.

Differential Diagnosis. Cellular schwannoma must be distinguished from sarcoma, particularly *well-differentiated MPNST*. Salient features distinguishing these lesions are summarized in Table 7-2. Unlike patients with cellular schwannoma, over half of those with MPNST have NF1 or tumors arising within a neurofibroma. The gross appearance of MPNSTs also differs from that of cellular schwannoma in that MPNSTs more often originate in large nerves, are often fusiform rather than globular, typically possess a pseudocapsule rather than a well-formed fibrous capsule, and are gray-tan on cut surface, often showing obvious areas of necrosis. Microscopic foci of necrosis are typically geographic and are bordered by palisaded, poorly differentiated cells. Vascular hyalinization, perivascular lymphocytic

Table 7-2

CONVENTIONAL SCHWANNOMA, CELLULAR SCHWANNOMA, AND MPNST: DIFFERENTIAL DIAGNOSIS

Findings	Conventional Schwannoma	Cellular Schwannoma	MPNST
Gross	Usually globoid encapsulated tumor that has abundant homogeneous light tan tissue, and may be cystic or hemorrhagic and show yellow patches. No gross necrosis.	Usually globoid encapsulated tumor, firmer than classic schwannoma and homogeneously tan. Occasional patches of yellow, but no gross necrosis.	Fusiform or globoid, pseudocapsulated (infiltrative of surrounding tissues), firm, cream-tan, usually grossly necrotic tumor.
Microscopic	Antoni A and B areas with Verocay bodies; commonly find hyalinized thick-walled blood vessels and lipid-laden histiocytes. Mitotic figures infrequent. Rarely see malignant transformation.	Mainly hypercellular Antoni A tissue. Cells are arranged in fascicles or whorls and may show marked hyperchromasia and nuclear pleomorphism. Notable are lymphoid deposits in capsule or perivascular area. Commonly find thick-walled blood vessels and collections of lipid-laden histiocytes. Rare foci of necrosis. Mitoses not uncommon but usually numbers no more than 4/10 HPF.	Markedly hypercellular, fasciculated, spindle cell tumor generally consisting of cells of a uniform size and pronounced hyperchromasia. Geographic necrosis and mitotic counts in excess of 4/10 HPF are common. Epithelioid cells predominate in about 5 percent of tumors and 15 percent show heterologous glandular or sarcomatous elements.
Immunohistochemical	Diffuse and strong expression of S-100 protein.	Diffuse and strong expression of S-100 protein.	S-100 protein expression in scattered cells of 50-70 percent of cases.
Electron Microscopy	Well-differentiated cells with long, often interlacing cytoplasmic processes coated by basement membrane on their free surfaces. Intercellular long-spacing collagen common.	Similar to classic schwannoma. Increased cellularity. More nuclear atypia and occasional residual arrays of long, basement membrane-coated cytoplasmic processes. Long-spacing collagen less common.	Poorly differentiated cells with more pleomorphic nuclei, thick cytoplasmic processes, and sometimes patchy basement membrane. Long-spacing collagen rarely seen.
Clinical Behavior	May cause bone erosion and can recur if incompletely excised. Thus far 5 reported examples with malignant transformation that followed a malignant clinical course.	May cause bone erosion and recur if incompletely excised. Thus far no clinically malignant examples.	Has a proclivity to invade and destroy nearby soft tissues, recur locally, and metastasize distantly (usually to lung). About 90 percent are high-grade lesions.

infiltrates, collections of lipid-laden histiocytes, hemosiderin deposits, and minor Antoni B components are common in cellular schwannoma but are lacking in MPNSTs. Mitotic activity is far higher in MPNSTs than in cellular schwannomas, often in excess of 10 per 10 high-power fields. Divergent differentiation, a rare occurrence in schwannomas of any type, is evident in nearly 10 percent of MPNSTs. The uniform S-100 protein reactivity of cellular schwannomas also differs from that of MPNST which is often scattered or patchy at best. Only the occasional well-differentiated MPNST shows significant S-100 protein immunoreactivity. Whereas such rare tumors may also exhibit limited GFAP reactivity (109). Staining for GFAP is far more often seen in benign rather than malignant nerve sheath tumors (115). The same is true of staining for collagen 4 or laminin. Ultrastructurally, the uniform Schwann cell differentiation seen in cellular schwannoma is lacking in most MPNSTs, wherein cells are usually poorly differentiated and show only patchy basement membrane formation (107,110,111).

Cellular schwannomas on occasion exhibit foci resembling *neurofibroma*. Such lesions pose a diagnostic problem, given the fact that neurofibromas can give rise to MPNST. The distinction from neurofibroma rests with the higher cellularity of cellular schwannoma, and the larger, less uniform size and shape of its nuclei. Unlike in neurofibroma, S-100 protein reactivity in cellular schwannoma is present in virtually all cells, even those in neurofibroma-like areas. Lastly, neurofilament protein stains generally show more residual axons with neurofibromas than schwannomas.

To date, no bona fide examples of cellular schwannoma have been shown to undergo malignant change or to metastasize. Indeed, those rare schwannomas having done so have been conventional forms of the tumor. Furthermore, *schwannomas with malignant transformation* do not histologically resemble ordinary MPNST, but assume an epithelioid or a primitive neuroectodermal tumor (PNET)-like appearance (119,120). The subject is further discussed in chapter 11.

Unlike cellular schwannoma, *leiomyosarcoma* lacks a fibrous capsule, and on cut surface often exhibits a distinctive whorled pattern. No associated nerve involvement is evident. Nuclei often are blunt-ended rather than tapered like those of Schwann cells. The cells of leiomyosarcoma are somewhat better defined and, with optimal fixation, their cytoplasm is seen to be fibrillar. Such fibrils are highlighted on trichrome or PTAH stains by which they appear red or blue, respectively. Immunostains for actin are frequently positive, but desmin stains are less often so. With rare exception (117), S-100 protein reactivity is lacking in leiomyosarcoma. Ultrastructurally, the cytoplasm of leiomyosarcoma cells may be microfilament (actin) rich, especially in well-differentiated examples. On careful study, fusiform dense bodies, subplasmalemmal attachment plaques, and pinocytotic vesicles may be found. Basement membrane formation is common to both Schwann cell and smooth muscle tumors, but the latter lack long-spacing collagen (Luse bodies).

Unlike cellular schwannomas, *fibrosarcomas* exhibit linear rather than curved or sinuous nuclear and cytoplasmic outlines. The cells form parallel arrays which contribute to the formation of a fascicular, often "herringbone" pattern. They also have more distinct cytoplasmic borders. Like most soft tissue tumors, fibrosarcomas are strongly vimentin reactive, but do not stain for Schwann cell markers, including S-100 protein, Leu-7, and myelin basic protein. Ultrastructurally, the cytoplasm of fibrosarcomas contains an often well-developed, branching rough endoplasmic reticulum as well as a prominent Golgi apparatus. Basement membrane formation is absent in fibrosarcoma, but may be focally present in myofibroblastic tumors.

Cellular schwannomas must also be distinguished from *meningioma*, particularly ones occurring in the posterior fossa, at the skull base, or in the intraspinal space. Unlike schwannoma, a nerve-associated tumor, meningiomas are dura based. Enlargement of the spinal foramen is a common feature of schwannoma, but is infrequent in meningioma. At the microscopic level, meningiomas lack the hyaline capsule of a schwannoma as well as Antoni A and B pattern variation. Although a hyaline vasculature is common to both, schwannomas more often show perivascular macrophage and hemosiderin deposition. Collagen disposition in schwannoma is generally reticular, diffuse, and intercellular, whereas in meningioma it takes the form of bands or blocks. A dense intercellular pattern of reticulin staining is characteristic of schwannoma, but not of ordinary meningioma; only the uncommon fibrous variant of meningioma shows such extensive stroma formation. Although schwannomas may show whorled cells, such whorls are vague rather than discrete and tightly wound as in meningioma. Psammoma bodies, a common feature of meningioma, are largely limited to the melanotic variant of schwannoma. At the immunohistochemical level, schwannomas are readily recognized by their diffuse, strong S-100 protein reaction. In contrast, only 20 percent of meningiothelial or transitional meningiomas exhibit patchy S-100 protein reactivity (118). Extensive staining may, however, be seen in fibrous meningiomas (101). A membrane pattern of staining for epithelial membrane antigen is characteristic of meningiomas; instead, the occasional staining seen in schwannomas is patchy and cytoplasmic in distribution (118). Reactivity for GFAP may be seen in central and peripheral nervous system schwannomas (102,103) but is not observed in meningioma. Ultrastructure readily distinguishes schwannoma from meningioma in that the former exhibits long entangled processes enshrouded by basement membranes. In contrast meningioma shows interdigitation of cell membranes and well-formed desmosomes, but lacks basement membranes.

Treatment and Prognosis. Given the benign nature of cellular schwannoma, therapy should be conservative and directed towards sparing the parent nerve. Depending upon tumor location, the extent of tumor resection achieved varies considerably among reported series. In those series dealing primarily with peripherally situated tumors, 90 percent were amenable to gross total removal, with a recurrence rate of 5 percent (119). In contrast, cellular schwannomas affecting the intracranial space, spinal canal, and paravertebral region are more often debulked; their frequency of gross total removal falls to 10 percent (103). The rate of recurrence in one series in which central lesions were numerous averaged 16 percent; recurrence is particularly high in intraspinal (33 percent), sacral (37 percent), and intracranial (40 percent) lesions (103). The rate of tumor growth, whether of primary or recurrent lesions, is slow. In some cases the interval to recurrence may be as long as two decades; in the three largest series the mean time to recurrence was 7 years (103,112,119). Occasional tumors undergo multiple recurrences. Although there is no statistically significant association between recurrence and PCNA or MIB-1 labeling indices, a statistically significant association with mitotic index has been reported (103). To date, no cellular schwannoma has metastasized, nor have patients died of tumor.

PLEXIFORM SCHWANNOMA

Definition. This tumor is composed exclusively of Schwann cells and exhibits plexiform, most often intraneural, growth.

General Comments. Schwannomas of the conventional or cellular variety are occasionally multinodular or plexiform in configuration (122,

123–127,129–131,135). Such tumors primarily arise in dermal and subcutaneous tissue of young adults and are usually unassociated with NF1 or 2.

Clinical Features. Of the approximately 50 cases of plexiform schwannoma thus far reported, patient ages have ranged from 50 days to 80 years (mean, 34 years). About 75 percent occur in the first four decades. Both sexes are equally represented. Three patients had NF1 (129,131,132) and a number have had associated NF2 (128a,133). Only three congenital cases have been reported (122,126,131). Commonly, the mass had been present for years before diagnosis. Occasional tumors are painful or tender (129). At least 90 percent of plexiform schwannomas arise in the dermis or in subcutaneous tissue. Most often affected is an extremity, followed by the trunk and the head and neck. Rare examples present in the oral mucosa (123), vulva (135), and penis (130); visceral examples are very rare (fig. 7-44) (128). Multicentricity is infrequent (129,132,133).

Gross Findings. Plexiform schwannomas often are relatively circumscribed, gray-yellow or tan lesions composed of nodules representing segments of enlarged contorted nerve (figs. 7-44, 7-45). Few are grossly obvious; most are best appreciated at low magnification microscopy (fig. 7-46). The reported average dimensions range from 1.2 to 2.4 cm. Large tumors (over 10 cm) are rare (fig. 7-44) or involve viscera (fig. 7-45) (128, 135). Occasional soft tissue schwannomas assume a somewhat but not fully developed plexiform configuration (see fig. 7-8C). Unless such lesions are traumatized, neither hemorrhage nor necrosis are grossly evident. As in conventional schwannoma, the occasional finding of compressive erosion of adjacent bone is of no prognostic significance (fig. 7-44, bottom). Particularly in children, occasional examples are poorly circumscribed and infiltrative (131).

Histologic Findings. Microscopically, the tumors consist of round to oval nodules of varying size (fig. 7-47). Large nodules are often surrounded by a thin fibrous capsule (fig. 7-47, right) or are unencapsulated. The number of nodular profiles comprising a tumor ranges from 2 to at least 50 (126,135). In many instances, serial sections show that the nodular, puzzle piece–shaped profiles are interconnecting (fig. 7-46). A majority of tumors are composed entirely of compact

Figure 7-44
PLEXIFORM SCHWANNOMA
This unusually large, recently growing example (top) from the skin and subcutaneous tissue of the hip of a 78-year-old man had been present for over 50 years, and had been the basis of a draft deferment. Note the plexiform, nodular appearance of the lesion, as well as its focal yellow color, a reflection of lipid accumulation. (Fig. 1 from Hirose T, Scheithauer BW, Sano T. Giant plexiform schwannoma: report of two cases with soft tissue and visceral involvement. Mod Pathol 1997;11: 1075–81.) As in the case of conventional schwannoma (see fig. 7-5), plexiform tumors abutting bone may cause osseous erosion (bottom). In this case the site of erosion was the cortex of the tibial bone. Thirteen months earlier, a plexiform schwannoma had been resected from the leg of this 18-month-old boy (see ref. 122).

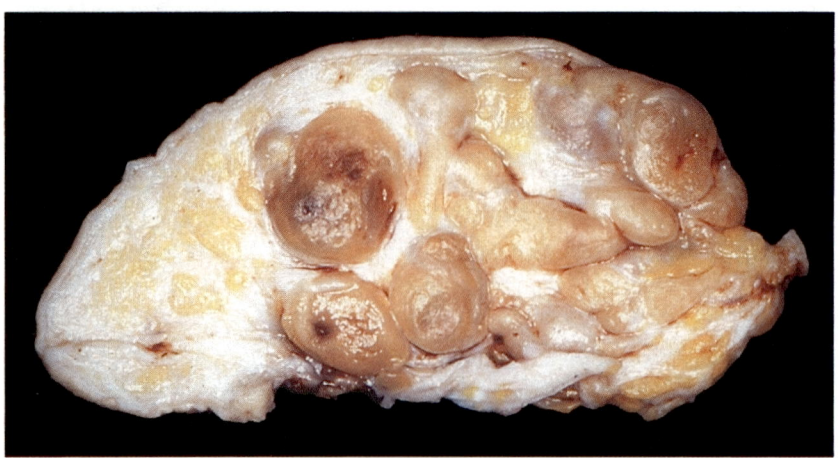

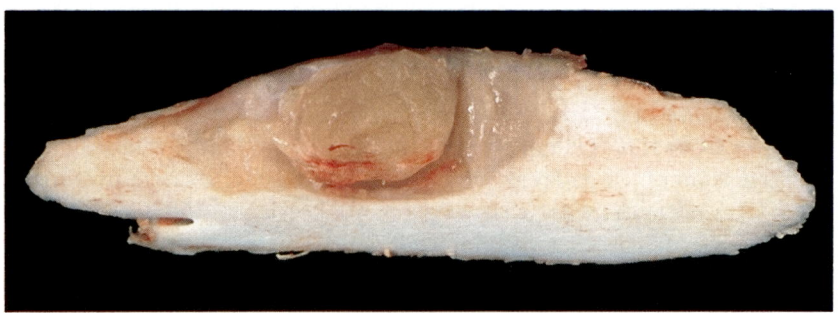

cellular Antoni A tissue (fig. 7-46); only a few feature Antoni B tissue, and even fewer show Verocay body formation. More common than the latter are solitary, simple arrays of palisaded nuclei (nuclear palisades) (fig. 7-48A), sweeping arrays of cells (fig. 7-48B), or cloverleaf-like clusters of nuclei (fig. 7-48C). The cytologic features are typical of schwannoma (fig. 7-49). Degenerative nuclear atypia may be seen but, as a rule, mitoses are rare (fig. 7-49) and necrosis is absent. Some tumors are sufficiently cellular to be placed in the cellular schwannoma category (fig. 7-50).

A subset of plexiform schwannoma recently reported by Meis-Kindblom and Enzinger (131) and designated "plexiform malignant peripheral nerve sheath tumors of infancy and childhood," includes some examples featuring infiltrative growth resembling entangled hypercellular nerves. The tumors in this subgroup are usually markedly hypercellular, with hyperchromatic nuclei and a somewhat increased mitotic index (mean, 4 per 10 high-power fields). We have independently studied some of the cases reported by these authors: ultrastructurally, one of

the tumors was composed of differentiated Schwann cells (122), and all were strongly immunoreactive for S-100 protein. Based on this, we consider these tumors, with the possible exception of one congenital orbital lesion, to be plexiform cellular schwannomas (134).

Immunohistochemical Findings. Plexiform schwannomas are reactive for S-100 protein (fig. 7-51, left) (129,130) and in most cases for GFAP (129). As in other Schwann cell tumors, reactivity for S-100 protein is present in both nuclei and cytoplasm (130). Consistent but weak reactivity for neuron-specific enolase has been reported, but none stained for myelin basic protein (129). Neurofilament protein stains show small numbers of residual axons coursing within the plexiform structures (fig. 7-51, right).

Ultrastructural Findings. The fine structural features of plexiform schwannoma are identical to those of conventional schwannoma (figs. 7-52, 7-53) (124,128,135).

Differential Diagnosis. The differential diagnosis includes plexiform neurofibromas, palisaded encapsulated neuroma, traumatic neuroma, and

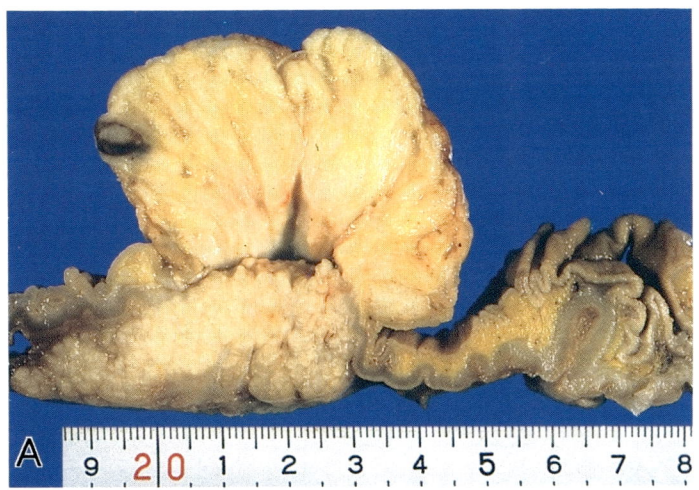

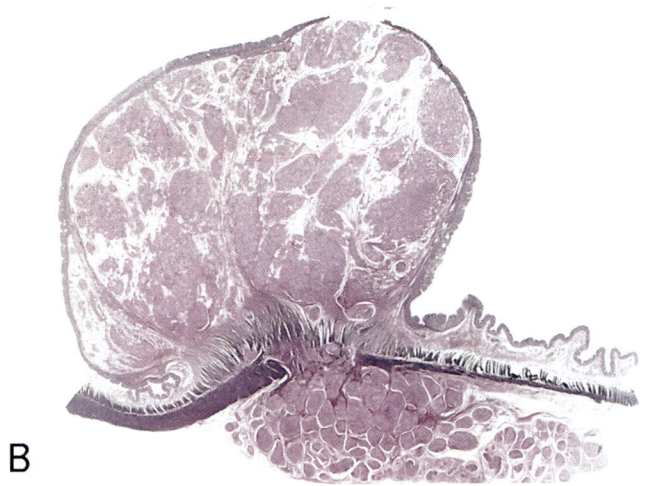

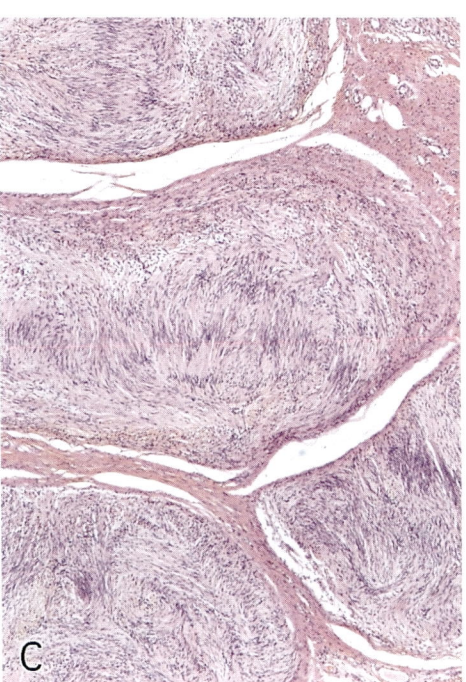

Figure 7-45
PLEXIFORM SCHWANNOMA
This giant visceral example (A) arose in the colon of a 54-year-old male without neurofibromatosis. Note the polypoid intraluminal and serosal components (B). Microsections show typical schwannoma features including Verocay bodies (C). (Fig. 2 from Hirose T, Scheithauer BW, Sano T. Giant plexiform schwannoma: report of two cases with soft tissue and visceral involvement. Mod Pathol 1997;11:1075–81.)

cutaneous leiomyoma. The distinction from *plexiform neurofibroma* is based upon the uniform appearance of ovoid to spindled nuclei in neurofibromas, ones smaller and more widely spaced than those of plexiform schwannoma. The cells of neurofibroma are often separated by large collagen bundles and an abundant mucinous matrix. Unlike the uniform staining of schwannoma, S-100 protein preparations are reactive in only a portion of neurofibroma cells. Plexiform schwannomas are most closely simulated by *palisaded encapsulated neuroma (PEN)*. The latter, although usually uninodular, may occasionally have a somewhat multinodular configuration, and features vague microfasciculation, little or no well-formed nuclear palisades, and far more abundant axonal processes. Numerous intralesional axons are an even more prominent feature in

traumatic neuroma, a process lacking the circumscription and nuclear palisading of plexiform schwannoma. In addition, an obvious parent nerve is often seen in traumatic neuroma. *Cutaneous leiomyoma* is composed of cells with more dense, fibrillated cytoplasm, and may readily be distinguished from plexiform schwannoma by staining for muscle markers such as HHF35 (muscle common actin) and smooth muscle actin.

Treatment and Prognosis. The prognosis for patients with plexiform schwannoma is excellent following simple excision alone. Only one of the well-circumscribed tumors reported in adults recurred locally; this, the largest plexiform schwannoma yet reported, was a 15 x 10 x 4 cm tumor removed from the vulva of a 26-year-old woman (135). The tumor focally had a mitotic count of 8 per 10 high-power fields. There were

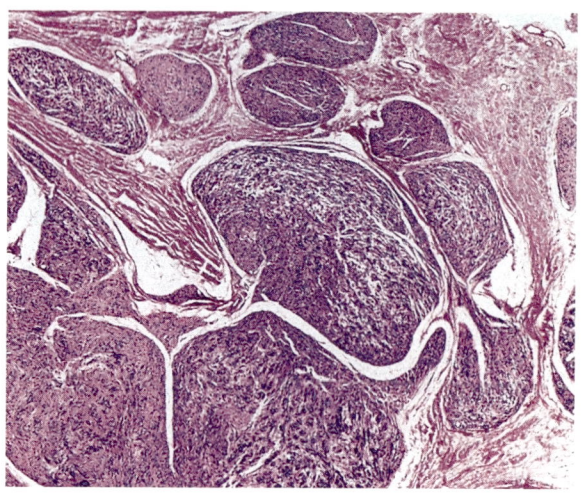 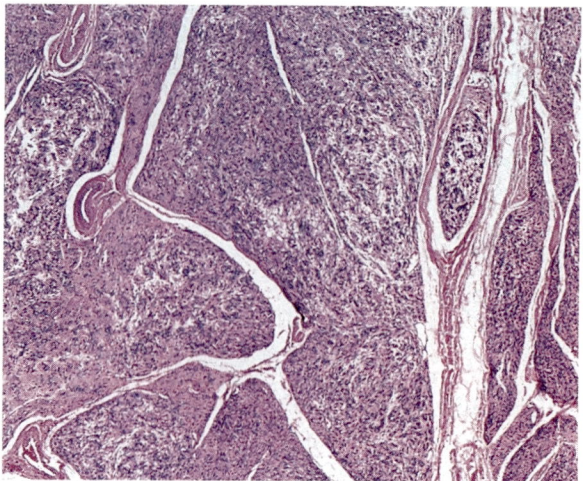

Figure 7-46
PLEXIFORM SCHWANNOMA
Cellular, worm-like expansions of dermal nerves appear oval (left) or geometric in contour (right). Like puzzle pieces, the profiles are separated one from the other and from surrounding connective tissue by cracking artifact.

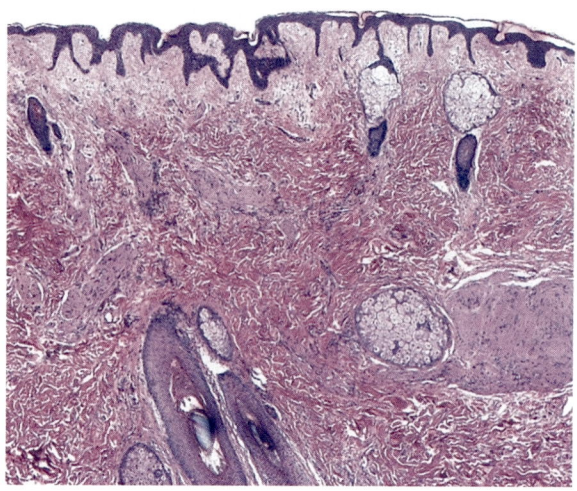 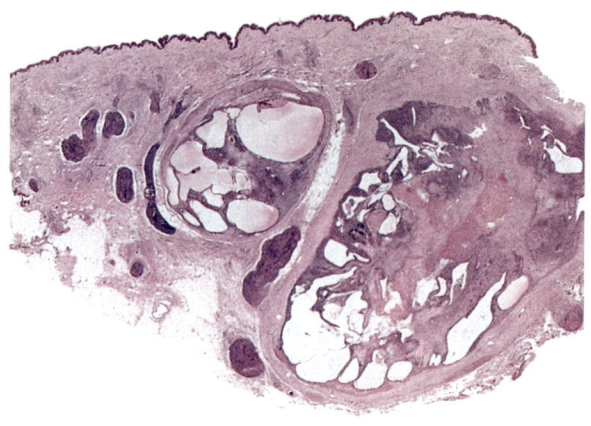

Figure 7-47
PLEXIFORM SCHWANNOMA
Whole mount sections of two cutaneous examples. The profile of a small tumor (left) lies among skin adnexae. A larger tumor (right) affects dermal and subcutaneous nerves and shows cystic change.

two local recurrences, the first measuring 3 mm and the second 5 mm in greatest dimension. This patient was alive and well after 3 years.

In contrast, five of the nine plexiform schwannomas of infants and children reported by Meis-Kindblom and Enzinger (131) recurred locally 8 to 31 months following initial excision. Some of these were originally infiltrative, noncircum-scribed tumors. Of the nine patients, the tumor of one recurred to invade bone. Yet another patient, a newborn with an orbital lesion, died of locally invasive tumor within 1 year. Because of the presence of high cellularity, a mean mitotic rate of 4 per 10 high-power fields, local recurrence in four cases, locally aggressive behavior in two of six cases with follow-up, and death of the one

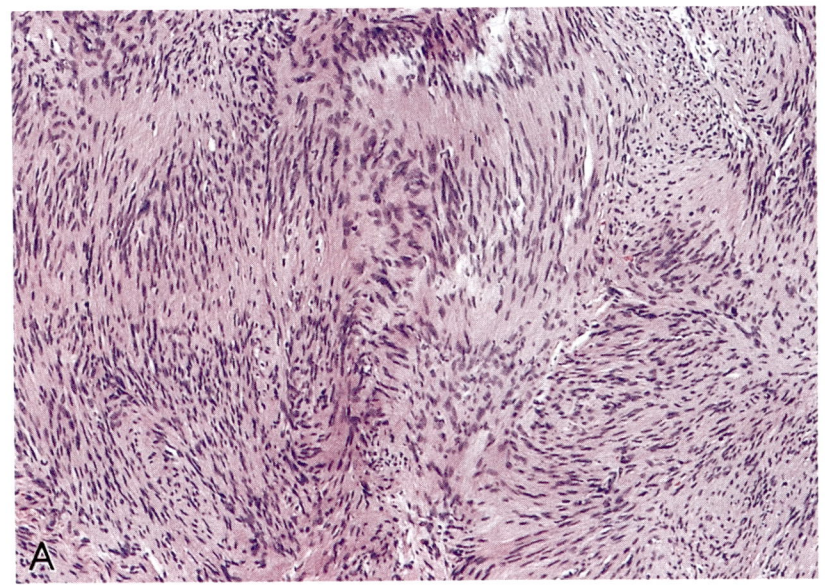

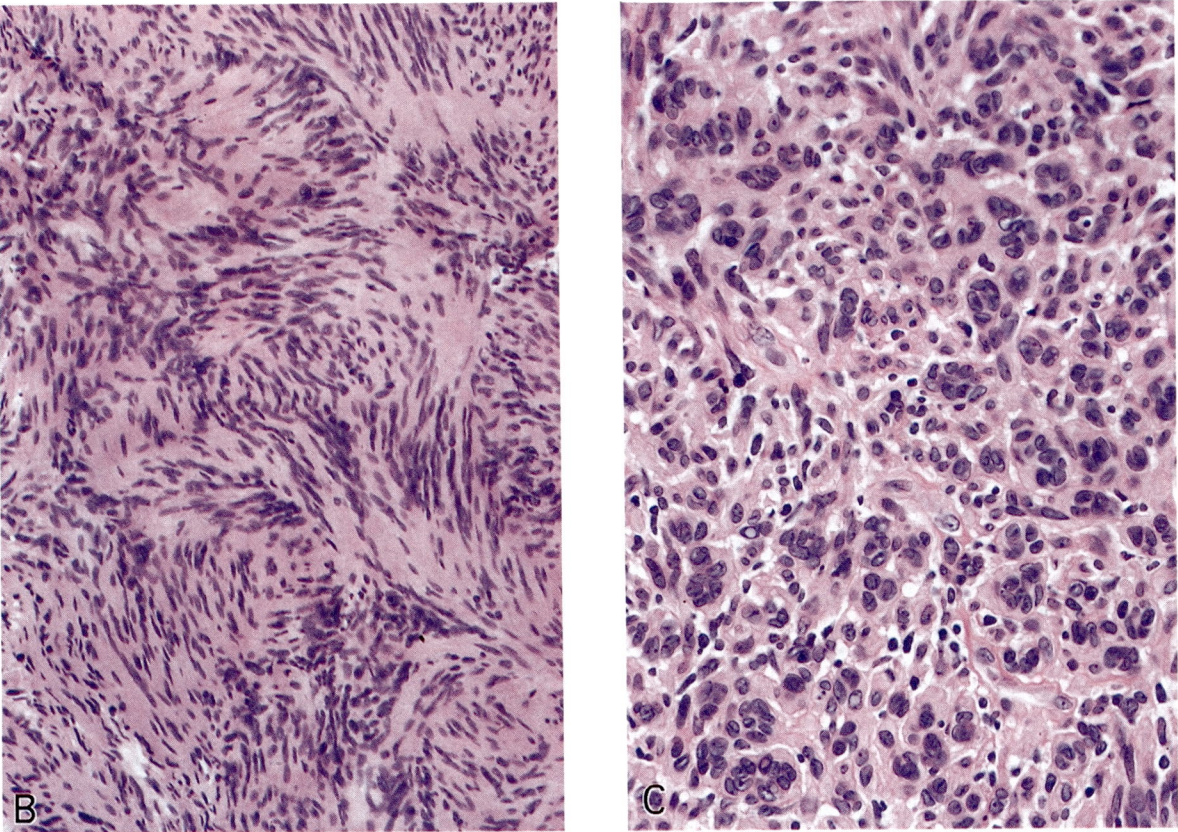

Figure 7-48
PLEXIFORM SCHWANNOMA

In addition to nuclear palisading (A) and vague Verocay body formation (B), this uncommon example features epithelioid cells in a cloverleaf-like arrangement (C).

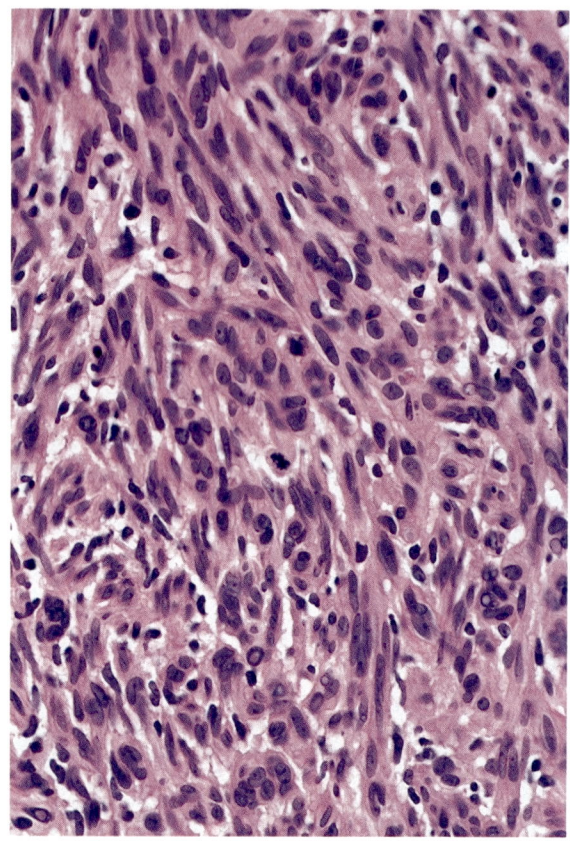

Figure 7-49
PLEXIFORM SCHWANNOMA
The cytologic features, which include spindle cells with dense eosinophilic cytoplasm, are those of conventional schwannoma.

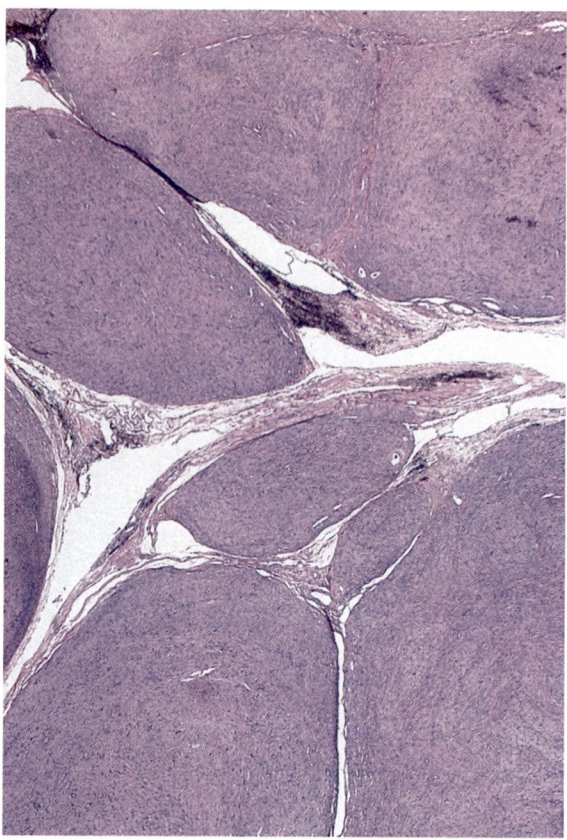

Figure 7-50
PLEXIFORM CELLULAR SCHWANNOMA
Due to high cellularity a minority of tumors qualify for the designation "cellular."

patient with an orbital lesion, Meis-Kindblom and Enzinger considered these tumors to be low-grade MPNSTs. We differ in opinion. With the exception of the orbital lesion, we consider them to represent a variant of plexiform schwannoma. In our experience, marked hypercellularity, mitotic activity, local recurrence, and even bone involvement may be seen in plexiform schwannomas of the cellular type (134).

MELANOTIC SCHWANNOMA

Definition. This is an often circumscribed nerve sheath tumor composed of melanin-producing cells with ultrastructural features of Schwann cells. The large majority are benign. Synonyms include *pigmented schwannoma, melanogenic schwannoma,* and *melanotic nerve sheath tumor.*

General Comments. Since Millar's 1932 description of a pigmented tumor of a sympathetic ganglion (183) and Hodson's 1961 report of a somatic nerve example and his correct identification of it as a schwannoma (163), over 70 patients with one or more melanotic schwannomas have been reported (136–143,146,148–151,153,155–164,166–174,176–182,184–189,193–198,200–203, 205,206). Melanotic schwannomas are classifiable as peripheral nerve sheath tumors due to the often accompanying neurological signs and symptoms, and to the tendency of these tumors to involve identifiable somatic and autonomic nerves. Unique by virtue of often heavy pigmentation, their basic features are nonetheless those of schwannoma. The cells are predominately spindled, often exhibit cellular whorl formation and palisading of nuclei, and are consistently immunoreactive for S-100 protein. Ultrastructural findings

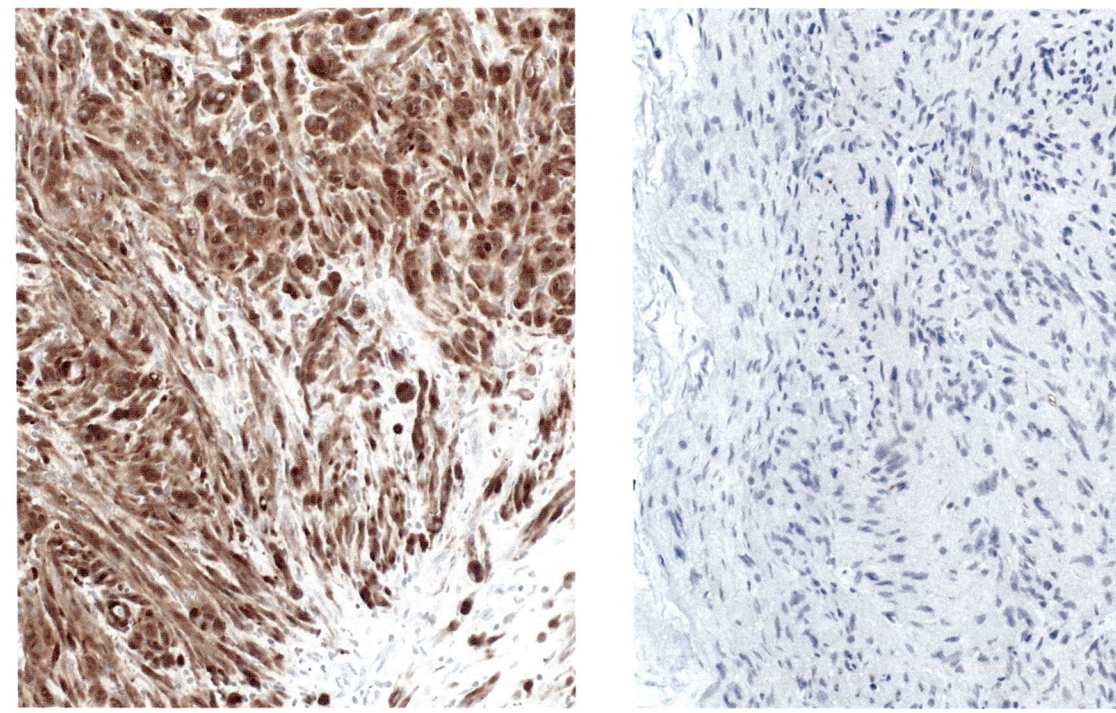

Figure 7-51
PLEXIFORM SCHWANNOMA
Left: As in conventional schwannoma, the tumor cells are S-100 protein positive.
Right: Occasional nerve fibers may be seen on neurofilament protein stain.

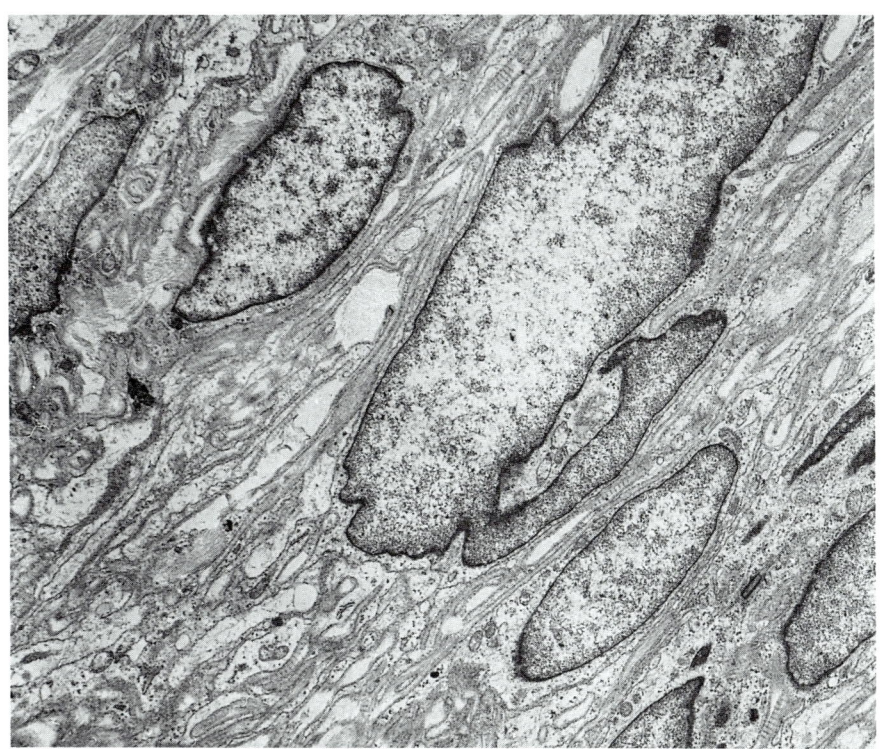

Figure 7-52
PLEXIFORM
SCHWANNOMA
At the ultrastructural level, this tumor (same case as fig. 7-45, top) shows the features of typical Schwann cells, including cytoplasmic intermediate filaments and processes covered by basement membrane (X5,000).

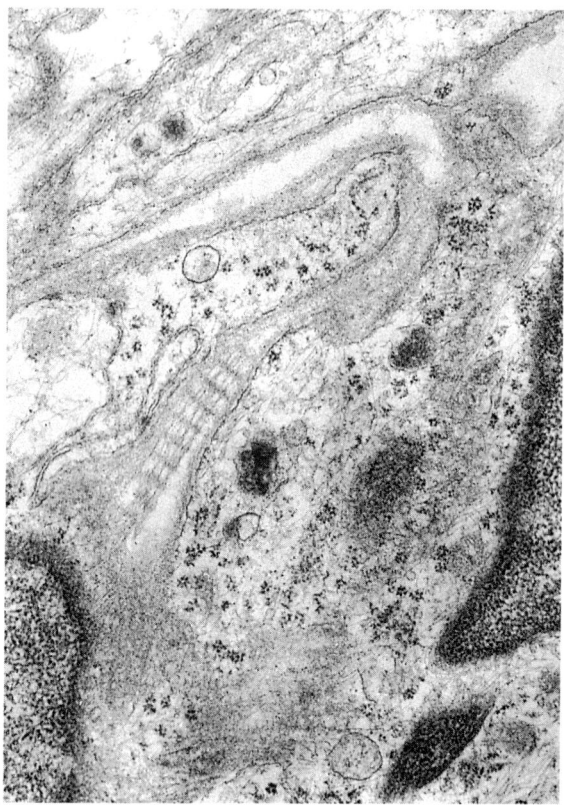

Figure 7-53
PLEXIFORM SCHWANNOMA
Note occasional Luse bodies (long-spacing collagen) in an intercellular space (X10,025).

also indicate Schwann cell differentiation and include elongate cell processes lined by continuous or discontinuous basement membrane, as well as intercellular aggregates of long-spacing collagen (Luse bodies). Dissimilarities with conventional schwannoma include the absence of clear-cut Antoni A and B tissue as well as Verocay bodies, the frequent presence of epithelioid cells, occasional psammoma bodies and adipose tissue components, and ultrastructural evidence of melanin synthesis by tumor cells.

Psammoma bodies are observed in approximately 40 to 50 percent of melanotic schwannomas. Over half of patients with such *"psammomatous melanotic schwannomas"* have Carney's complex, a dominantly transmitted autosomal disorder (143–145). The nonoccurrence of conventional schwannoma in patients with Carney's complex and of melanotic schwannoma in patients with NF2 underscores the fundamental

difference between these two principal forms of schwannoma. In further contrast to classic schwannoma, among which examples showing malignant change are rare, approximately 10 percent of all melanotic schwannomas are malignant.

Clinical Features. Melanotic schwannomas have occurred in patients 10 to 84 years of age, but their peak incidence is in the fourth decade (mean age, 37 years). A slight female predominance is noted at a ratio 1.4 to 1. While widely distributed, the tumor shows a predilection for spinal nerve involvement (46 percent of patients), particularly at the cervical and thoracic levels (fig. 7-54). A small minority involve autonomic nerves of the alimentary tract (stomach, sigmoid colon, rectum, and esophagus). Spinal nerves are more commonly involved by *nonpsammomatous* tumors, whereas the majority of alimentary tract tumors are of the *psammomatous* type. Tumors of the trigeminal ganglion, acoustic nerve, sympathetic ganglia, and the eye have been reported. Unusual sites include the heart, liver, bronchus, soft tissues, bone, and soft palate. Symptoms at presentation relate to involvement of a nerve (pain or sensory abnormality) or to mass effect within an organ or soft tissue. Bone erosion may be noted, particularly in spinal nerve root tumors, the expansile growth of which affects vertebral foramina. Frank destruction of bone is more often a feature of malignant examples.

Fifty-five percent of patients with psammomatous melanotic schwannoma have *Carney's complex* (143), an often familial disorder transmitted as an autosomal dominant trait (144,145). The mean age at diagnosis of patients with Carney's complex and melanotic schwannoma, 27 years, is a full decade earlier than that of patients with ordinary melanotic schwannoma. In addition to the melanotic schwannomas, which affect primarily posterior spinal nerve roots, upper alimentary tract, bone, and skin, the principal features of the complex are quite characteristic (fig. 7-55) (143–145,145a) and include: lentiginous pigmentation (65 percent); myxomas of the heart (65 percent), skin (25 percent), or breast (20 percent); endocrine overactivity (10 percent); and blue nevi (10 percent). Pigmentation (fig. 7-55A) involves primarily the face (lips, lacrimal caruncle, conjunctival semilunar fold) and, in females, the external genitalia. Endocrinopathy includes Cushing's syndrome (25 percent) associated with pigmented

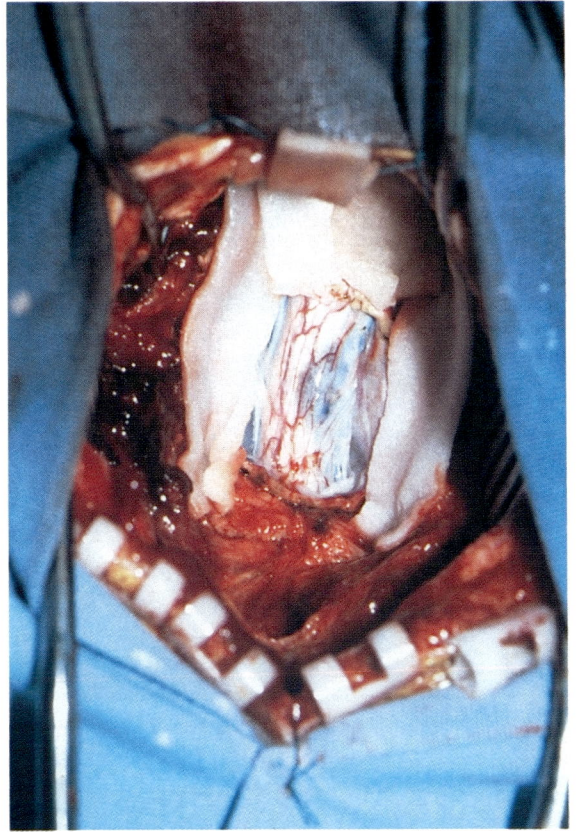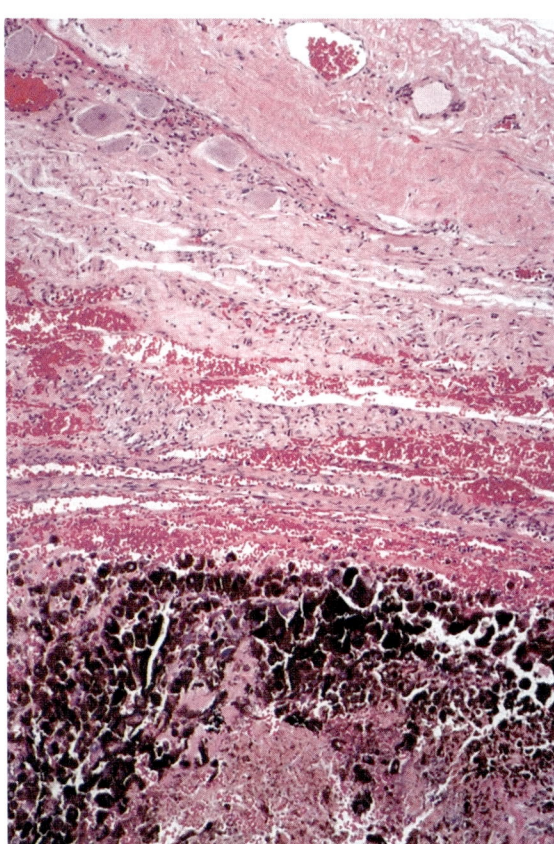

Figure 7-54
SPINAL MELANOTIC SCHWANNOMA
At surgery, this deeply pigmented spinal tumor (left) arose in relation to a T5 nerve root, but was seen to be partially embedded within the spinal cord. More common are examples arising nearby sympathetic ganglia; seen here (right) is an affected ganglion adjacent to a heavily pigmented tumor which grossly resembled tar.

nodular adrenocortical disease (fig. 7-55C,D), sexual precocity (30 percent) resulting from large cell Sertoli cell tumors of the testis, and acromegaly (8 percent) due to pituitary adenoma. The blue nevi affect primarily the extremities and trunk, are typically multiple and small, and may be either of the conventional or epithelioid type (145a).

In a small minority of instances, melanotic schwannomas may be multiple; at least three individuals have been reported to have four or more tumors (143,148,158). Whereas the incidence of multiplicity of nonpsammomatous melanotic schwannomas is unknown, that of psammomatous tumors is 19 percent (143). The majority of patients with multiple psammomatous melanotic schwannomas, 83 percent in one series (143), have Carney's complex.

Gross Findings. Melanotic schwannomas range from 0.5 to 26 cm (143,205); most are 5 cm in diameter or larger. Most tumors are circumscribed. Their configuration varies from round to ovoid or sausage shaped. Lesions affecting spinal nerve roots are often dumbbell shaped (143). Large tumors are occasionally lobulated (143) or cystic (143,146,205). Their consistency is variously described as soft, firm, or rubbery, although infrequent examples are friable or hard (143,155,172). Encapsulation, a cardinal feature of conventional schwannoma, is not seen in melanotic schwannoma. Instead, they are enveloped by a thin connective tissue layer, which is occasionally interrupted by infiltration of surrounding soft tissue (fig. 7-56, left) (143). When seen, bone destruction is generally associated with malignant examples (fig. 7-56, right). On cut surface the tumors are

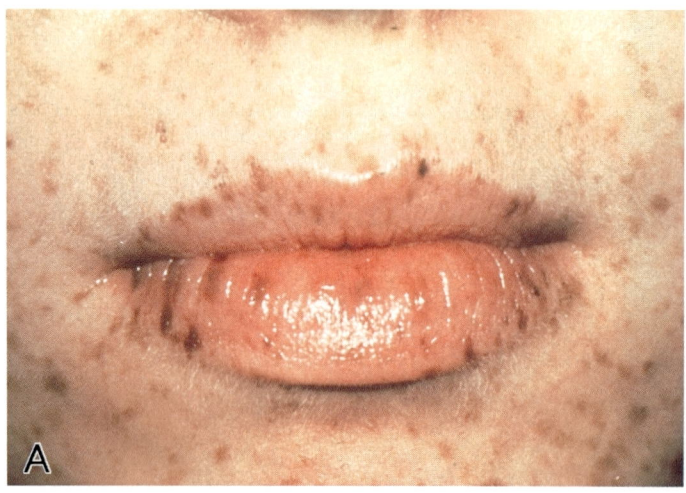

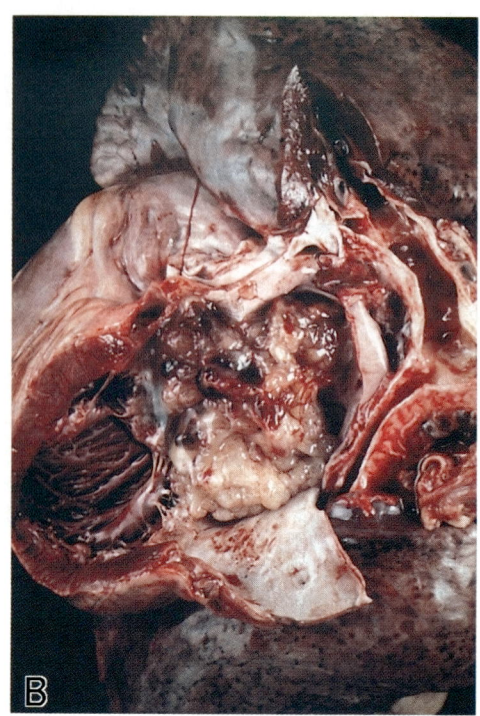

Figure 7-55
CARNEY'S COMPLEX

Aside from psammomatous melanotic schwannoma, a feature of many but not all cases of Carney's complex, the disorder includes lentiginous pigmentation, here seen to conspicuously involve the face and lips (A), myxoma of the heart (B) or other sites, and endocrine overactivity, often Cushing's syndrome due to pigmented multinodular adrenocortical disease (C,D). (Courtesy of Dr. J. A. Carney, Rochester, Minnesota.)

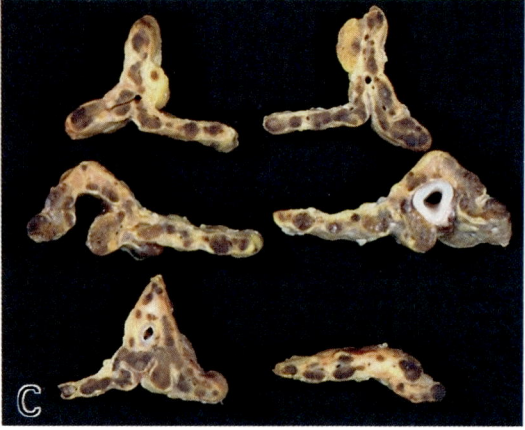

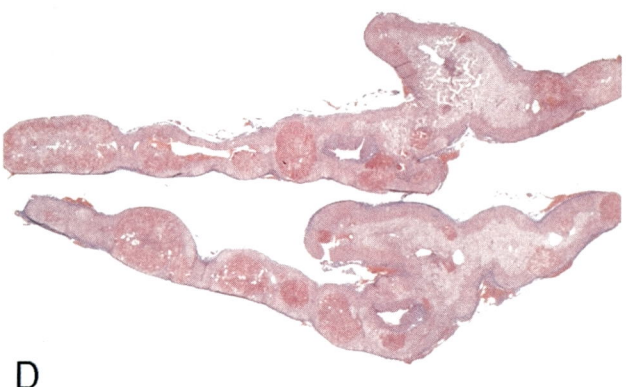

typically solid. Their tar black, blue, brown, or gray pigmentation may be uniform or unevenly distributed (figs. 7-56, 7-63). Some tumors exhibit areas of hemorrhage (142,143,172,205) or necrosis (143,146). Occasional psammomatous tumors show gross subcapsular calcification and metaplastic bone formation (143).

Microscopic Findings. Most melanotic schwannomas are highly cellular and are composed of spindle-shaped and epithelioid cells (figs. 7-57–7-59). Closely packed, such cells are usually arranged in lobules, fascicles, or cellular whorls (fig. 7-57). Palisades and Verocay body–like structures are uncommon. The same is true of microcyst formation (fig. 7-58). The cells possess eosinophilic to amphophilic cytoplasm. The outlines of spindle cells may be indistinct, whereas the cell borders of epithelioid cells are well-defined. Scattered multinucleated cells are often present (fig. 7-57F). Far less frequent are cells with vacuolated cytoplasm (fig. 7-61A,C) or clear cells (fig. 7-62E) (143). Nuclei are often round

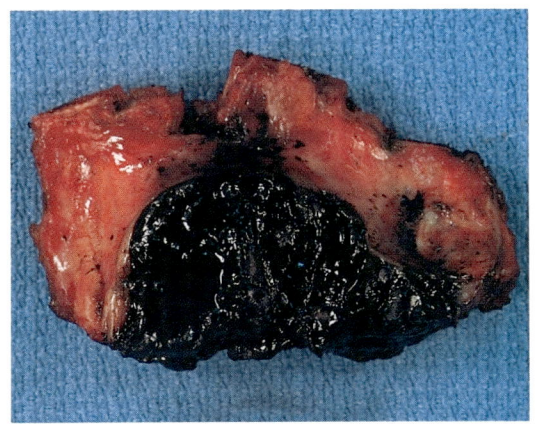 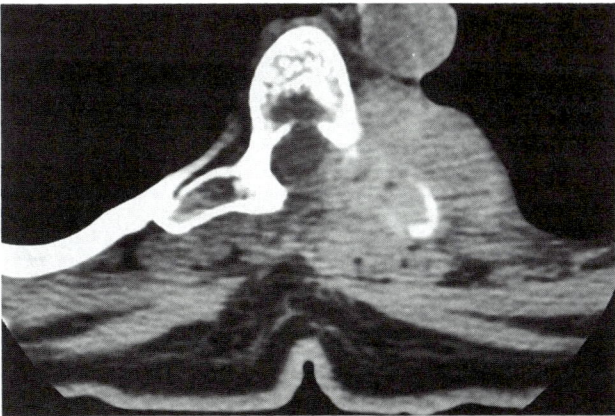

Figure 7-56
MALIGNANT PSAMMOMATOUS MELANOTIC SCHWANNOMA
This unencapsulated, paravertebral tumor (left) arose in the T6 nerve root, destroyed adjacent vertebral bone and a rib (right), and gave rise to multifocal pulmonary metastases.

and contain delicate, evenly distributed chromatin as well as a small, distinct nucleolus. Pink nuclear-cytoplasmic pseudoinclusions are commonly seen (figs. 7-60C, 7-63C). Melanin pigment in the form of brown to black granules is deposited in greatly varying amounts within the cytoplasm of both spindled and epithelioid cells (figs. 7-59–7-63). In some instances the Fontana-positive pigment obscures nuclear details. Often encountered are heavily pigmented macrophages (melanophages) (figs. 7-57A–C, 7-61B) and small clusters of lymphocytes (fig. 7-60C). Use of the potassium permanganate bleaching reaction for melanin may be required in order to reveal the cytologic features of the pigmented cells (199). In contrast, rare examples contain only patches of pigmented cells. Some tumors show myxoid change or stromal fibrosis (fig. 7-59, right).

Psammomatous Melanotic Schwannoma. In addition to showing the cytologic features noted above, psammomatous melanotic schwannomas are characterized by the presence of laminated calcospherites (fig. 7-60A,B) (143). Often a focal finding, these spherical to oval, PAS-positive bodies range from very few (fig. 7-61A) to numerous (143). Another remarkable feature, one evident in nearly 60 percent of psammomatous melanotic schwannomas, is the presence of cytoplasmic vacuoles, large examples of which result in an appearance of mature adipose tissue (fig. 7-60B). Unlike in conventional and cellular schwannomas, vessels are thin-walled rather

than thickened and hyalinized. Local hemorrhage is noted in many instances, and focal necrosis in some. Infrequently, osseous metaplasia may be seen at the periphery of the tumor.

Malignancy in Melanotic Schwannomas. Unlike conventional schwannoma, melanotic schwannomas may follow a malignant course, usually after local recurrence (figs. 7-61–7-64). Although histologic criteria for malignancy in melanotic schwannomas have not been clearly formulated, features common to clinically malignant tumors include large, vesicular nuclei with scant chromatin and very prominent eosinophilic or violaceous macronucleoli; increased mitotic activity including abnormal mitoses; and broad zones of necrosis (figs. 7-61–7-63). While these features are seen in varying combination in tumors that metastasize, none in isolation permits a diagnosis of malignancy. For example, macronucleoli may be seen in tumors that do not metastasize (143). Cytologic preparations may be of diagnostic assistance (fig. 7-64).

Immunohistochemical Findings. The often bipolar, spindled and epithelioid Schwann cells comprising both benign and malignant melanotic schwannomas are immunoreactive for vimentin, S-100 protein, and HMB-45 (fig. 7-65A,B) (142, 143,155,166,182,185,204). Immunoreactivity is also noted for the basement membrane markers laminin (182) and collagen type 4 (fig. 7-65C). To date, no examples of melanotic schwannoma have been reported to stain for GFAP (143).

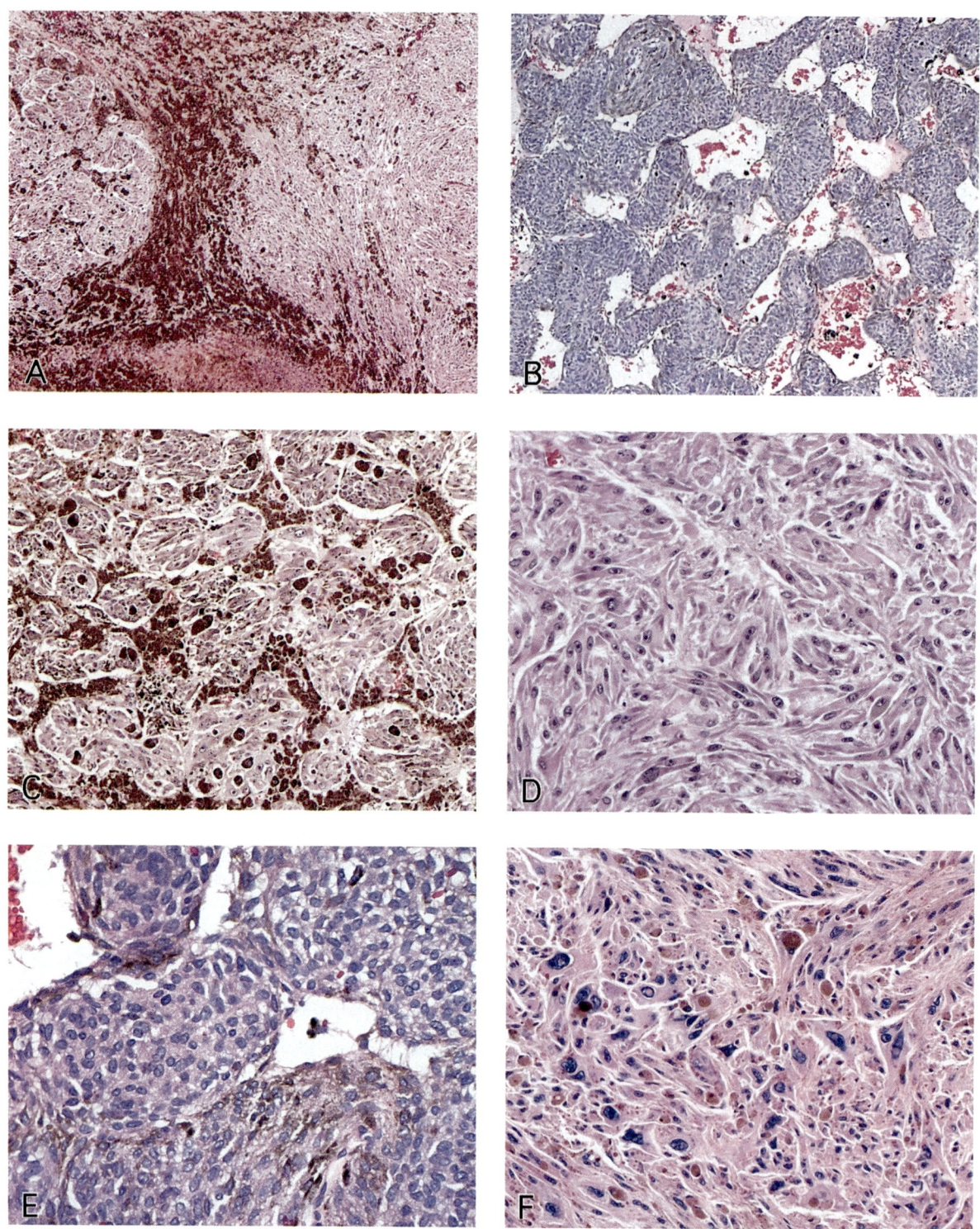

Figure 7-57
MELANOTIC SCHWANNOMA

The architecture may vary, but most tumors form sheets (A) or lobules (B). Although pigmentation is generally obvious, maximal accumulation being seen in macrophages (A center, C), sampling may show portions of the tumor to be nearly devoid of melanin (D). As a rule, uniform spindle to epithelioid cells predominate (E), but bizarre hyperchromatic multinucleate cells may be seen (F). The latter are not indicative of malignancy.

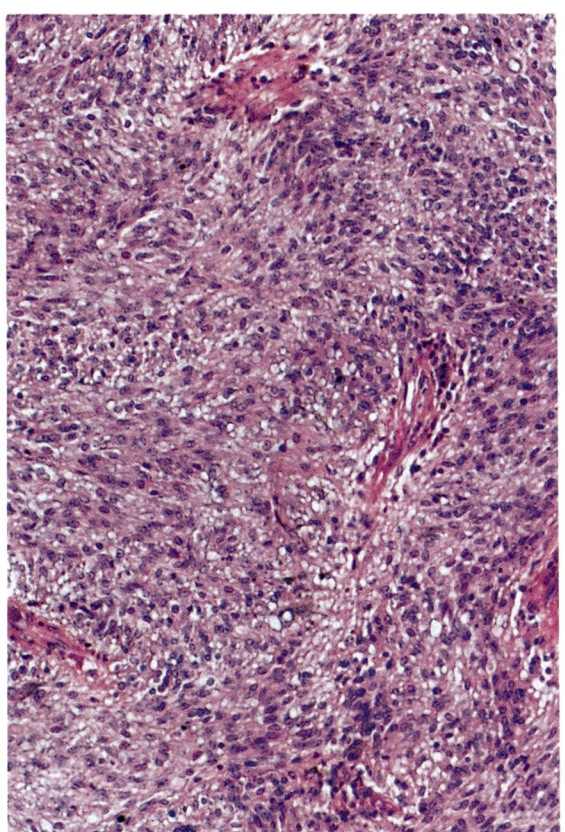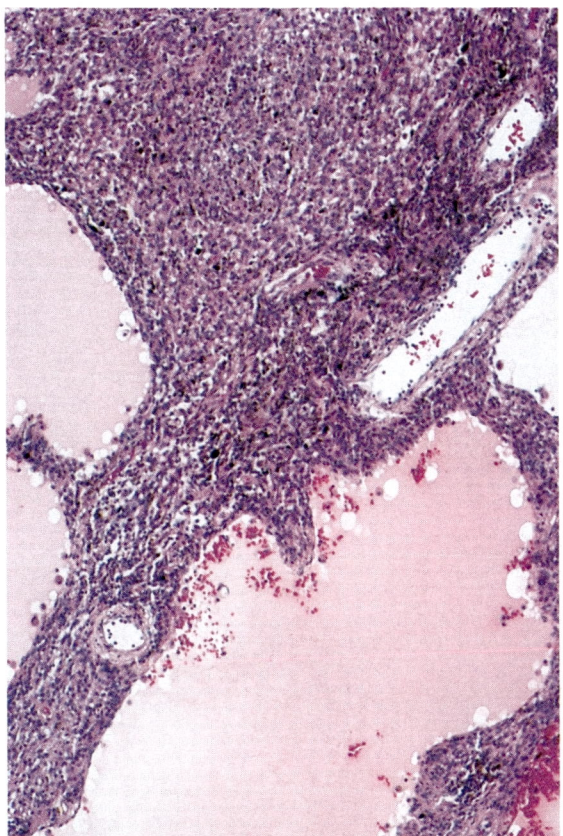

Figure 7-58
MELANOTIC SCHWANNOMA
Left: This gastric example featured plump spindle cells with scant pigmentation.
Right: Portions of the tumor showed microcystic change.

Ultrastructural Findings. Studies of melanotic schwannoma, primarily spinal nerve or sympathetic ganglion examples, have shown them to be composed of clusters of spindle-shaped or plump cells with long, often interdigitating cytoplasmic processes. The latter are joined by occasional rudimentary cell junctions and coated on their free surfaces by a continuous, often reduplicated basement membrane (figs. 7-66, 7-67). In addition to these typical schwannian features, conspicuous melanosomes in all stages of maturation, usually stages II to IV, are readily found within the cytoplasm of tumors cells (figs. 7-66, 7-67) (142,155,164,166,170,173, 181,182,185,204). Nonspecific ultrastructural features of melanotic schwannomas include extracellular long-spacing collagen (Luse bodies) (142,173), variable numbers of surface micropinocytotic vesicles (166,173,181), cytoplasmic intermediate filaments (166), and glycogen particles (figs. 7-66, 7-67).

Differential Diagnosis. The differential diagnosis of melanotic schwannoma includes conventional schwannoma and pigmented lesions, such as pigmented neurofibroma, meningeal melanocytoma, metastatic melanoma, and clear cell sarcoma of soft parts.

As a rule, melanotic schwannomas are readily distinguished from *conventional schwannoma*. Melanotic schwannomas lack a distinct capsule, well-formed Verocay bodies, and clear-cut Antoni A and B areas, whereas conventional schwannomas lack melanin, psammoma bodies, and fat. The gray-brown granular pigment occasionally seen in ordinary schwannomas represents not true melanin but lipofuscin. Unlike melanotic schwannomas, conventional schwannomas rarely involve the gastrointestinal tract.

163

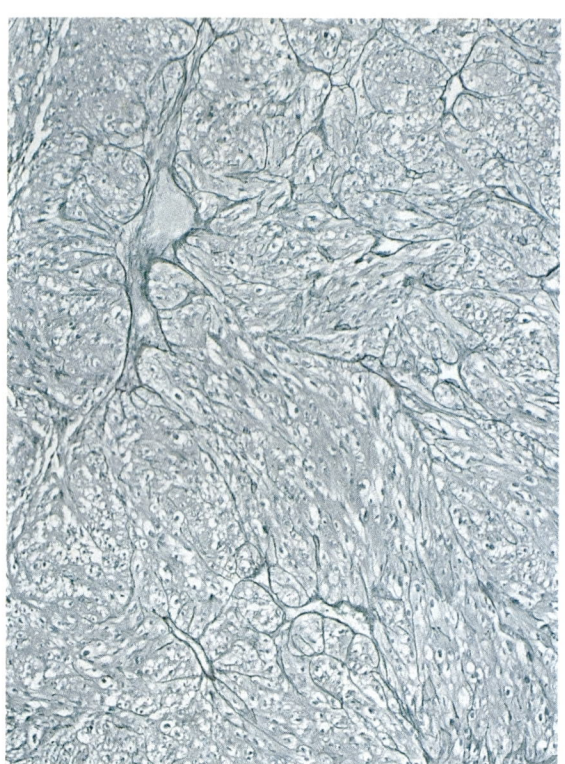 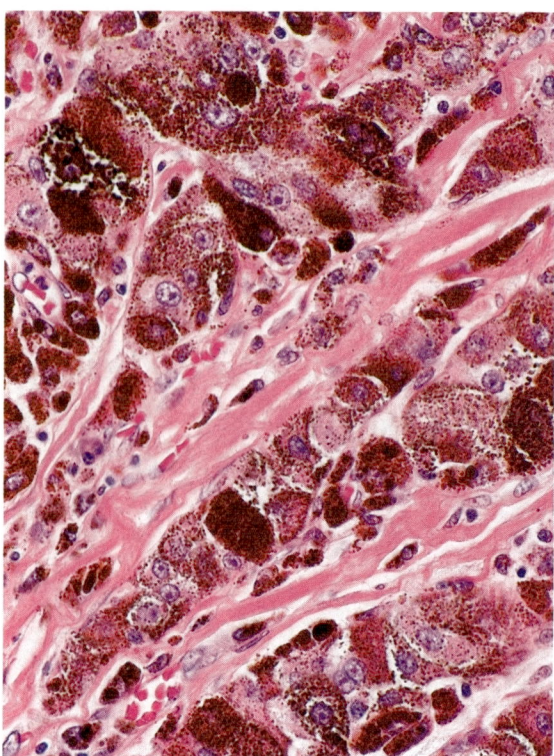

Figure 7-59
MELANOTIC SCHWANNOMA

Left: Most lesions show tumor cells with delicate intercellular reticulin staining disposed in islands surrounded by a distinct vascular connective tissue stroma (same case as fig. 7-63).

Right: Less often, as in this spinal nerve root example, the tumors show extensive collagen deposition.

The distinction of melanotic schwannoma from "pigmented neurofibroma" (155a) and other pigmented PNSTs (190) is more difficult. Such neurofibromas are often of the diffuse type, vary in size, show only microscopic pigmentation, and lack both psammoma bodies and fat. Their nuclei are small and often elongate, whereas those of melanotic schwannoma tend to be round with delicate chromatin and a distinct central nucleolus. The cytoplasm of melanotic schwannoma cells is generally abundant whereas that of neurofibroma is scant. Immunostaining for S-100 protein is not uniform in neurofibroma. The ultrastructural heterogeneity of cell types in neurofibroma also contrasts with the uniform morphology of melanotic schwannoma cells.

Also in the differential of melanotic schwannoma are *melanocytomas*, central nervous system tumors showing mainly melanocytic features. As more of these two tumors are critically studied, they may be found to represent a lesion continuum.

Melanocytomas typically arise in the cranial or spinal leptomeninges (141a,165,175,191,207), are usually demarcated and compressive of their surroundings, and consist of often heavily pigmented, polygonal to somewhat elongate or occasionally dendritic cells with vesicular nuclei and prominent nucleoli. Mitoses are scant to absent. Their immunoprofile is very similar to that of pigmented schwannoma, although staining for collagen type 4 is often less abundant. The distinction may require electron microscopy. Features common to both tumors include variably pigmented melanosomes, occasional intermediate junctions, and basement membrane production. Not only are melanocytomas devoid of psammoma bodies and adipose-like cells, but in our experience, they ultrastructurally lack both pericellular basement membrane as well as long-spacing collagen.

Of greatest clinical importance is a distinction of melanotic schwannoma from *metastatic melanoma*. In this regard, Carney (143) refers to the

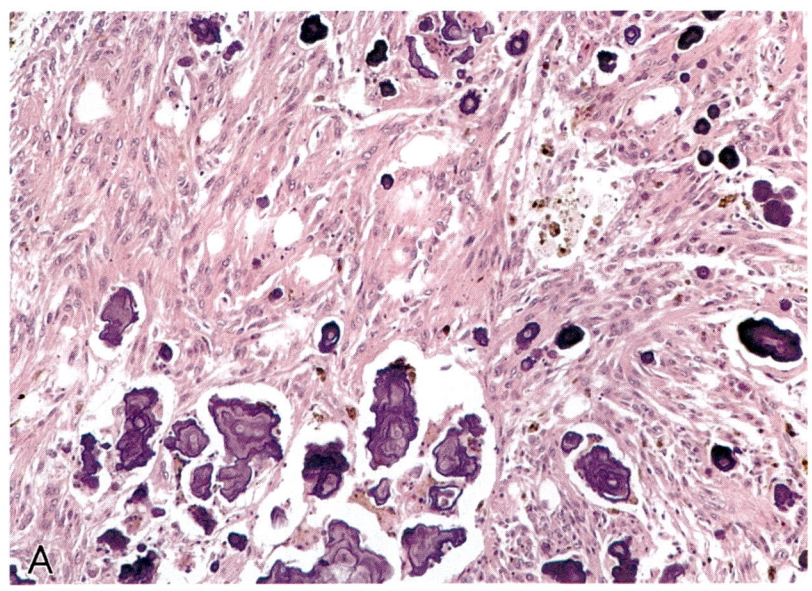

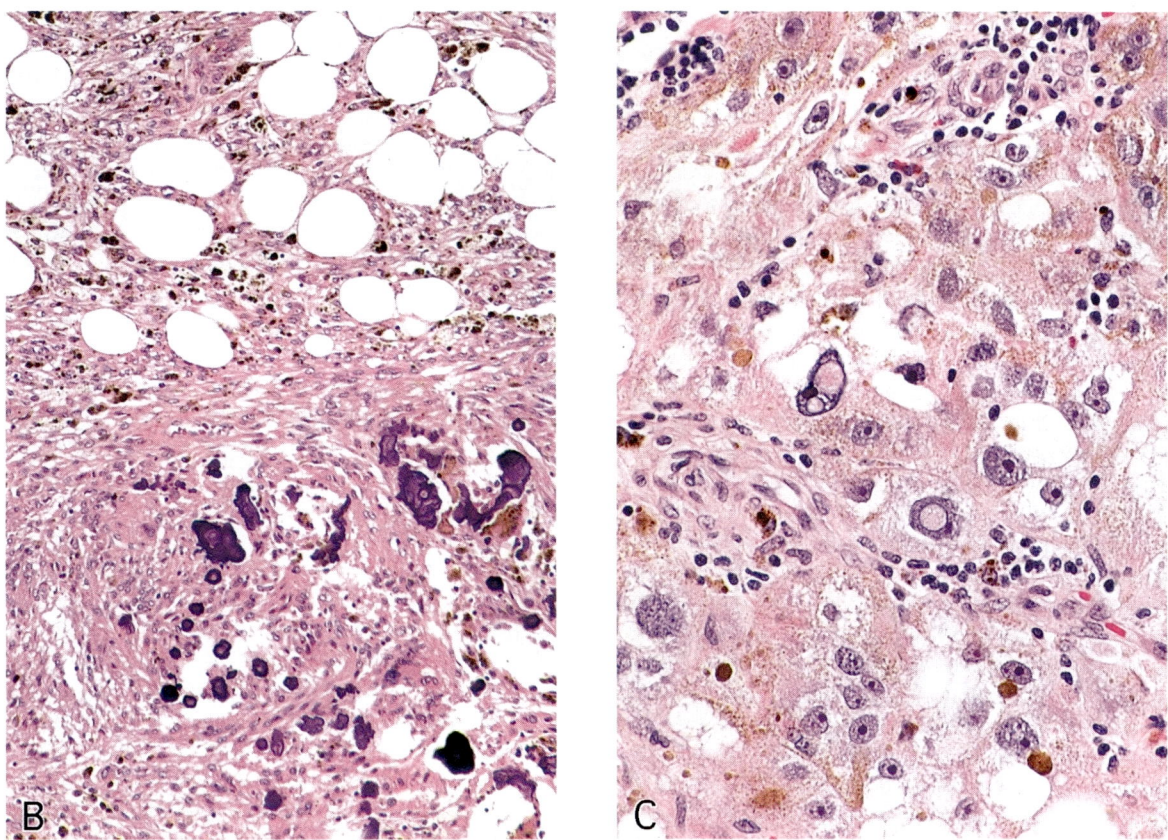

Figure 7-60

PSAMMOMATOUS MELANOTIC SCHWANNOMA

This example, occurring in the setting of Carney's complex, shows psammoma bodies of varying shape (A) as well as adipose-like cells (B). Like conventional melanotic schwannomas, such tumors show cytologic variation ranging from spindle to epithelioid, with open chromatin, nucleolar prominence, and degenerative nuclear atypia with the formation of nuclear-cytoplasmic pseudoinclusions (C).

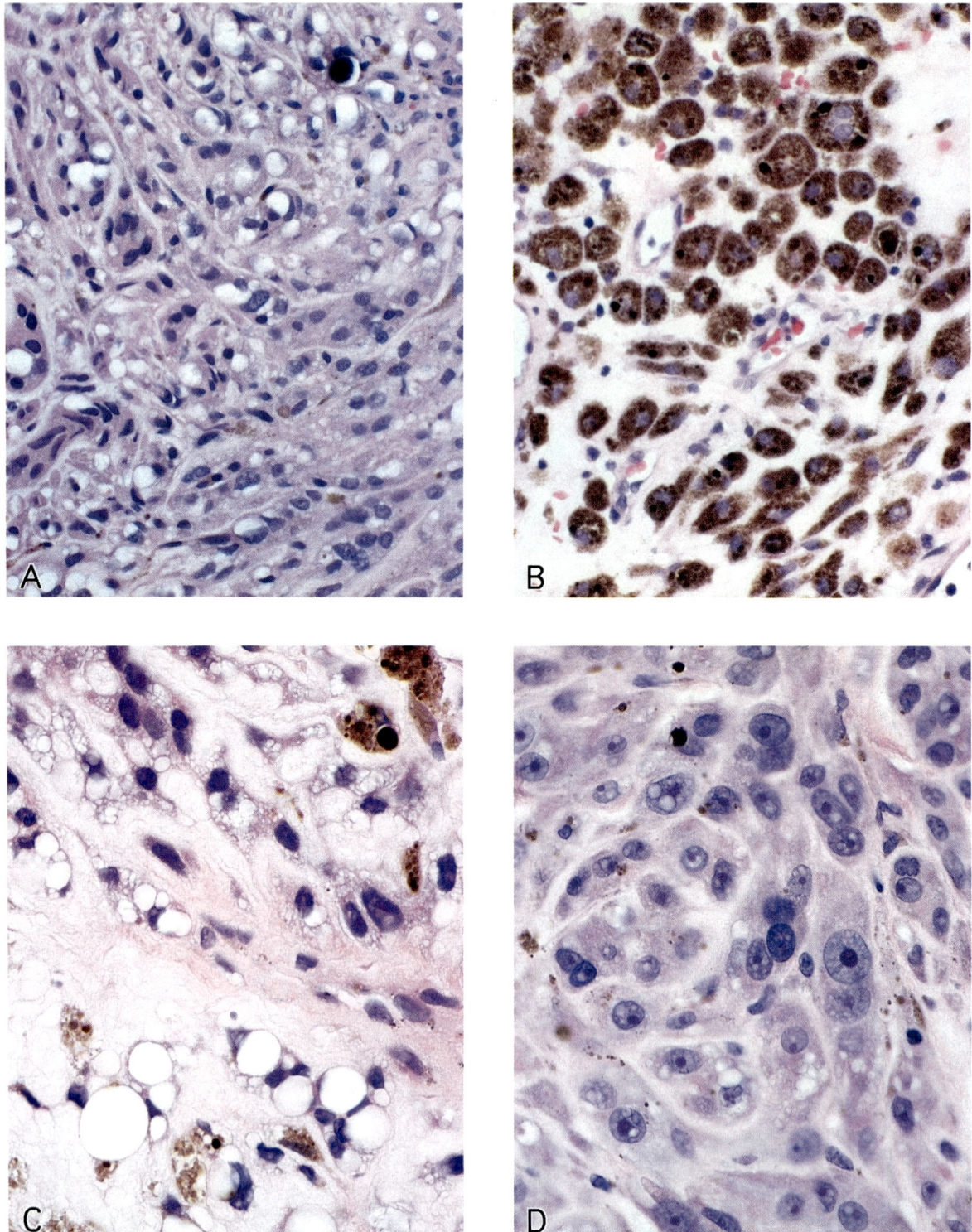

Figure 7-61
MALIGNANT PSAMMOMATOUS MELANOTIC SCHWANNOMA
This tumor featured mild pigmentation (A), accumulations of melanophages (B), the formation of cytoplasmic lipid-like vacuoles displacing nuclei (C), and only scant psammoma bodies (A). Portions of the tumor showed macronucleoli (D) as well as abnormal mitotic figures.

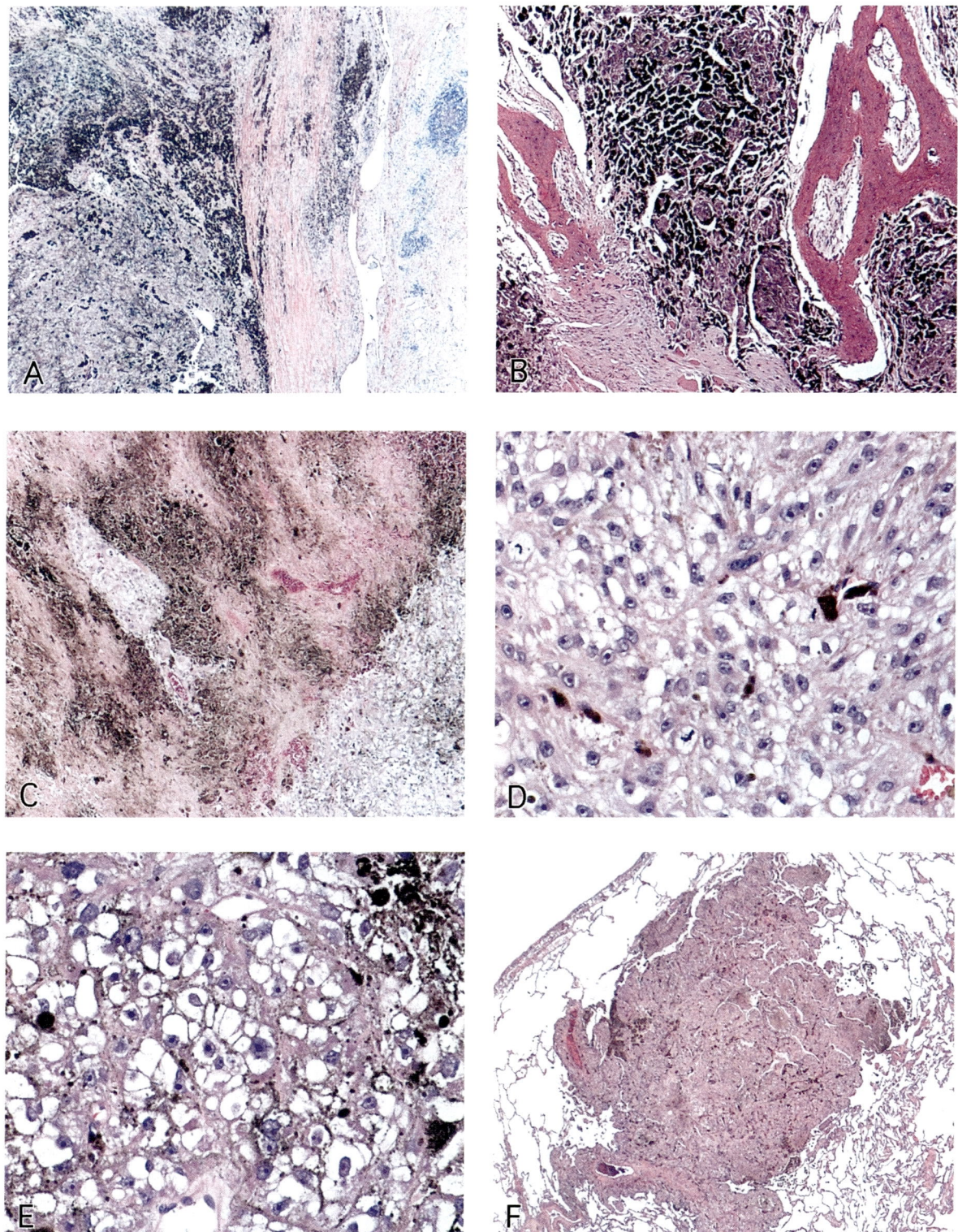

Figure 7-62
MALIGNANT PSAMMOMATOUS MELANOTIC SCHWANNOMA
This example showed invasion of peritumoral soft tissue (A), bone infiltration (B), necrosis (C), mitotic activity (D), clear cell change (E), and pulmonary metastases (F).

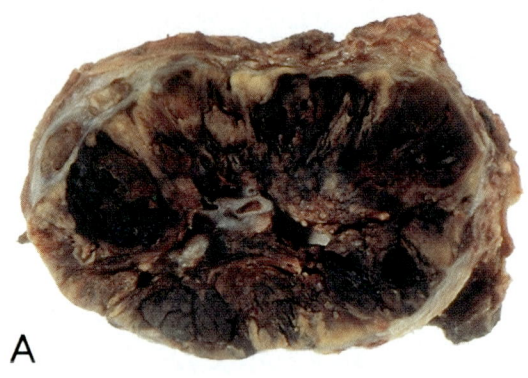

A

Figure 7-63
MALIGNANT MELANOTIC SCHWANNOMA

This large example arising in a spinal sympathetic ganglion near an adrenal gland of a 36-year-old female shows the typical pitch black appearance of such tumors (A). The histology varied from plump spindle cells (B) with prominent nuclear pseudoinclusions (C), to a necrotic, epithelioid, and heavily pigmented malignant lesion exhibiting large violaceous nucleoli (D). The tumor metastasized widely and resulted in death 2 years after its resection. For further details see reference 1. (Courtesy of Dr. S. McClure, Akron, Ohio.)

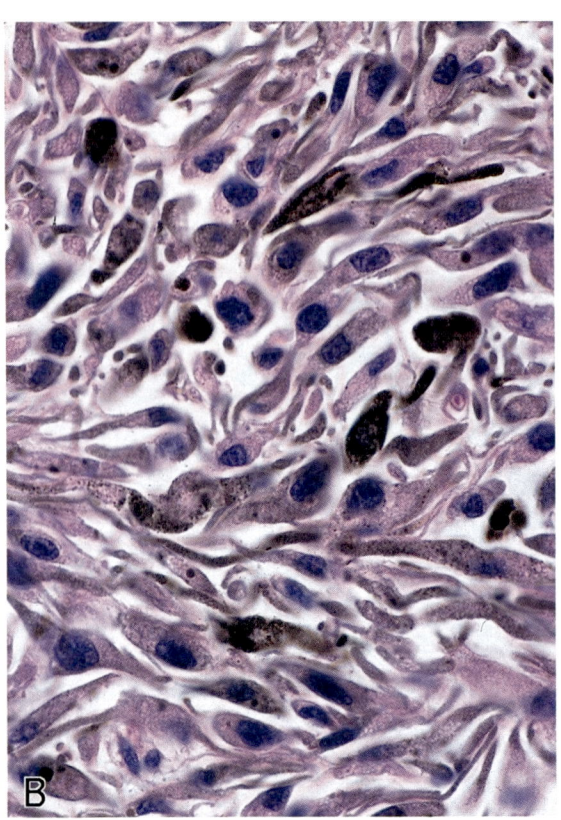

B

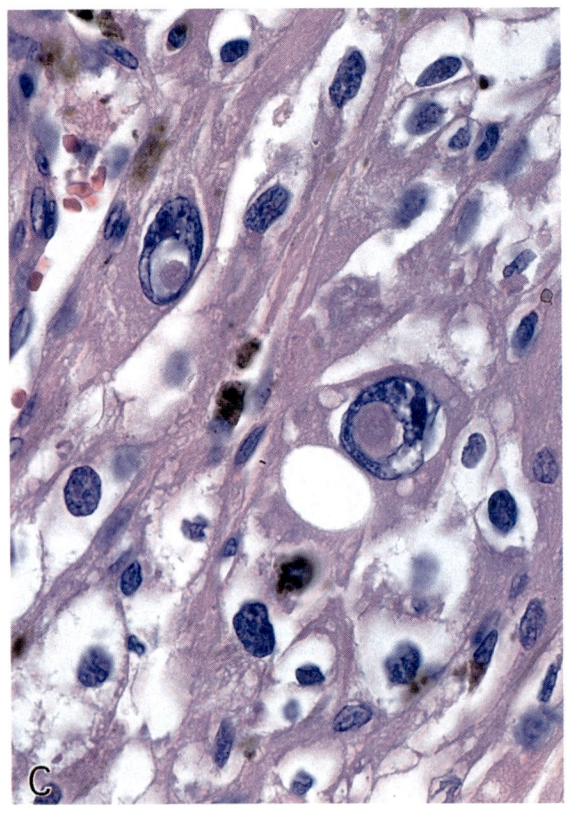

C

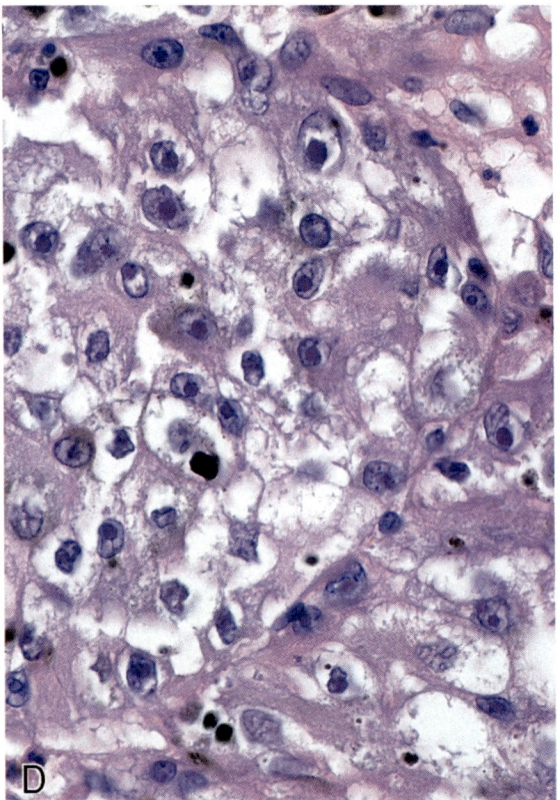

D

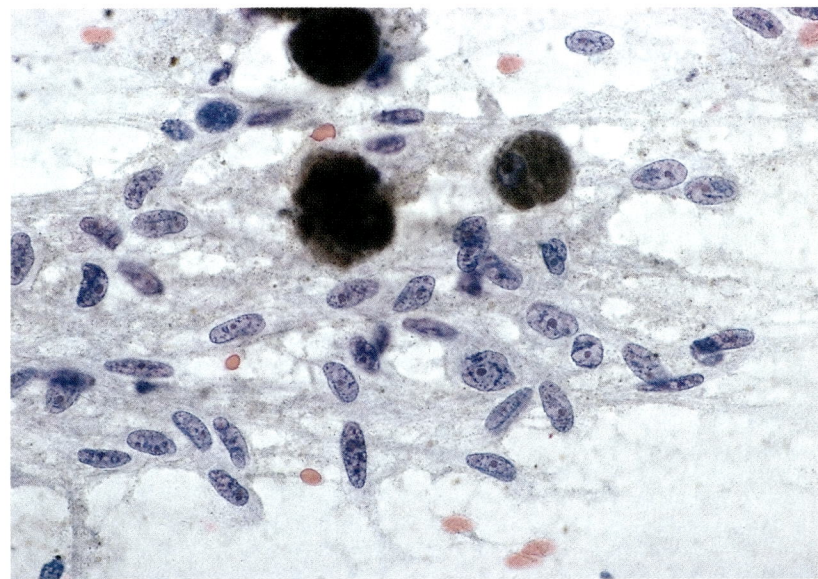

Figure 7-64
MALIGNANT PSAMMOMATOUS
MELANOTIC SCHWANNOMA:
CYTOLOGY
This Papanicolaou-stained smear
shows cytologic malignancy, particu-
larly macronucleoli. Pigmentation
varies and is most abundant in
melanophages. (Courtesy of Dr. P. B.
Illei, New York, NY.)

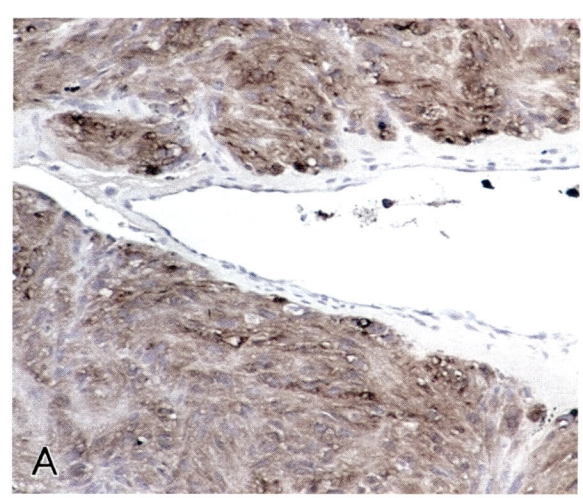

Figure 7-65
MELANOTIC SCHWANNOMA
Since this tumor is immunoreactive for S-100 protein (A),
HMB 45 (B), and type 4 collagen (C), it shares some features
of both schwannoma and melanoma. Although this example
had a more prominent lobular collagen 4 staining pattern,
ultrastructure typically shows pericellular basement membrane formation (see figures 7-66, 7-67).

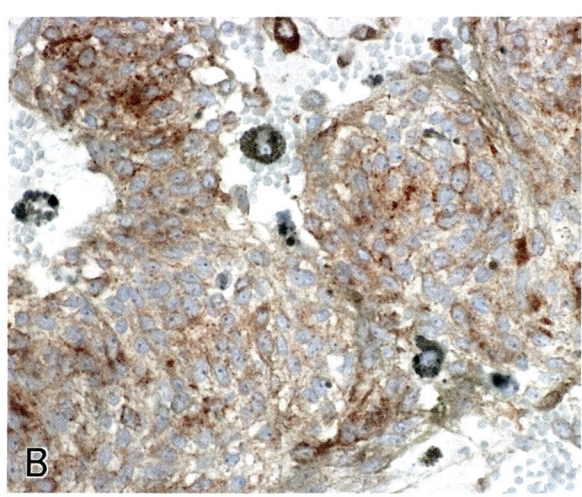

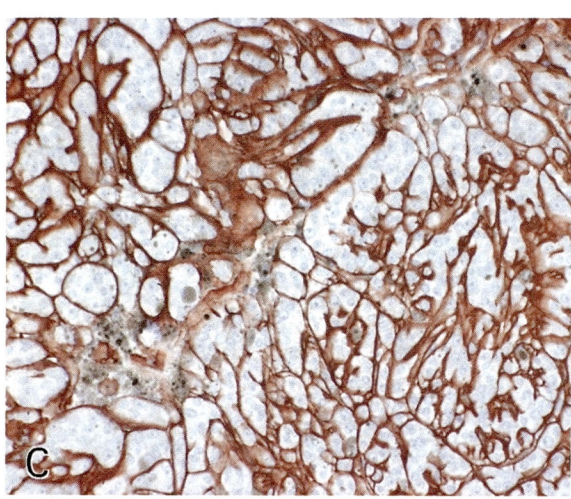

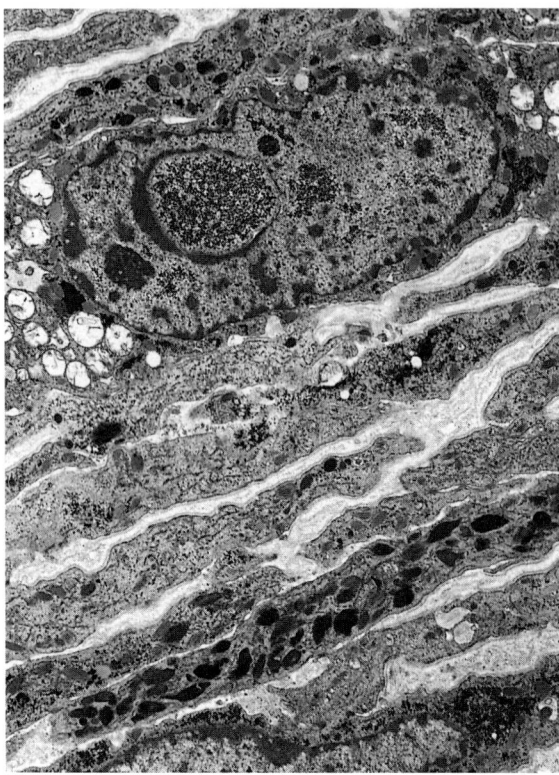

Figure 7-66
MELANOTIC SCHWANNOMA
The spindle-shaped neoplastic Schwann cells contain numerous electron-dense melanosomes as well as clusters of glycogen particles. Note the reduplicated basement membranes in the intercellular spaces (X6,900).

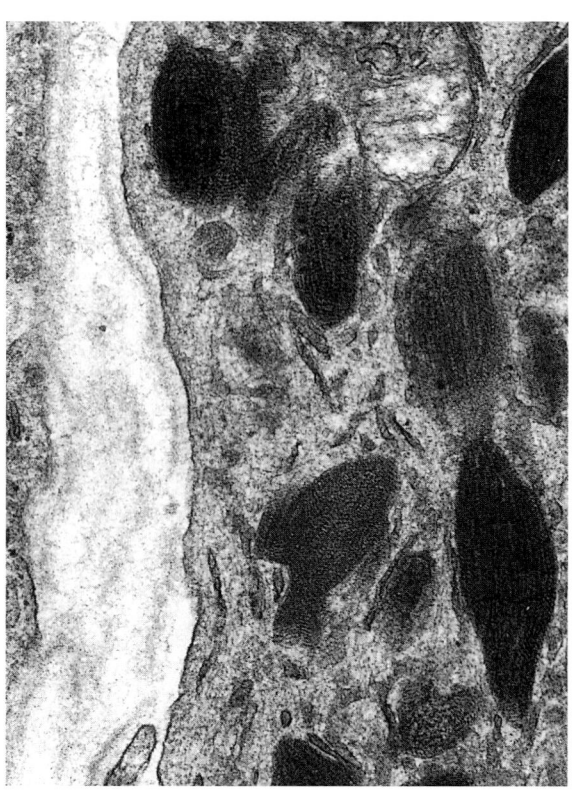

Figure 7-67
MELANOTIC SCHWANNOMA
Detail of a melanosome-containing Schwann cell process. Basement membrane substance is present in the intercellular space (X38,900).

dendritic appearance of cells in melanotic schwannoma, a feature rarely seen in metastatic melanoma. Unlike the majority of melanotic schwannomas, most melanomas are cytologically malignant. Furthermore, melanomas are devoid of psammoma bodies and fat. At the immunohistochemical and ultrastructural levels, melanomas only rarely exhibit basement membrane formation (152,192).

Clear cell sarcomas (soft tissue melanoma) (147,154) show a predilection for soft tissues, are both macroscopically and microscopically invasive, and are composed of cytologically malignant cells with little or no pigment production. Such tumors are devoid of psammoma bodies and fat, and lack evidence of basement membrane formation.

Treatment and Prognosis. Most melanotic schwannomas are benign, slowly growing tu-

mors, albeit ones that may erode bone. Among malignant examples, death due to disease, often metastatic tumor, is as frequent in conventional melanotic schwannomas as in psammomatous tumors. Of all reported patients with melanotic schwannoma, approximately 15 percent with conventional tumors (148,150,157,159,164,196) and 15 percent with psammomatous tumors have died of tumor (143). Since melanotic schwannomas may be multiple, distinguishing between a second primary lesion and a metastasis may be difficult (143). Some patients with Carney's complex experience additional morbidity and mortality due to associated cardiac myxomas or endocrinopathy. Surgical excision with tumor-free margins is the treatment of choice for primary melanotic schwannoma of either conventional or psammomatous type.

REFERENCES

Schwannoma

1. Abernathy CD, Onofrio BM, Scheithauer BW, Pairolero PC, Shives TC. Surgical management of giant sacral schwannomas. J Neurosurg 1986;65:286–95.

2. Ackerman LV, Taylor FH. Neurogenous tumors within the thorax. A clinicopathological evaluation of forty-eight cases. Cancer 1951;4:669–91.

3. Allegranza A, Ferraresi S, Luccarelli G. Malignant glandular schwannoma: a case with favorable prognosis. Histopathology 1988;12:549–52.

4. Beatty CW, Scheithauer BW, Katzmann JA, Roche PC, Kjeldahl KS, Ebersold MJ. Acoustic schwannoma and pregnancy: a DNA flow cytometric, steroid hormone receptor, and proliferation marker study. Laryngoscope 1995;105:693–700.

5. Bello MJ, de Campos JM, Kusak ME, et al. Clonal chromosome aberrations in neurinomas. Genes Chromosomes Cancer 1993;6:206–11.

6. Bijlsma EK, Brouwer-Mladin R, Bosch DA, Westerveld A, Hulsebos TJ. Molecular characterization of chromosome 22 deletions in schwannomas. Genes Chromosomes Cancer 1992;5:201–5.

7. Brooks JJ, Draffen RM. Benign glandular schwannoma. Arch Pathol Lab Med 1992;116:192–5.

7a. Brouchet A, Delisle MB, Bonafe A, Flores P, Lombard L, Fraysse B. Accoustic schwannomas: magnetic resonance imaging and histopathology. Laryngoscope (In press).

8. Burger PC, Scheithauer BW. Tumors of the central nervous system. Atlas of Tumor Pathology, 3rd series, Fascicle 10. Washington, D.C.: Armed Forces Institute of Pathology, 1994.

9. Carney JA. Psammomatous melanotic schwannoma. A distinctive heritable tumor with special associations, including cardiac myxoma and the Cushing syndrome. Am J Surg Pathol 1990;14:206–22.

10. Casadei GP, Komori T, Scheithauer BW, Parisi JE, Miller GM, Kelly PJ. Intracranial parenchymal schwannoma. J Neurosurg 1993;79:217–22.

11. Celli P, Acqui M, Ferrante L, Mastronardi L, Fortuna A, Palma L. Neuroma of the third, fourth, and sixth cranial nerves: a survey and report of a new fourth nerve case. Surg Neural 1992;38:216–24.

12. Cervùs-Navarro J, Matakas F, Lazardo MC. Das Bauprinzip der Neurinome. Ein Beitrag Zur Histogenese der Nerrentumonen. Virchows Arch [A] 1968;345:276–91.

13. Chan JK, Fok KO. Pseudoglandular schwannoma. Histopathology 1996;29:481–3.

13a. Chaubal A, Paetau A, Zoltic KP, Miettinen M. CD34 immunoreactivity in nervous system tumors. Acta Neuropathol 1994;88:454–8.

14. Clark HB, Minesky JJ, Agrawal D, Agrawal HC. Myelin basic protein and P2 protein are not immunohistochemical markers for Schwann cell neoplasms. A comparative study using antisera to S-100, P2, and myelin basic proteins. Am J Pathol 1985;121:96–101.

15. Couturier J, Delattre O, Kujas M, et al. Assessment of chromosome 22 anomalies in neurinomas by combined karyotype and RFLP analyses. Cancer Genet Cytogenet 1990;45:55–62.

16. Daimaru Y, Hideki K, Hashimoto H, Enjoji M. Benign schwannoma of the gastrointestinal tract: a clinicopathologic and immunohistochemical study. Hum Pathol 1988;19:257–64.

17. Das Gupta TK, Brasfield RD, Strong EW, Hajdu SI. Benign solitary schwannoma (neurilemomas). Cancer 1969;24:355–66.

18. Davis K, MacCollin M, Jacoby LB, et al. The molecular basis of schwannomatosis [Abstract]. American Society of Human Genetics, June 7, 1996.

19. DelaMonte SM, Dorfan HD, Chandra R, Malawer M. Intraosseous schwannoma: histopathologic features, ultrastructure and review of the literature. Hum Pathol 1984;15:551–8.

20. Dickersin GR. The electron microscopic spectrum of nerve sheath tumors. Ultrastruct Pathol 1987;11:103–46.

21. Elston DM, Bergfeld WF, Biscotti CV, McMahon JT. Schwannoma with sweat duct differentiation. J Cutan Pathol 1993;20:254–8.

22. Emory TS, Unni KK. Intraosseous neurilemmoma: a clinicopathologic study of 26 cases [Abstract]. Am J Clin Pathol 1993;100:328–9.

23. Erlandson RA. Diagnostic transmission electron microscopy of tumors. New York: Raven Press, 1994:447–54.

24. Erlandson RA. Melanotic schwannoma of spinal nerve origin. Ultrastruct Pathol 1985;9:123–9.

25. Erlandson RA, Woodruff JM. Peripheral nerve sheath tumors: an electron microscopic study of 43 cases. Cancer 1982;49:273–87.

26. Escalona-Zapata J, Diez Nau MD. The nature of macrophages (foam cells) in neurinomas. Tissue culture study. Acta Neuropathol 1978;44:71–5.

27. Evans DG, Huson SM, Donnai D, et al. A genetic study of type 2 neurofibromatosis in the United Kingdom. I. Prevalence, mutation rate, fitness and confirmation of maternal transmission effect on severity. J Med Genet 1992;29:841–6.

28. Factor S, Turi G, Biempica L. Primary cardiac neurilemoma. Cancer 1976;37:883–90.

29. Fawcett DW. Skin. In: Bloom and Fawcett. A textbook of histology. New York: Chapman and Hall, 1994:548–50.

30. Ferry JA, Dickersin GR. Pseudoglandular schwannoma. Am J Clin Pathol 1988;89:546–52.

31. Fisher C, Chappell ME, Weiss SW. Neuroblastoma-like epithelioid schwannoma. Histopathology 1995;26:193–4.

32. Fletcher CD, Davies SE. Benign plexiform (multinodular) schwannoma: a rare tumor unassociated with neurofibromatosis. Histopathology 1986;10:971–80.

33. Fletcher CD, Madziwa D, Heyderman E, McKee PH. Benign dermal schwannoma with glandular elements—true heterology or a local "organizer" effect. Clin Exp Dermatol 1986;11:475–85.

34. Geddes JF, Sutcliffe JC, King TT. Mixed cranial nerve tumors in neurofibromatosis type 2. Clin Neuropathol 1995;14:310–3.

35. Giangaspero F, Fratamico FC, Ceccarelli C, Brisigotti M. Malignant peripheral nerve sheath tumors and spindle cell sarcomas: an immunohistochemical analysis of multiple markers. Appl Pathol 1989;7:134–44.

36. Goebel HH, Shimokawa K, Schaake TH, Kremp A. Schwannoma of the sellar region. Acta Neurochirurgica 1979;48:191–7.

37. Goetting MG, Swanson SE. Massive hemorrhage into intracranial neurinomas. Surg Neurol 1987;27:168–72.

38. Goldblum JR, Beals TF, Weiss SW. Neuroblastoma-like neurilemoma. Am J Surg Pathol 1994;18(3):266–73.

39. Gould VE, Moll R, Moll I, Lee I, Schwechheimer K, Franke WW. The intermediate filament complement of the spectrum of nerve sheath neoplasms. Lab Invest 1986;55:463–74.

40. Graham DI, Bond MR. Intradural spinal ossifying schwannoma. Case report. J Neurosurg 1972;36:487–89.

41. Gray MH, Rosenberg AE, Dickersin GR, Bhan AK. Glial fibrillary acidic protein and keratin expression by benign and malignant nerve sheath tumors. Hum Pathol 1989;20:1089–96.

42, Halliday AL, Sobel RA, Martuza RL. Benign spinal nerve sheath tumors: their occurrence sporadically and in neurofibromatosis types 1 and 2. J Neurosurg 1991;74:248–53.

43. Harkin JC, Reed RJ. Tumors of the peripheral nervous system. Atlas of Tumor Pathology, 2nd Series, Fascicle 3. Washington, D.C.: Armed Forces Institute of Pathology, 1969.

44. Hasegawa SL, Mentzel T, Fletcher CD. Schwannomas of the sinonasal tract and nasopharynx. Mod Pathol 1997;10:777–84.

45. Hirano A, Dembitzer HM, Zimmerman HM. Fenestrated blood vessels in neurilemoma. Lab Invest 1972;27:305–9.

46. Hirose T, Scheithauer BW, Sano T. Giant plexiform schwannoma: report of two cases with soft tissue and visceral involvement. Mod Pathol 1997;11:1075–81.

47. Inoue T, Fukui M, Matsushima T, Hasuo K, Matsunaga M. Neurinoma in the cavernous sinus: report of two cases. Neurosurgery 1990;27:986–90.

48. Izumi AK, Rosato FE, Wood MG. Von Recklinghausen's disease associated with multiple neurilemomas. Arch Dermatol 1971;104:172–6.

49. Jacoby LB, MacCollin M, Louis DN, et al. Exon scanning for mutation in the NF2 gene in schwannomas. Hum Molec Genet 1994;3:413–9.

50. Johnson MD, Glick AD, Davis BW. Immunohistochemical evaluation of Leu-7, myelin basic-protein, S-100 protein, glial-fibrillary acidic-protein, and LN3 immunoreactivity in nerve sheath tumors and sarcomas. Arch Pathol Lab Med 1988;112:155–60.

51. Kasantikul V, Brown WJ, Netsky MG. Mesenchymal differentiation in trigeminal neurilemoma. Cancer 1982;50:1568–71.

52. Kasantikul V, Glick AD, Netsky MG. Light and electron microscopic observations of blood vessels in neurilemoma. Arch Pathol Lab Med 1979;103:683–7.

53. Kasantikul V, Netsky MG. Combined neurilemmoma and angioma. Tumor of ectomesenchyme and a source of bleeding. J Neurosurg 1979;50:81–7.

54. Kawahara E, Oda Y, Ooi A, Katsuda S, Nakanishi I, Umeda S. Expression of glial fibrillary acidic protein (GFAP) in peripheral nerve sheath tumors. A comparative study of immunoreactivity of GFAP, vimentin, S-100 protein, and neurofilament in 38 schwannomas and 18 neurofibromas. Am J Surg Pathol 1988;12:115–20.

54a. Kindblom L, Meis G, Kindblom JM, Hovel G, Busch C. Benign epithelioid schwannoma. Am J Surg Pathol 1998;22:762–70.

54b. Klekamp J, Samii M. Surgery of spinal nerve sheath tumors with special reference to neurofibromatosis. Neurosurgery 1998;42:279–90.

54c. Kurtin PJ, Bonin DM. Immunohistochemical demonstration of the lysosome associated glycoprotein CD 68 (KP-1) in granular cell tumors and schwannoma. Hum Pathol 1994;25:1172–8.

55. Lassmann H, Jurecka W, Lassmann G, Grechart W, Matras H, Watzek G. Different types of benign nerve sheath tumors. Light microscopy, electron microscopy and autoradiography. Virchows Arch [Pathol Anat] 1977;375:197–210.

56. Louis DN, Ramesh V, Gusella JF. Neuropathology and molecular genetics of neurofibromatosis 2 and related tumors. Brain Pathol 1995;5:163–72.

57. MacCollin M, Ramesh V, Jacoby LB, et al. Mutational analysis of patients with neurofibromatosis 2. Am J Hum Genet 1994;55:314–20.

58. MacCollin M, Woodfin W, Kronn D, Short MP. Schwannomatosis: a clinical and pathologic study. Neurology 1996;46:1072–9.

59. McComb RD, Bigner DD. Immunolocalization of laminin in neoplasms of the central and peripheral nervous systems. J Neuropathol Exp Neurol 1985;44:242–53.

60. Melvin WS, Wilkinson MG. Gastric schwannoma. Clinical and pathologic considerations. Am Surg 1993;59:293–6.

61. Memoli V, Brown EF, Gould VE. Glial fibrillary acidic protein (GFAP) immunoreactivity in peripheral nerve sheath tumors. Ultrastruct Pathol 1984;7:269–75.

62. Murray MR, Stout AP. Schwann cell versus fibroblast as the origin of the specific nerve sheath tumor: observations upon normal nerve sheaths and neurilemomas in vitro. Am J Pathol 1940;16:41–60.

63. Neely JG. Hearing conservation surgery for acoustic tumors—a clinical-pathologic correlative study. Am J Otol 1985;(Suppl):143–6.

64. Oda Y, Kawahara E, Minamoto T, et al. Immunohistochemical studies on the tissue localization of collagen types I, III, IV, V and VI in schwannomas. Correlation with ultrastructural features of the extracellular matrix. Virchows Arch [Pathol Anat] 1988;56:153–63.

64a. Ogose A, Hotta T, Morita T, Otsuka H, Hirata Y. Multiple schwannomas in the peripheral nerves. J Bone Joint Surg 1998;80:657–61.

65. Ou YC, Yang DY, Chang CG. Ossification within a thoracic neurilemmoma—a case report. Chin Med J 1988;42:143–6.

66. Parry DM, Eldridge R, Kaiser-Kupfer MI, Bouzas EA, Pikus A, Patronas N. Neurofibromatosis 2 (NF2): clinical characteristics of 63 affected individuals and clinical evidence for heterogeneity. Am J Med Genet 1994;52:450–61.

67. Penneys NS, Adachi K, Zeigels-Weissman J, Nadji M. A survey of cutaneous neural lesions for the presence of myelin basic protein. An immunohistochemical study. Arch Dermatol 1984;120:210–3.

68. Pfeiffer SE, Sundarraj N, Dawson G, Kornblith PL. Human vestibular neurinomas: nervous system specific biochemical parameters. Acta Neuropathologica 1979;47:27–31.

69. Polkey CE. Intraosseous neurilemoma of the cervical spine causing paraparesis and treated by resection and grafting. J Neurol Neurosurg Psychiatry 1975;38:776–81.

70. Purcell M, Dixon M. Schwannomatosis. An unusual variant of neurofibromatosis or a distinct clinical entity? Arch Dermatol 1989;125:390–3.

71. Reith J, Goldblum J. Multiple cutaneous plexiform schwannomas. Report of a case and review of the literature with particular reference to the association with types 1 and 2 neurofibromatosis and schwannomatosis. Arch Pathol Lab Med 1996;120:399–401.

72. Rongioletti F, Drago F, Rebora A. Multiple cutaneous plexiform schwannomas with tumors of the central nervous system [Letter]. Arch Dermatol 1989;125:431–2.

72a. Rosenberg AE, Nielsen GP, Keel SB, Jacoby LB, Mac-Collin M. The pathology of schwannomatosis: a study of 20 tumors from 11 patients with molecular analysis of the NF2 gene [Abstract]. Mod Pathol 1999;12:14A.

73. Ross DA, Edwards MS, Wilson CB. Intramedullary neurilemomas of the spinal cord: report of two cases and review of the literature. Neurosurgery 1986;19:458–64.

74. Rouleau GA, Wertelecki W, Haines JL, Hobbs WJ, Trofatter JA, Seizinger BR. Genetic linkage of bilateral vestibular neurofibromatosis to a DNA marker on chromosome 22. Nature 1987;329:246–8.

75. Salvati M, Ciapetta P, Raco A, Capone R, Artico M, Santoro A. Radiation-induced schwannomas of the neuraxis. Report of three cases. Tumori 1992;78:143–6.

76. Sainz J, Huynh PD, Figueroa K, Ragge NK, Baser ME, Pulst SM. Mutations of the neurofibromatosis type 2 gene and lack of the gene product in vestibular schwannomas. Hum Mol Genet 1994;3:885–91.

77. Santoreneos S, Hanieh A, Jorgensen RE. Trochlear nerve schwannomas occurring in patients without neurofibromatosis: case report and review of literature. Neurosurgery 1997;41:282–7.

78. Sarlomo-Rikala M, Miettinen M. Gastric schwannoma—a clinicopathological analysis of six cases. Histopathology 1995;27:355–60.

79. Seizinger BR, Martuza RL, Gusella JF. Loss of genes on chromosome 22 in tumorigenesis of human vestibular neuroma. Nature 1986;322:644–7.

80. Shishiba T, Niimura M, Ohtsuka F, Tsuru N. Multiple cutaneous neurilemmomas as a skin manifestation of neurilemmomatosis. J Am Acad Dermatol 1984;10:744–54.

81. Shore-Freedman E, Abrahams C, Recant W, Schneider AB. Neurilemomas and salivary gland tumors of the head and neck following childhood irradiation. Cancer 1983;51:2159–63.

82. Sian CS, Ryan SF. The ultrastructure of neurilemmoma with emphasis on Antoni B tissue. Hum Pathol 1981;12:145–60.

83. Silverman JF, Leffers BR, Kay S. Primary pulmonary neurilemoma. Arch Pathol Lab Med 1976;100:644–8.

84. Sobel RA, Wang Y. Vestibular (vestibular) schwannomas: histologic features in neurofibromatosis 2 and in unilateral cases. J Neuropathol Exp Neurol 1993;52:106–13.

85. Spjut J, Dorfman HD, Fechner RE, Ackerman LV. Tumors of bone and cartilage. Atlas of Tumor Pathology. Fascicle 5. Washington D.C.: Armed Forces Institute of Pathology, 1971.

86. Stefanko SZ, Vuzevski VD, Maas AI, van Vroonhoven CC. Intracerebral malignant schwannoma. Acta Neuropathol 1986;71:321–5.

87. Stout AP. Case 5. Neurilemoma of the sciatic nerve. Cancer Seminar (Penrose Cancer Hospital) 1950;1:8–9.

88. Stout AP. The peripheral manifestations of specific nerve sheath tumor (neurilemoma). Am J Cancer 1935;24:751–96.

89. Suster S, Rosai J. Intranodal hemorrhagic spindle-cell tumor with "amianthoid" fibers. Report of six cases of a distinctive mesenchymal neoplasm of the inguinal region that simulates Kaposi's sarcoma. Am J Surg Pathol 1989;13:347–57.

90. Swanson PE, Manivel JC, Wick MR. Immunoreactivity for Leu-7 in neurofibrosarcoma and other spindle cell sarcomas of soft tissue. Am J Pathol 1987;126:546–60.

91. Swanson PE, Stanley MW, Scheithauer BW, Wick MR. Primary cutaneous leiomyosarcoma. A histologic and immunohistochemical study of 9 cases, with ultrastructural correlation. J Cutan Pathol 1988;15:129–41.

92. Sznajder L, Abrahams C, Parry DM, Gierlowski TC, Shore-Freedman E, Schneider AB. Multiple schwannomas and meningiomas associated with irradiation in childhood. Arch Intern Med 1996;156:1873–8.

93. Verocay J. Multiple Geschwülste als Systemerkrankung am nervösen Apparate. Festschrift Hans Chiari aus Anlasz Seines 25 Jèhrigen Professoren-Jubilaüms Gewidmet. W Braumüller, Wein and Leipzig, 1908:378–415

94. Verocay J. Zur Kenntnis der "Neurofibrome." Beitr path Anat allg Path 1910;48:1–69.

95. Waggener JD. Ultrastructure of benign peripheral nerve sheath tumors. Cancer 1966;19:699–709.

96. Weiss SW, Gnepp DR, Bratthauer GL. Palisaded myofibroblastoma. A benign mesenchymal tumor of lymph node. Am J Surg Pathol 1989;13:341–6.

97. Weiss SW, Langloss JM, Enzinger FM. Value of S-100 protein in the diagnosis of soft tissue tumors with particular reference to benign and malignant Schwann cell tumors. Lab Invest 1983;49:299–308.

98. Woodruff JM, Christensen WN. Glandular peripheral nerve sheath tumors. Cancer 1993;72:3618–28.

99. Woodruff JM, Marshall ML, Godwin TA, Funkhouser JW, Thompson NJ, Erlandson RA. Plexiform (multinodular) schwannoma: a tumor simulating the plexiform neurofibroma. Am J Surg Pathol 1983;7:691–7.

100. Yoshida SO, Toot BV. Benign glandular schwannoma. Am J Clin Pathol 1993;100:167–70.

Cellular Schwannoma

101. Carneiro SS, Scheithauer BW, Nascimento AG, Davis DH. Solitary fibrous tumor of the meninges: a lesion distinct from fibrous meningioma—a clinicopathologic and immunohistochemical study [Abstract]. Mod Pathol 1995;8:135A.

102. Casadei GP, Komori T, Scheithauer BW, Miller GM, Parisi JE, Kelly PJ. Intracranial parenchymal schwannoma: a clinicopathologic and neuroimaging study of nine cases. J Neurosurg 1993;79:217–22.

103. Casadei GP, Scheithauer BW, Hirose T, Manfrini M, Van Houton C, Wood MB. Cellular schwannoma: a clinicopathologic, DNA flow cytometric and proliferation marker study of 71 cases. Cancer 1995;75:1109–19.

104. Deruaz JP, Janzer RC, Costa J. Cellular schwannoma of the intracranial and intraspinal compartment: morphological and immunological characteristics compared with classical benign schwannomas. J Neuropathol Exp Neurol 1993;52:114–8.

105. Dickersin GR. The electron microscopic spectrum of nerve sheath tumors. Ultrastruct Pathol 1987;11:103–46.

106. Ducatman BS, Scheithauer BW, Piepgras DG, Reman HM, Ilstrup DM. Malignant peripheral nerve sheath tumors. A clinicopathologic study of 120 cases. Cancer 1986;57:2006–21.

107. Erlandson RA. Diagnostic transmission electron microscopy of tumors. Raven Press: New York, 1994:616–22.

108. Fletcher CD, Davies SE, McKee PH. Cellular schwannoma: a distinct pseudosarcomatous entity. Histopathology 1987;11:21–35.

109. Giangaspero F, Fratamico FC, Ceccarelli C, Brisigotti M. Malignant peripheral nerve sheath tumors and spindle cell sarcomas: an immunohistochemical analysis of multiple markers. Appl Pathol 1989;7:134–44.

110. Hirose T, Hasegawa T, Kudo E, Seki K, Sano T, Hizawa K. Malignant peripheral nerve sheath tumors: an immunohistochemical study in relation to ultrastructural features. Hum Pathol 1992;23:865–70.

111. Hirose T, Sano T, Mori K, et al. Paraganglioma of the cauda equina: an ultrastructural and immunohistochemical study of two cases. Ultrastruct Pathol 1988;12:235–43.

112. Kindblom LG, Ahlden M, Meis-Kindblom JM, Stenman G. Immunohistochemical and molecular analysis of p53, MDM2, proliferating cell nuclear antigen and Ki67 in benign and malignant peripheral nerve sheath tumors. Virchows Arch 1995;427:19–26.

113. Lodding P, Kindblom LG, Angervall L, Stenman G. Cellular schwannoma. A clinicopathologic study of 29 cases. Virchows Arch [A] 1990;416:237–48.

114. Megahed M, Ruzicka T. Cellular schwannoma. Am J Dermatopathol 1994;16(4):418–21.

115. Memoli V, Brown EF, Gould VE. Glial fibrillary acidic protein (GFAP) immunoreactivity in peripheral nerve sheath tumors. Ultrastruct Pathol 1984;7:269–75.

116. Russell DS, Rubinstein LJ. Tumours of the cranial, spinal, and peripheral nerve sheaths. Pathology of tumours of the nervous system. 5th ed. Baltimore: William & Wilkins, 1989:533–71.

117. Swanson PE, Stanley MW, Scheithauer BW, Wick MR. Primary cutaneous leiomyosarcoma. A histologic and immunohistochemical study of 9 cases, with ultrastructural correlation. J Cutan Pathol 1988;15:129–41.

118. Winek RR, Scheithauer BW, Wick MR. Meningioma, meningeal hemangiopericytoma (angioblastic meningioma), peripheral hemangiopericytoma, and vestibular schwannoma. A comparative immunohistochemical study. Am J Surg Pathol 1989;13:251–61.

119. White W, Shiu MH, Rosenblum MK, Erlandson RA, Woodruff JM. Cellular schwannoma. A clinicopathologic study of 57 patients and 58 tumors. Cancer 1990;66:1266–75.

120. Woodruff JM, Selig AM, Crowley K, Allen PW. Schwannoma with malignant transformation. A rare distinctive peripheral nerve tumor. Am J Surg Pathol 1994;18:882–95.

121. Woodruff JM, Susin M, Godwin TA, Martini N, Erlandson RA. Cellular schwannoma. A variety of schwannoma sometimes mistaken for a malignant tumor. Am J Surg Pathol 1981;5:733–44.

Plexiform Schwannoma

122. Argenyi ZB, Goodenberger ME, Strauss JS. Congenital neural hamartoma ("fascicular schwannoma"). A light microscopic, immunohistochemical and ultrastructural study. Am J Dermatopathol 1990;12:283–93.

123. Barbosa J, Hansen LS. Solitary multinodular schwannoma of the oral cavity. J Oral Med 1984;39:232–5.

124. Casadei GP, Scheithauer BW, Hirose T, Manfrini M, Van Houton C, Wood MB. Cellular schwannoma. A clinicopathologic, DNA flow cytometric and proliferation marker study of 71 cases. Cancer 1995;75:1109–19.

125. Enzinger FM, Weiss SW. Soft tissue tumors. St. Louis: C.V. Mosby, 1983:587.

126. Fletcher CD, Davies SE. Benign plexiform (multinodular) schwannoma: a rare tumor unassociated with neurofibromatosis. Histopathology 1986;10:971–80.

127. Harkin JC, Arrington JH, Reed RJ. Benign plexiform schwannoma. A lesion distinct from plexiform neurofibroma [Abstract]. J Neuropathol Exp Neurol 1978;37:622.

128. Hirose T, Scheithauer BW, Sano T. Giant plexiform schwannoma: report of two cases with soft tissue and visceral involvement. Mod Pathol 1997;11:1075–81.

128a. Ishida T, Kuroda M, Motoi T, Oka T, Imamura T, Machinami R. Phenotypic diversity of neurofibromatosis 2: association with plexiform schwannoma. Histopathology 1998;32:264–70.

129. Iwashita T, Enjoji M. Plexiform neurilemoma: a clinicopathological and immunohistochemical analysis of 23 tumors from 20 patients. Virchows Arch [A] 1987;411:305–9.

130. Kao GF, Laskin WB, Olsen TG. Solitary cutaneous plexiform neurilemoma (schwannoma): a clinicopathologic, immunohistochemical, and ultrastructural study of 11 cases. Mod Pathol 1989;2:20–6.

131. Meis-Kindblom JM, Enzinger FM. Plexiform malignant peripheral nerve sheath tumor of infancy and childhood. Am J Surg Pathol 1994;18:479–85.

132. Reith JD, Goldblum JR. Multiple cutaneous plexiform schwannomas. Report of a case and review of the literature with particular reference to the association with types 1 and 2 neurofibromatosis and schwannomatosis. Arch Pathol Lab Med 1996;120:399–401.

133. Shishiba T, Niimura M, Ohtsuka F, Tsuru N. Multiple cutaneous neurilemmomas as a skin manifestation of neurilemmomatosis. J Am Acad Dermatol 1984;10:744–54.

134. Woodruff JM, Erlandson R, Scheithauer BW. Letter to the editor. Am J Surg Pathol 1995;19:608–9.

135. Woodruff JM, Marshall ML, Godwin TA, Funkhouser JW, Thompson NJ, Erlandson RA. Plexiform (multinodular) schwannoma. A tumor simulating the plexiform neurofibroma. Am J Surg Pathol 1983;7:691–7.

Melanotic Schwannoma

136. Abbott AE Jr, Hill RE, Flynn MA, McClure S, Murray GF. Melanotic schwannoma of the spinal sympathetic ganglia: pathologic and clinical characteristics. Ann Thoracic Surg 1990;49:1006–8.

137. Anderson B, Robertson DM. Melanin containing neurofibroma: case report with evidence of Schwann cell origin of melanin. Can J Neurol Sci 1979;6:139–43.
138. Assor D. A melanotic tumor of the esophagus. Cancer 1975;35:1438–43.
139. Bagchi AK, Sarkar SK, Chakraborti DP, Roy CK. Melanotic spinal schwannoma. Surg Neurol 1975;3:79–81.
140. Bain J. "Carney's complex" [Letter]. Mayo Clin Proc 1986;61:508.
141. Bigotti G, Familiari V. Schwannoma melanocitico: descrizione di un caso e revisione della letteratura. Riv Anat Pat Oncol 1986;45:279–84.
141a. Brat DJ, Giannini C, Scheithauer BW, Burger PC. Primary melanocytic neoplasms of the central nervous system. Am J Surg Pathol (in press).
142. Burns DK, Silva FG, Forde KP, Mount PM, Clark HB. Primary melanotic schwannoma of the stomach. Evidence of dual melanocytic and schwannian differentiation in an extra-axial site in a patient without neurofibromatosis. Cancer 1983;52:1432–41.
143. Carney JA. Psammomatous melanotic schwannoma. A distinctive, heritable tumor with special associations, including cardiac myxoma and the Cushing syndrome. Am J Surg Pathol 1990;14:206–22.
144. Carney JA, Gordon H, Carpenter PC, Shenoy V, Go VL. The complex of myxomas, spotty pigmentation, and endocrine overactivity. Medicine 1985;64:270–83.
145. Carney JA, Hruska LS, Beauchamp GD, Gordon H. Dominant inheritance of the complex of myxomas, spotty pigmentation, and endocrine overactivity. Mayo Clin Proc 1986;61:165–72.
145a. Carney JA, Stratakis CA. Epithelioid blue nevus and psammomatous melanotic schwannoma: the unusual pigmented skin tumors of the Carney complex. Semin Diag Pathol 1998;15:216–24.
146. Christensen C. Malignant melanocytic schwannoma. A case report. Acta Chir Scand 1986;152:385–6.
147. Chung EB, Enzinger FM. Malignant melanoma of soft parts. A reassessment of clear cell sarcoma. Am J Surg Pathol 1983;7:405–13.
148. Cras P, Ceuterick-Groote CH, Van Vyve M, Vercruyssen A, Martin JJ. Malignant pigmented spinal nerve root schwannoma metastasizing in the brain and viscera. Clin Neuropathol 1990;9:290–4.
149. Danoff A, Jormark S, Lorber D, Fleischer N. Adrenocortical micronodular dysplasia, cardiac myxomas, lentigines, and spindle cell tumors. Report of a kindred. Arch Intern Med 1987;147:443–8.
150. Dastur DK, Sinh G, Pandya SK. Melanotic tumor of the acoustic nerve. Case report. J Neurosurg 1967;27:166–70.
151. DiGregorio C, Fano RA, Criscuolo M. Melanotic schwannoma: a case report. Appl Pathol 1984;2:110–5.
152. Dimaio SM, Mackay B, Smith JL, Dickersin GR. Neurosarcomatous transformation in malignant melanoma: an ultrastructural study. Cancer 1982;50:2345–54.
153. Ducastelle T, Ducastelle CH, Hemet J, Lefort J, Borde J. Schwannome mÄlanotique (neurilemmome pigmentÄ). Etude en microscopie optique et electronique d'un cas, avec double localisation tumorale d'implantation pÄriostÄe. Ann Pathol (Paris) 1981;1:205–13.
154. Enzinger FM. Clear cell sarcoma of tendons and aponeuroses. An analysis of 21 cases. Cancer 1965;18:1163–74.
155. Erlandson RA. Melanotic schwannoma of spinal nerve origin. Ultrastruct Pathol 1985;9:123–9.
155a. Fetsch JF, Michal M, Miettinen M. Pigmented (melanotic) neurofibroma: a clinicopathologic and immunohistochemical analysis of 19 lesions from 17 patients. Am J Surg Pathol (in press).
156. Font RL, Truong LD. Melanotic schwannoma of soft tissues. Electron-microscopic observations and review of the literature. Am J Surg Pathol 1984;8:129–38.
157. Fu YS, Kaye GI, Lattes R. Primary malignant melanocytic tumors of the sympathetic ganglia, with an ultrastructural study of one. Cancer 1975;36:2029–41.
158. Gelfand ET, Taylor RF, Rao S, Hendin D, Akabutu J, Callaghan JC. Melanotic malignant schwannoma of the right atrium. J Thorac Cardiovasc Surg 1977;74:808–12.
159. Graham DI, Paterson A, McQueen A, Milne JA, Urich H. Melanotic tumours (blue naevi) of spinal nerve root. J Pathol 1976;118:83–9.
160. Graziani N, Gambarelli D, Bartoli JM, Dechambenoit G, Bellard S, Grisoli F. Tumeur melanique intradurale extramedullarie: a propos d'un cas de neurinome pigmente dorsal. Revue de la literature. Neurochirurgie 1988;33:210–7.
161. Gregorios JB, Chou SM, Bay J. Melanotic schwannoma of the spinal cord. Neurosurgery 1982;11:57–60.
162. Hisaoka M, Ohta H, Haratake J, Horie A. Melanotic schwannoma in the spinal canal. Acta Pathol Jpn 1991;41:685–8.
163. Hodson JJ. An intra-osseous tumor combination of biological importance–invasion of a melanotic schwannoma by an adamantinoma. J Pathol Bact 1961;82:257–66.
164. Janzer RC, Makek M. Intraoral malignant melanotic schwannoma. Ultrastructural evidence for melanogenesis by Schwann's cells. Arch Pathol Lab Med 1983;107:298–301.
165. Jellinger K, Bock F, Breener H. Meningeal melanocytoma: report of a case and review of the literature. Acta Neurochir 1988;94:78–87.
166. Jensen OA, Bretlau P. Melanotic schwannoma of the orbit. Immunohistochemical and ultrastructural study of a case and survey of the literature. Acta Pathol Microbiol Immunol Scand [A] 1990;98:713–23.
167. Jones H, Theaker JM, Kelly PM, Woods CG, Greenall MJ. Melanotic schwannomas arising within localized pigmented neurofibromatosis of the sympathetic chain. Histopathology 1990;17:567–82.
168. Kai Y, Park JH, Nakamura M, Osada H, Sawada T, Sakurai I. Melanotic schwannoma: a case report. Jap J Clin Pathol 1987;37:823–8.
169. Katenkamp D, Filippowa N, Raikhlin NT. Das melanozytische Schwannom. Licht-und Elektronenmikroskopische Befunde zur Morphologie Diagnose und Differential diagnose. Zentralbe allg Pathol Anat 1986;137:107–18.
170. Kayano H, Katayama I. Melanotic schwannoma arising in the sympathetic ganglion. Hum Pathol 1988;19:1355–8.
171. Kellert E, Woodruff R. Pigmented ganglionic tumor of the thorax. Cancer 1956;9:300–5.
172. Killeen RM, Davy CL, Bauserman SC. Melanotic schwannoma. Cancer 1988;62:174–83.
173. Krausz T, Azzorpardi JG, Pearse E. Malignant melanoma of the sympathetic chain: with a consideration of pigmented nerve sheath tumors. Histopathology 1984;8:881–94.

174. Leedman PJ, Cohen AK, Matz LR. The complex of myxomas, spotty pigmentation and endocrine overactivity. Clin Endocrinol 1986;25:527–34.

175. Limas C, Tio FO. Meningeal melanocytoma ("melanotic meningioma"). Its melanocytic origin as revealed by electron microscopy. Cancer 1972;30:1286–94.

176. Lowman RM, Livolsi VA. Pigmented (melanotic) schwannomas of the spinal canal. Cancer 1980;46:391–7.

177. Mandybur TI. Melanotic nerve sheath tumors. J Neurosurg 1974;41:187–92.

178. Marchese MJ, McDonald JV. Intramedullary melanotic schwannoma of the cervical spinal cord. Report of a case. Surg Neurol 1990;33:353–5.

179. McGavran WL, Sypert GW, Ballinger WE. Melanotic schwannoma. Neurosurgery 1978;2:47–51.

180. Meier RJ, Altermatt HJ, Musy JP, Gebbers JO. Melanotisches Schwannom. Fallbericht und Literaturubersicht. Pathologie 1987;8:282–90.

181. Mennemeyer RP, Hallman KO, Hammar SP, Raisis JE, Tytus JS, Bockus D. Melanotic schwannoma. Clinical and ultrastructural studies of three cases with evidence of intracellular melanin synthesis. Am J Surg Pathol 1979;3:3–10.

182. Miettinen M. Melanotic schwannoma coexpression of vimentin and glial fibrillary acidic protein. Ultrastruct Pathol 1987;11:39–46.

183. Millar WG. A malignant melanotic tumor of ganglion cells arising from a thoracic sympathetic ganglion. J Pathol Bact 1932;35:351-7.

184. Miller RT, Sarikaya H, Sos A. Melanotic schwannoma of the acoustic nerve. Arch Pathol Lab Med 1986;110:153–4.

185. Myers JL, Bernreuter W, Dunham W. Melanotic schwannoma of bone. Clinicopathologic, immunohistochemical and ultrastructural features of a rare primary bone tumor. Am J Clin Pathol 1990;93:424–9.

186. Napoli P, De Domenico P. Primary melanotic schwannoma of the spinal canal. Appl Pathol 1987;5:253–60.

187. Parent M, Beyls-Noel I, Lecomte-Houcke M, Fontaine C, Dupont A. Schwannome melanotique. Etude anatomo-clinique d'une observation et revue de la literature. Semin Hop Paris 1987;63:3287–92.

188. Paris F, Cabanes J, Munoz C, Tamarit L. Melanotic spinothoracic schwannoma. Thorax 1979;34:243–6.

189. Parker JB, Marcus PB, Martin JH. Spinal melanotic clear-cell sarcoma: a light and electron microscopic study. Cancer 1980;46:718–24.

190. Payan MJ, Gambarelli D, Keller P, et al. Melanotic neurofibroma: a case report with ultrastructural study. Acta Neuropathol (Berlin) 1986;69:148–52.

191. Prabhu SS, Lynch PG, Keogh AJ, Parekh HC. Intracranial meningeal melanocytoma: a report of two cases and a review of the literature. Surg Neurol 1993;40:516–21.

192. Prieto VG, Woodruff JM. Expression of laminin, type 4 collagen, S-100 protein, and HMB 45 antigens in spindle cell melanoma. J Cutan Pathol 1998;25:297–300.

193. Quencer RM, Stokes NA, Wolfe D, Page LK. Melanotic nerve sheath tumor of the gasserian ganglion and trigeminal nerve. AJR Am J Roentgenol 1979;133:142–4.

194. Robertson DM, Ghadially FN. Case 15. Ultrastruct Pathol 1983;5:369–74.

195. Rowlands D, Edwards C, Collins F. Malignant melanotic schwannoma of the bronchus. J Clin Pathol 1987;40:1449–55.

196. Roytta M, Elfversson J, Kalimo H. Intraspinal pigmented schwannoma with malignant progression. Acta Neuro Chir (Wien) 1988;95:147–54.

197. Schulz H, Haneke C, Caleff N. Ein gutartiges melanotic Neurinom der Mundschleimhaut. Dtsch Zahn Mund Kieferheilkunde 1965;44:369–73.

198. Scully S, MacPherson SG, Reid R, Dagg JH, Critchlow H, McGowan D. Melanotic nerve sheath tumor in the neck. Int J Oral Surg 1981;10:376–9.

199. Sheehan DC, Hrapchak BB. Pigments and minerals. In: Theory and practice of histotechnology. 2nd ed. St. Louis: C.V. Mosby, 1980:214–32.

200. Shields JA, Font RL, Eagle RC Jr, Shields CL, Gass JD. Melanotic schwannoma of the choroid. Immunohistochemistry and electron microscopic observations. Ophthalmology 1994;101:843–9.

201. Shilitoe AJ. Melanotic schwannoma. J Pathol Bacteriol 1965;90:667–8.

202. Sokolova IN, Parshikova SM. Melanotic schwannoma. Arch Pathol (Moscow) 1986;48:57–63.

203. Solomon RA, Handler MS, Sedelli RV, Stein BM. Intramedullary melanotic schwannoma of the cervicomedullary junction. Neurosurgery 1987;20:36–8.

204. Terzakis JA, Opher E, Melamed J, Santagada E, Sloan D. Pigmented melanotic schwannoma of the uterine cervix. Ultrastruct Pathol 1990;14:357–66.

205. Theodossiou A, Segditsas T. Uber ein intraabdominal gelegenes melanotisches Schwannoma. Zentralbl Allg Path Bd 1971;114:168–72.

206. Webb JN. The ultra-structure of a melanotic schwannoma of the skin. J Pathol 1982;137:25–36.

207. Winston KR, Sotrel A, Schnitt SJ. Meningeal melanocytoma. Case report and review of the clinical and histological features. J Neurosurg 1987;66:50–7.

✧✧✧

8

NEUROFIBROMA

Definition. Neurofibroma is a benign nerve sheath tumor composed of a variable mixture of Schwann, perineurial-like, and fibroblastic cells, as well as ones with features intermediate between these various cells. Residual interspersed myelinated and unmyelinated nerve fibers often are present.

General Comments. Whereas the term "solitary benign nerve sheath tumor" was at one time applied to both schwannoma and neurofibroma, the designation is now avoided. The distinction of the two tumors is possible in almost all instances, and is clinically important, not only for diagnosing neurofibromatosis but, on occasion, for excluding a diagnosis of malignant peripheral nerve sheath tumor (MPNST). The principal clinicopathologic features distinguishing schwannoma from neurofibroma are summarized in Table 7-1.

The nature of neurofibroma, whether a neoplasm or a hyperplastic process, remains unsettled. The development of myriads of lesions in patients with neurofibromatosis type 1 (NF1) as well as their cytologic, immunohistochemical, and ultrastructural heterogeneity are used to support the hyperplasia concept, whereas the almost imperceptible transition of neurofibromas to MPNST suggests they are neoplastic. Assuming that Schwann cells are the key constituent of neurofibromas, most experimental studies have, rightly or wrongly, focused upon this cell. The Schwann cells of neurofibromas differ from normal ones by their ability to promote angiogenesis and invade basement membrane (51). On the other hand, neurofibroma Schwann cells respond normally by proliferation when exposed to specific Schwann cell mitogens (44) and growth factors present in neurofibroma tissue. These findings and the finding that neurofibroma-derived Schwann cells do not form progressive tumors when injected into mice (51), have lent support to the concept that it is the physiologic milieu of neurofibromas that stimulates proliferation of nerve sheath cells and perhaps the development of subpopulations prone to neoplastic transformation. Recent evidence

based upon studies of X chromosome inactivation suggests that neurofibromas are monoclonal lesions (54). As currently understood, all NF1 patients harbor one nonfunctional NF1 gene (germline mutation) in every cell in the body (18), and it is assumed that neurofibromas arise as a result of a second, somatic mutation (18,53). Although yet to be demonstrated, the pathogenesis of non-NF1-related neurofibromas is probably due to alterations of the NF1 gene. Thereafter, the occasional transformation of neurofibroma to MPNST (17) appears to involve loss or mutation of one or more tumor suppressor genes. We believe that more complete characterization of the constituent cells of neurofibromas will shed light upon their cytogenesis and further support the concept that neurofibromas are neoplastic in nature.

Whereas von Recklinghausen (61) considered neurofibromas to be fibrous tumors, Verocay (60) in 1910 postulated that they arose instead from neuroectodermal nerve sheath elements, such as Schwann cells, or from embryonal neuroectodermal cells. Although the subsequent demonstration of nonspecific cholinesterase activity in neurofibromas supports their neuroectodermal nature (65), it now appears that several different types of cells are present. Ultrastructural and immunohistochemical studies show that they are composed of Schwann cells, perineurial-like cells, fibroblasts, and cells with features intermediate between perineurial-like cells and the others. At the ultrastructural level, typical well-differentiated Schwann cells predominate in a majority of neurofibromas, a finding supported by immunostains for S-100 protein which label these cells. The extent to which normal residual Schwann cells are represented is unclear, however. Perineurial-like cells are defined as ones possessing the ultrastructural characteristics, but not the immunoprofile, of normal perineurial cells. With the exception of occasional peripherally situated perineurial cells, remnants of the parent nerve, intraneural neurofibromas show no staining for epithelial membrane antigen (EMA), the principal marker of such cells. In addition, diffuse neurofibromas occasionally show perineurial cells to surround pseudomeissnerian corpuscles (see fig. 8-28D). Nonetheless, virtually all neurofibromas do contain perineurial-like cells. In a minority of tumors, such cells predominate. Thus, the constant presence of perineurial-like cells in neurofibromas makes them an important marker of this tumor. Myelinated and unmyelinated axons ensheathed by normal Schwann cells are frequently seen in tumors, although not widely dispersed.

Clinicopathologic and Gross Findings. Neurofibromas develop either in patients with NF1 (peripheral neurofibromatosis, von Recklinghausen's disease) or more commonly as solitary sporadic lesions unassociated with the disorder. They are very uncommon in the setting of NF2. The present discussion focuses primarily upon those neurofibromas encountered in skin and soft tissue. Visceral neurofibromas and ganglioneuromatous lesions of NF1 are discussed in chapters 5 and 13.

Several forms of neurofibroma have been described. Despite morphologic overlap, their clinicopathologic features differ considerably. These variants are considered below. The discussion of neurofibromas arising in small cutaneous nerves (localized and diffuse cutaneous neurofibromas) precedes that of tumors originating in larger nerves, including roots, trunks, and branches (localized intraneural and plexiform neurofibromas). We take this approach because the gross appearances of neurofibroma variants reflect their manner of growth and spread. For instance, in neurofibromas arising in small to minute nerves, such as those of skin, permeative growth in nerve quickly gives way to diffuse infiltration of surrounding soft tissue, and parent nerves are inconspicuous. In localized neurofibromas arising in sizable nerves, endoneurial spread of neurofibroma cells results in symmetric, typically fusiform enlargement of fascicles (localized neurofibroma) (22,66). Lastly, in addition to widespread endoneurial growth, plexiform lesions frequently exhibit diffuse soft tissue infiltration as well.

Localized Cutaneous Neurofibroma. This most common form of neurofibroma occurs either as single or multiple lesions. They often affect the dermis and subcutis and show no particular site predilection. Soft, slightly elevated, nodular or polypoid (figs. 8-1, 8-2), such tumors are painless, slow growing, freely moveable, and uncommonly exceed 1 to 2 cm in maximum dimension. Most (90 percent) are solitary, unassociated with NF1, and present in young adults between age 20 and 30 years. In individuals with NF1, neurofibromas are typically multiple (fig. 8-1) and may be overlain by a hyperpigmented epidermal macule, the café-au-lait spot (see below). Most patients with NF1 have developed cutaneous neurofibromas by the time of puberty; thereafter, the tumors simply increase in number and often in size. Only on rare occasion does their continued proliferation result in the patient being quite literally covered by innumerable cutaneous nodules, many of which are polypoid (fig. 8-1C,D). On cut section localized cutaneous neurofibromas are homogeneously gray or gray-tan and lack the degenerative changes that typify schwannomas. Although relatively circumscribed, they are not encapsulated (fig. 8-2). Many but not all are separated from epidermis by a grenz zone (fig. 8-2B). Deeper portions are often less defined from surrounding dermis or subcutaneous fat. Whether solitary or multiple, the microscopic features of cutaneous neurofibromas are essentially the same. As a rule, no underlying involved nerve is apparent, since the proliferation is extraneural. We have not seen a localized cutaneous neurofibroma that underwent malignant change.

Diffuse Cutaneous Neurofibroma. The distinction between localized and diffuse tumors is usually easy, since the term diffuse neurofibroma is generally applied to only large lesions. Nonetheless, mixed patterns may be observed, particularly in the setting of NF1 (fig. 8-3). Once termed "paraneurofibroma," the diffuse cutaneous variant is uncommon and presents primarily in children and young adults. The association is not strong, but fully 10 percent arise in the setting of NF1. Diffuse neurofibromas form ill-defined, plaque-like thickenings of the dermis and subcutaneous tissue (figs. 8-4, 8-5), usually of the head and neck. Although the content of overrun adipose tissue renders them yellow-white (fig. 8-4), the texture of the neurofibromatous tissue resembles that of localized cutaneous neurofibroma. Diffuse tumors are nondestructive of their surroundings. Instead, they permeate the dermis, wherein they entrap adnexae (fig. 8-5C), and spread freely along connective tissue septa as well as within subcutaneous adipose tissue (figs. 8-4, 8-5D). Pseudo-meissnerian corpuscles may be seen. Diffuse neurofibromas only rarely undergo malignant change.

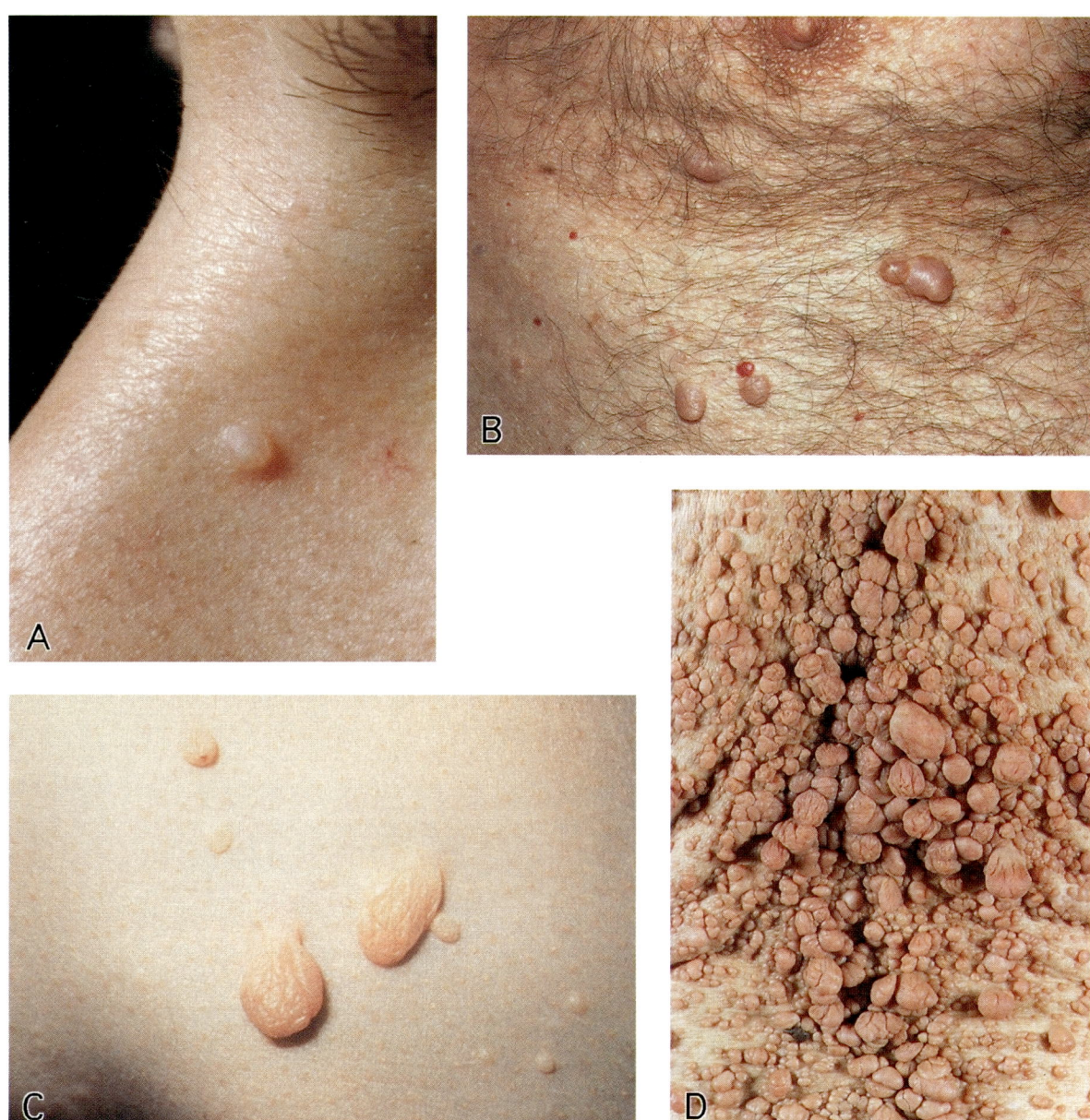

Figure 8-1
LOCALIZED CUTANEOUS NEUROFIBROMA
Such tumors may be solitary (A) or multiple and often NF1 associated (B-D). The latter may be dome shaped (B) or polypoid (C). On occasion they lie densely clustered (D) as on the lower back of this markedly affected patient. (C, courtesy of Dr. H. Goebel, Mainz, Germany.)

Localized Intraneural Neurofibroma. Second in frequency and the result of permeative intraneural growth of tumor cells, this variant of neurofibroma causes segmental, fusiform nerve enlargement (figs. 8-7, 8-9). Examples range from less than one to many centimeters in greatest dimension (fig. 8-10). Multiple lesions occur primarily in the setting of NF1. Localized intraneural neurofibromas come to clinical attention either as a lump in superficial soft tissues or, if arising at a deep site, by causing tingling or pain along the course of a nerve. A number are incidental findings

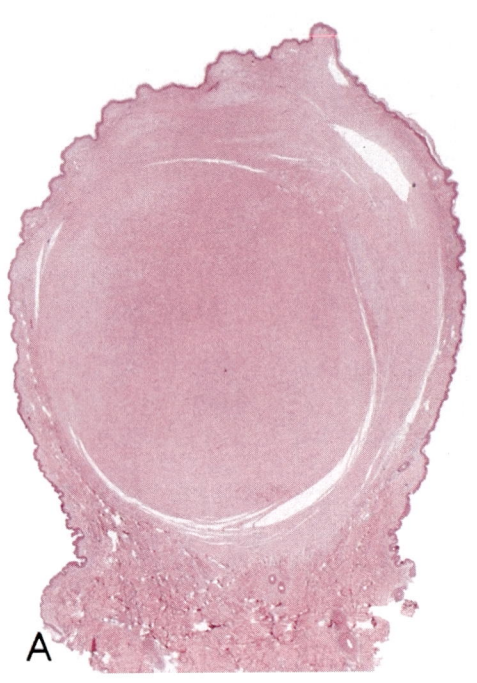

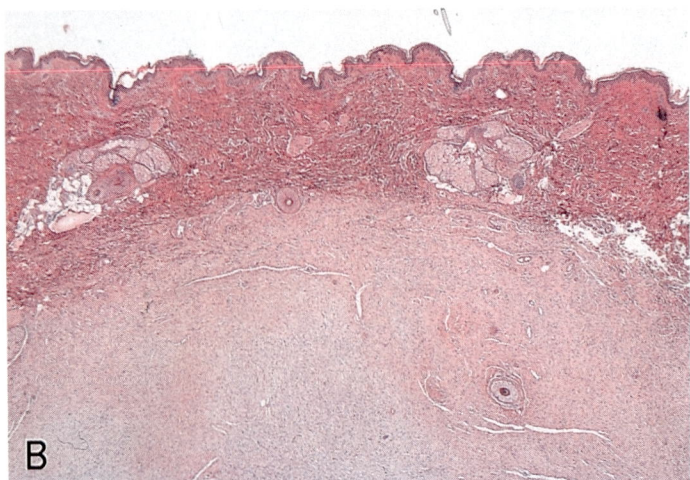

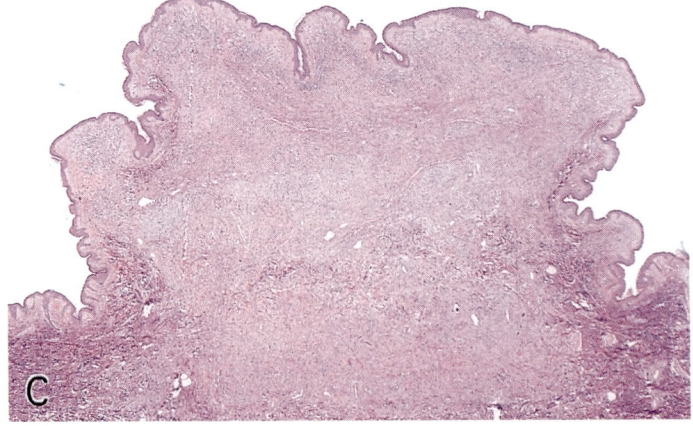

Figure 8-2
LOCALIZED CUTANEOUS
NEUROFIBROMA

These three examples, all occurring in patients with NF1, show variation in microarchitecture, particularly their relation to surrounding tissue, which ranges from discrete and compressive (A,B) to infiltrative (C).

Figure 8-3
DIFFUSE CUTANEOUS
NEUROFIBROMA

Such plaque-like lesions are typically larger than localized tumors. This example, occurring in a patient with NF1, also features nodules much like those comprising localized neurofibromas.

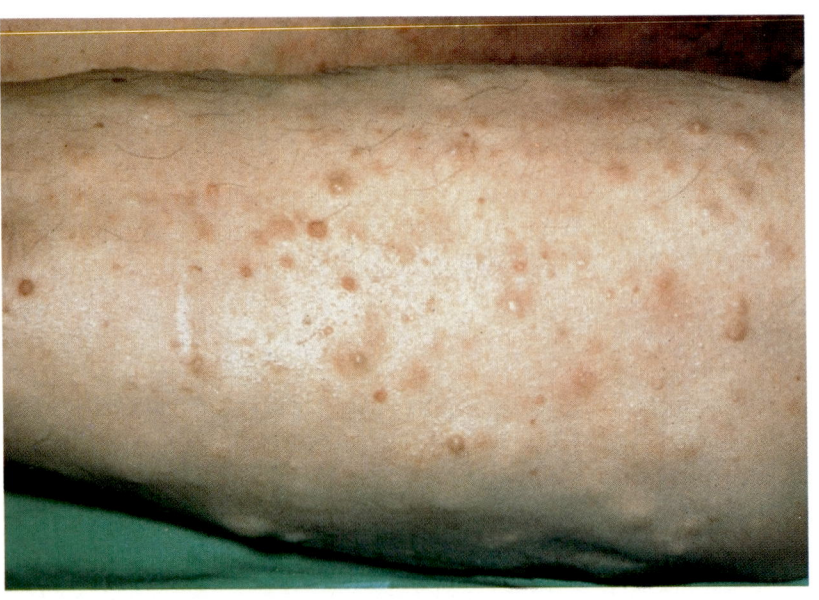

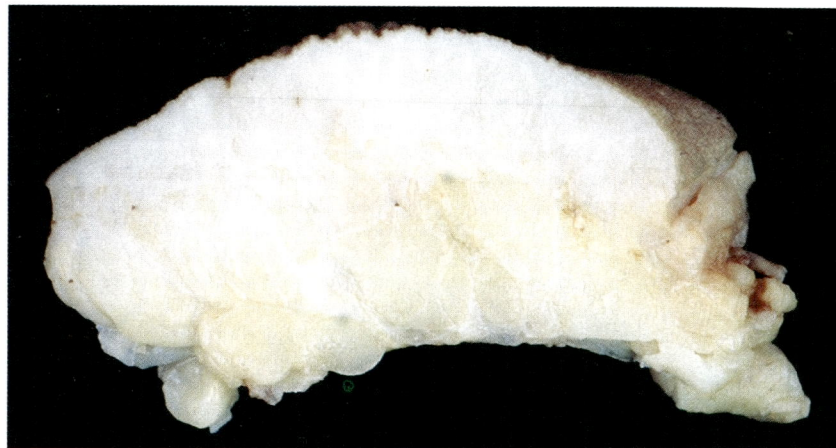

Figure 8-4
DIFFUSE CUTANEOUS
NEUROFIBROMA
This brawny, NF1-associated example massively involves subcutaneous fat. Strands of tumor separate lobules of fat. Its white rather than gray-tan color is an artifact of fixation. (Fig. 3.444 from Okazaki H, Scheithauer BW. Atlas of neuropathology, 1988. With permission from the Mayo Foundation.)

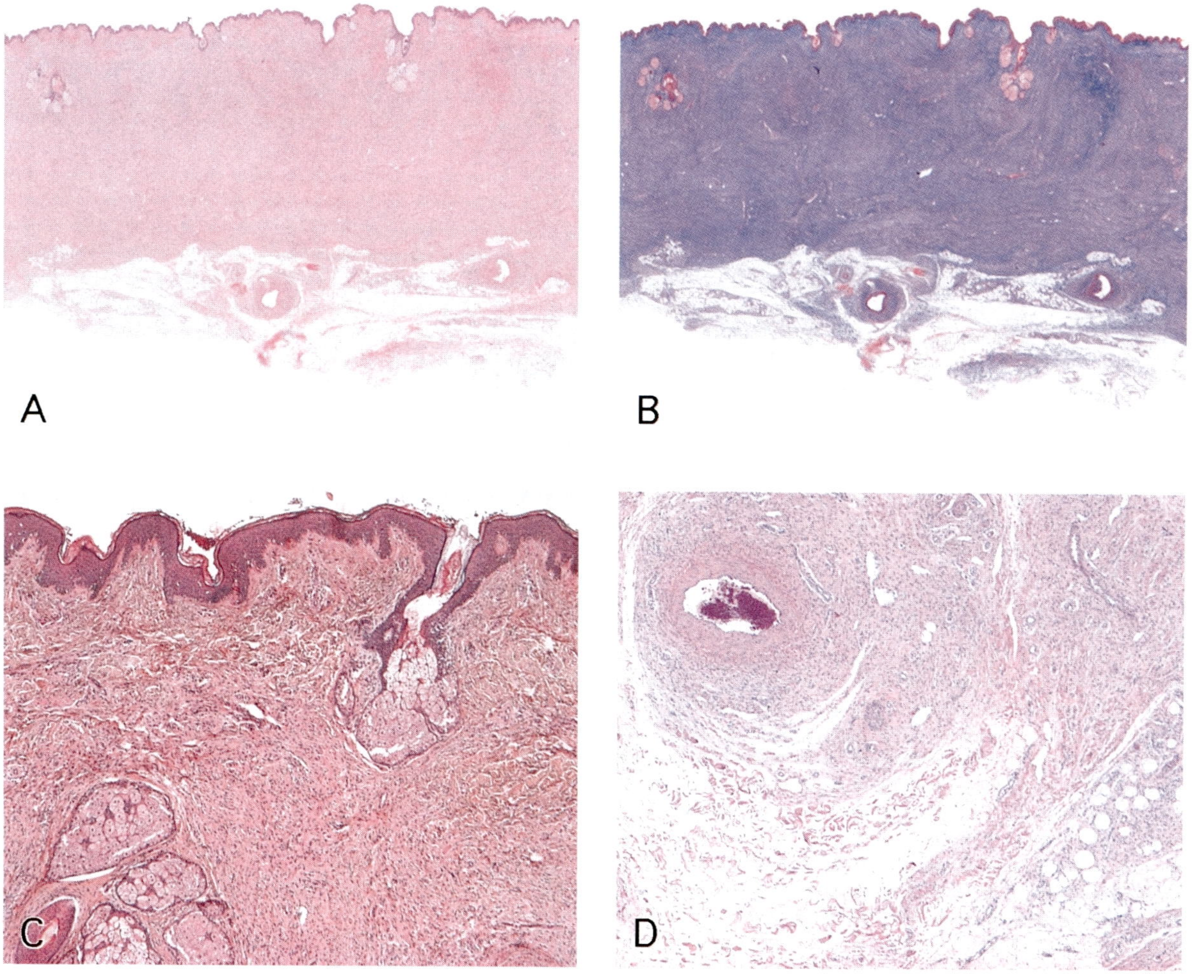

A

B

C

D

Figure 8-5
DIFFUSE CUTANEOUS NEUROFIBROMA
Such tumors permeate dermal and subcutaneous tissues (A,B), surround adnexae (C), and infiltrate fat (D).

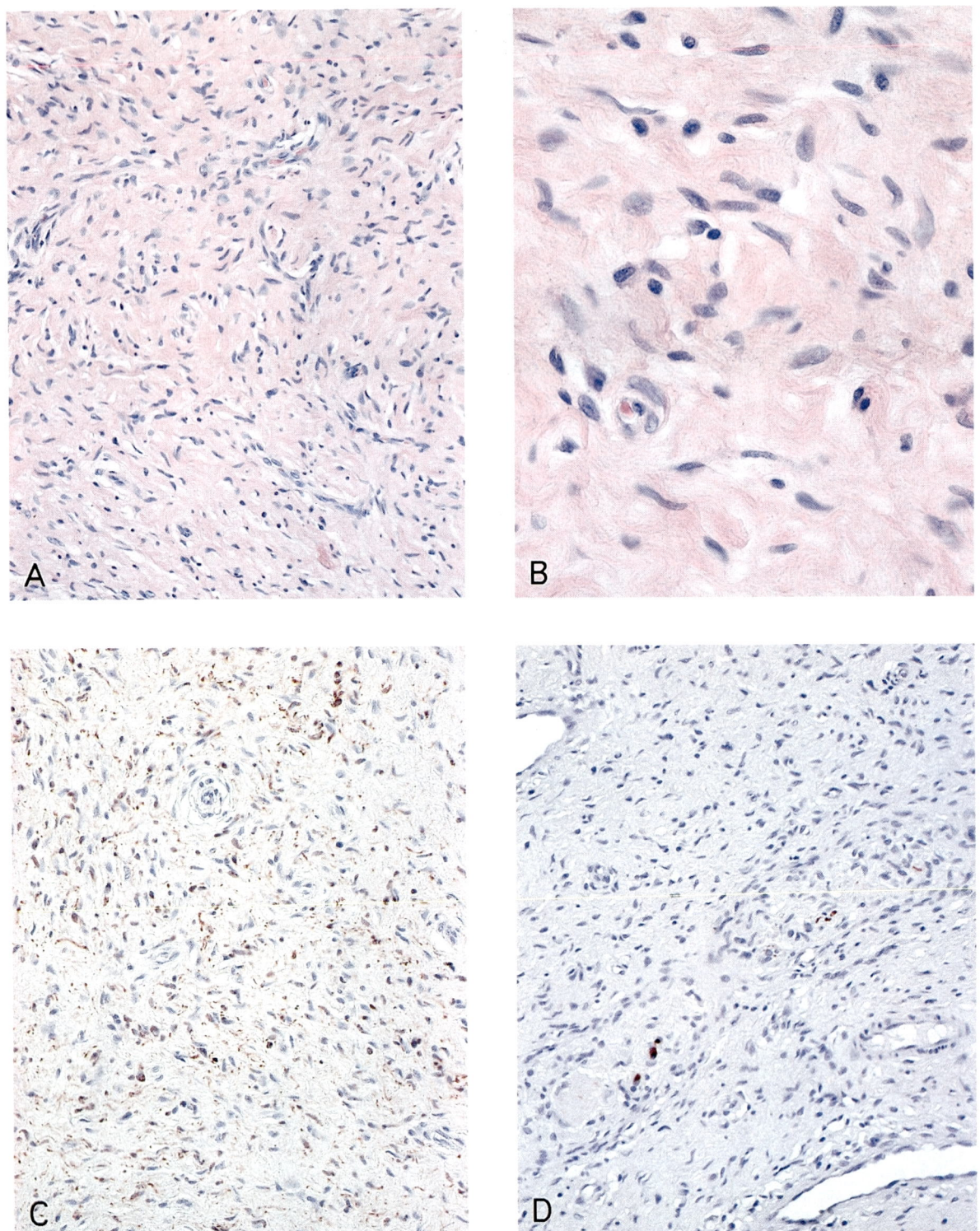

Figure 8-6
DIFFUSE CUTANEOUS NEUROFIBROMA

Note the diffuse infiltration by uniform neurofibroma cells (A). At high power, the delicate processes of these cells are usually not apparent (B). Many but not all cells are S-100 protein immunoreactive (C). In that such lesions are largely extraneural, neuritic processes are scant on neurofilament protein stain (D).

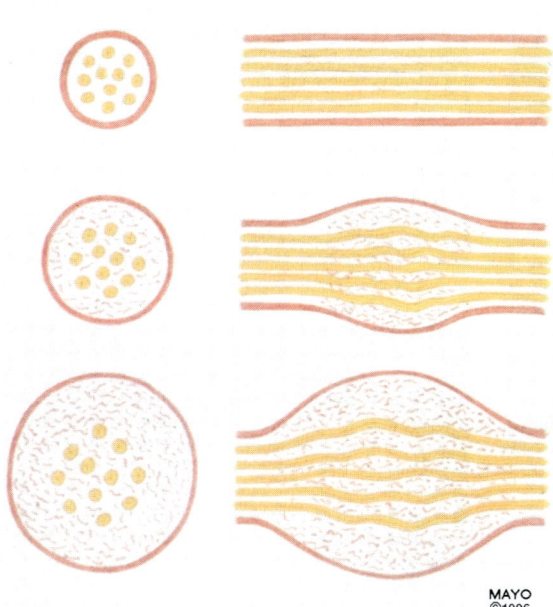

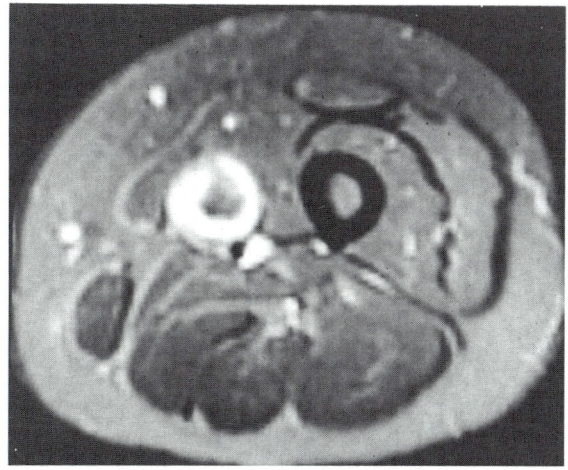

Figure 8-8
LOCALIZED INTRANEURAL NEUROFIBROMA
This axial T2-weighted MRI image shows the target config-
uration characteristic of neurofibroma.

Figure 8-7
LOCALIZED INTRANEURAL NEUROFIBROMA
A schematic illustrates the slow development of neurofibroma to a fusiform, mucin-rich lesion traversed by normal
residual axons.

on imaging studies. Localized intraneural neurofibromas may affect any nerve, spinal or cranial, from the root level to the smallest branch.
NF1-associated spinal root tumors preferentially
affect the cervical level, as do spinal root
schwannomas in NF2 (19). Tumors arising in
proximal spinal nerves may have both an intraspinal and extraspinal component. Such
"dumbbell-shaped" neurofibromas occur both
sporadically and in association with NF1. Neurofibromas also affect the autonomic nervous system. Gross examination of localized intraneural
neurofibromas show them to be fusiform, diffuse
enlargements of the affected nerve (fig. 8-9A,B,
E). On cut section, they appear translucent and
gray to tan (figs. 8-9C, 8-10). Texture and color
variations reflect differences in collagen content
which may be focally accentuated (fig. 8-10F).
Favorably oriented sections often demonstrate
underlying residual nerve fibers (fig. 8-11). By
way of comparison, intraneural neurofibromas
lack the globular paraneural configuration,
thick capsule, lipid-related bright yellow coloration, cystic changes, and occasional hemorrhagic

foci that characterize schwannomas. These differences are also radiologically evident (figs. 8-8,
8-9D; see also figs. 7-3–7-7) and of use in differential diagnosis with MPNST (9a). Localized
intraneural neurofibromas infrequently undergo malignant change.

Plexiform Neurofibroma. Grossly and microscopically, this uncommon but highly characteristic variant of neurofibroma shows a tendency to
affect sizable nerves (22,66). Its recognition is important since it occurs almost exclusively in patients with NF1 and is significantly prone to undergo malignant change (see below). A diagnosis of
plexiform neurofibroma in a patient with no other
features of the disorder therefore requires a genetic workup. Although we have seen only a rare
plexiform neurofibroma in patients with no family history and in whom no other features of NF1
were found, it has recently been suggested that
a significant minority lack the association (37).

The varied clinical manifestations of plexiform neurofibroma are discussed in detail in
chapter 13. Severely deforming affected tissues,
their architectural features and gross appearance cover a spectrum (figs. 8-18–8-21). Most
involve either a plexus of nerves, with a resultant
tree-like pattern in which innumerable branches
and twigs form a complex tangle (figs. 8-18, 8-19),
or multiple fascicles of a medium to large nerve
with preservation of its general configuration

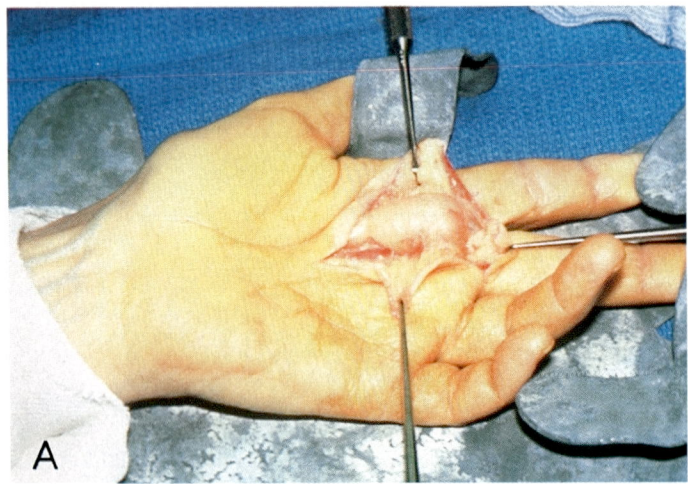
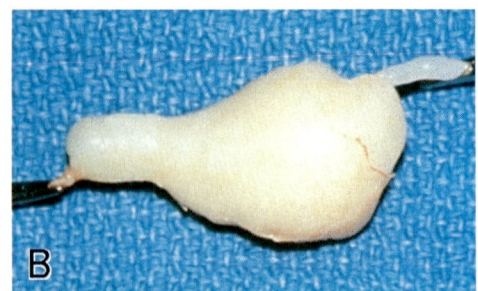
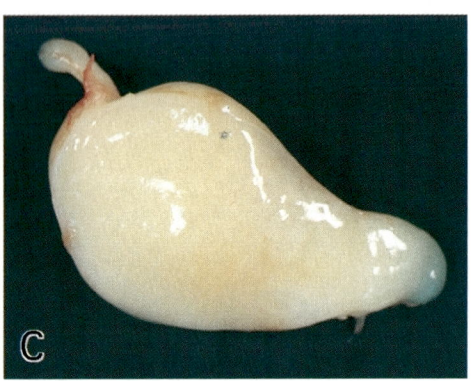

Figure 8-9
LOCALIZED INTRANEURAL NEUROFIBROMA

Resection of neurofibroma, illustrated by an operative photo (A). The resection of this tumor involved its removal with proximal and distal segments of the parent nerve (B). The cross section of this specimen shows the typical translucency and gray-tan color of such tumors (C). Yet another example affecting a sensory nerve of the popliteal region in an NF1 patient shows typical T2-weighted MRI features (D). Its resection (E) permitted sparing of uninvolved fascicles and no significant neurological deficit.

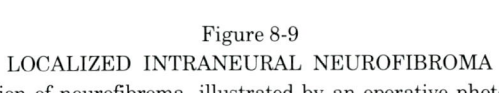
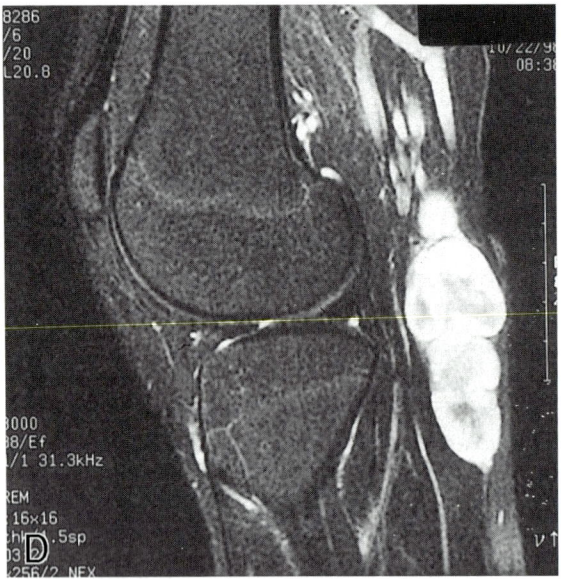
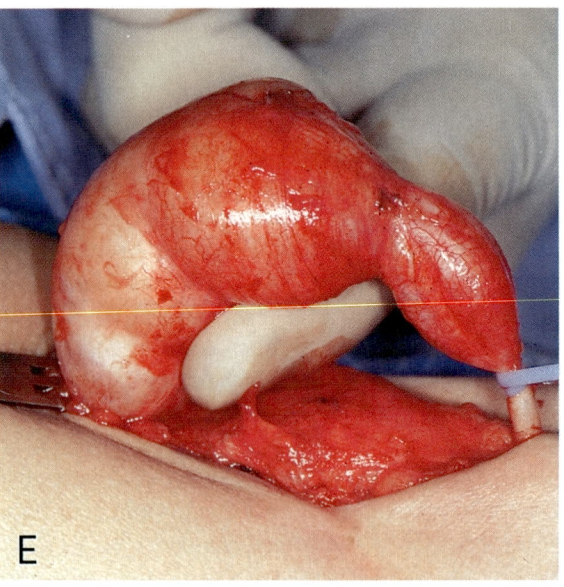

(fig. 8-20). The configuration of plexiform neurofibromas thus reflects the normal anatomy of the affected nerve. Highly branching nerves, such as the trigeminal and the brachial or the sacral plexus, are converted into a complex, worm-like tangle (figs. 8-18, 8-19A–C). In contrast, examples affecting large, relatively nonbranching nerves, such as the sciatic, convert the nerve into a firm, ropy cylinder (fig. 8-20A,B) composed of crude strands. Such tumors may appear less plexiform but, when closely examined, show neurofibromatous involvement of multiple fascicles, each several times the normal diameter. Involvement of organs or viscera is best seen in

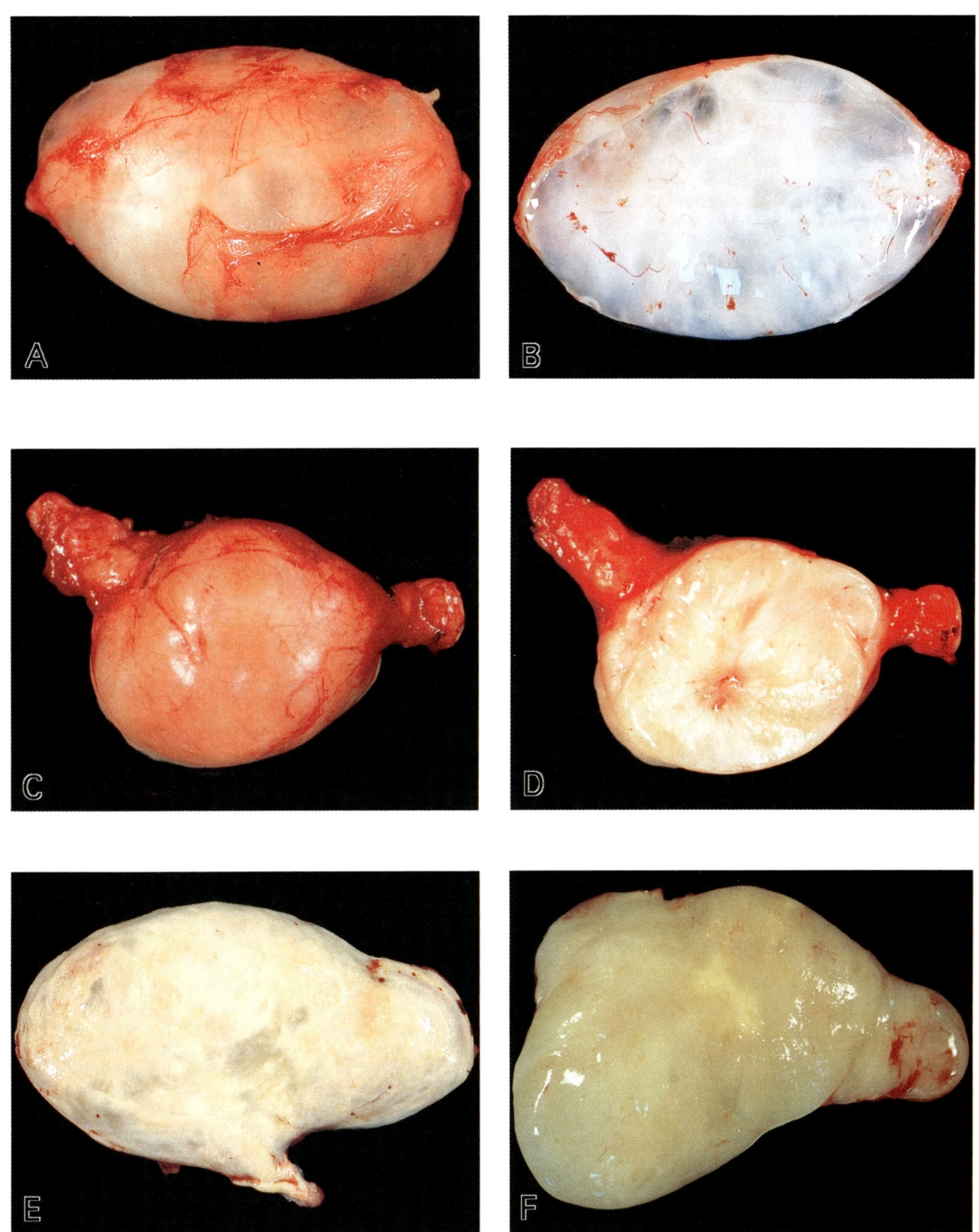

Figure 8-10
LOCALIZED INTRANEURAL NEUROFIBROMA

Classic examples are ovoid or fusiform in configuration, delicately encapsulated, and feature a gray-white or gray-tan, translucent cut surface (A,B,D,F). Large tumors, such as these vagus nerve (C,D), pelvic plexus (E), and sciatic nerve (F) examples, are often variegated gray-tan due to variation in collagen content.

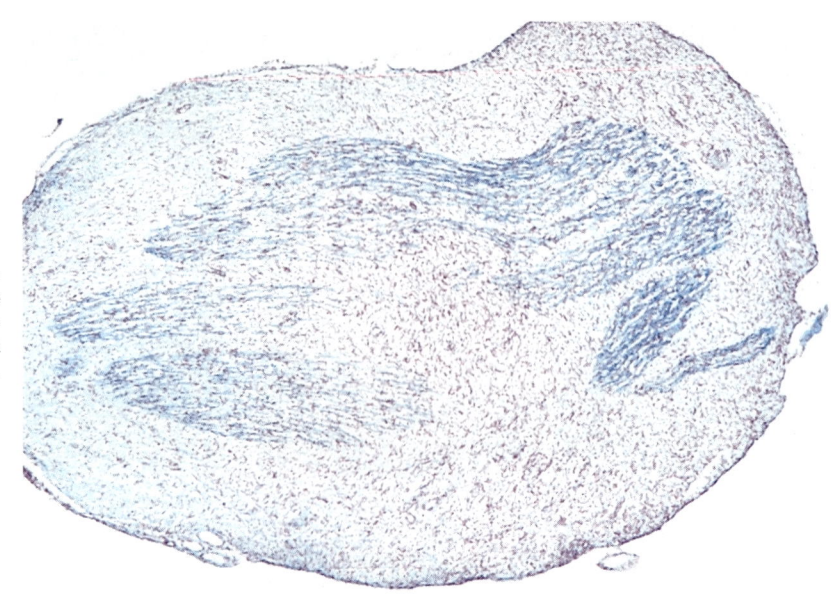

Figure 8-11
LOCALIZED INTRANEURAL
NEUROFIBROMA
Residual nerve tissue is most apparent in neurofibromas of large nerves, such as this ovoid tumor involving an intradural spinal root in a patient with NF1. (Courtesy of Dr. H. Okazaki, Rochester, MN.)

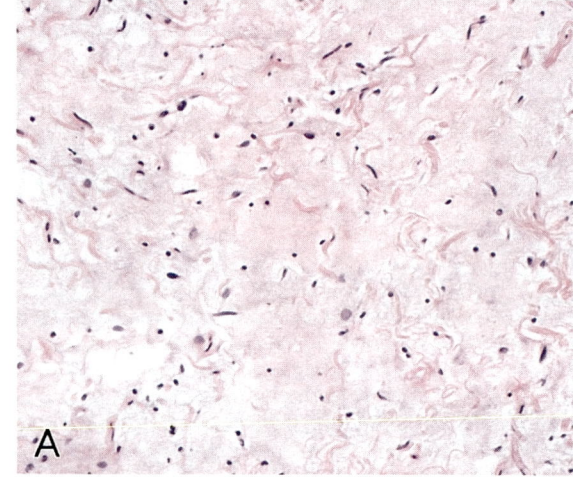

Figure 8-12
LOCALIZED INTRANEURAL NEUROFIBROMA
The relative proportion of stromal mucin and collagen, the basis of the tan color, is highly variable (A-C).

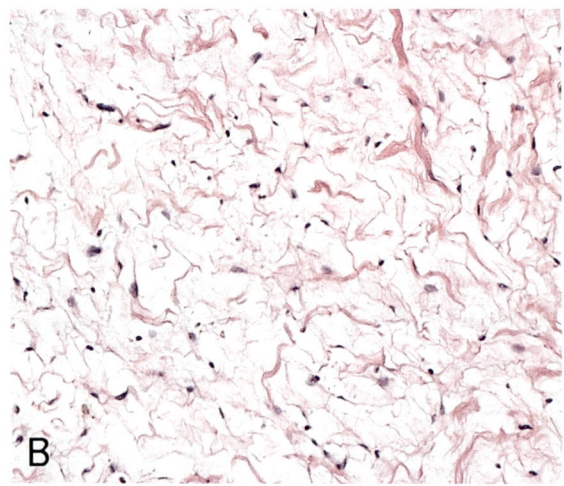

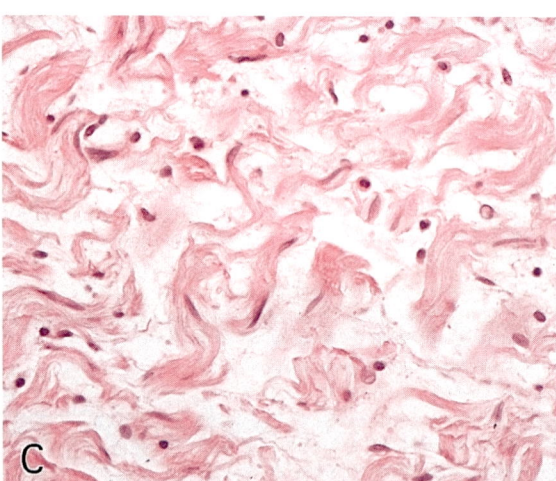

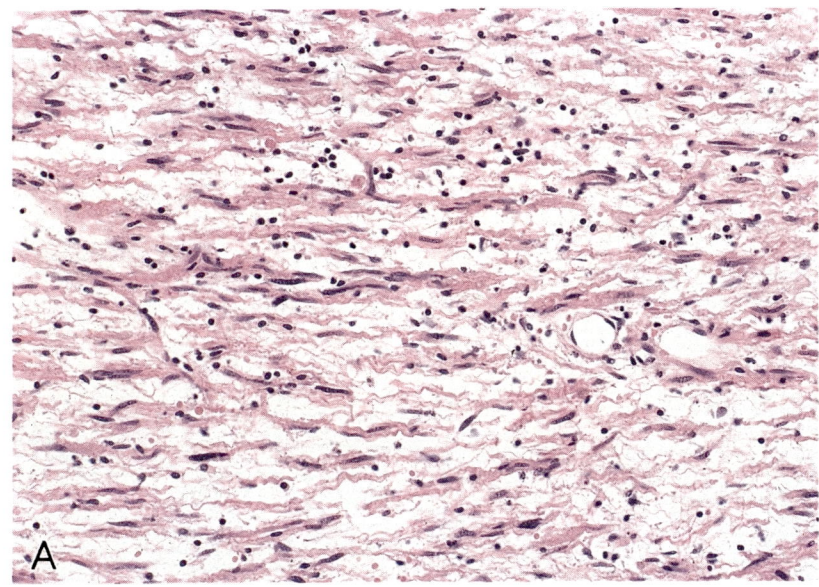

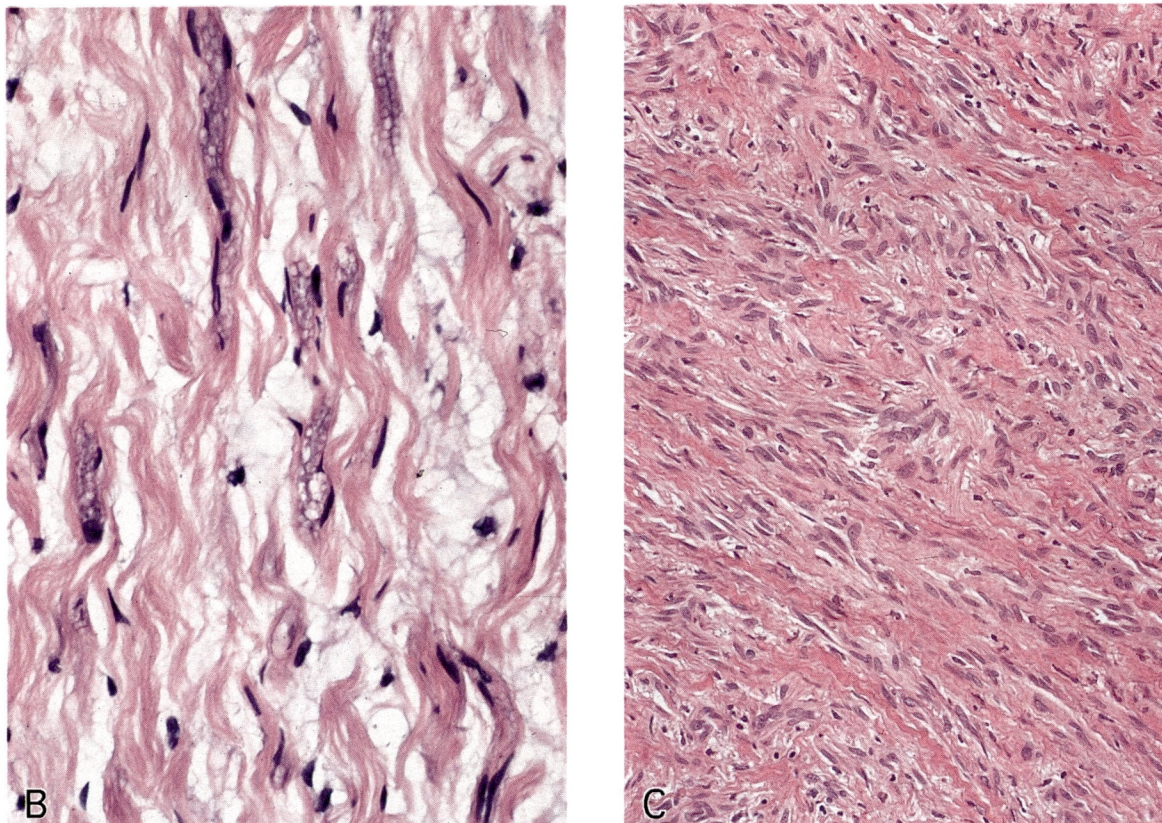

Figure 8-13
LOCALIZED INTRANEURAL NEUROFIBROMA

The cytology of such lesions varies from cells with dense, spindle-shaped curved nuclei (A,B) to ones in which nuclei are relatively plump with open chromatin (C). There may be scattered residual myelinated nerve fibers.

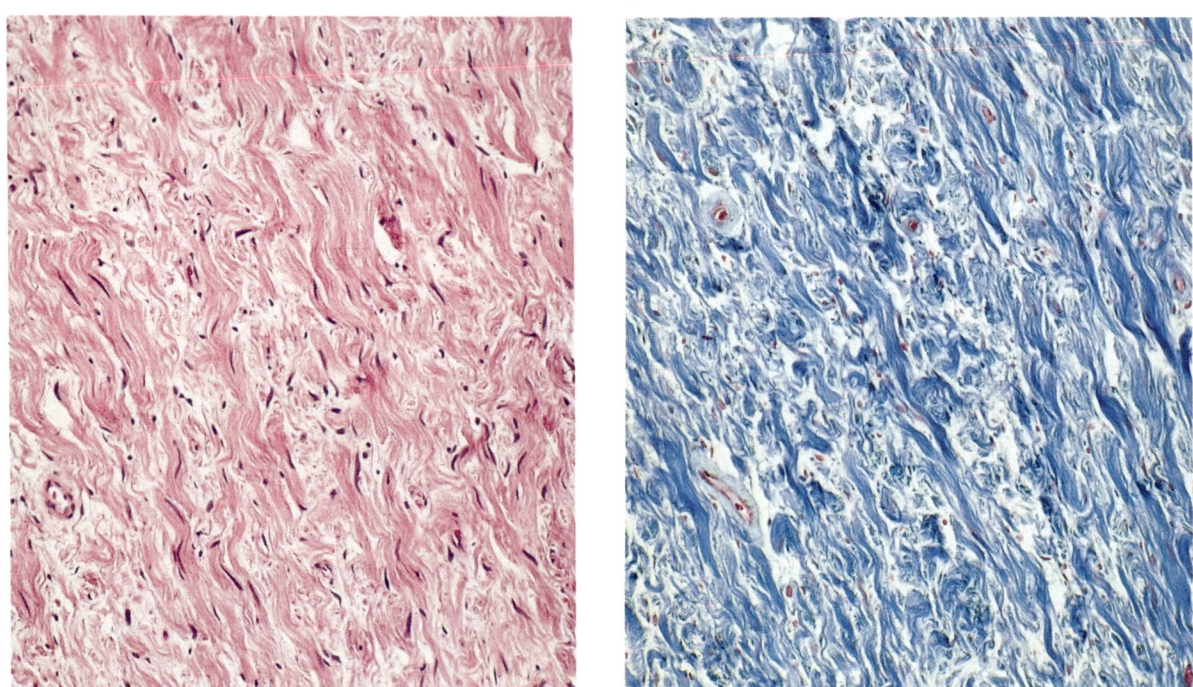

Figure 8-14
LOCALIZED INTRANEURAL NEUROFIBROMA
In tumors of long standing, the collagen deposition may be massive (left), as is evident on trichrome stain (right).

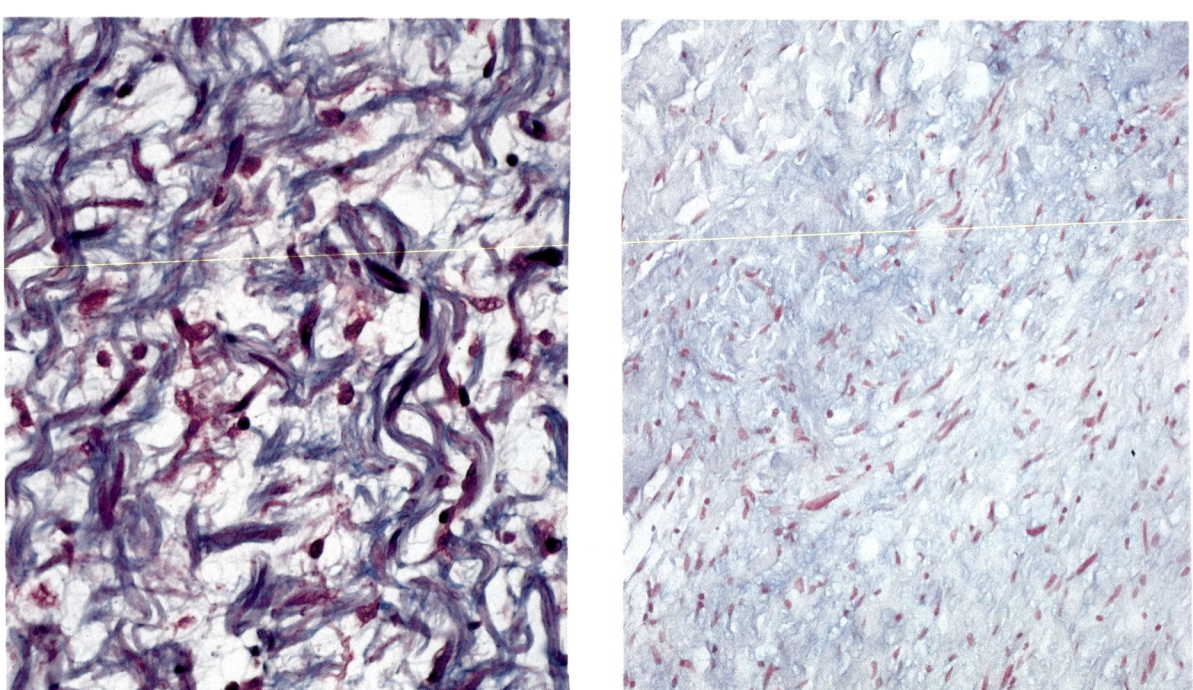

Figure 8-15
LOCALIZED INTRANEURAL NEUROFIBROMA
Left: Stromal collagen often takes the form of compact, sinuous bundles.
Right: Stromal mucin is readily demonstrated on Alcian blue stain.

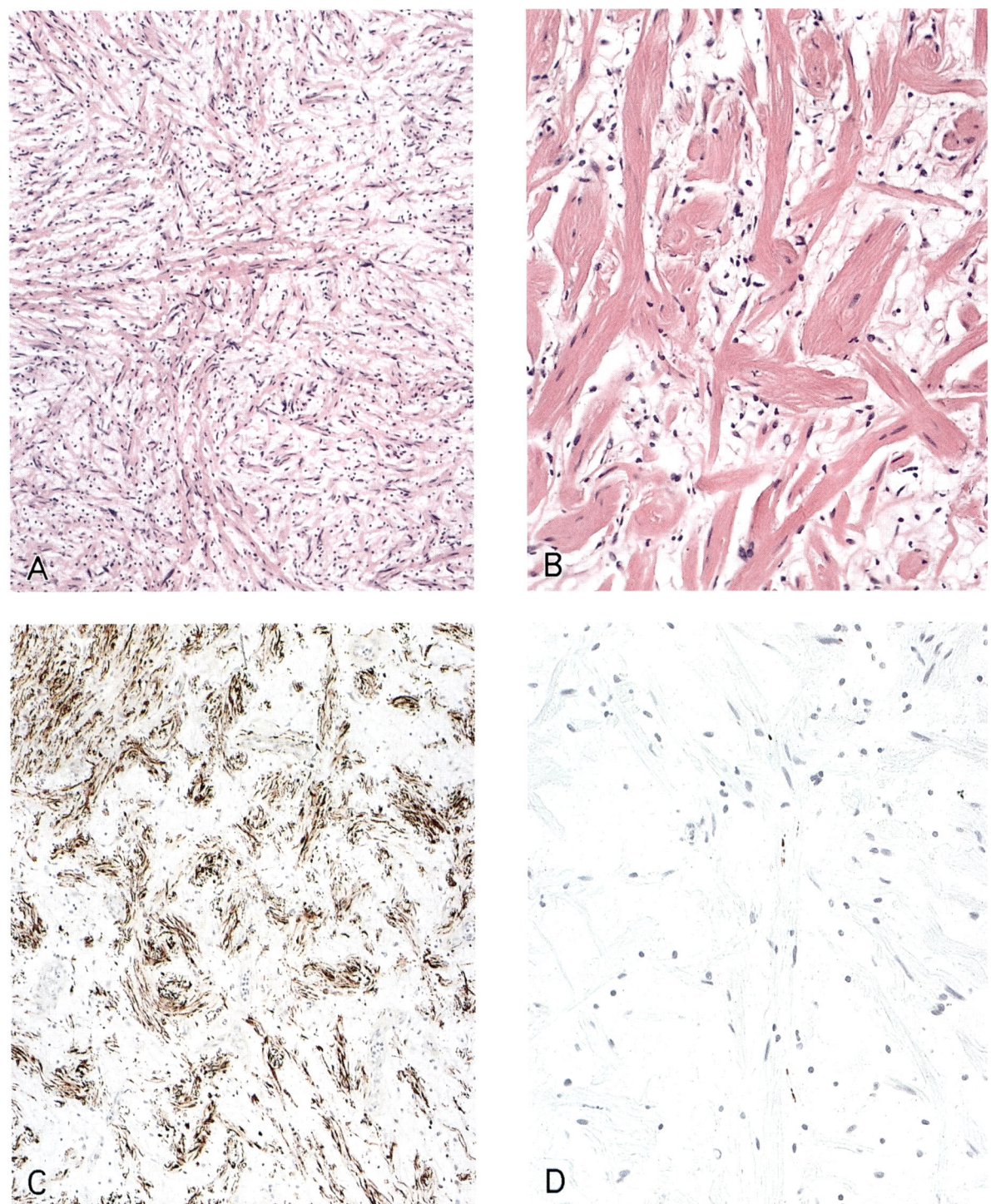

Figure 8-16
LOCALIZED INTRANEURAL NEUROFIBROMA
Collagen deposition is often progressive in neurofibroma, being laid down along the course of preexisting nerve fibers (see fig. 8-6). The collagen bundles vary from long and narrow (A) to blocky in configuration (B), the latter being likened to "shredded carrots." Immunostains of a neurofibroma wherein collagen deposition is just beginning shows the residual nerve fiber sheaths to be abundant (C, S-100 protein immunostain). In advanced collagen deposition, the blocky collagen arrays contain few residual neurofilament-positive axons (D).

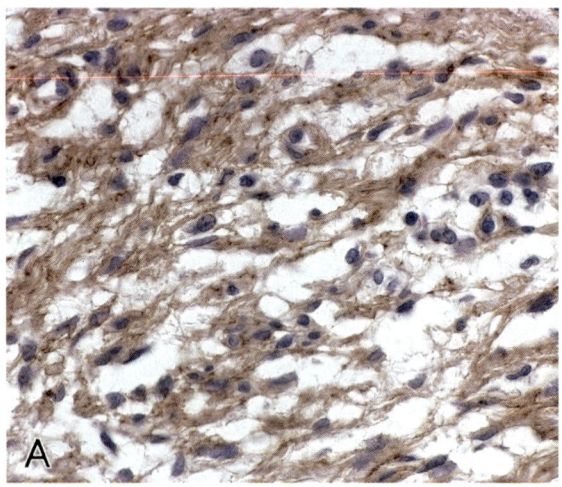

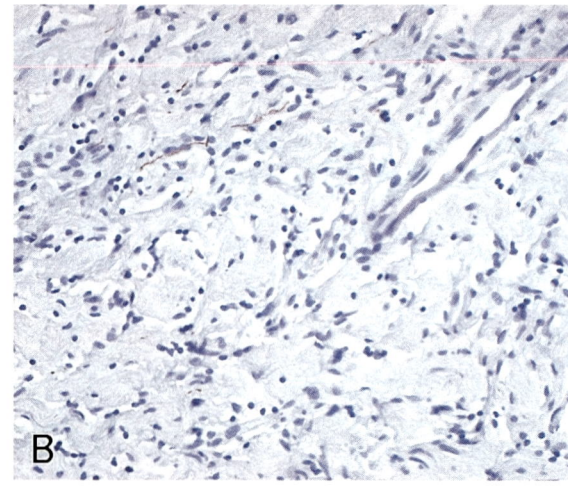

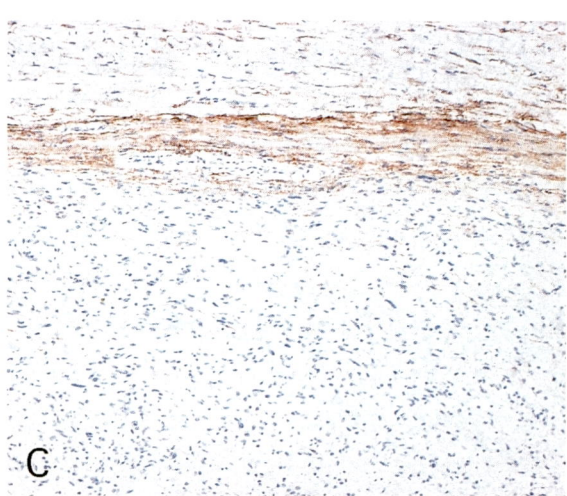

Figure 8-17
LOCALIZED INTRANEURAL NEUROFIBROMA

As in all forms of neurofibroma, the lesions contain numerous S-100 protein-positive cells (A). Note that not all cells within such neurofibromas are reactive. Scattered axons are most easily demonstrated on stains for neurofilament protein (B). The delicate "capsule" of intraneural tumors consists in part of the residual EMA-immunoreactive perineurium (C). Note the usual lack of tumor cell staining.

microsections (fig. 8-22). Plexiform components are often found in massive soft tissue neurofibromas (fig. 8-31A,C). Since the fascicles of plexiform tumors contain a mucin-rich stroma, their translucent appearance and rubbery texture have been likened to a "bag of worms." Due to collagen deposition, large, often longstanding lesions may be firm. Plexiform neurofibromas involve the same nerves as do localized intraneural tumors. The majority of neurofibromas affecting visceral autonomic nerves and the mesentery are of plexiform type (fig. 8-22; see also figs. 5-15, 13-12–13-18) (26). Although this variant is most prone to undergo malignant change, the latter only rarely occurs in viscera. The subject of plexiform neurofibromas affecting viscera, particularly the gastrointestinal tract, is discussed in chapters 5 and 13.

Massive Soft Tissue Neurofibroma. This least common form of neurofibroma is restricted to patients with NF1. A large, diffuse tumor, it often features a plexiform component and causes either "localized gigantism" of an extremity (fig. 8-30B) (66) or simply massive enlargement of regional soft tissues (fig. 8-30A). Infiltration of soft tissue is widespread and includes muscle invasion (fig. 8-30C). Progressive growth results in folds of redundant soft tissue extending cape-like, as over the shoulder (see fig. 13-10), or in pendulous bag-like masses of neurofibromatous tissue unilaterally enlarging the pelvic girdle and lower extremity (figs. 8-30B, 13-1). The now antiquated term "elephantiasis neuromatosa" was once applied to such tumors. Massive soft tissue neurofibromas only rarely undergo malignant change.

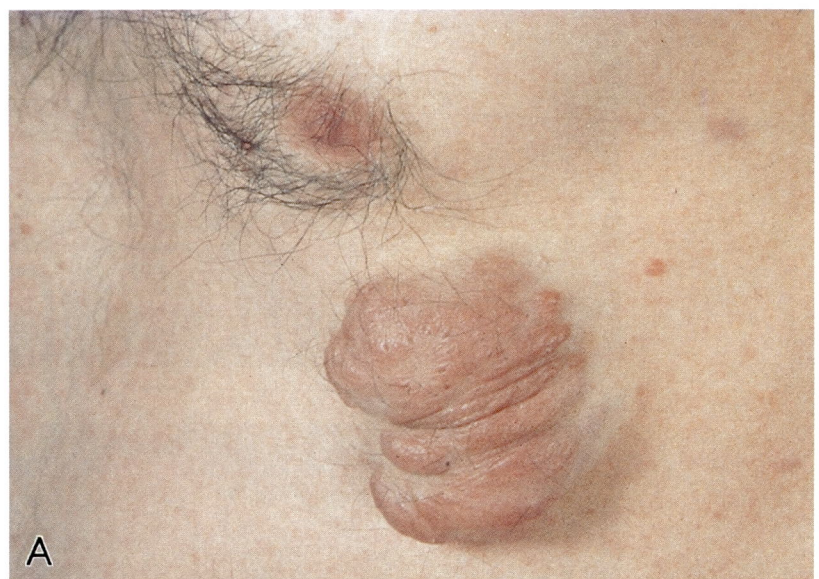

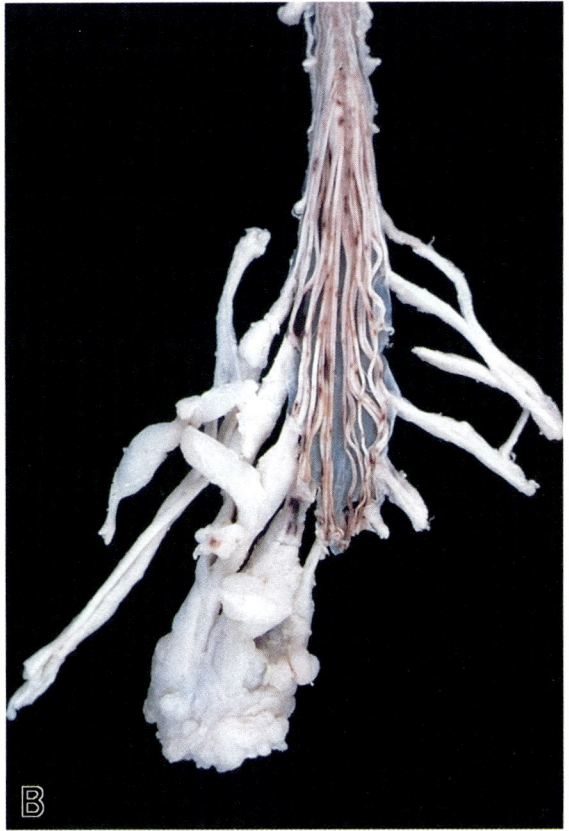

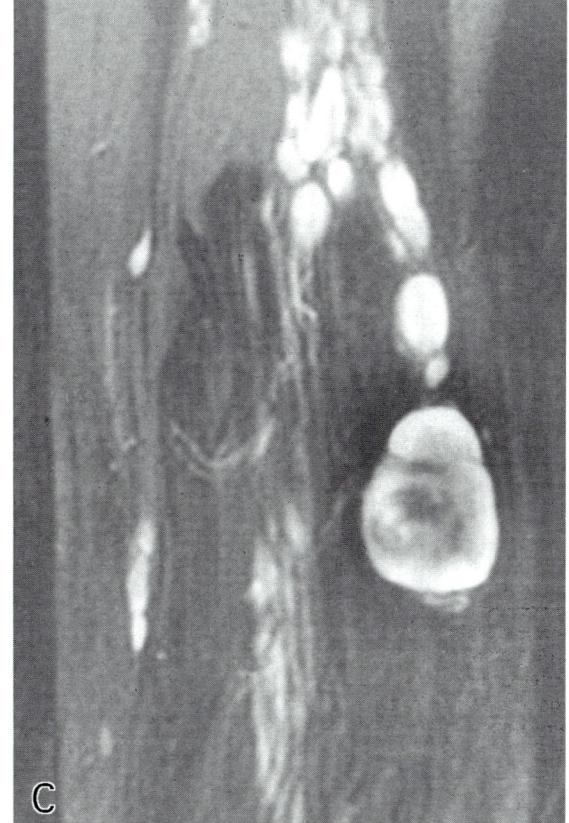

Figure 8-18

PLEXIFORM NEUROFIBROMA

This highly characteristic lesion is pathognomonic of NF1 and forms a lumpy, often bag-like mass which disfigures underlying tissue (A). Formed of multiple, entangled and enlarged nerve fascicles, such cutaneous lesions typically affect small nerves. Alternatively, large lesions, such as of the lumbosacral plexus may be sizeable (B). The imaging characteristics of plexiform neurofibroma are characteristic. A coronal T2-weighted MRI image of the thigh (C) shows multiple, interconnected lesions with increased signal, the largest of which has a target configuration.

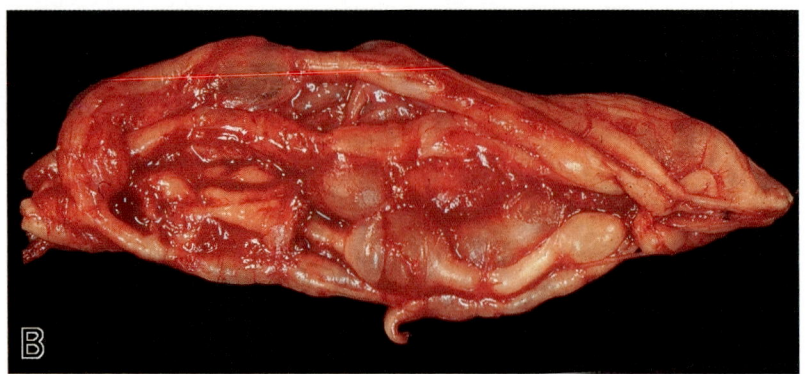

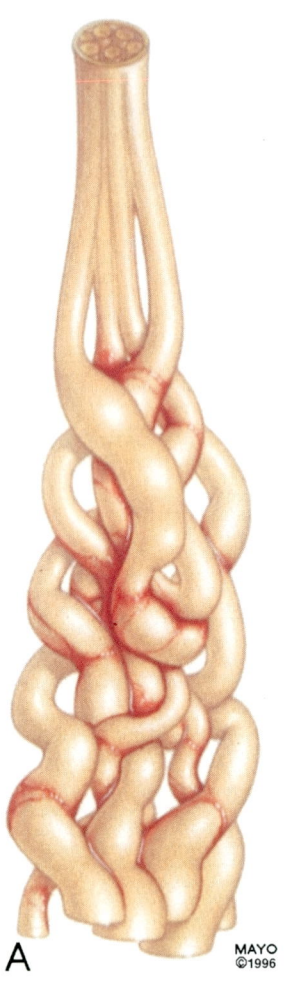

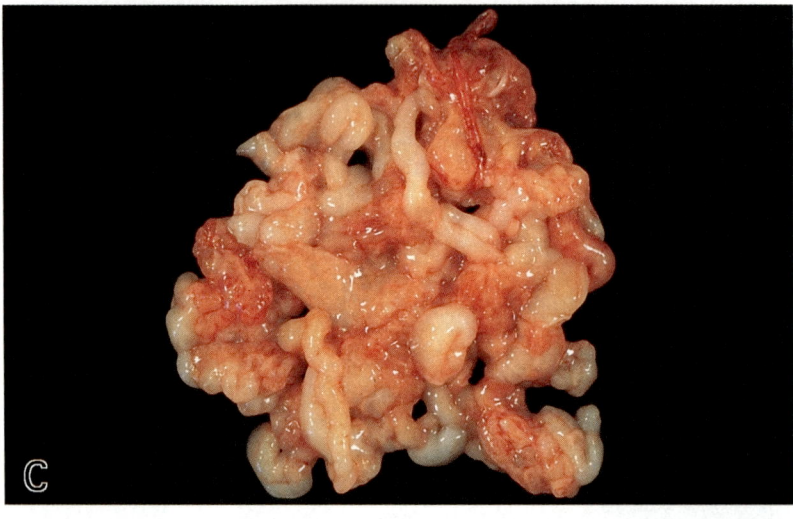

Figure 8-19
PLEXIFORM NEUROFIBROMA
These distinctive lesions consist of neurofibromatous change in multiple nerve fascicles (A,B). Unfortunately, surgical specimens often consist of only fragmented nerve segments (C). Whereas occasional tumors consist of abnormal fascicles of uniform diameter, others show them to be transformed into segmental, jelly-like expansions (D,E).

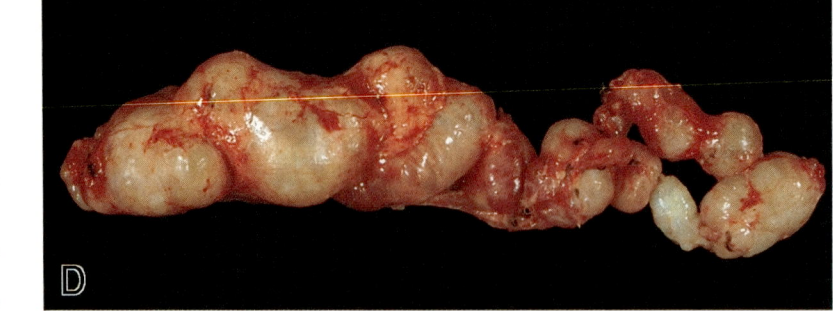

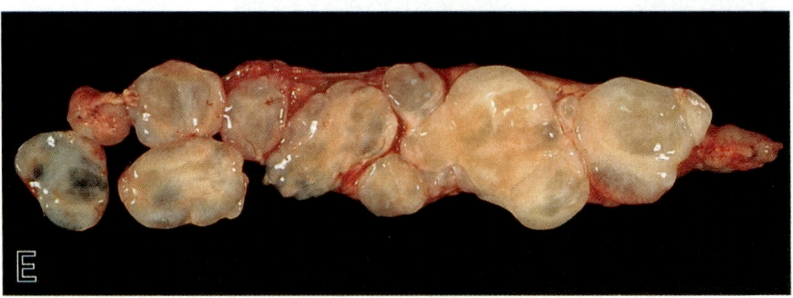

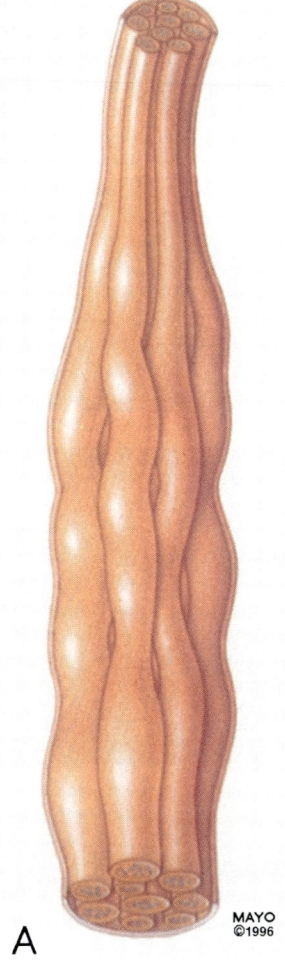

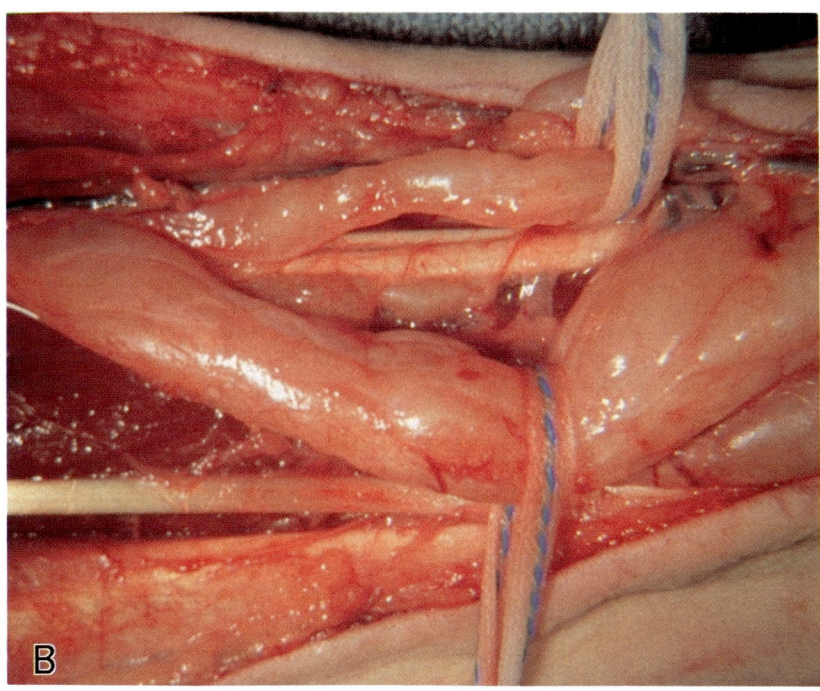

Figure 8-20
PLEXIFORM NEUROFIBROMA
Although such tumors are typically envisioned as "bags of worms," when large and relatively nonbranching nerves are affected the lesion frequently forms a rope-like mass (A). Careful inspection of one such tumor of the ulnar nerve demonstrates multiple fascicle involvement in each of two branches (B). Multifascicle involvement is better seen in yet another ulnar nerve lesion in which affected fascicles lie separated (C).

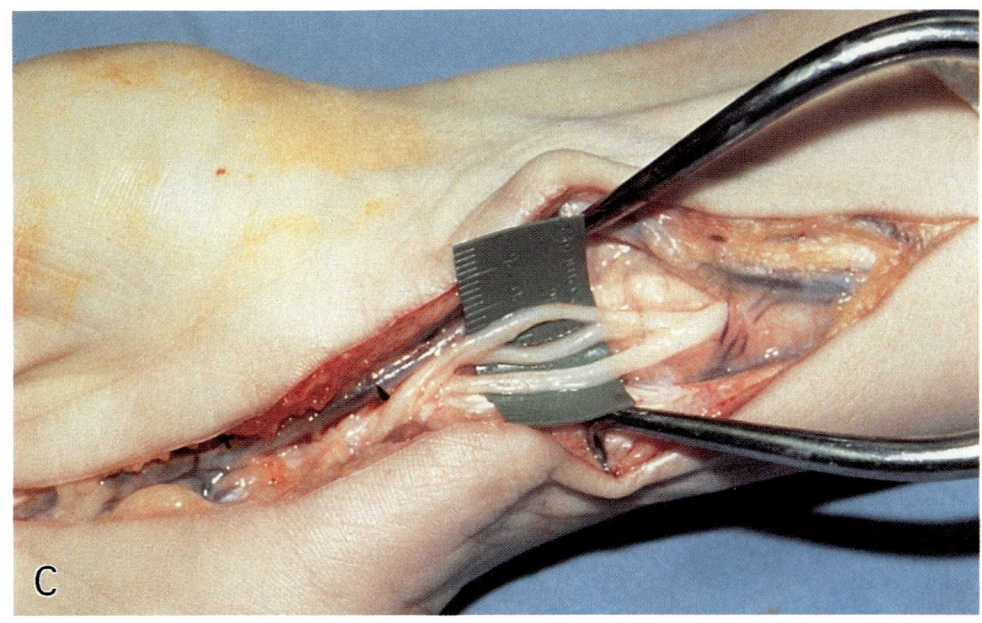

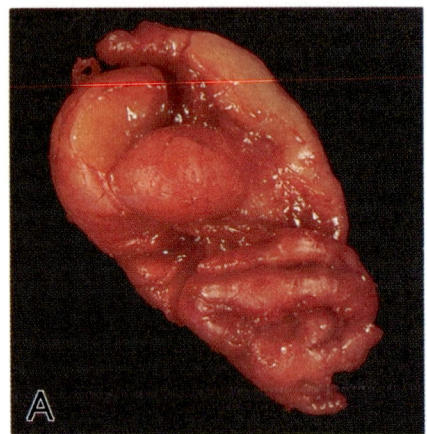

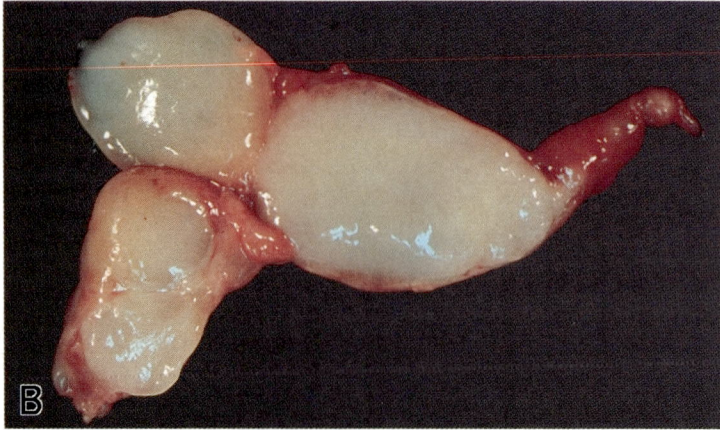

Figure 8-21
PLEXIFORM
NEUROFIBROMA
Occasional tumors show unusual configurations including clustered tangles (A), multinodular lesions within a multifascicle nerve (B), and delicate fusiform expansions along a thin, branching, multifascicle nerve (C).

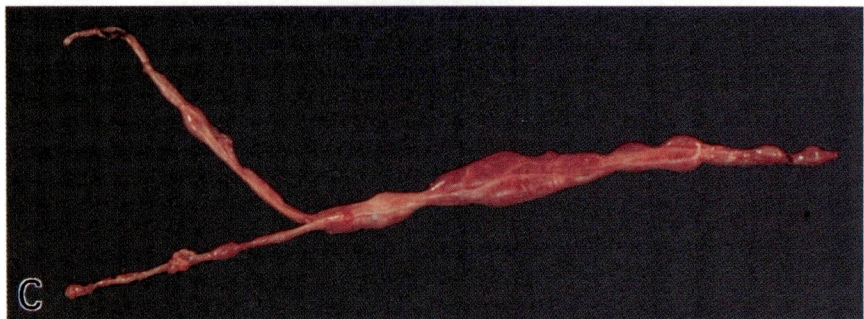

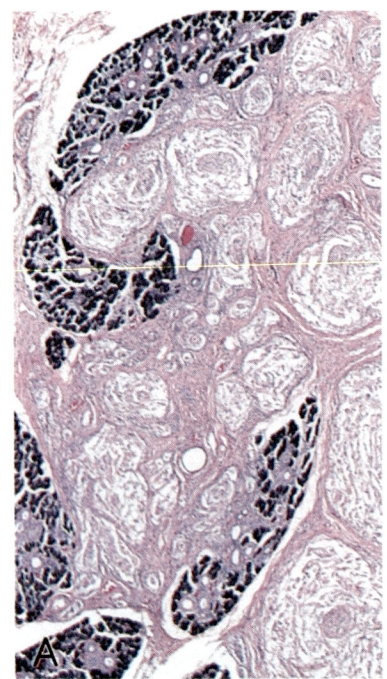

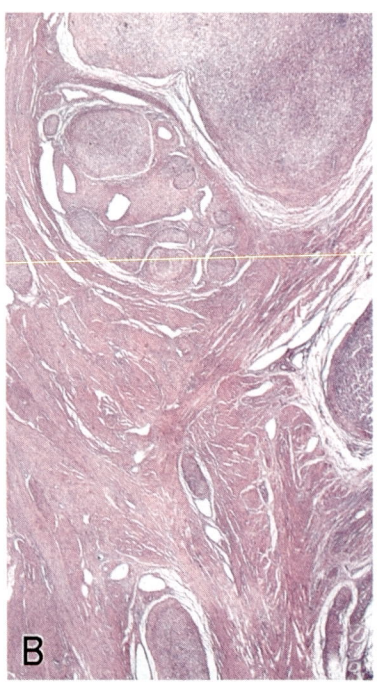

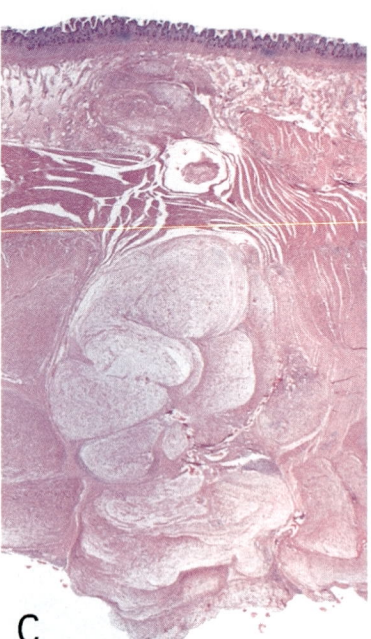

Figure 8-22
PLEXIFORM NEUROFIBROMA
Involvement of superficial organs such as the parotid gland is frequently seen in tumors affecting the trigeminal nerve (A). In deep-seated tumors, involvement of viscera such as the uterus (B) or the small bowel (C) may also be observed.

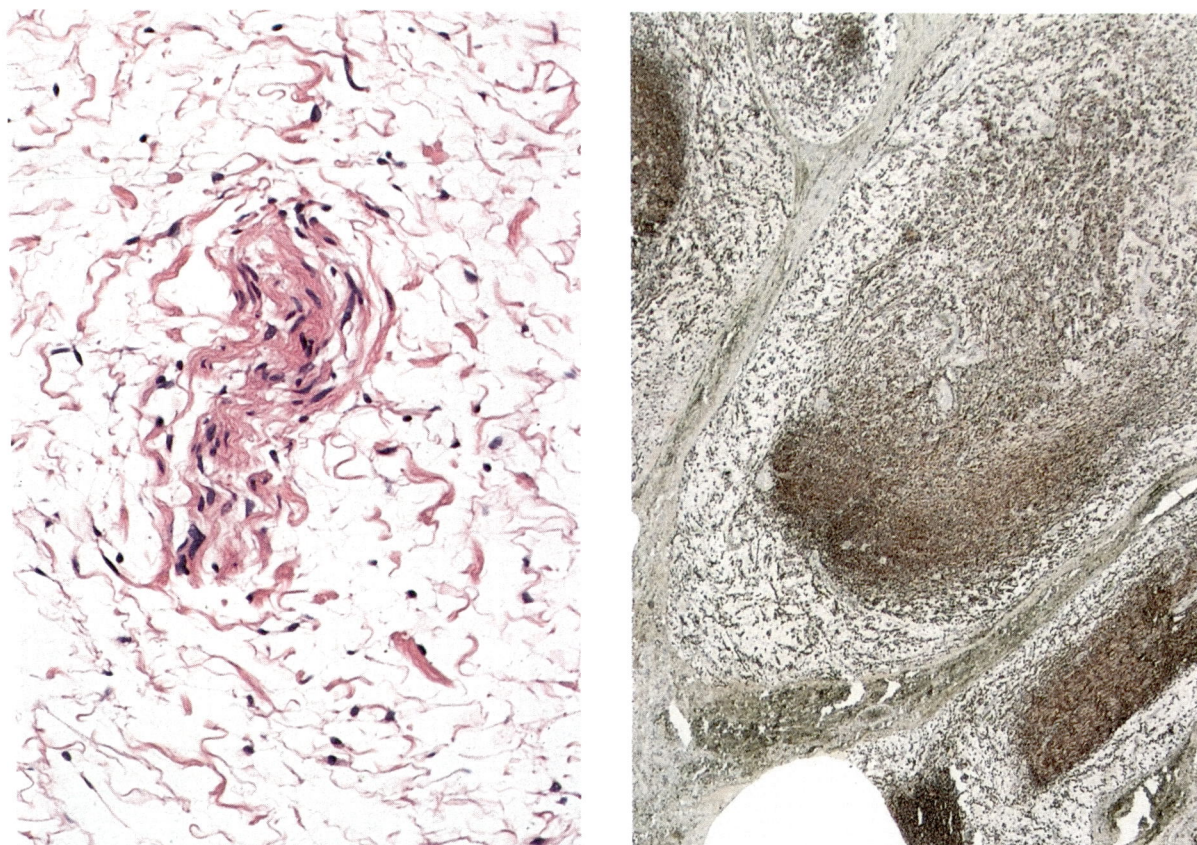

Figure 8-23
PLEXIFORM NEUROFIBROMA OF SOFT TISSUE
Left: At higher power, the affected fascicles may be seen to contain centrally placed nerve fibers.
Right: These are readily highlighted with immunostains for S-100 protein.

Microscopic Findings. Several basic microscopic features are shared by most types of neurofibroma. In their simplest form, they are hypocellular and composed of widely spaced cells with ovoid to thin, elongate nuclei and scant cytoplasm embedded in a mucopolysaccharide-rich, variably collagenous matrix (fig. 8-12). In lesions in which residual nerve is apparent, the neurofibroma cells are usually aligned along the course of nerve fibers traversing the lesion (figs. 8-11, 8-13). Tumor cell nuclei are roughly one third to half the size of those of schwannoma cells and three times the size of lymphocyte nuclei (fig. 8-13). In most instances, their cytoplasmic processes are indiscernible (figs. 8-6, 8-13) without recourse to immunohistochemistry or electron microscopy. The relative proportion of stromal mucin and collagen is highly variable (figs. 8-12, 8-14–8-16). Whereas lymphocytes and histiocytes are uncommon, mast cells are often

present in significant number. In cutaneous tumors they may comprise up to 5 percent of all cells. Rarer yet are melanin-containing cells (fig. 8-31E) (6,41) which are never as numerous as in melanotic variants of schwannoma.

In all forms of neurofibroma the neoplastic cells are diffusely infiltrative of nerve, soft tissue, or both. Even localized intraneural tumors may show a limited degree of soft tissue infiltration. Accumulation of neoplastic cells is typically associated with a faintly mucoid matrix containing wavy collagen fibers (figs. 8-12, 8-15). As neurofibromatous tissue increases, an affected nerve is transformed from a cylindrically enlarged segment to a fusiform mass surrounded by attenuated perineurium and epineurium (figs. 8-7, 8-11, 8-19, 8-21, 8-26). Nondestructive entrapment of cutaneous adnexae (fig. 8-5C) or permeation of adipose tissue (figs. 8-5D, 8-25) and skeletal muscle (figs. 8-30, 8-31F)

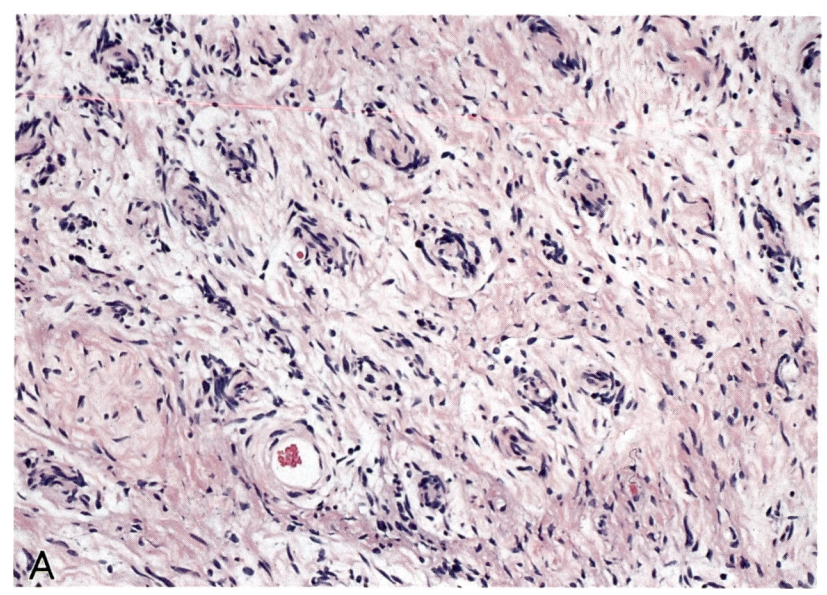

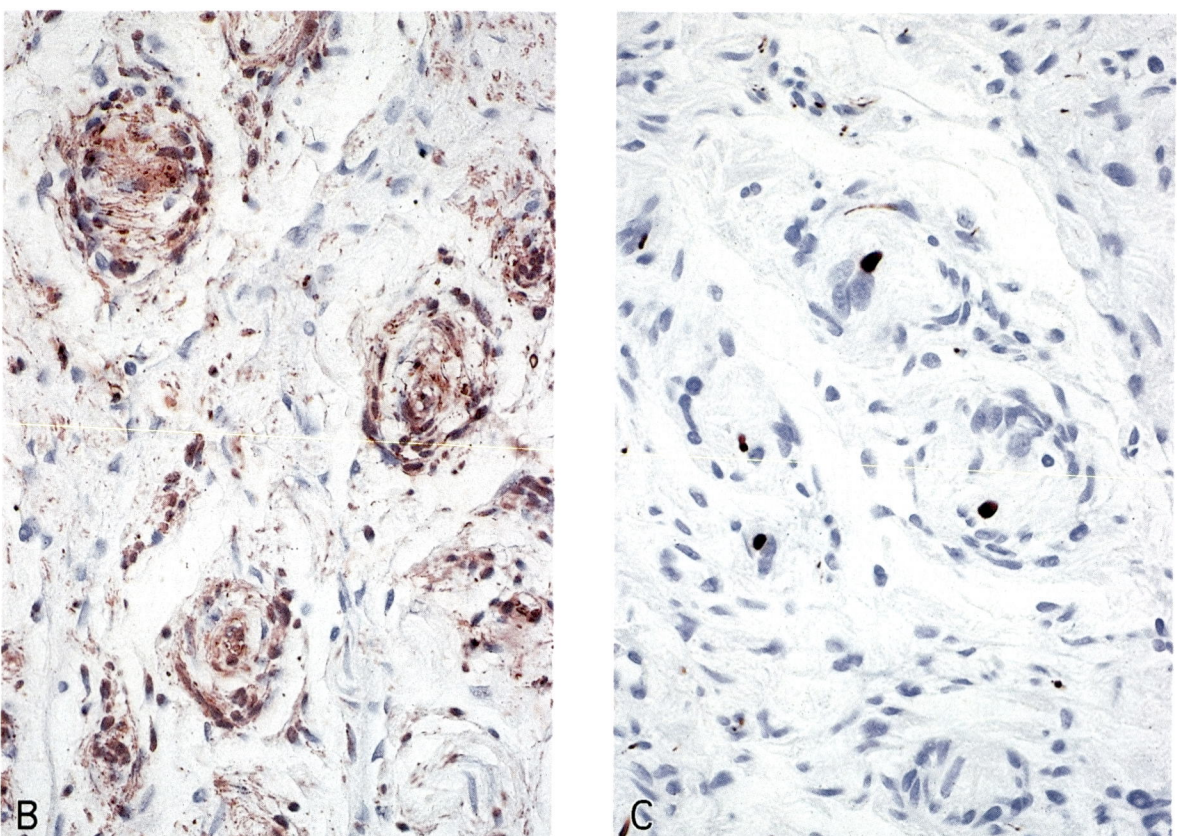

Figure 8-24
PLEXIFORM NEUROFIBROMA
Onion bulb-like arrangement of neoplastic cells is rarely seen (A). Note the whorls of S-100 protein–immunoreactive Schwann cells (B) around residual NF protein-positive axons (C).

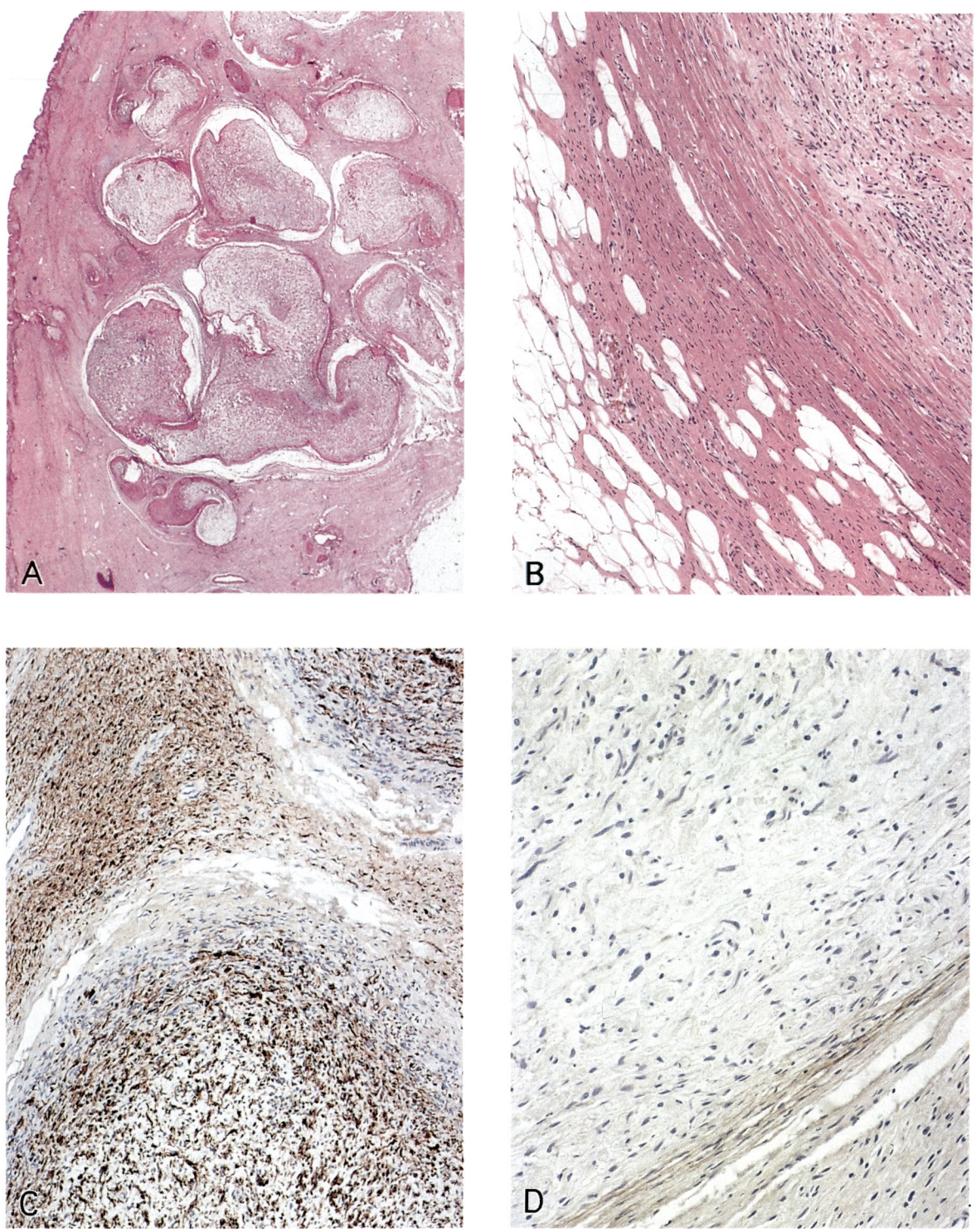

Figure 8-25
PLEXIFORM NEUROFIBROMA

This rather superficially situated example had an accompanying diffuse dermal and subcutaneous component (A). At higher power the extension of neurofibroma cells into surrounding adipose tissue is well seen (B). Immunostains for S-100 protein show both the intraneural and extraneural components to be reactive (C). Immunoreactivity for epithelial membrane antigen (D) is limited to residual perineurial sheaths surrounding affected fascicles.

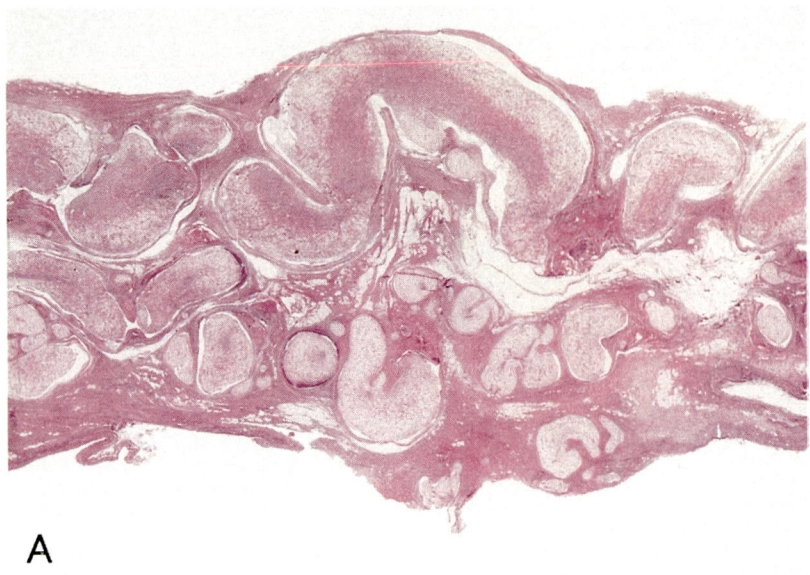

A

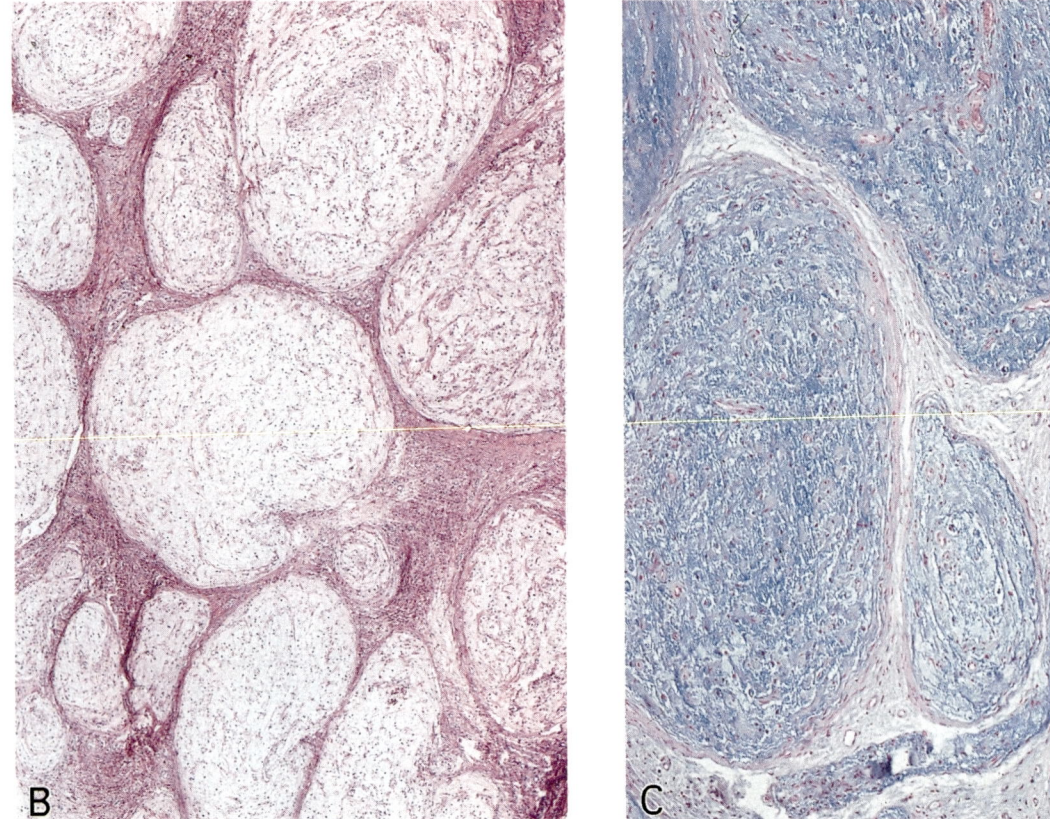

Figure 8-26
PLEXIFORM NEUROFIBROMA

Whole mount sections of this example show multiple fascicles to be enlarged by neurofibroma tissue (A). The fascicles vary from pale and mucin rich to ones in which the configuration of the underlying nerve fibers can still be seen (A, top). At higher power, the crowded fascicles contain and are seen to lie within a matrix (B) which is mucinous and strongly reactive on Alcian blue stain (C).

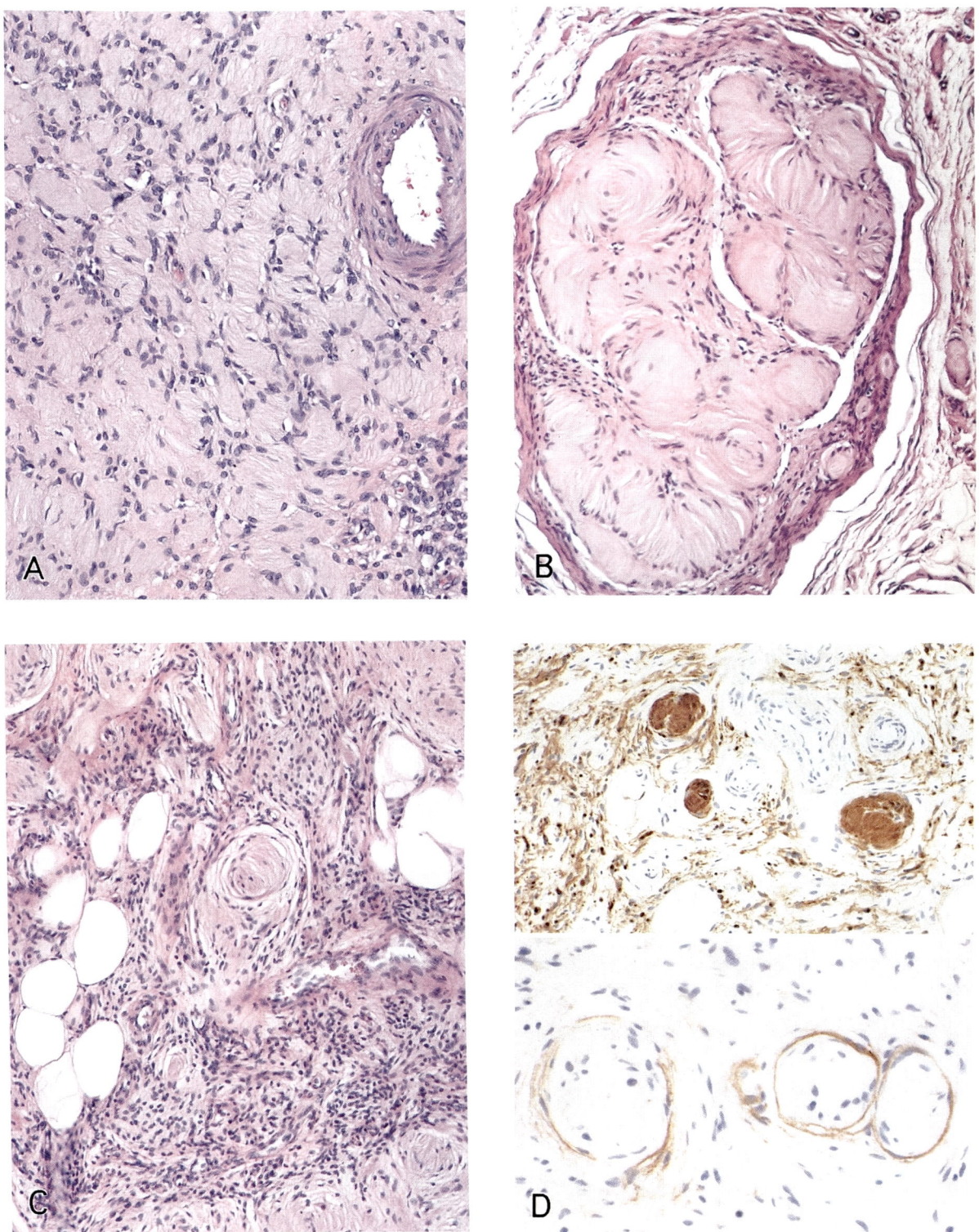

Figure 8-27
PLEXIFORM NEUROFIBROMA

Apparent "tactile differentiation" may be noted. Examples include pseudo-meissnerian corpuscles (A) which may occasionally be spherical and aggregated (A, bottom; B). Whorls vaguely reminiscent of pacinian corpuscles may also be seen (C). These structures are S-100 protein immunoreactive (D, top), and some examples have a peripheral rim of EMA-reactive cells (D, bottom).

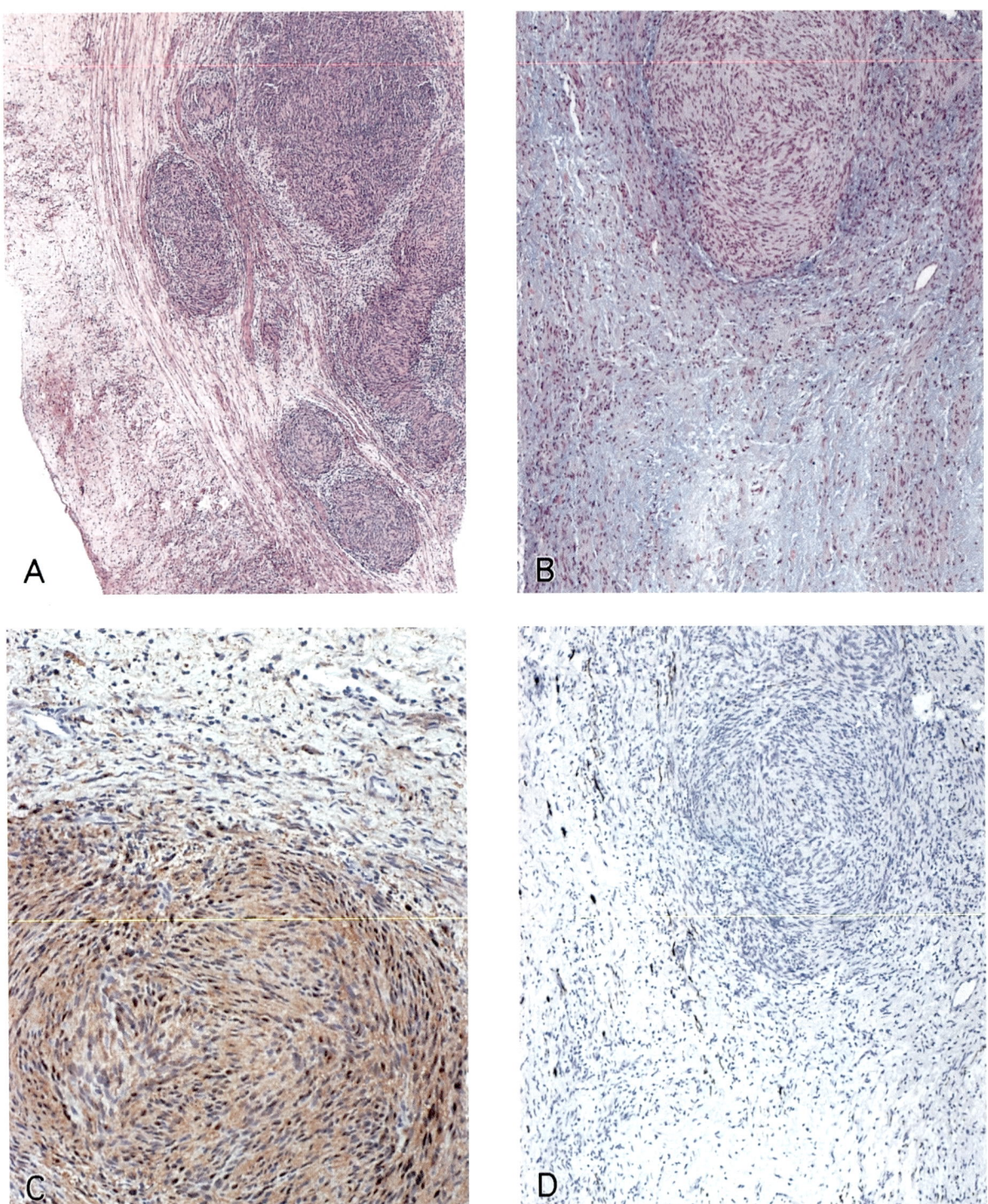

Figure 8-28
PLEXIFORM NEUROFIBROMA WITH MULTIFOCAL SCHWANNOMA-LIKE NODULES
Such nodules are typically a microscopic finding in association with more typical neurofibromatous tissue (A). The surrounding matrix, unlike the nodules, contains mucin (B, Alcian blue). The neurofibroma component has scattered S-100-positive neurofibroma cells, whereas the schwannoma-like component is uniformly reactive for this marker (C). Unlike ordinary schwannomas, the loose textured tissue surrounding the nodules often contains residual nerve fibers (D, neurofilament protein immunostain).

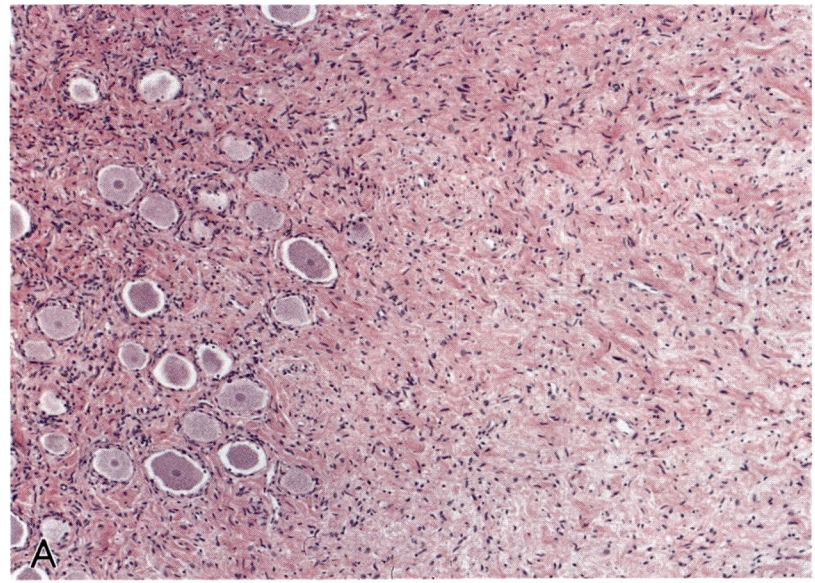

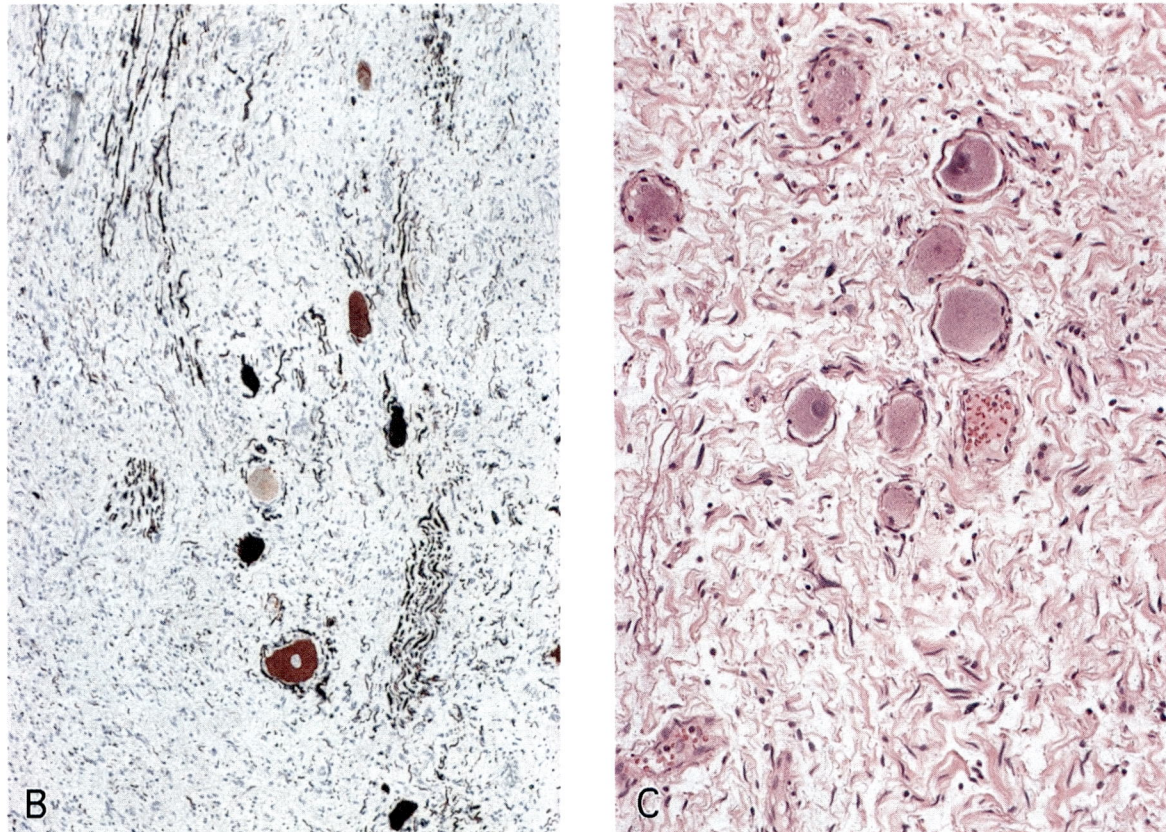

Figure 8-29
PLEXIFORM NEUROFIBROMA INVOLVING DORSAL ROOT GANGLION
This lesion shows gradual transition of tumor to dorsal root ganglion tissue (A, left). The ganglion cells are a local finding within the tumor (A) and are accompanied by neurofilament protein–immunopositive nerve fiber bundles (B). Unlike the ganglion cells of ganglioneuroma, nearly all are seen to be surrounded by a uniform layer of satellite cells (C) (see figs. 9-51, 9-53, 9-54, and 9-59).

are conspicuous features of diffuse cutaneous and massive soft tissue tumors, respectively.

Some histologic differences do exist between the various forms of neurofibroma. For example, collagen fibers in localized and diffuse *cutaneous neurofibromas* as well as in diffuse soft tissue neurofibromas are typically delicate (figs. 8-2, 8-6) and lie within a variably abundant mucopolysaccharide-rich matrix. The latter accounts for the gray, translucent appearance of many localized intraneural and plexiform tumors (figs. 8-9, 8-19, 8-21). *Intraneural neurofibromas* frequently exhibit an abundance of coarse, refractile collagen fibers (figs. 8-12, 8-14–8-16), a feature that explains their often tan color (fig. 8-10). In many instances, the dominant microscopic finding is shreds of collagen bundles disposed in parallel arrangement or jumbled (figs. 8-14, 8-15). Dense collections of sizeable collagen bundles bear a striking resemblance to "shredded carrots" (fig. 8-16) (66). Both in skin and at noncutaneous sites, collagen deposition may result in frank hyalinization of portions of a tumor (fig. 8-14). This is particularly true at the periphery.

The histologic features of *plexiform neurofibroma* are highly distinctive. Early in their development, involved fascicles are hypocellular and feature prominent endoneurial mucin deposition (fig. 8-26). The faintly basophilic neurofibroma tissue consists in large part of a hyaluronidase-sensitive mucopolysaccharide-rich matrix which appears watery gray-blue on hematoxylin and eosin (H&E) stain, is weakly periodic acid–Schiff (PAS) positive, and reacts strongly in Alcian blue preparations (fig. 8-26). Although present to some degree in all neurofibromas, mucoid matrix is particularly abundant in plexiform tumors, the fascicles of which show considerable variation in mucin content (figs. 8-25, 8-26). Over time, as the tumors enlarge and become more cellular, collagen becomes more abundant. Neurofibroma tissue surrounds nerve fiber bundles (fig. 8-20) which, as a rule, lie at the center of affected fascicles where their accompanying Schwann sheaths appear as bundles of wavy, spindle cells (figs. 8-23, 8-26).

Characteristic variations in cell pattern occur in neurofibromas. Although infrequent, they are sufficiently distinctive as to be diagnostically useful. These cell formations primarily resemble Wagner-Meissner corpuscles (figs. 8-27A,B, 8-31D). Less often they vaguely simulate pacinian corpuscles (figs. 8-24, 8-27C). Since such cell arrangements often show strong S-100 protein immunoreactivity (fig. 8-27D) and the peripheral cells express EMA staining (fig. 8-27D), these structures are mere caricatures of tactile bodies. Normal Wagner-Meissner corpuscles do not have a peripheral rim of EMA-positive cells and pacinian corpuscles stain predominantly for EMA, not S-100 protein. Therefore, it is inappropriate to refer to neurofibromas with tactile body-like structures as "pacinian neurofibromas" (28). Tactile-like bodies are most commonly seen in diffuse and massive soft tissue neurofibromas as well as in plexiform tumors. Occasional neurofibromas, mainly plexiform lesions, contain microscopic nodules composed entirely of Schwann cells, some featuring Verocay bodies (fig. 8-28). When sizable, these may resemble small schwannomas. Such tumors pose a problem in differential diagnosis between neurofibroma and schwannoma. This issue, as well as the distinction of neurofibroma overrunning ganglia from ganglioneuroma (fig. 8-29), is further discussed below.

Melanin production in neurofibromas is very uncommon. Although the term "pigmented neurofibroma" is often applied, we do not consider such tumors a distinct neurofibroma variant. The only sizable series, that of Fetsch et al. (15a), critically reviews the literature, eliminating other pigmented PNSTs (41). Their study indicates a predilection for males and blacks as well as a broad age range. Approximately 50 percent occurred in patients with NF1. The tumors involved primarily skin and subcutaneous tissue, varied greatly in size, and were typically of the diffuse type. Pigmentation was generally patchy. Dendritic, spindle, or epithelioid in cytology, the pigmented cells were scattered or loosely clustered, often in superficial subcutaneous tissue (fig. 8-31E), and were immunoreactive for melanocytic markers. No tendency to malignant transformation was noted.

Divergent Differentiation. We have studied one example of a plexiform neurofibroma demonstrating epithelial differentiation (fig. 8-32).

Atypical and Cellular Neurofibroma. Two microscopic features commonly displayed by neurofibromas may fool the unwary and lead to an erroneous diagnosis of malignancy: the presence of atypical cells and diffuse hypercellularity. For the former we use the term *"atypical" neurofibroma* (66), denoting tumors often but not invariably large

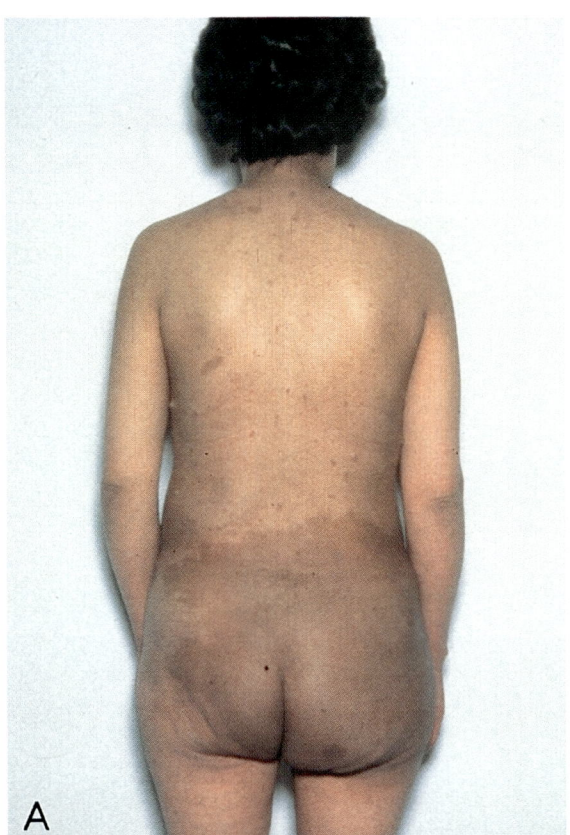
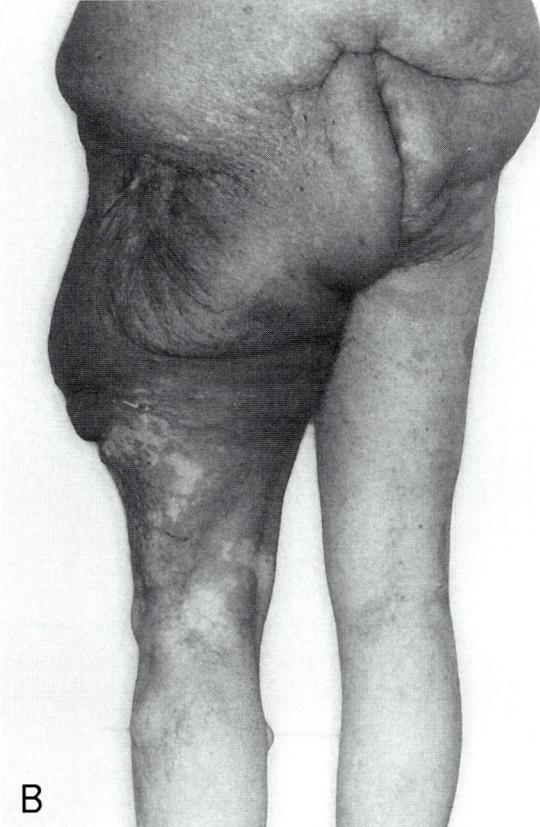
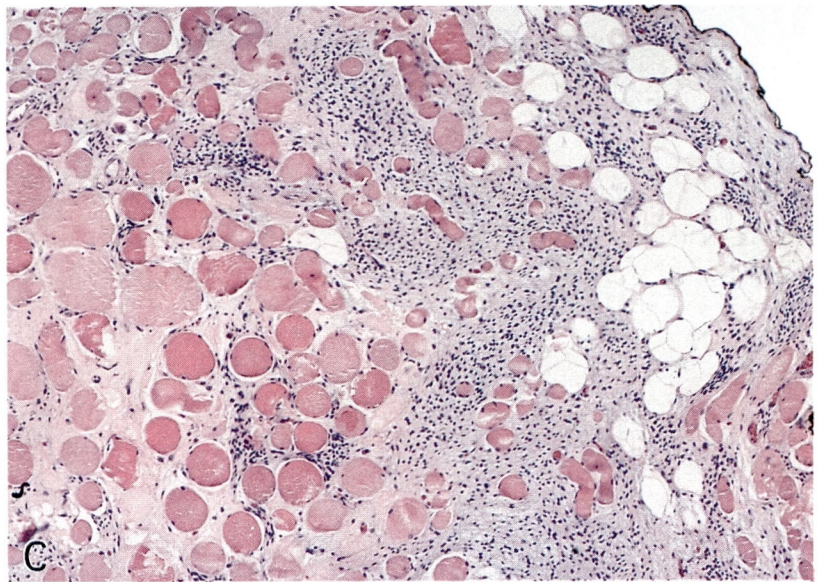

Figure 8-30
MASSIVE SOFT TISSUE NEUROFIBROMA
A: This diffuse lesion involved the buttocks and was associated with widespread cutaneous hyperpigmentation.
B: Another impressive example shows involvement not only of the hip girdle but of a leg as well ("elephantiasis neuromatosa"). The underlying lesion also included a large plexiform neurofibroma.
C: Diffuse components of such tumors freely infiltrate fat and skeletal muscle.

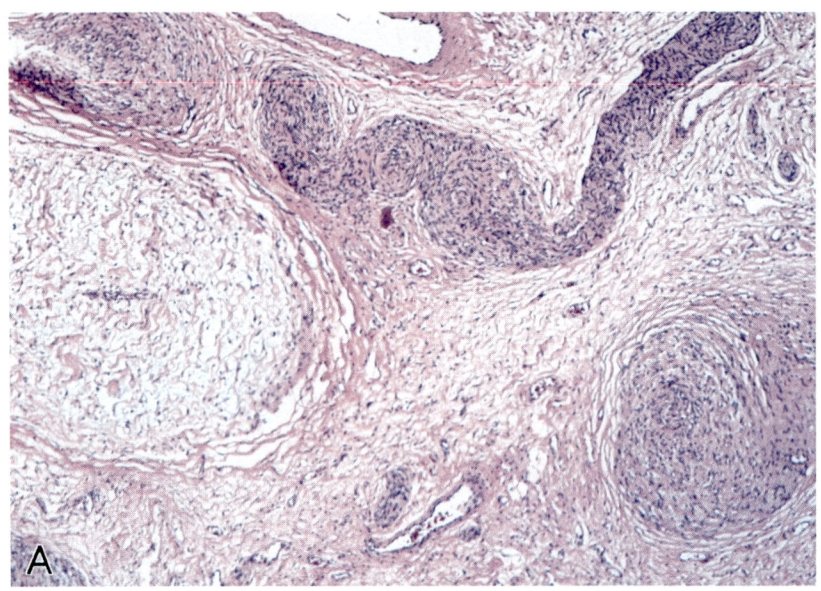

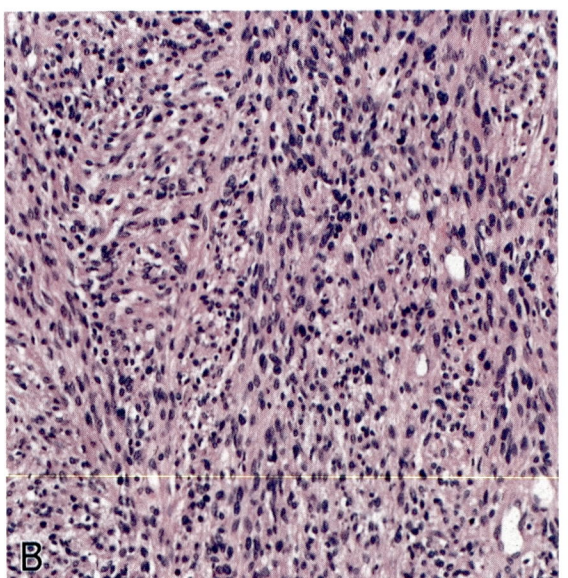
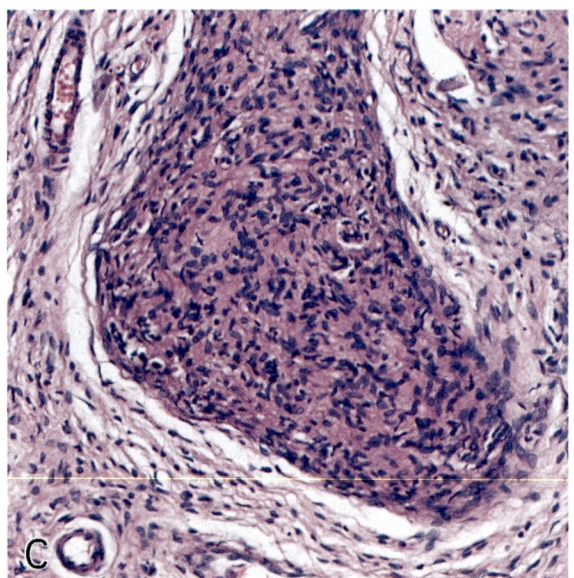

Figure 8-31
MASSIVE SOFT TISSUE NEUROFIBROMA

The proliferation is typically monomorphous cellular (A). The constituent cells vary in cytology from ones with ovoid nuclei and scant cytoplasm to others with frankly spindled cytology (B). Such tumors frequently exhibit plexiform components (A,C) which lie jumbled within the proliferation.

or of long standing with nuclear atypia akin to that seen in "ancient schwannoma" (2). Cells with such large, pleomorphic nuclei, cytoplasmic nuclear inclusions, smudgy chromatin, and inconspicuous nucleoli are accompanied by more typical neurofibroma cells and do not comprise the entire lesion (fig. 8-33). Unlike the bizarre

malignant cells of MPNST, the pleomorphic cells of atypical neurofibroma lack mitotic activity and show no appreciable MIB-1 labeling. We apply the term *"cellular" neurofibroma* to tumors with increased cellularity with or without low level mitotic activity (fig. 8-34). Our concept of when neurofibroma becomes cellular neurofibroma,

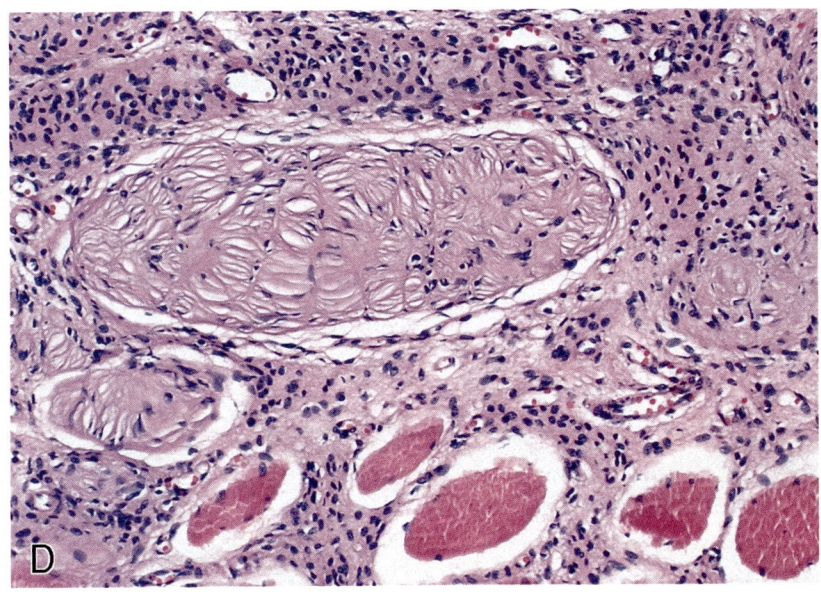

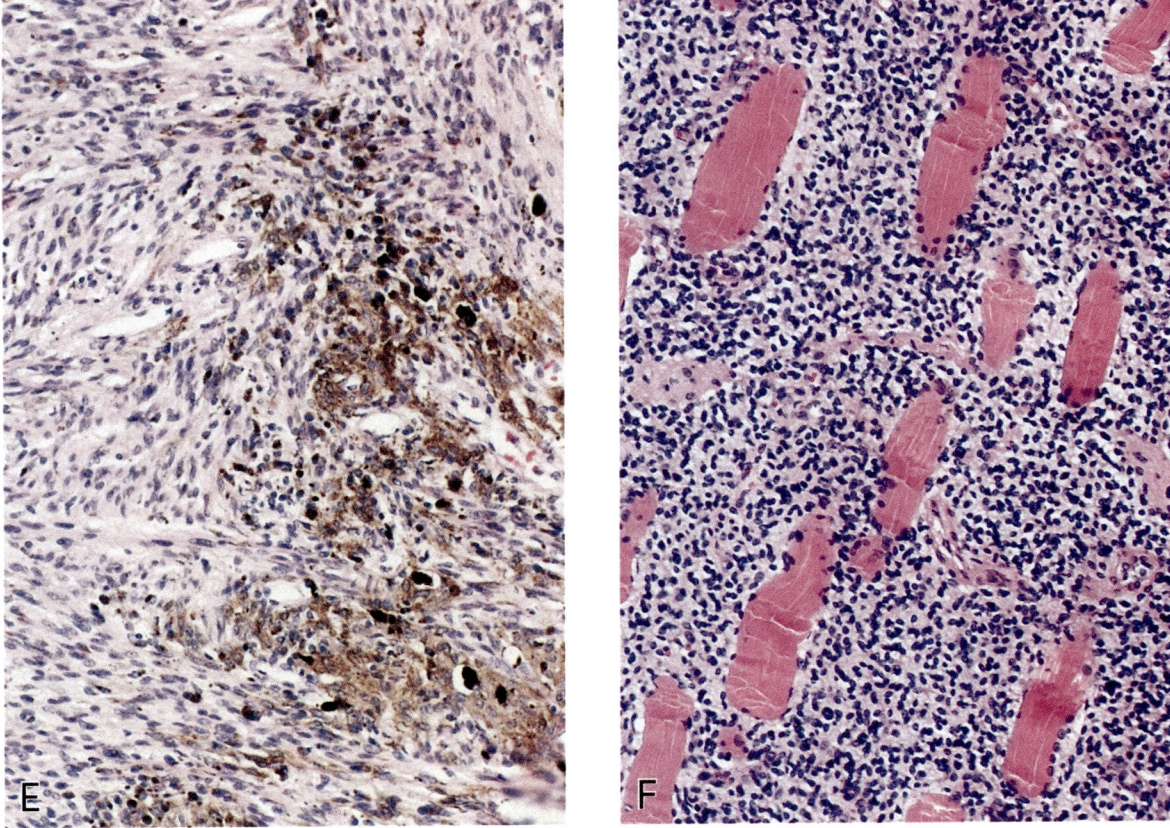

Figure 8-31 (Continued)

Pseudo-meissnerian corpuscles (D) are also a common feature. Less frequent is the finding of melanin pigmentation (E). These neurofibromas typically invade surrounding soft tissues, as evidenced by extensive skeletal muscle infiltration (F). The cellularity of this example results from relative lack of stromal collagen and should not be mistaken for a malignant small cell neoplasm.

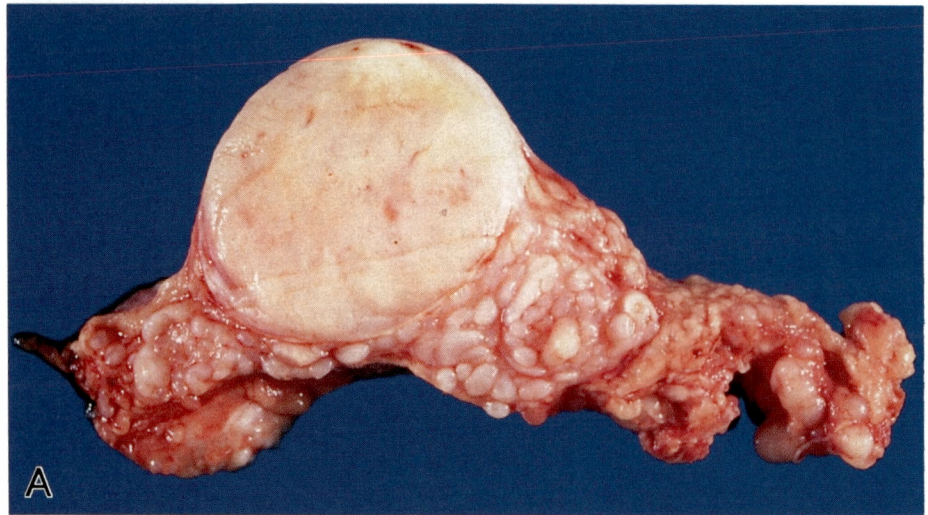

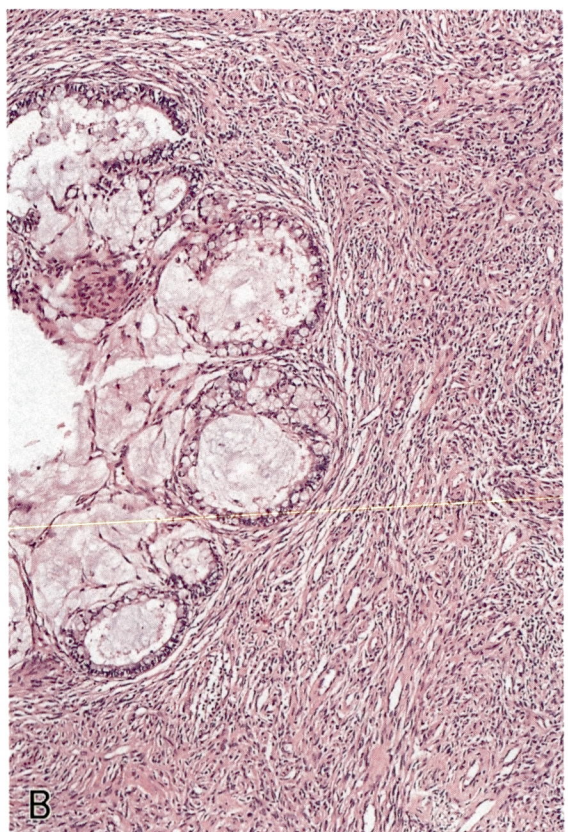

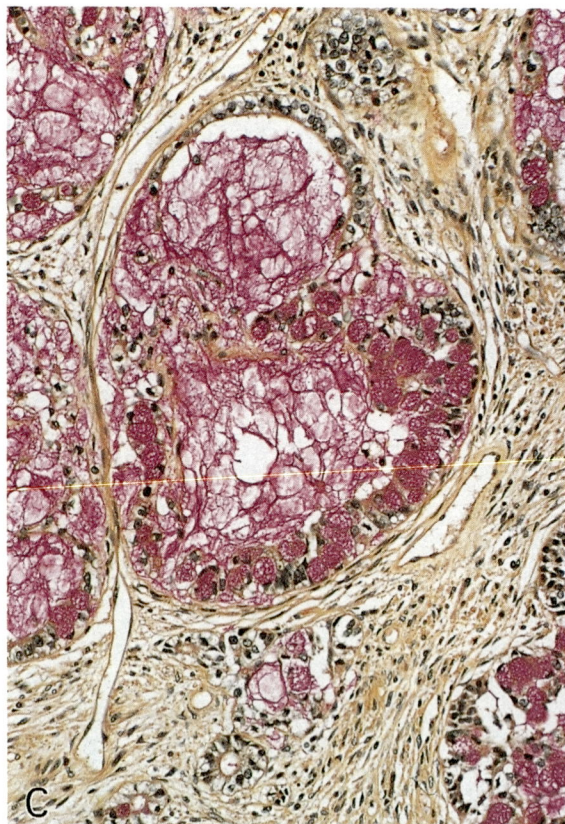

Figure 8-32

DIVERGENT DIFFERENTIATION IN A PLEXIFORM NEUROFIBROMA

This unique example from the retroperitoneum of a patient with NF1 showed the localized formation of a nodule (A) within which neurofibroma tissue was accompanied by a variety of epithelia. Microsections showed cytologically benign glands in a neurofibromatous stroma (B), mucin-producing goblet cells (C), immunoreactivity for cytokeratin as well as carcinoembryonic antigen (D), and neuroendocrine epithelium (E) showing chromogranin immunoreactivity (F). The neurofibromatous stroma appeared cytologically benign throughout the gland-containing area, although early malignant transformation was noted elsewhere. (Courtesy of Dr. S. Wester, Lacrosse, WI.)

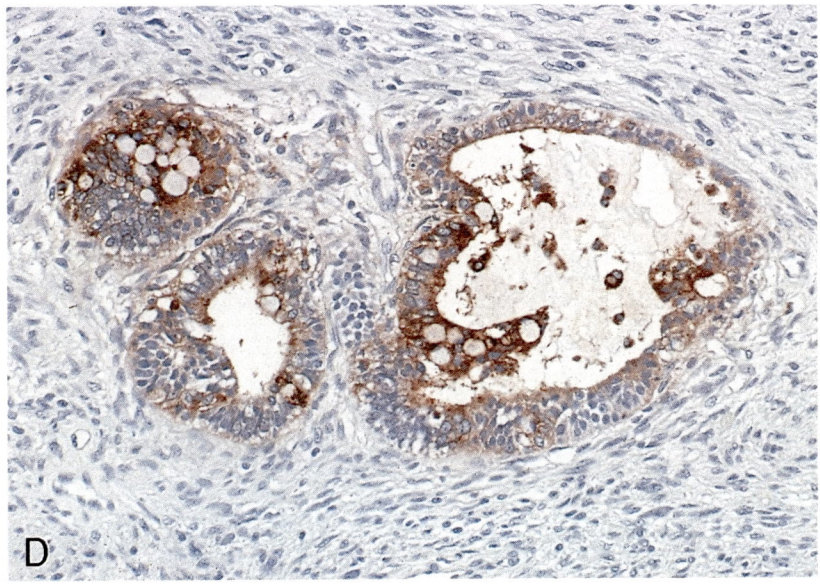

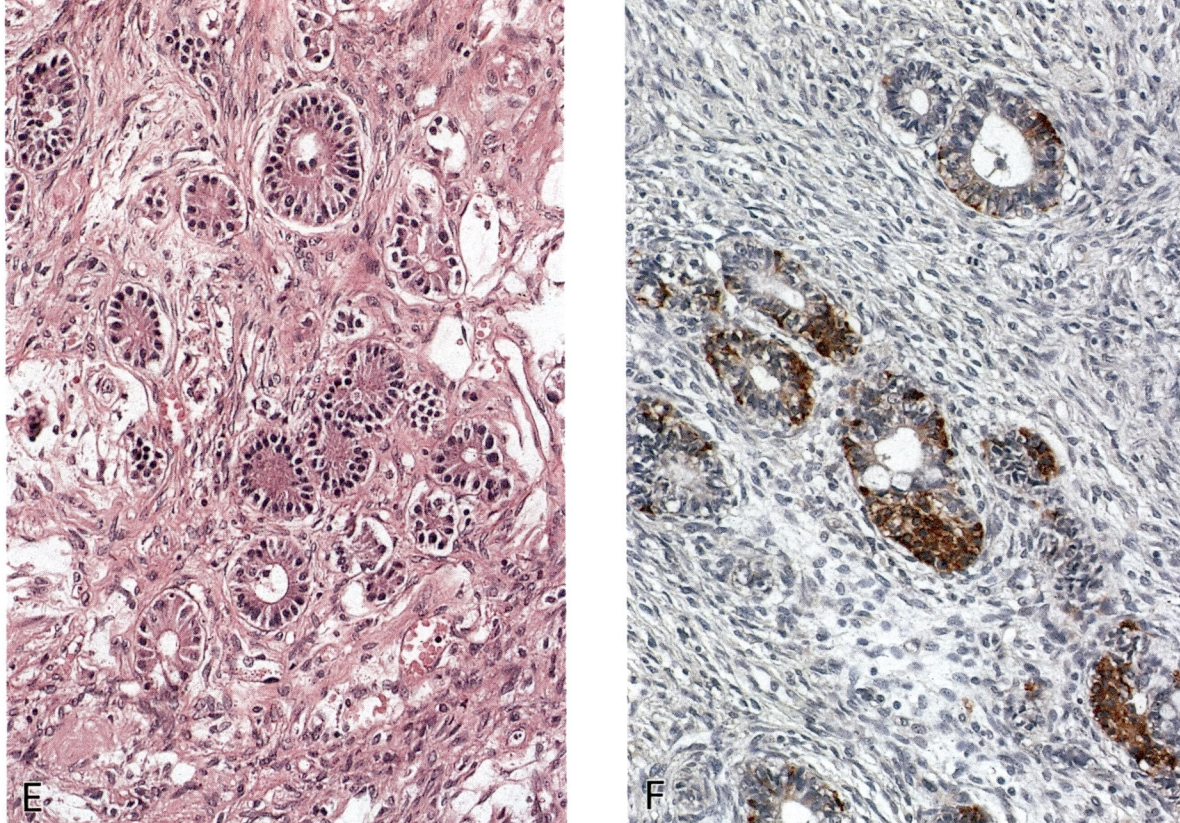

Figure 8-32 (Continued)

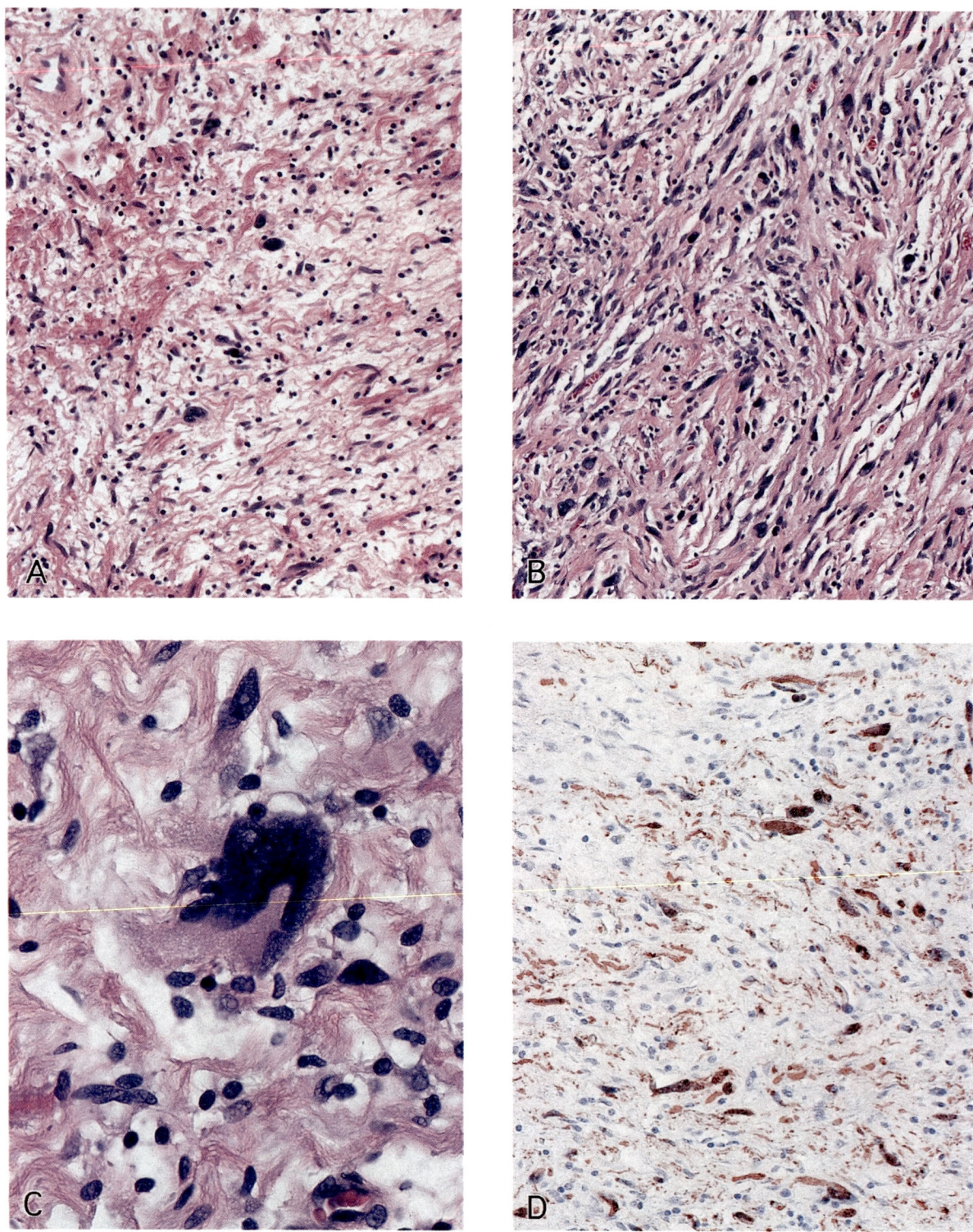

Figure 8-33

INTRANEURAL NEUROFIBROMA WITH DEGENERATIVE NUCLEAR ATYPIA ("ATYPICAL NEUROFIBROMA")

Pleomorphic nuclei with smudgy chromatin and occasional nuclear inclusions (A) are considered a degenerative change. When occurring in more cellular tumors, this feature may prompt consideration of MPNST (B,C). Such cells are S-100 protein positive (D), but proliferation marker studies (MIB-1) show their nuclei to be unlabeled.

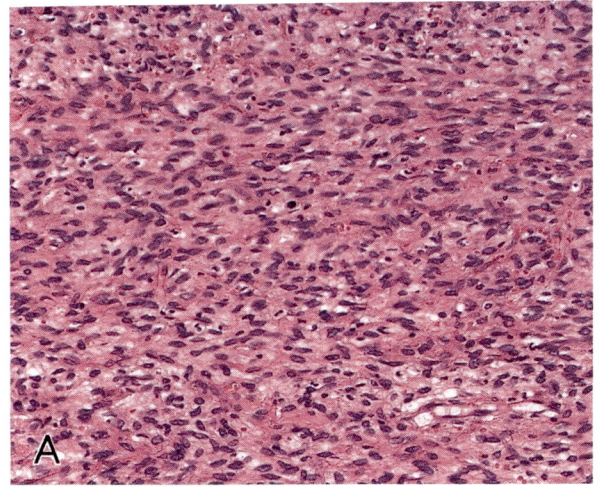

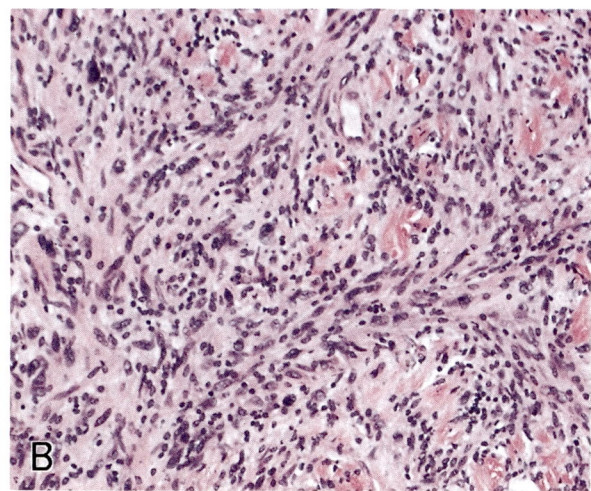

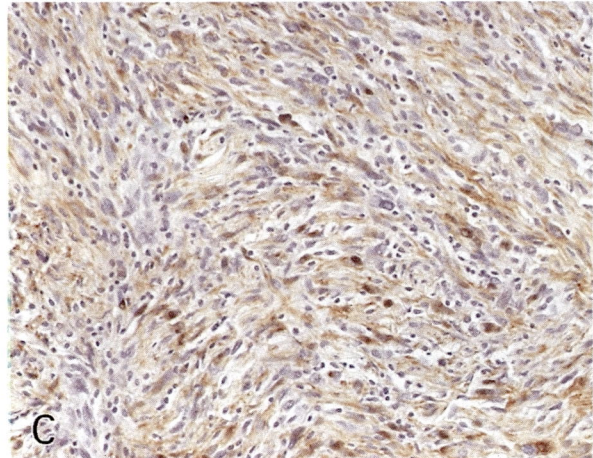

Figure 8-34
"CELLULAR NEUROFIBROMA"
When neurofibromas (A) become hypercellular, the designation "cellular neurofibroma" is appropriate. Such tumors may also feature occasional mitotic figures. Cellular neurofibroma components (B,C) may be seen in MPNSTs arising in transition from neurofibroma. Like conventional neurofibromas they show S-100 protein immunoreactivity (C). The point at which such lesions in transit to MPNST are to be considered malignant is discussed in detail in chapter 9 and is illustrated in photographic sequence (see fig. 11-17).

and when the latter gives way to MPNST is presented in chapter 11. Since MPNSTs frequently arise in neurofibroma and the various patterns of this continuum may coexist in a single specimen, extensive sampling of cellular neurofibromas is required. On the basis of one limited study, it appears that neither atypical nor cellular neurofibromas tend to recur (35a).

Immunohistochemical Findings. Although immunostains are usually not needed for diagnosis, neurofibromas of all types routinely stain for S-100 protein (figs. 8-6C, 8-16C, 8-17A, 8-23B, 8-24B, 8-25C, 8-33D, 8-34C). The proportion of immunoreactive cells is highly variable but does not approach that seen in schwannoma (25). Tactile-like bodies are also S-100 protein immunoreactive (fig. 8-27D). Staining for Leu-7 is observed in greater than half of neurofibromas (43). Despite

the presence of cells with ultrastructural features of perineurial-like cells, neurofibromas do not, as a rule, contain epithelial membrane antigen (EMA)-reactive cells (8-17C). Instead, the only reactivity for this antigen is seen in residual, often compressed normal perineurium surrounding involved nerve fascicles (figs. 8-17C, 8-25D) (7) and at the periphery of some tactile-like bodies (fig. 8-27D). A reported exception is that of Perentes et al. (42) who found focal weak EMA staining in two neurofibromas. Neurofibromas also stain variably for CD34 (9c,11,47,64). Since in most instances such cells differ from other nerve sheath cells by having dendritic processes and round or oval, rather than spindle-shaped nuclei, Weiss and Nickoloff (64) concluded that CD34 reactivity resides in cells other than those expressing S-100 protein. The authors suggested that such

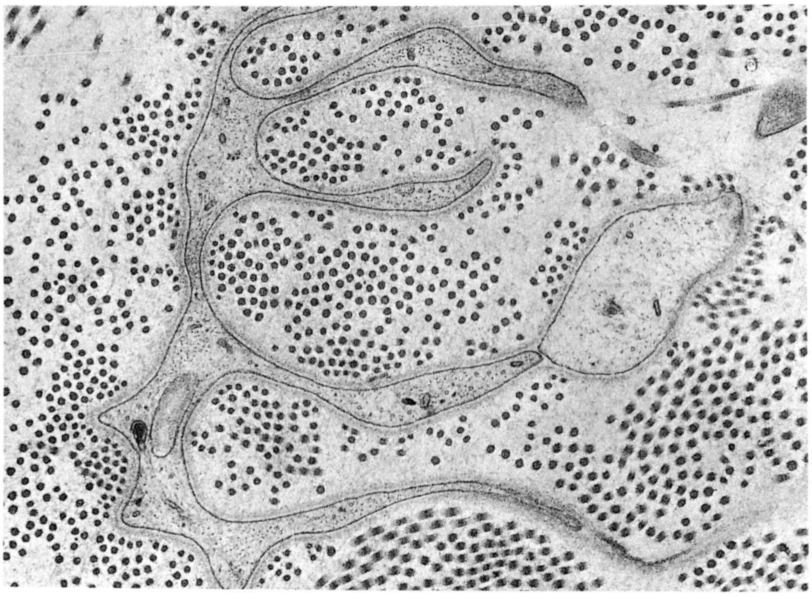

Figure 8-35
DIFFUSE NEUROFIBROMA
Detail of a Schwann cell with numerous thin processes that appear to be enveloping collagen fibrils. Note the continuous basement membrane on the cell surface (X26,400).

cells may represent an as yet undescribed nerve sheath element, one playing a supportive role relative to the Schwann cell. An alternative explanation (10,11) is that CD34-immunoreactive cells represent monocytes present in normal nerves, perhaps the ones involved in experimental neuritis (39,57). Collagen IV staining in neurofibromas is typically pericellular and involves many cells (9b). Residual axons are neurofilament protein immunoreactive (figs. 8-6D, 8-16D, 8-24C, 8-28D, 8-29B).

Two immunohistochemical studies of proliferation marker expression by neurofibromas have been undertaken (32,49). In the largest, a study of 26 cases (49), the Ki-67 (MIB-1) labeling indices ranged from 1 to 13 percent (mean, 4.7 percent). So-called atypical neurofibromas had indices one standard deviation (3.2 percent) higher than typical tumors. In comparison, 28 MPNSTs had indices of 5 to 38 percent (mean, 18.5 percent; standard deviation, 9.6 percent). A smaller study of five cutaneous and four plexiform tumors (Kindblom) found MIB-1 labeling indices of less than 1 percent in all cases. For comparison, all but 3 of 26 MPNSTs had values greater than 5 percent, and half were greater than 30 percent.

Staining for p53 protein is seen in less than 5 percent of neurofibromas, including plexiform examples (20,37).

Ultrastructural Findings. Although electron microscopy is rarely required to make the diagnosis of neurofibroma, it nonetheless plays a role in the assessment of the cellular composition and the complex cell/stroma interactions that characterize these lesions. Regardless of the type of neurofibroma under consideration, individual cases as well as different areas of a single tumor are characterized by variation in cell makeup (15,31,59).

Schwann Cells. Most cells encountered in neurofibromas, irrespective of tumor subtype, are Schwann cells (figs. 8-35, 8-36). Their frequency varies from less than to greater than 50 percent of the constituent cells. Often lying singly, they are primarily found among aggregates of collagen (fig. 8-40), their variously sectioned processes enwrapping collagen fibrils (figs. 8-35, 8-40). Schwann cells are recognized by their thin arborizing cytoplasmic processes, their content of intermediate filaments and occasional microtubules, and their continuous basement membrane (external lamina) (figs. 8-35, 8-40). Pinocytotic vesicles are inconspicuous or absent. Scattered myelinated and unmyelinated nerve fibers are also evident (fig. 8-40) but are markedly reduced in number as compared to normal nerve.

Perineurial-like Cells and Cell Nests with Tactile-like Differentiation. Cells with the ultrastructural features of perineurial cells are variably distributed within neurofibromas: they are at the periphery of unmyelinated and myelinated nerves, in the vicinity of Schwann cells (fig. 8-36), and loosely

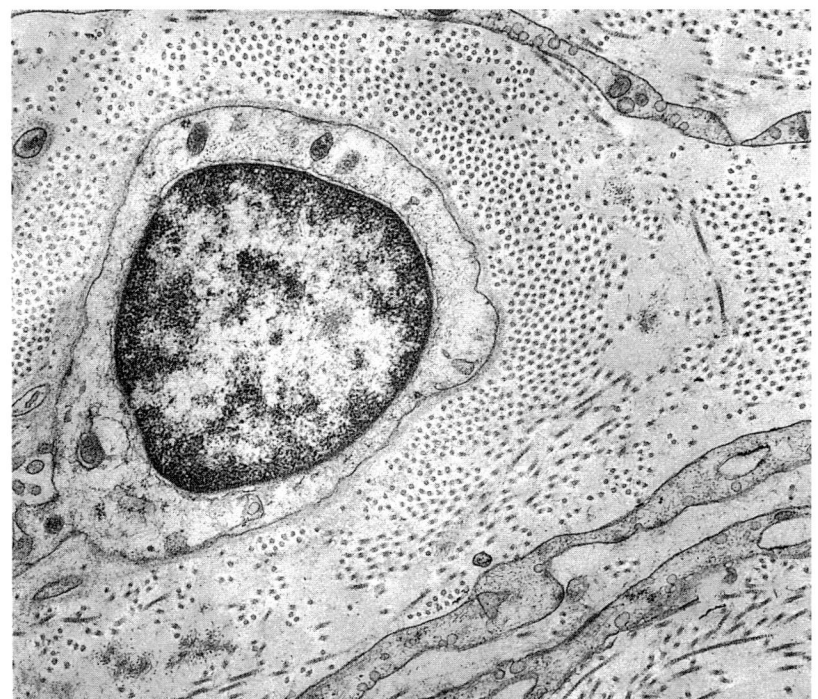

Figure 8-36
CUTANEOUS
NEUROFIBROMA
A Schwann cell (center left) with a
continuous basement membrane is
surrounded by collagen fibrils. Portions of three perineurial-like cell processes, one at the top right and two at
the bottom right, with distinctive pinocytotic vesicles, are also evident
(X25,000).

Figure 8-37
CUTANEOUS
NEUROFIBROMA
Detail of a perineurial-like cell process with pinocytotic vesicles, scattered
intermediate filaments, and remnants
of basement membrane substance in
the acellular myxocollagenous matrix
(by light microscopy) (X69,300).

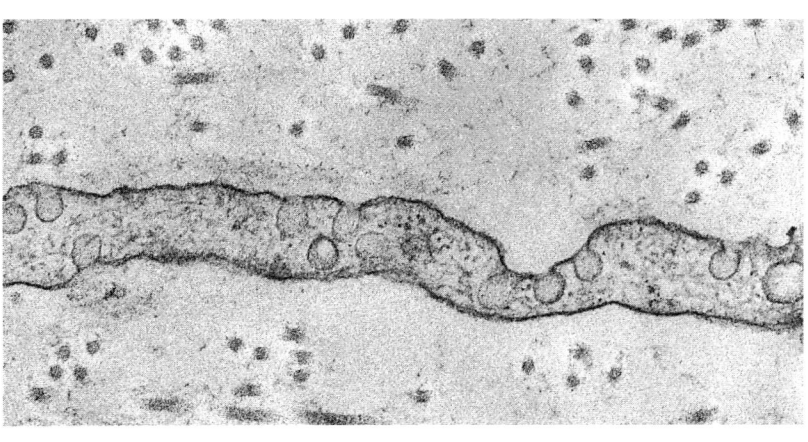

scattered within myxocollagenous matrix (fig.
8-37). Such cells feature long, straight or gently
curved, very thin cytoplasmic processes with abundant pinocytotic vesicles and a discontinuous coat
of basement membrane. They are referred to as
perineurial-like cells since, to date, they have not
been shown to express EMA immunoreactivity.
Immunoelectron microscopy is necessary to determine whether EMA is present in the very thin,
widely separated processes of these cells.

Tactile corpuscle-like cell arrangements in neurofibroma, ones consisting of cells with processes
either stacked or arranged in circular lamellae, are
generally likened to meissnerian and pacinian
corpuscles, respectively (5,12,29,50,52,55). Some
neurofibromas with these features have loosely
been referred to as pacinian neurofibromas (46,
63). Other examples of so-called pacinian neurofibroma either lacked features which, on critical
review, would have supported that diagnosis (9,
35,37,45,58), or are best interpreted as examples
of nerve sheath myxoma (36,40). Whereas normal
meissnerian and pacinian corpuscles are composed mainly of Schwann and perineurial cells,
respectively (see chapter 2), ultrastructural (fig.
8-38) (28,29,55,62,63) and immunohistochemical

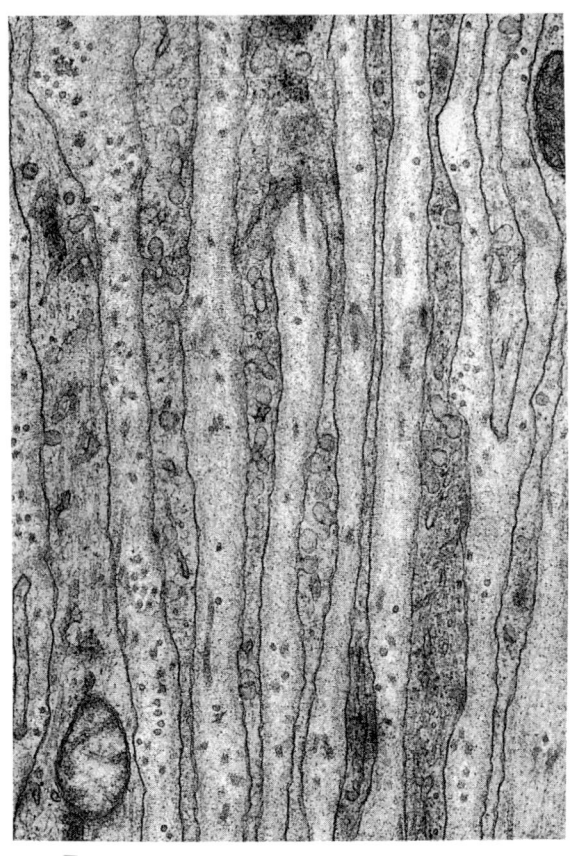

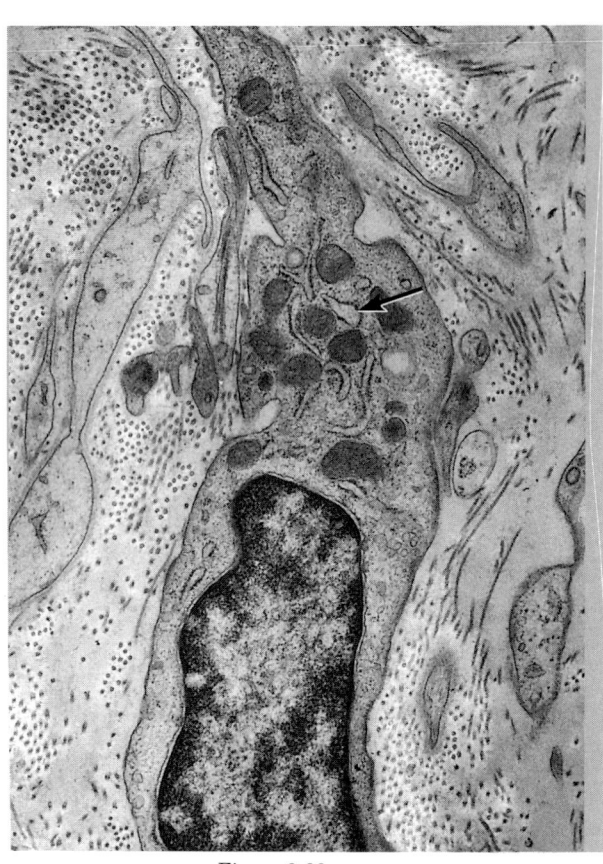

Figure 8-38
CUTANEOUS NEUROFIBROMA IN NF1
A portion of a lamellar structure resembling a pacinian-like corpuscle consisting of parallel arrays of perineurial-like cell processes. Note the pinocytotic vesicles and the discontinuous basement membranes (X36,400).

Figure 8-39
CUTANEOUS NEUROFIBROMA IN NF1
Shown is a fibroblastic cell with a moderately well-developed rough endoplasmic reticulum (arrow), few pinocytotic vesicles, and no basement membrane surrounded by collagen fibrils. Schwann cell processes are coated by a distinct basement membrane (X16,300).

Figure 8-40
PLEXIFORM NEUROFIBROMA
An aggregate of collagen fibrils is intermixed with two myelinated axons (top), two unmyelinated axons (arrow), and numerous complex Schwann cell processes that entrap collagen fibrils (X8,800).

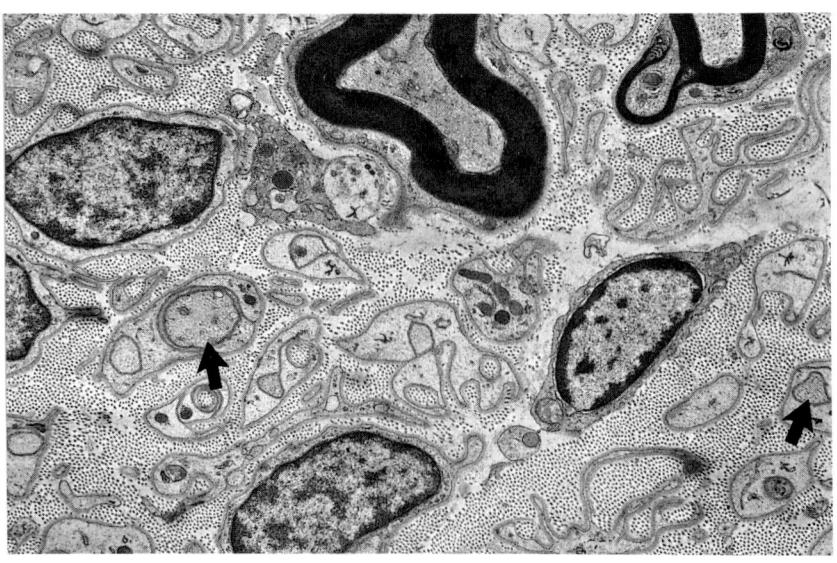

findings (28,52,62) are discordant with respect to the constituent cells of tactile-like structures in neurofibromas. Even though they are immunoreactive for S-100 protein, a Schwann cell marker, their fine structure is that of perineurial-like cells (30,62).

Fibroblasts. Fibroblasts, characterized by ample, branching rough endoplasmic reticulum, a well-developed Golgi apparatus, sparse pinocytotic vesicles, and lack of basement membrane coating (fig. 8-39), are found in greatest number in cutaneous and sclerotic neurofibromas. As previously noted, studies have suggested that neurofibroma fibroblasts may differ from normal fibroblasts (24,44).

Transitional Cells. Cells with features of both perineurial cells and fibroblasts or of Schwann and perineurial cells are found in varying number in neurofibromas. Such cells are termed transitional cells and appear to be hybrids in terms of their ultrastructural features. For example, the perineurial fibroblast is characterized by a moderately well-developed rough endoplasmic reticulum and bipolar cytoplasmic processes somewhat thicker than those of normal perineurial cells, but featuring scattered pinocytotic vesicles and occasional short segments of surface basement membrane.

DNA Flow Cytometry. On the basis of one flow cytometric study of 26 neurofibromas, 66 percent were diploid and the remainder were aneuploid; 1 to 8 percent of cells were in S phase (mean 3.4 percent) (49). Of 28 MPNSTs similarly studied, 64 percent were aneuploid; 2 to 46 percent of cells were in S phase (mean, 12.4 percent). A smaller image analysis study of Feulgen-stained sections found one of five neurofibromas to have a hyperdiploid DNA histogram, with the remainder diploid (48).

Differential Diagnosis. The differential diagnosis of neurofibroma includes schwannoma, low-grade MPNST, ganglioneuroma, dermatofibrosarcoma protuberans of ordinary and pigmented types (Bednar tumor), nerve sheath myxoma, myxoma, and neuronevus.

A detailed summary of the features distinguishing localized intraneural neurofibroma from *schwannoma,* the principal lesion in the differential diagnosis, appears in Table 7-1. Neurofibromas are more often fusiform than globular, and do not lie eccentric to the parent nerve.

Furthermore, they lack both a thick hyaline capsule, hyalinized vasculature, degenerative cyst formation, and usually, Antoni A and B growth patterns with Verocay body formation. As previously noted, nodules of Antoni A tissue are rarely seen in neurofibroma (fig. 8-28). The nuclei of neurofibroma cells are approximately one third to half the size of those found in schwannoma cells. Unlike schwannomas, neurofibromas often feature conspicuous, broad bands of collagen ("shredded carrots"). Neurofibromas contain collagen fibers of types 1 and 3, whereas those in schwannomas are predominantly of type 3 (27). Pools of mucinous matrix are far more often seen in neurofibromas. Since immunoreactivity for S-100 protein is a feature of some but not all neurofibroma cells, staining is less uniform and pronounced than in schwannoma. Lastly, unlike the cellular heterogeneity that ultrastructurally characterizes neurofibromas (see above), schwannomas consist of a uniform population of well-differentiated Schwann cells.

The distinction of neurofibroma from *low-grade MPNST* usually poses no problem, but atypical neurofibromas (fig. 8-33) and cellular neurofibromas (fig. 8-34) may (66). The spectrum of cellular neurofibromas and our "cut off" for a diagnosis of low-grade MPNST is discussed in detail and illustrated elsewhere (see chapter 11; fig. 11-17). Degenerative nuclear atypia, i.e., pleomorphism, smudgy hyperchromasia, and nuclear cytoplasmic pseudoinclusions, when associated with no or only rare mitotic activity, is of no clinical significance (fig. 8-33). Such cells are typically S-100 protein immunoreactive (fig. 8-32) and lack staining for proliferation markers. The nuclear changes in atypical neurofibromas are, therefore, similar to those in ancient schwannoma, a tumor noted for its degenerative nuclear atypia.

The distinction of *ganglioneuroma* from neurofibroma rests upon the identification of ganglion cells and abundant nerve fibers, definitive features of the former and ones not seen in ordinary neurofibroma. Both features may, however, be seen in neurofibromas overrunning dorsal root or autonomic ganglia (fig. 8-29). In such cases the ganglion cells are not distributed throughout the lesion, but rather are localized. Furthermore, they lie among aligned nerve fiber bundles uniformly oriented traversing the overrun ganglion (fig. 8-29B). Unlike the majority of dorsal root nerve fibers, those

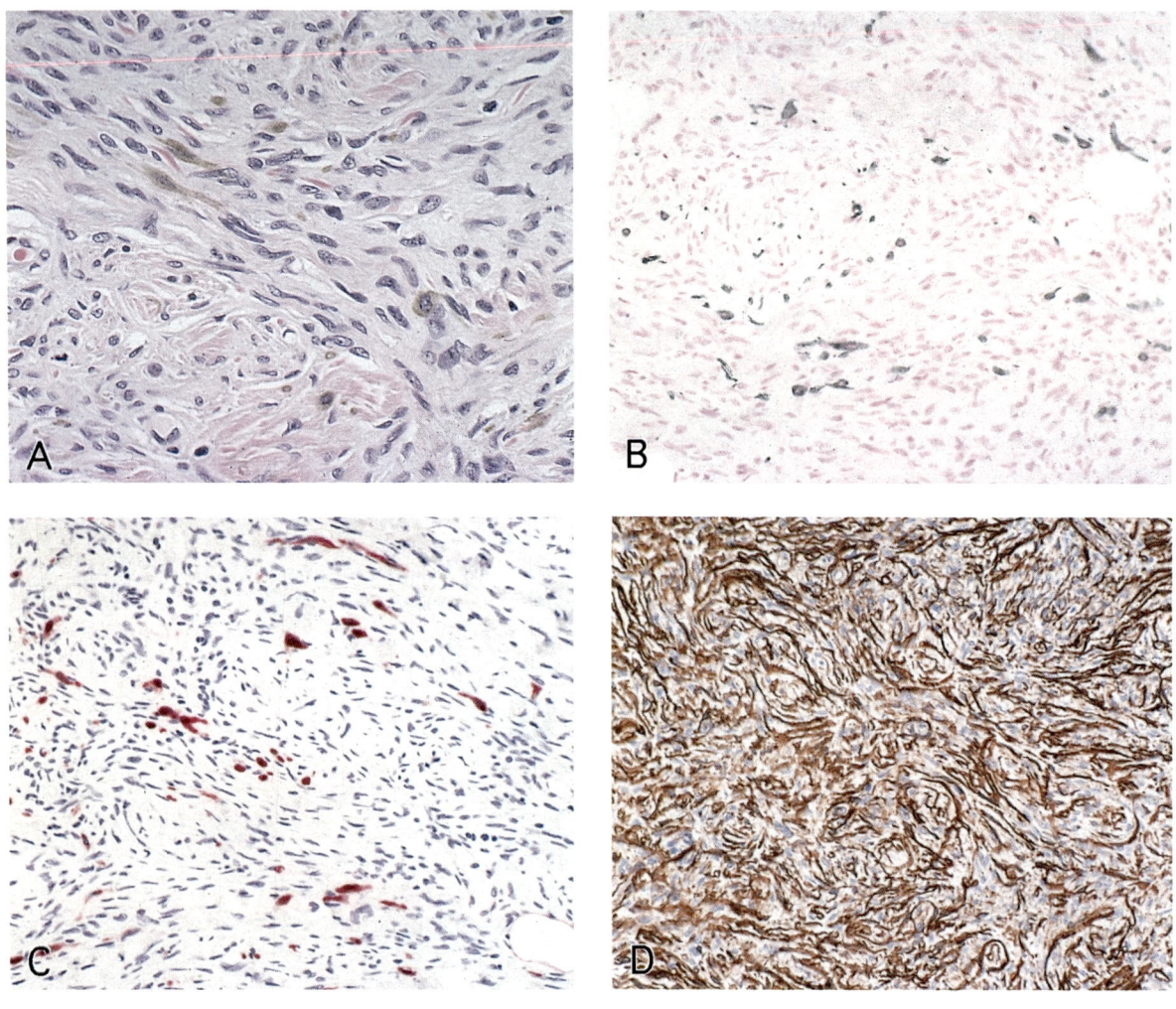

Figure 8-41
BEDNAR TUMOR
Unlike neurofibroma, such lesions are composed of S-100 protein–negative spindle cells in a storiform arrangement. Lying among them are pigmented spindle cells (A). Such cells are positive on melanin stain (B, Fontana) and are S-100 protein immunoreactive (C). Bednar tumors, like ordinary dermatofibrosarcoma protuberans, show strong CD34 immunoreactivity (D).

of ganglioneuroma are unmyelinated. Although normal and ganglioneuromatous ganglion cells are surrounded by satellite cells, such cells are less numerous and uniformly arranged in ganglioneuromas (fig. 8-29C).

Due to the propensity of *dermatofibrosarcoma protuberans (DFSP)* to infiltrate dermal and adipose tissue and its capacity to undergo myxoid change, it may be mistaken for diffuse neurofibroma. In contrast to the latter, DFSP is more cellular, consists of larger cells resembling fibroblasts, usually shows a storiform pattern, and lack both pseudo-meissnerian corpuscles and S-

100 protein immunoreactivity. Like neurofibroma (1,3,4,11,23,33,47), the cells of DFSP express CD34 (11,64), however, the pattern of CD34 staining in neurofibroma is variable and never affects all the cells. In DFSP virtually every cell is CD34 immunoreactive (64). Neurofibromas with pigmented cells must be distinguished from the so-called *Bednar tumor* (fig. 8-41) (8), some examples of which were wrongly termed "storiform neurofibroma." It is thought by some that this slow-growing, focally pigmented dermal tumor is a DFSP secondarily colonized by dendritic melanocytes (16). Unlike

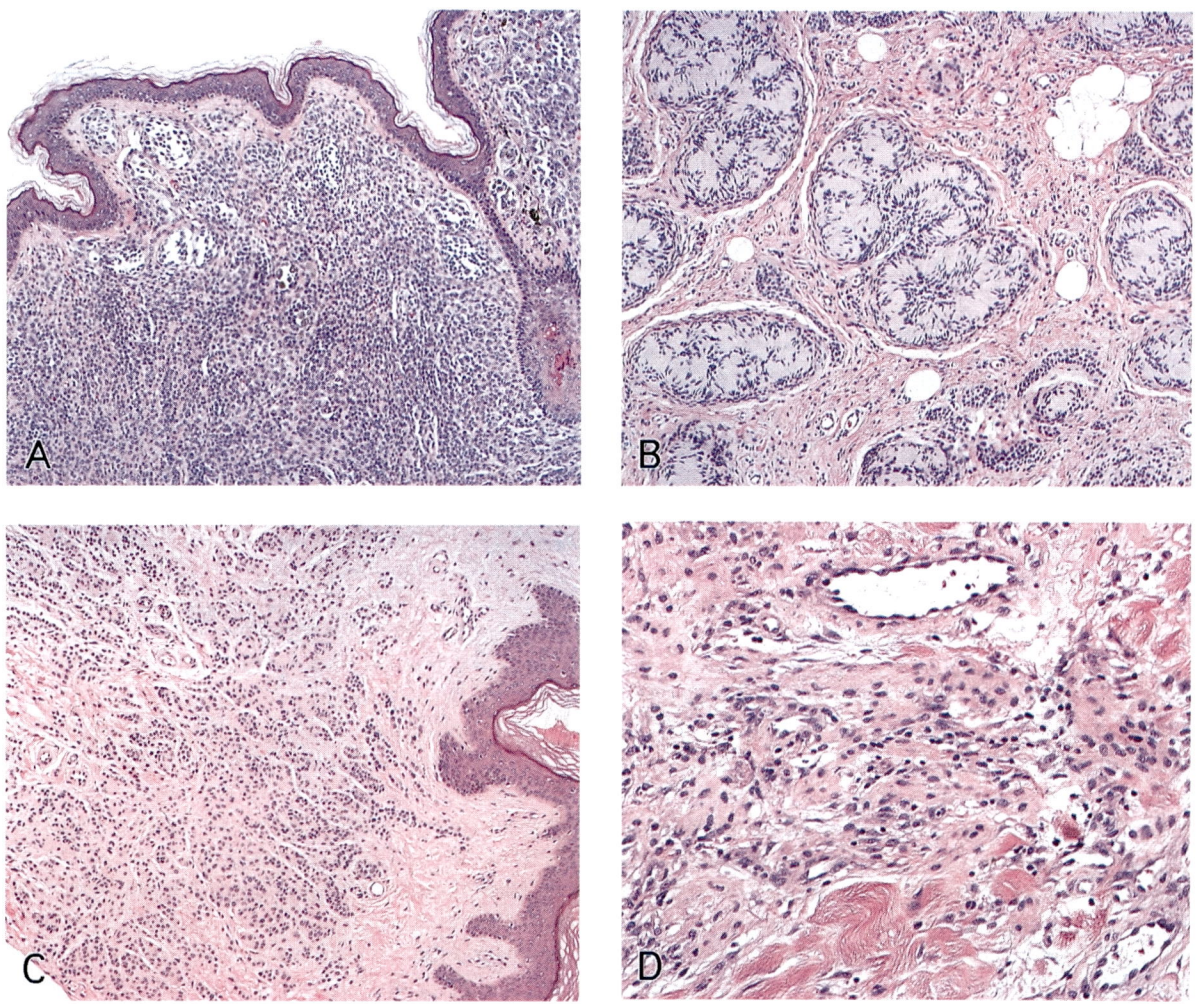

Figure 8-42
CONGENITAL NEVUS AND NEURONEVUS
Both lesions may show conspicuous schwannian differentiation. Readily recognized by its superficial component of ordinary nevus cells (A), the congenital nevus may exhibit well-formed pseudo-meissnerian corpuscles in an obviously schwannian background (B). Neuronevus similarly consists of a superficial nevus cell component (C) and a deeper portion with schwannian features (D).

neurofibroma cells, the predominant spindle cells of Bednar tumor lack S-100 protein immunoreactivity (fig. 8-41D) and ultrastructurally resemble fibroblasts (14,34).

Differing from most neurofibromas, *nerve sheath myxoma* exhibits a distinctly lobulated architecture, marked hypocellularity, the presence of "stringy"-appearing spindle and occasionally epithelioid cells, multinucleation, vacuolation of both nuclei and cytoplasm, and no nerve association. Immunostaining for S-100 protein is seen in both lesions and does not reliably distinguish the two tumors. At the ultra-structural level, nerve sheath myxomas lack the heterogeneity of neurofibroma, since they are composed mainly of Schwann cells.

The distinction of neurofibroma from *spindle cell lipoma* rests upon the frequent occurrence of the latter in deep soft tissue of the posterior neck in elderly patients, and its delicate encapsulation, often conspicuous vascularity, content of fat, lack of degenerative atypia, and occasional floret cell formation. Its spindle cells are CD34 immunoreactive, and lack staining for both S-100 protein and the basement membrane markers, collagen type 4 and laminin.

Due to its lack of extensive collagen fiber formation, *myxoma* is usually readily distinguished from myxoid neurofibromas. A firmer distinction rests upon demonstrating lack of S-100 reactivity in myxoma.

It may be very difficult to distinguish cutaneous neurofibroma from deep portions of *congenital* or *neuronevi* (fig. 8-42). The finding of classic nevus cells in superficial portions of a neuronevus is, of course, the most helpful diagnostic feature. Most neuronevus cells have conspicuous cytoplasm, whereas that of neurofibroma cells is often inapparent in conventionally stained material. An additional distinguishing feature is the strong pattern of diffuse S-100 protein expression in neuronevus as opposed to less uniform staining in neurofibroma.

Few lesions enter into the differential diagnosis of plexiform neurofibroma. These variously affect skin, subcutaneous tissue, and superficial soft tissue and include primarily plexiform schwannoma and plexiform fibrohistiocytic tumor. Unlike plexiform neurofibroma, *plexiform schwannoma* consists of a uniform proliferation of Schwann cells occasionally forming Verocay bodies (21) and lacking a significant stromal mucopolysaccharide matrix. The cells of plexiform schwannoma are larger than those of neurofibroma, are uniformly and strongly S-100 protein immunoreactive, and represent well- differentiated Schwann cells. Both lesions may contain scant residual neurofilament protein–immunoreactive axons and a delicate investment of EMA-positive perineurial cells. Whereas plexiform neurofibromas often have a diffusely extraneural component, the cells of plexiform schwannoma are limited to nerves. Plexiform schwannomas are unaccompanied by overlying cutaneous pigmentation, a feature of some plexiform neurofibromas. Unlike plexiform neurofibroma, the dermal variant of *plexiform fibrohistiocytic tumor* occurs predominantly in females, generally measures only 1 to 2 cm, and is hard in texture (67). This tumor is skin-colored and not associated with hyperpigmentation. The "bag of worms" appearance so characteristic of plexiform neurofibroma is only rarely seen (67). In contrast to plexiform neurofibroma, fibrohistiocytic tumors exhibit a biphasic histology which includes a major component of spindle to stellate myofibroblasts with accompanying stromal collagen and scattered osteoclast-like giant cells as well as epithelioid mononuclear cells. The myofibroblasts are HHF35 immunoreactive and the osteoclast-like giant cells are positive for KP-1 (CD68) (67). Plexiform fibrohistiocytic tumors lack a nerve association and are immunonegative for S-100 protein.

Treatment and Prognosis. Resection of localized or diffuse cutaneous neurofibroma is curative and unassociated with neurologic deficits. Large lesions of the diffuse or massive soft tissue type may be amenable to only subtotal removal. As previously noted, diffuse cutaneous neurofibromas rarely undergo malignant change.

Although curative treatment of localized intraneural neurofibroma consists of resection, a procedure which necessarily requires sacrifice of the parent nerve, excision of major, still functional nerves may not be warranted. The same is true in the case of large plexiform neurofibroma which, if entirely resected, can produce devastating neurologic sequelae. In addition to alleviating the mechanical disability that accompanies large neurofibromas, some are resected because of pain or rapid increase in size. Both these manifestations may herald malignant transformation, an uncommon occurrence in localized intraneural neurofibroma (56), but one that may occur in up to 5 percent of plexiform tumors (13). In one recent large series of plexiform neurofibromas (37), patients whose tumors showed MPNST transformation were older than those with benign lesions (38 versus 22 years); the rate of tumor recurrence also differed substantially (47 versus 23 percent).

REFERENCES

1. Abenoza P, Lillemoe T. CD34 and factor XIIIa in the differential diagnosis of dermatofibroma and dermatofibrosarcoma protuberans. Am J Dermatopathol 1993;15:429–34.
2. Ackerman LV, Taylor FH. Neurogenous tumors within the thorax. A clinical pathological evaluation of forty-eight cases. Cancer 1951;4:669–91.
3. Aiba S, Tabata N, Ishii H, Ootani H, Tagami H. Dermatofibrosarcoma protuberans is a unique fibrohistiocytic tumour expressing CD34. Br J Dermatol 1992;127:79–84.
4. Altman DA, Nickoloff BJ, Fivenson DP. Differential expression of factor XIIIa and CD34 in cutaneous mesenchymal tumors. J Cutan Pathol 1993;20:154–8.
5. Altmeyer P. Histologie eines rankenneuroms mit vaterpacini-lamellen korper-ahnlichen strukturen. Hautarzt 1979;30:248–52.
6. Anderson B, Robertson DM. Melanin containing neurofibroma: case report with evidence of Schwann cell origin in melanin. Can J Neurol Sci 1979;6:139–43.
7. Ariza A, Bilboa JM, Rosai J. Immunohistochemical detection of epithelial membrane antigen in normal perineurial cells and perineurioma. Am J Surg Pathol 1988;12:678–83.
8. Bednar B. Storiform neurofibromas of the skin, pigmented and nonpigmented. Cancer 1957;10:368–76.
9. Bennin B, Barsky S, Salgia K. Pacinian neurofibroma. Arch Dermatol 1976;112:1558.
9a. Bhargava R, Parham DM, Lasater OE, Chari RS, Chen G, Fletcher BD. MR imaging differentiation of benign and malignant peripheral nerve sheath tumors: use of the target sign. Pediatr Radiol 1997;27:124–9.
9b. Chanoki M, Ishii M, Fukai K, et al. Immunohistochemical localization of type I, III, IV, V, and IV collagens and laminin in neurofibroma and neurofibrosarcoma. Am J Dermatol 1991;13:365–73.
9c. Choubal A, Paetau A, Zoltic KP, Miettinen M. CD34 immunoreactivity in nervous system tumors. Acta Neuropathol 1994;88:454–8.
10. Cohen PR, Rapini RP, Farhood AI. CD34 expression in neural and fibrohistiocytic lesions [Letter]. Am J Surg Pathol 1995;19:115–6.
11. Cohen PR, Rapini RP, Farhood AI. Expression of the human hematopoietic progenitor cell antigen CD34 in vascular and spindle cell tumors. J Cutan Pathol 1993;20:15–20.
12. Dible JH. Verocay bodies and pseudo-Meissnerian corpuscles. J Pathol Bacteriol 1963;85:425–33.
13. Ducatman BS, Scheithauer BW, Piepgras DG. Malignant peripheral nerve sheath tumors. A clinicopathologic study of 120 cases. Cancer 1986;57:2006–21.
14. Dupree WB, Langloss JM, Weiss SW. Pigmented dermatofibrosarcoma protuberans (Bednar tumor). A pathologic ultrastructural and immunohistochemical study. Am J Surg Pathol 1985;9:630–9.
15. Erlandson RA. Diagnostic transmission electron microscopy of tumors. New York: Raven Press, 1994:571–5.
15a. Fetsch JF, Michal M, Miettinen M. Pigmented (melanotic) neurofibroma: a clinicopathologic and immunohistochemical analysis of 19 lesions from 17 patients. Am J Surg Pathol (in press).
16. Fletcher CD, Theaker JM, Flanagan A, Krausz T. Pigmented dermatofibrosarcoma protuberans (Bednar tumor): melanocytic colonization or neuroectodermal differentiation? A clinicopathological and immunohistochemical study. Histopathology 1988;13:631–43.
17. Friedman JM, Fialkow PJ, Greene CL, Weinberg MN. Probable clonal origin of neurofibrosarcoma in a patient with hereditary neurofibromatosis. JNCI 1982;69:1289–92.
18. Gutmann DH, Collins FS. The neurofibromatosis type 1 gene and its protein product, neurofibromin. Neuron 1993;10:335–43.
19. Halliday AL, Sobel RA, Martuza RL. Benign spinal nerve sheath tumors: their occurrence sporadically and in neurofibromatosis types 1 and 2. J Neurosurg 1991;74:248–53.
20. Halling KC, Scheithauer BW, Halling AC, et al. p53 expression in neurofibroma and malignant peripheral nerve sheath tumor. An immunohistochemical study of sporadic and NF1-associated tumors. Am J Clin Pathol 1996;106:282–8.
21. Harkin JC, Arrington JH, Reed RJ. Benign plexiform schwannoma. A lesion distinct from plexiform neurofibroma [Abstract]. J Neuropathol Exp Neurol 1978;37:622.
22. Harkin JC, Reed RJ. Tumors of the peripheral nervous system. Atlas of Tumor Pathology, 2nd Series, Fascicle 3. Armed Forces Institute of Pathology, 1969.
23. Hashimoto K, Fujiwata K, Mehregan A. Current topics of immunohistochemistry as applied to skin tumors. J Dermatol (Tokyo) 1993;20:521–32.
24. Hayashi S, Kubota Y, Shimada S, Hori Y. Characterization of cultured neurofibroma cells derived from von Recklinghausen's disease. Clin Exp Dermatol 1990;15:217–21.
25. Hirose T, Sano T, Hizawa K. Ultrastructural localization of S-100 protein in neurofibroma. Acta Neuropathol 1986;69:103–10.
26. Hochberg FH, Dasila AB, Galdabini J, Richardson EP Jr. Gastrointestinal involvement in von Recklinghausen's neurofibromatosis. Neurology 1974;24:1144–51.
27. Junqueira LC, Montes GS, Kaupert D, Shigihara KM, Bolonhani TM, Krisztçn RM. Morphological and histochemical studies on the collagen in neurinomas, neurofibromas, and fibromas. J Neuropathol Exp Neurol 1981;40:123–33.
28. Jurecka W. Tactile corpuscle-like structures in peripheral nerve sheath tumors in plastic embedded material. Am J Dermatopathol 1988;10:74–9.
29. Jurecka W, Lassman H, Lassmann G, Matras H, Watzek G, Hollmann K. Tactile corpuscle-like structures in a case of plexiform neurofibromatosis. Arch Dermatol Res 1979;266:43–50.
30. Kaiserling E, Geerts ML. Tumour of Wagner-Meissner touch corpuscles. Wagner-Meissner neurilemmoma. Virchows Arch [A] 1986;409:241–50.
31. Kimura M, Kamatu Y, Matsumoto K, Takaya H. Electron microscopic study on the tumor of von Recklinghausen's neurofibromatosis. Acta Pathol Jpn 1974;24:79–91.
32. Kindblom LG, Ahlden M, Meis-Kindblom JM, Stenman G. Immunohistochemical and molecular analysis of p53, MDM2, proliferating cell nuclear antigen and Ki-67 in benign and malignant peripheral nerve sheath tumors. Virchows Arch 1995;427:19–26.
33. Kutzner H. Expression of the human progenitor cell antigen CD34 (HPCA-1) distinguishes dermatofibrosarcoma protuberans from fibrous histiocytoma in formalin-fixed, paraffin-embedded tissue. J Am Acad Dermatol 1993;28:613–7.

217

34. Lautier R, Wolff HH, Jones RE. An immunohistochemical study of dermatofibrosarcoma protuberans supports its fibroblastic character and contradicts neuroectodermal or histiocytic components. Am J Derm Pathol 1990;12:25–30.

35. Levi L, Curri SB. Multiple pacinian neurofibroma and relationship with the finger-tip arteriovenous anastomoses. Brit J Dermatol 1980;102:345–9.

35a.Lin BT, Weiss LM, Medeiros LJ. Neurofibroma and cellular neurofibroma with atypia. 1997;21:1443–9.

36. MacDonald DM, Wilson-Jones E. Pacinian neurofibroma. Histopathology 1977;1:247–55.

37. McCarron KF, Goldblum JR. Plexiform neurofibroma with and without associated malignant peripheral nerve sheath tumor: a clinicopathologic and immunohistochemical analysis of 54 cases [Abstract]. Mod Pathol 1998;11:612–7.

38. McCormack K, Kaplan D, Murray JC, Fetter BF. Multiple hairy pacinian neurofibromas (nerve-sheath myxomas). J Am Acad Dermatol 1988;18:416–9.

39. Oldfors A. Macrophages in peripheral nerves. An ultrastructural and enzyme histochemical study on rats. Acta Neuropathol (Berl) 1980;49:43–9.

40. Owen DA. Pacinian neurofibroma [Letter]. Arch Pathol Lab Med 1979;103:99–100

41. Payan MJ, Gambarelli D, Keller P, et al. Melanotic neurofibroma: a case report with ultrastructural study. Acta Neuropathol (Berlin) 1986;69:148–52.

42. Perentes E, Nakagawa Y, Ross GW, Stanton C, Rubinstein LJ. Expression of epithelial membrane antigen in perineurial cells and their derivatives. An immunohistochemical study with multiple markers. Acta Neuropathol 1987;75:160–5.

43. Perentes E, Rubinstein LJ. Immunohistochemical recognition of human nerve sheath tumors by anti-Leu 7 (HNK-I) monoclonal antibody. Acta Neuropathol 1986;69:227–33.

44. Pleasure D, Kreider B, Sobue G, et al. Schwann-like cells cultured from human dermal neurofibromas. Immunohistological identification and response to Schwann cell mitogens. Ann NY Acad Sci 1986;486:227–40.

45. Prichard RW, Custer RP. Pacinian neurofibroma. Cancer 1952;5:297–301.

46. Prose PH, Gherardi GJ, Coblenz A. Pacinian neurofibroma. Arch Dermatol 1957;76:65–9.

47. Ramani P, Bradley NJ, Fletcher CD. QBEND/10, a new monoclonal antibody to endothelium: assessment of its diagnostic utility in paraffin sections. Histopathology 1990;17:237–42.

48. Salmon I, Kiss R, Segers V, et al. Characterization of nuclear size, ploidy, DNA histogram type and proliferation index in 79 nerve sheath tumors. Anticancer Res 1992;12:2277–83.

49. Scheithauer BW, Halling KC, Nascimento AG, Hill EM, Sim FH, Katzmann JA. Neurofibroma and malignant peripheral nerve sheath tumor: a proliferation index and DNA ploidy study [Abstract]. Path Res Pract 1995;19:177.

50. Schochet SS Jr, Barrett DA. Neurofibroma with aberrant tactile corpuscles. Acta Neuropathol 1974;28:161–5.

51. Sheela S, Riccardi VM, Ratner N. Angiogenic and invasive properties of neurofibroma Schwann cells. J Cell Biol 1990;111:645–53.

52. Shiurba RA, Eng LF, Urich H. The structure of pseudo-Meissnerian corpuscles. An immunohistochemical study. Acta Neuropathol 1984;63:174–6.

53. Skuse GR, Kosciolek BA, Rowley PT. Molecular genetic analysis of tumors in von Recklinghausen neurofibromatosis: loss of heterozygosity for chromosome 17. Genes Chromosom Cancer 1989;1:36–41.

54. Skuse GR, Kosciolek BA, Rowley PT. The neurofibroma in von Recklinghausen neurofibromatosis has a unicellular origin. Am J Hum Genet 1991;49:600–7.

55. Smith TW, Bhawan J. Tactile-like structures in neurofibromas. An ultrastructural study. Acta Neuropathol 1980;50:233–6.

56. Sorensen SA, Mulvihill JJ, Nielsen A. Long-term follow-up of von Recklinghausen neurofibromatosis: survival and malignant neoplasms. N Engl J Med 1986;314:1010–5.

57. Stevens A, Schabet M, Schott K, Wietholter H. Role of endoneurial cells in experimental allergic neuritis and characterization of a resident phagocytic cell. Acta Neuropathol (Berl) 1989;77:412–9.

58. Toth BB, Long WH, Pleasants JE. Central pacinian neurofibroma of the maxilla. Oral Surg 1975;39:630–4.

59. Ushigome S, Takakuwa T, Hyuga M, Tadokora M, Shinagawa T. Perineurial cell tumor and the significance of the perineurial cells in neurofibroma. Acta Pathol Jpn 1986;36:973–87.

60. Verocay J. Zur kenntnis der Neurofibrome. Beitr Pathol Anat Allg Pathol 1910;48:1–69.

61. von Recklinghausen FD. Über die multiplen Fibromeder Haut und ihre Beziehung zuden multiplen neuromen. Berlin: A. Hirschwald, 1882.

62. Watabe K, Kumanishi T, Ikuta F, Oyake Y. Tactile-like corpuscles in neurofibromas: immunohistochemical demonstration of S-100 protein. Acta Neuropathol 1983;61:173–7.

63. Weiser G. An electron microscopic study of "pacinian neurofibroma." Virchows Arch [A] 1975;366:331–40.

64. Weiss SW, Nickoloff BJ. CD-34 is expressed by a distinctive cell population in peripheral nerve, nerve sheath tumors, and related lesions. Am J Surg Pathol 1993;17:1039–45.

65. Winkelmann RK, Johnson LA. Cholinesterases in neurofibromas. Arch Dermatol 1962;85:106–14.

66. Woodruff JM, Horten BC, Erlandson RA. Pathology of peripheral nerves and paragangliomas. In: Principles and practice of surgical pathology. New York: John Wiley, 1983:1503–20.

67. Zelger B, Weinlich G, Steiner H, Zelger BG, Egarter-Vigl E. Dermal and subcutaneous variants of plexiform fibrohistiocytic tumor. Am J Surg Pathol 1997;21:235–41.

9
MISCELLANEOUS BENIGN NEUROGENIC TUMORS

PERINEURIOMA

The cytogenesis and histologic, immunohistochemical, and ultrastructural features of perineurial cells are discussed in chapter 1. Alone or with other nerve sheath elements, perineurial or perineurial-like cells contribute to the formation of a variety of nerve sheath lesions (6). These include reactive processes such as traumatic, plantar, and palisaded encapsulated neuroma, as well as benign nerve sheath tumors, particularly neurofibroma. Rare malignant peripheral nerve sheath tumors (MPNST) may also show perineurial cell differentiation (9,10). The term perineurioma, however, is reserved for two forms of PNST consisting of well-differentiated perineurial cells. One presents as a soft tissue tumor and the other as an intraneural tumor with distinctive clinicopathologic features. Both tumors have an abnormality of chromosome 22 (5,8).

Perineurial cell growth cannot be identified with certainty on conventionally stained material. This is obviated by their specific ultrastructural appearance and characteristic immunohistochemical staining profile. Thus, proof of the perineurial cell constitution of a tumor necessitates the demonstration of perineurial cell features using one or both of these specialized techniques.

Intraneural Perineurioma

Definition. This is an intraneural neoplasm composed exclusively of perineurial cells.

General Comments. Given the superficial microscopic resemblance of intraneural perineuriomas to reactive or hereditary lesions composed of Schwann cells (Charcot-Marie-Tooth disease, Déjerine-Sotas disease), it was not until the application of electron microscopy and thereafter immunohistochemistry that intraneural perineurial proliferations were recognized. Their essential nature, whether reactive and resembling a perineurial response to injury (12,25) or neoplastic (3,24), has been contested. Those favoring a reactive interpretation consider the lesion to be an exaggerated perineurial reaction to injury, such as repeated trauma or ischemia, with resultant breakdown of the perineurial-endoneurial barrier. The resultant microfasciculation produced by such injuries has been well studied. Whether spontaneous or experimentally induced (2,14,23), the microfasciculation is limited in extent and differs in cytoarchitecture. Recent cytogenetic demonstration of a clonal abnormality of chromosome 22 in intraneural perineurioma, one similar to that observed in meningioma and soft tissue perineurioma (8), argues strongly in favor of the lesion being a neoplastic process (5).

Over 30 cases of intraneural perineurioma have been reported to date (5), most under the umbrella term "localized hypertrophic neuropathy," a designation we reserve for localized, nonhereditary Schwann cell proliferations characterized by onion bulb formation (see chapter 5).

Clinical Features. Patients with intraneural perineurioma typically present in adolescence or early adulthood, and males and females are equally affected. An antecedent history of trauma is exceptional (3,20,22). The most common symptom is muscle weakness which is progressive over months to 15 years (16). Sensory disturbances are less often noted. On physical examination, localized muscle atrophy may be apparent. Electromyography demonstrates denervation. Although the affected nerve is only occasionally palpable, magnetic resonance imaging (MRI) scans generally show segmental enlargement. Cranial nerve involvement is rare (16).

Gross Findings. Intraneural perineuriomas produce symmetric tubular enlargement of the affected nerve, increasing its diameter several fold (fig. 9-1). When the epineurium is stripped, individual nerve fascicles often appear coarse and pale (fig. 9-1B–D), and firm in texture. As a rule, intraneural perineuriomas are localized. Most measure 2 to 10 cm in length, although one exceptional lesion was greater than 30 cm (fig. 9-1D) (5). The "bag of worms" appearance so characteristic of plexiform neurofibroma is not seen. With the exception of one case in which two adjacent spinal nerve roots were involved (5), intraneural perineuriomas are solitary lesions.

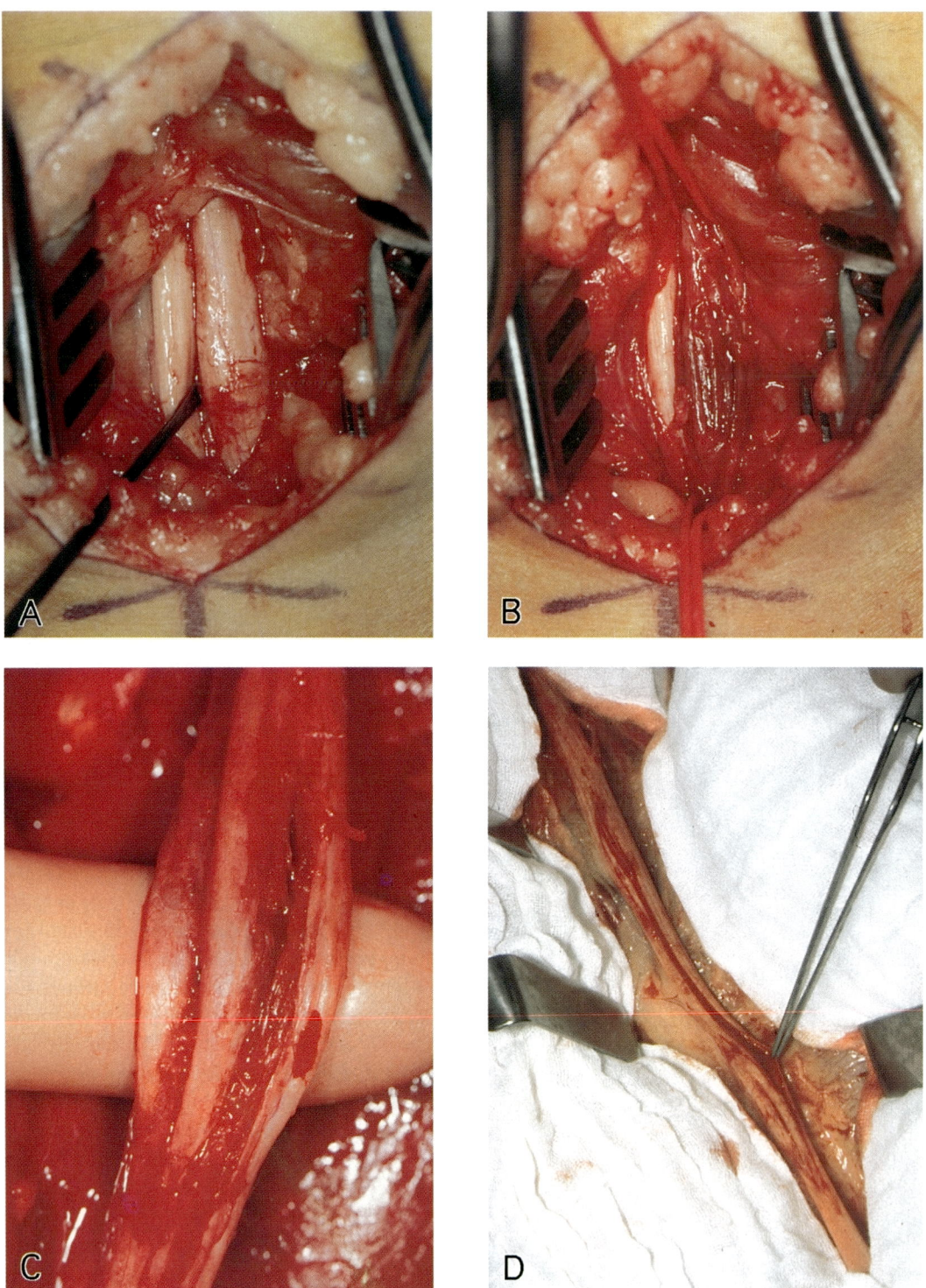

Figure 9-1
INTRANEURAL PERINEURIOMA

An operative photograph (A) of a peroneal nerve lesion shows the normal tibial nerve (left) beside the affected peroneal nerve (right) both before (A) and after (B) opening of the epineurium. Note the abnormal, somewhat nodular appearance of the enlarged fascicles. Fascicular thickening is even more apparent in a tibial example (C). One remarkably extensive tumor (D) involved the sciatic nerve from the level of the sciatic notch to the knee. The epineurium has been opened to demonstrate the enlarged fascicles.

Microscopic Findings. On cross section of an affected nerve, the recognition of intraneural perineurioma is based upon the finding of whorls of perineurial cells around nerve fibers (figs. 9-2–9-4). These circumferential arrangements have been termed "pseudo-onion bulbs," given their superficial resemblance to the better organized, Schwann cell–derived onion bulbs that typify hypertrophic neuropathies (see chapter 5). Whereas the telltale whorls of intraneural perineurioma are readily apparent on cross sections of the affected nerve, longitudinal sections show only ill-defined, parallel, rope-like bundles of perineurial cells surrounding nearly indiscernible nerve fibers (fig. 9-5). In most instances, well-oriented cross sections show most fascicles to be affected and to appear enlarged. On occasion, however, several fascicles in an otherwise heavily involved nerve may appear entirely spared (fig. 9-6A). Both the perineurium and perineurial septa of affected fascicles may be variably thickened by proliferating perineurial cells (fig. 9-6B,C). Although these cells may extend from the parent nerve perineurium into the endoneurium, they do not invade surrounding epineurial tissue.

Compared to normal nerve, perineuriomas are distinctly hypercellular. This is due entirely to the numerous overlapping perineurial cells disposed concentrically about axons (figs. 9-2–9-4). Despite their number, arrangement, and the occasional enlarged or hyperchromatic example (figs. 9-2B,C, 9-6C,D), most cells appear to be cytologically normal. Nuclei are elongate and chromatin is delicate (fig. 9-5A). Mitoses are absent or exceedingly rare (fig. 9-6D). Cell layers vary considerably in number but five or six laminae are often seen (fig. 9-2B,C). In optimal preparations or in plastic-embedded semi-thin sections, cells at the periphery of a whorl may occasionally sweep toward and contribute to the structure of an adjacent whorl (fig. 9-2B). Particularly large whorls may contain numerous nerve fibers (fig. 9-4B,C). Endoneurial capillaries may also be surrounded by whorls of perineurial cells (fig. 9-2D). In well-established or chronic lesions, stains for axons and myelin such as the Bielschowsky and Luxol-fast blue–periodic acid-Schiff (PAS) preparations, show them to be scant or absent despite the persistence of Schwann cells at the center of most whorls (fig. 9-4D). Collagen characterizes chronic lesions (fig. 9-7, right).

Immunohistochemical Findings. Similar to normal perineurial cells, the tumor cells forming pseudo-onion bulbs exhibit immunoreactivity for epithelial membrane antigen (EMA) (figs. 9-3A, 9-5B). The EMA staining pattern is membranous and widespread. Reactivity is limited to pseudo-onion bulbs, perineurial cells involving septa, and remaining normal perineurium. Lack of S-100 protein staining in the concentrically layered cells clearly distinguishes these lesions from a Schwann cell process. Residual axons and Schwann cells, whether myelinated or not, are immunoreactive for neurofilament protein and S-100 protein, respectively (fig. 9-3C,D).

One recent study reported significant nuclear immunoreactivity for proliferation markers, including proliferating cell nuclear antigen (PCNA) and MIB-1 (5); the MIB-1 labeling index ranged from 5 to 15 percent.

Immunoreactivity for p53 protein has been reported in a significant proportion of perineuriomas; its significance is uncertain (5).

Ultrastructural Findings. Unlike their solid, soft tissue counterparts, the essential architecture of intraneural perineuriomas consists of two components: one or more non-neoplastic, myelinated or unmyelinated axons and Schwann cells surrounded by multiple layers of neoplastic, but rather normal-appearing perineurial cells. The latter are separated by basement membrane substance and variable numbers of collagen fibrils (figs. 9-8, 9-9). The ultrastructural features of normal perineurium are described in chapter 2.

Differential Diagnosis. The differential diagnosis of intraneural perineurioma is limited because the uniform pseudo-onion bulbs noted on cross sections of affected nerve are mimicked only by the Schwann cell–derived, true onion bulbs occurring in *hypertrophic neuropathies.* Such disorders are either inherited and generalized (hereditary sensorimotor neuropathies) or are, on rare occasion, sporadic and focal (see chapter 5). The schwannian nature of these more discrete and uniform size onion bulbs is readily confirmed by S-100 protein immunostains which are positive; stains for EMA are negative.

Even infrequently occurring cylindrical *neurofibromas* involving a segment of nerve pose no problem in differential diagnosis. Their lesser cellularity and the way in which residual axons, unaccompanied by multilayer sheaths of encircling

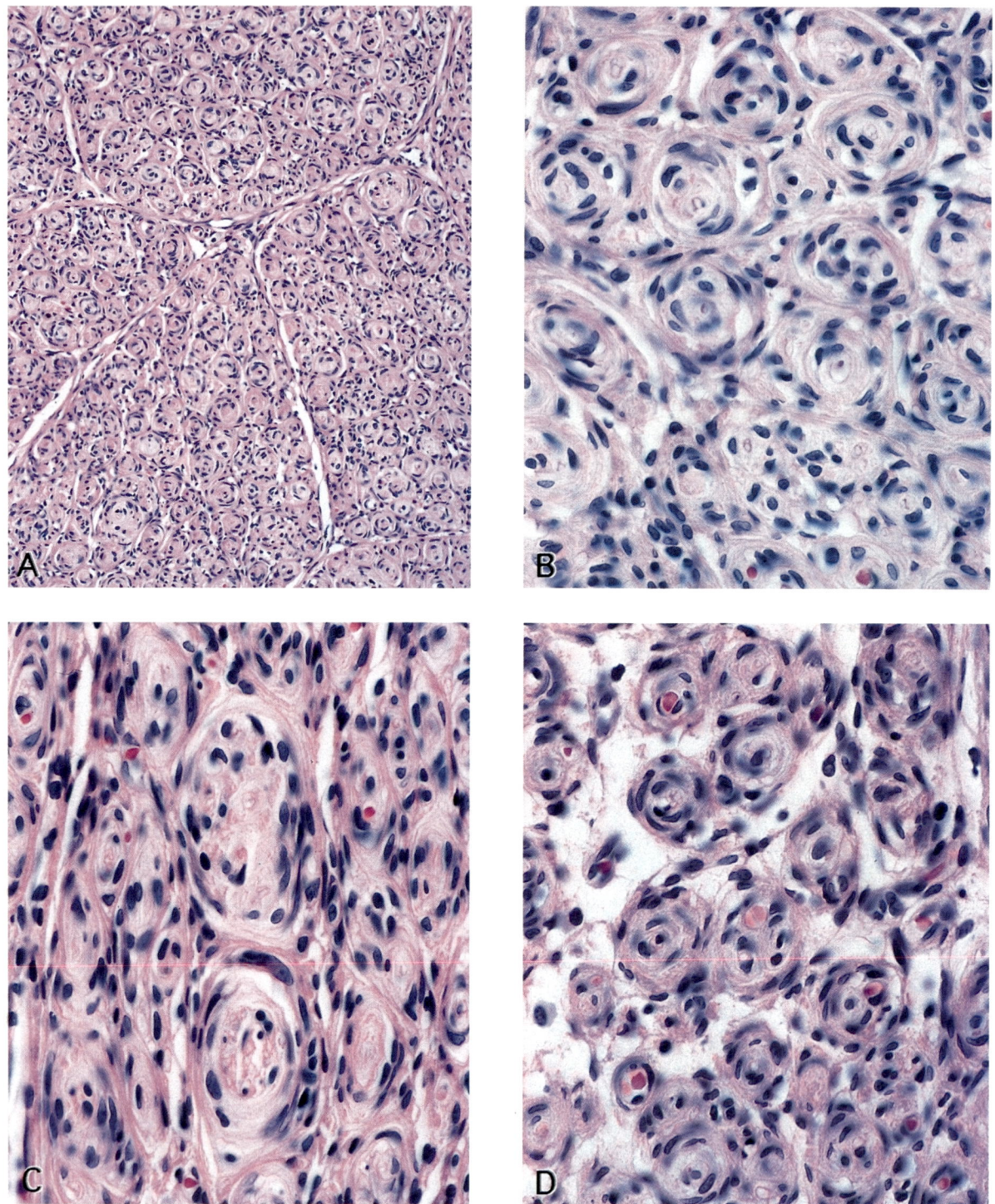

Figure 9-2

INTRANEURAL PERINEURIOMA

Making the correct diagnosis depends upon examination of cross sections of the nerve to demonstrate the hypercellular fascicles, approximately four of which appear in this field (A). At higher power, distinctive pseudo-onion bulbs (B) are seen to be composed of perineurial cells surrounding one or more nerve fibers and their accompanying Schwann sheaths. Note occasional "spinning off" of perineurial cells from one pseudo-onion bulb to another (C). Whorls may also form around endoneurial vessels (D).

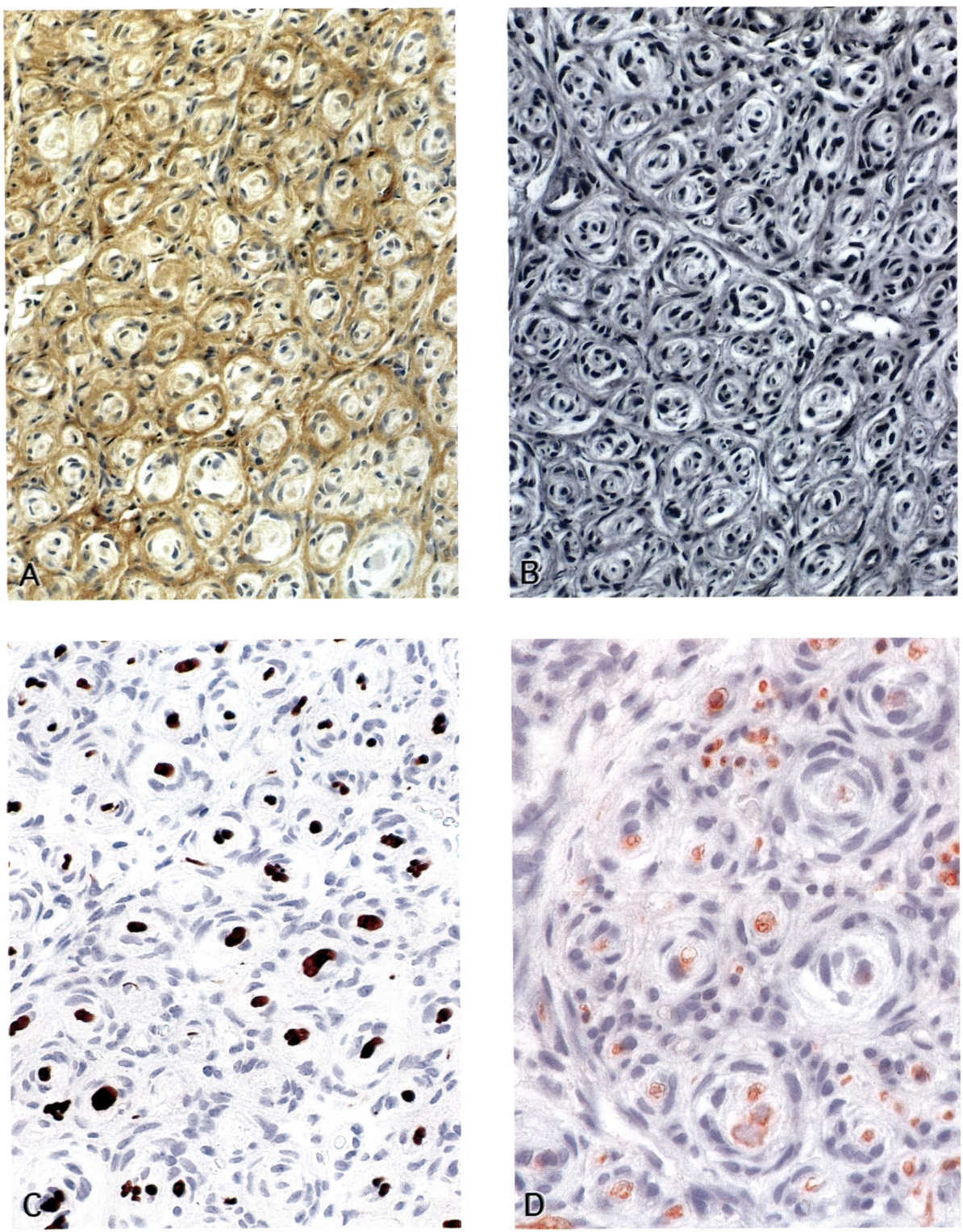

Figure 9-3
INTRANEURAL PERINEURIOMA
Pseudo-onion bulbs consist of multilayer wrappings of EMA-positive perineurial cells (A) around normal, Bielschowsky-positive (B), neurofilament-reactive axons (C) and their S-100 protein-positive Schwann sheaths (D).

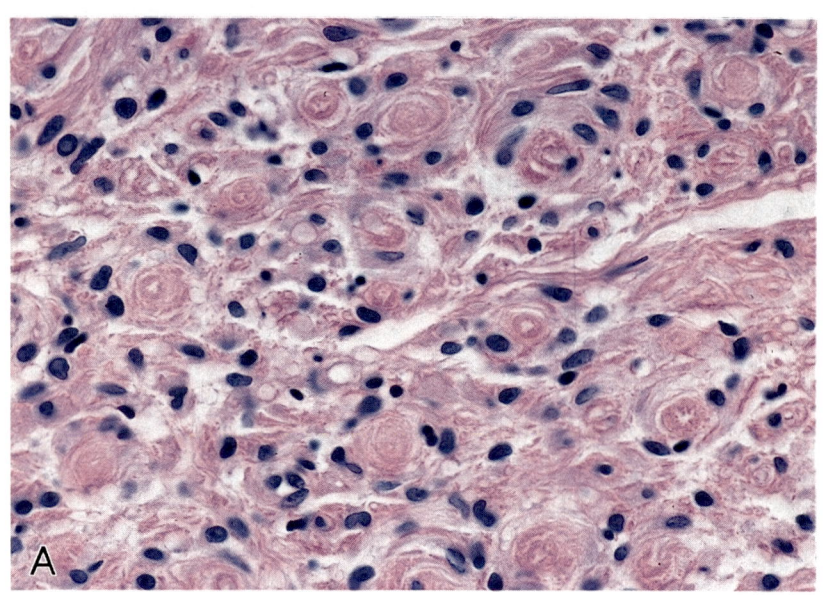

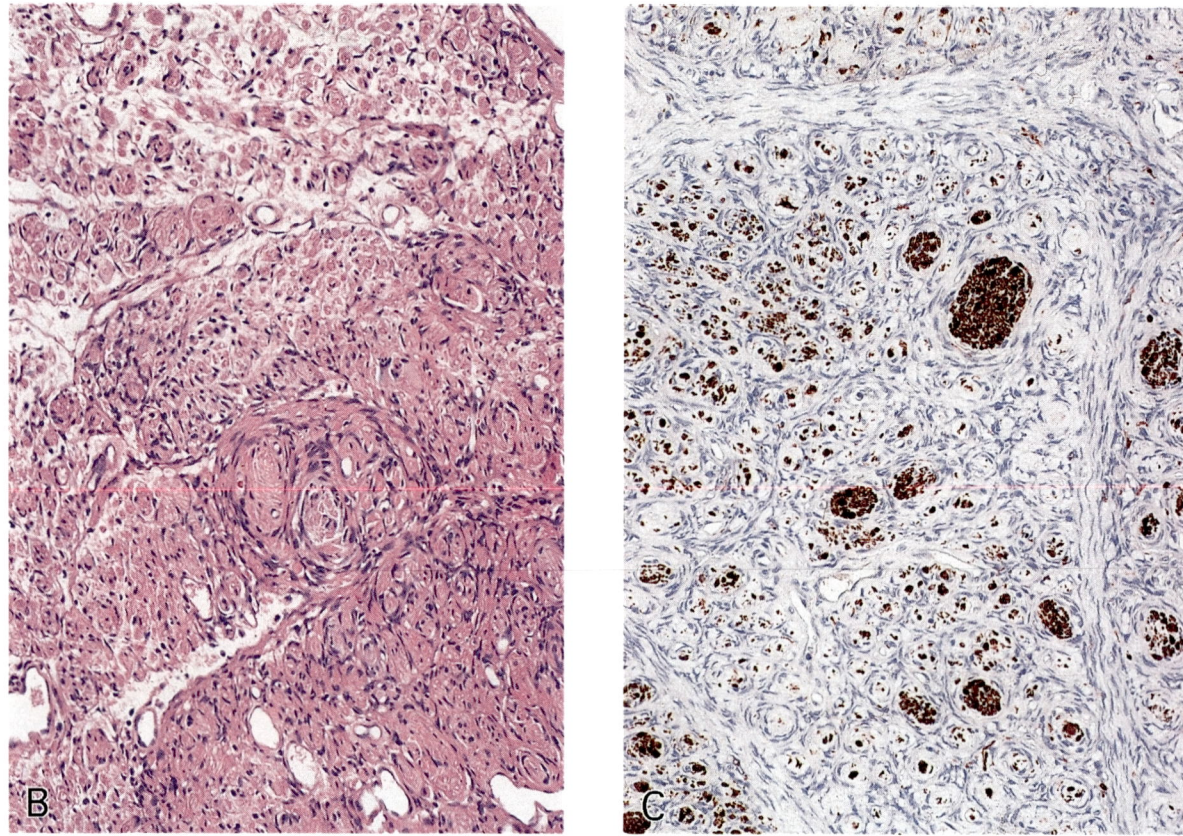

Figure 9-4
INTRANEURAL PERINEURIOMA

Microscopic variations include partial involvement of nerve fascicles. Some fibers are unaffected, others only show scant perineurial ensheathment (A). In some instances, large pseudo-onion bulbs are seen surrounding bundles of numerous nerve fibers (B), a finding best seen on neurofilament stain (C).

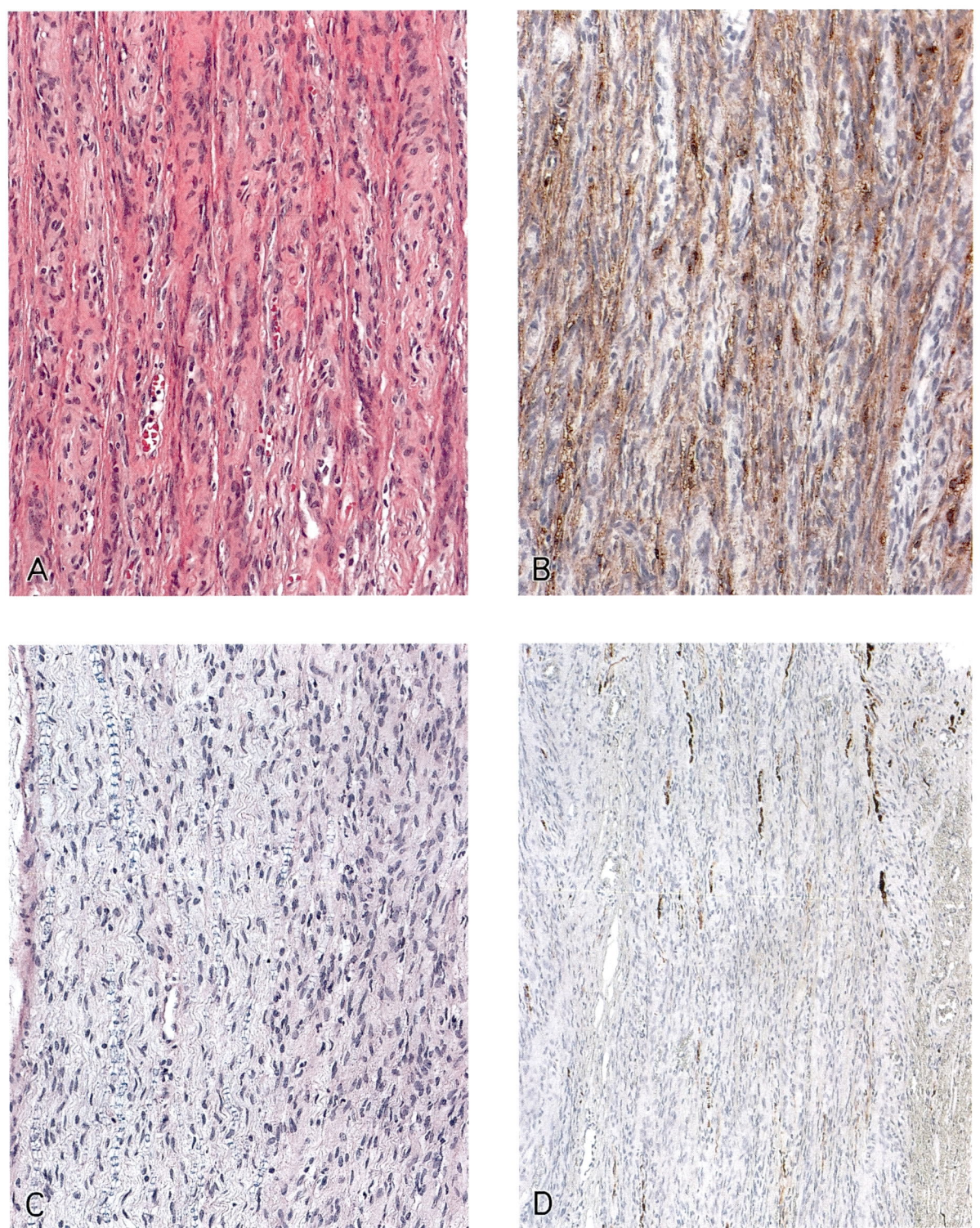

Figure 9-5
INTRANEURAL PERINEURIOMA

Although assessment of longitudinal sections makes the diagnosis more difficult, perineurial wrapping of fibers imparts a characteristic ropy appearance (A) which is accentuated on EMA stain (B). Luxol-fast blue–PAS preparation of a variably affected fascicle shows gradation of myelin loss (C). Axonal loss is well seen on neurofilament protein immunostains (D).

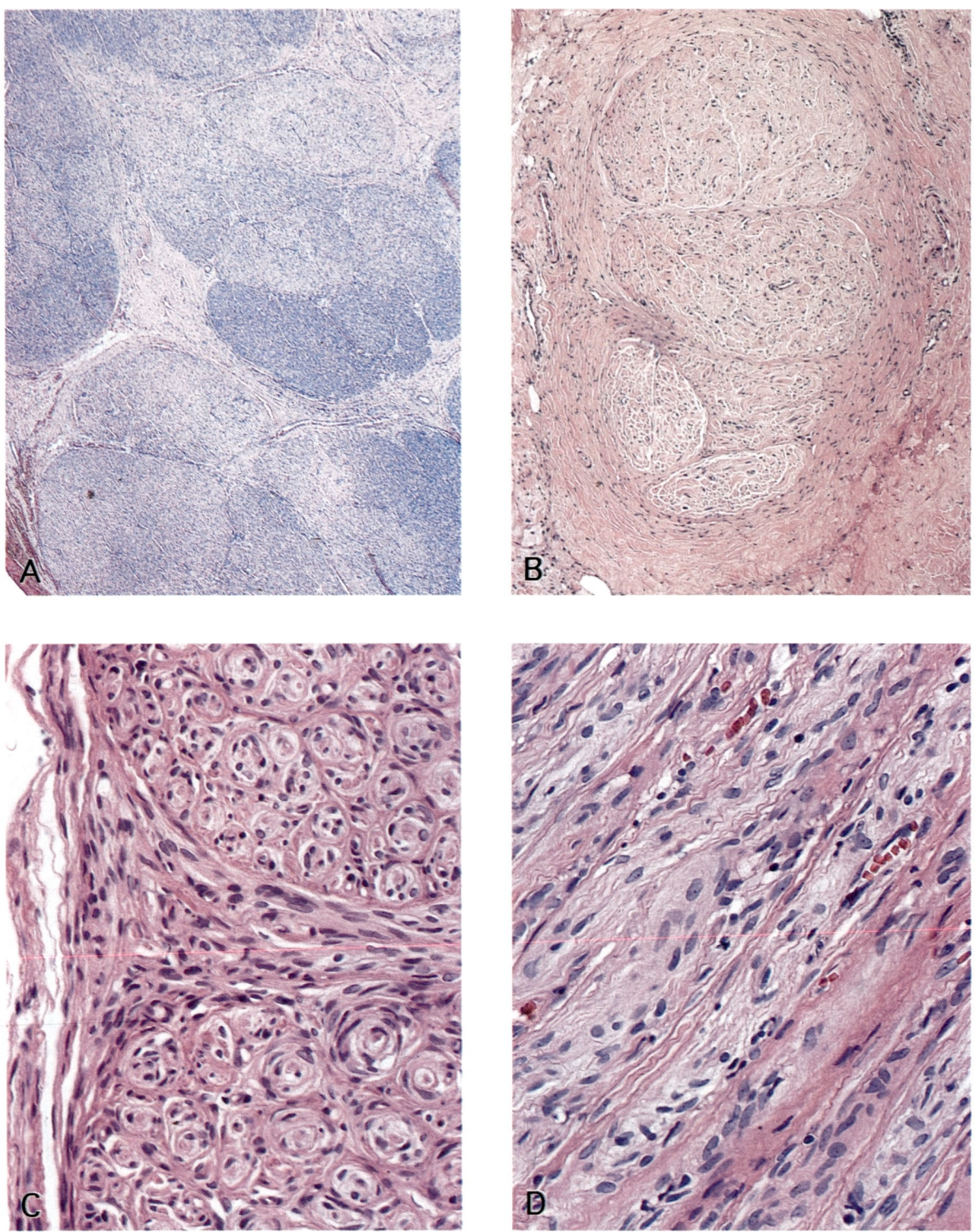

Figure 9-6
INTRANEURAL PERINEURIOMA
Although the gross appearance of such tumors does not suggest malignancy, some microscopic features may be misleading. These include marked variation in endoneurial cellularity (A), conspicuous involvement of the perineurium (B,C), and the occurrence of occasional mitoses, particularly when seen in longitudinal sections (D).

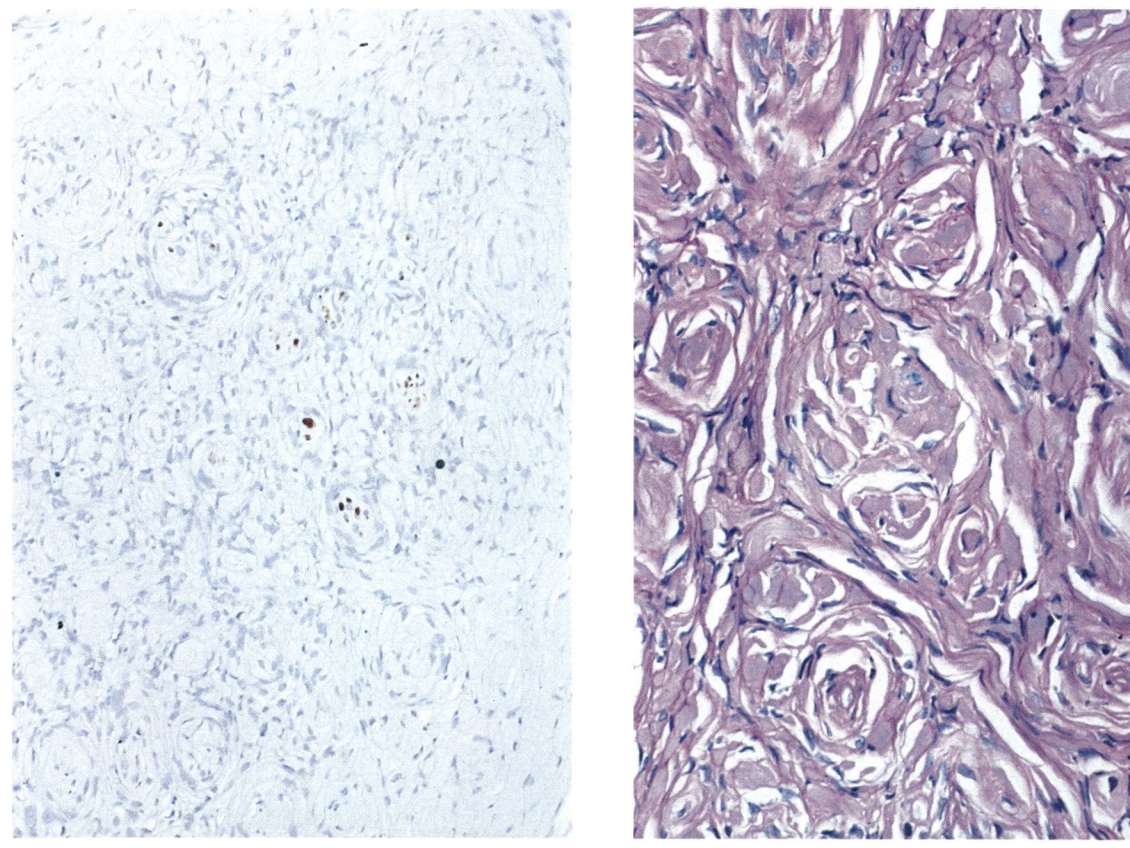

Figure 9-7
INTRANEURAL PERINEURIOMA
In longstanding cases, extensive collagen deposition is associated with near-total loss of nerve fibers and myelin, here illustrated on a neurofilament protein preparation (left) and a Luxol-fast blue–PAS stain for myelin (right). Note only rare blue myelin sheaths.

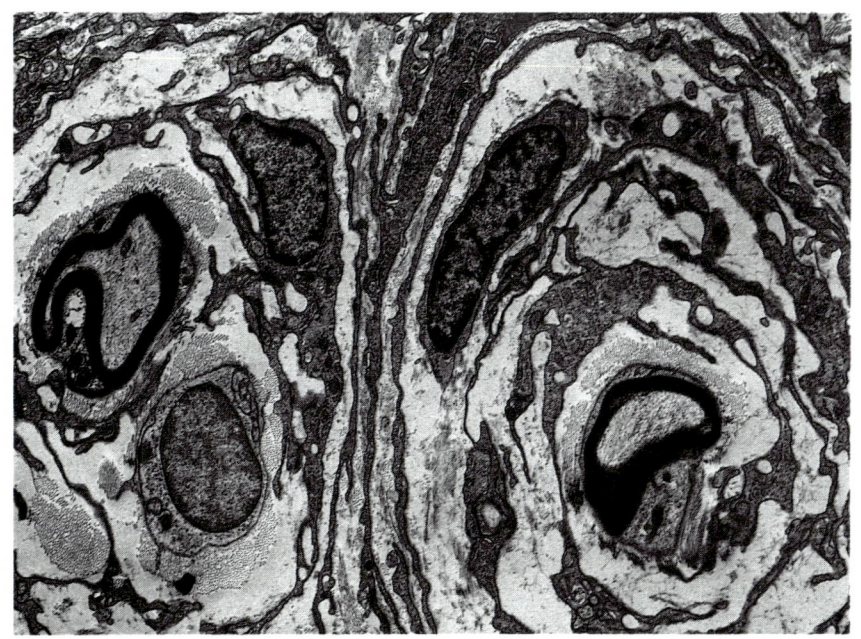

Figure 9-8
INTRANEURAL
PERINEURIOMA
Two myelinated nerve fibers are circumferentially surrounded by layers of perineurial cells (X7,500).

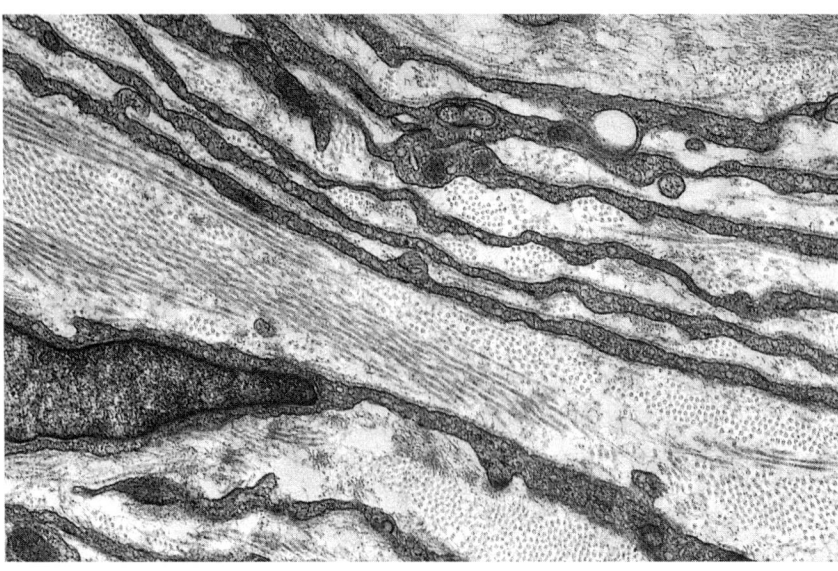

Figure 9-9
INTRANEURAL
PERINEURIOMA
Higher magnification of a
pseudo-onion bulb showing nine
thin perineurial cell cytoplasmic
processes and part of a nucleus.
Numerous pinocytotic vesicles,
surface basement membranes,
and abundant stromal collagen fibrils are evident (X18,500). (Figures 9-9, 9-12, 9-17, and 9-18 are
from the same patient.)

perineurial cells, appear to float in an Alcian
blue–positive mucopolysaccharide-rich stroma is
very different from perineurioma. Neurofibromas occasionally show onion bulb-like structures
superficially resembling those of perineurioma,
but the cells react for S-100 protein rather than for
EMA. In comparison, the neoplastic cells of intraneural perineuriomas encircle nerve fibers
and are EMA reactive, S-100 protein staining
being strictly limited to Schwann sheaths.

A particular concern is that intraneural perineurioma not be mistaken for *MPNST*. In view
of the uniform cylindrical shape, small diameter,
and generally limited extent to which intraneural
perineuriomas involve nerve, they are not likely to
be confused with MPNST. Nonetheless, the cellularity of intraneural perineurioma (fig. 9-6A), particularly when cut in longitudinal section (fig. 9-
5A), and the finding of the occasional mitotic figure
(fig. 9-6D) may cause concern. Careful inspection
of such longitudinal sections reveals a ropy appearance corresponding to the parallel sheaths of perineurial cells encircling axons. Should the differential arise at the time of frozen section, the simplest
solution is to examine a cross section of the lesion:
MPNSTs lack pseudo-onion bulb formation.
Lastly, the positive reaction of pseudo-onion bulbs
for EMA confirms the diagnosis of perineurioma.

Treatment and Prognosis. Long-term follow-up has confirmed the benign nature of intraneural perineurioma by showing there is neither a risk of recurrence nor of metastasis (5). Our
experience indicates that biopsy alone is sufficient for diagnosis. It is advised that fascicles
confirmed to be nonfunctional by direct nerve
stimulation be selected for biopsy. In our opinion,
even if only partially functional, affected nerves
should be preserved. Excision and nerve graft
reconstruction should only be considered in the
setting of a totally nonfunctional nerve with a
well-localized lesion. Even after reconstruction,
recovery of nerve function may not be obtained.

Resection, when undertaken, is curative. No
recurrences have been reported.

Soft Tissue Perineurioma

Definition. This is a soft tissue tumor consisting of differentiated perineurial cells.

General Comments. In recent years an extraneural soft tissue tumor composed of perineurial cells has been recognized (15). Since perineurial
cells are notoriously difficult to distinguish from
fibroblasts, it is no surprise that the tumor had
formerly been classified as "storiform perineural
fibroma" (21). With the application of electron microscopy and immunochemistry, the perineurial nature of this tumor has been confirmed.

Perineurial cells have characteristic ultrastructural features that provide a gold standard
for diagnosis. Indeed, the original description of
the tumor was based on such features (15). Immunohistochemical findings are less specific. Nevertheless, a tumor displaying histologic features

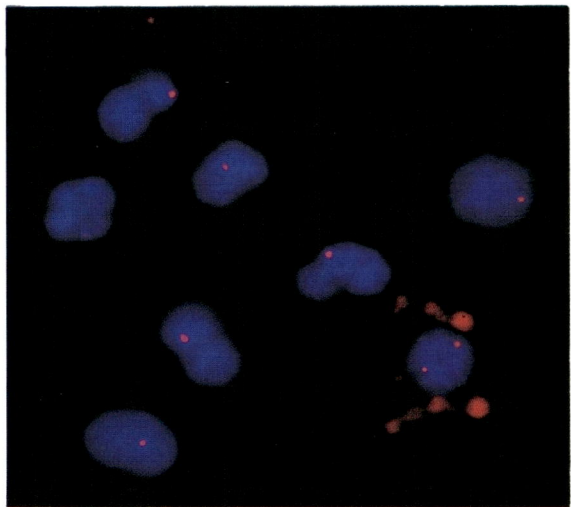

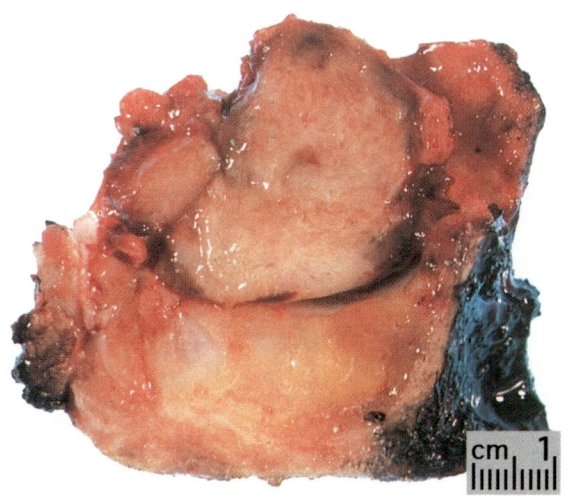

Figure 9-10
SOFT TISSUE PERINEURIOMA

The fluorescence in situ hybridization (FISH) preparation of isolated nuclei is shown. Of the seven nuclei, six show only one signal for M-bcr, a chromosome 22 marker, thus indicating monosomy.

resembling those described for ultrastructurally confirmed cases: diffuse immunoreactivity for EMA, varying degrees of collagen 4 or laminin staining, and absence of S-100 protein reactivity, is diagnosed as perineurioma. Using these criteria we have identified 19 well-documented examples of this tumor (1,4,8,11,13,15,17,25–27). Using fluorescence in situ hybridization (FISH) with a probe specific for the M-bcr locus which maps to chromosome band 22q11, we noted a high percentage of nuclei with at least partial deletion of chromosome 22 (fig. 9-10) (8).

Clinical Features. Soft tissue perineuriomas are generally found in subcutaneous sites and only infrequently affect deep soft tissues of the extremities or trunk. The hands are also a common site (2a,7), particularly in males. An origin in skin is uncommon (4b,17,22a). One example, originally considered a meningioma (14a), occurred in the mandible. Val-Bernal et al. (26a) recently reported a well-circumscribed soft tissue perineurioma located at the junction of the right renal capsule and kidney parenchyma of a 7-year-old girl. In addition, among two examples we recently studied, one involved the right nasal cavity and maxillary sinus of a 54-year-old woman (figs. 9-11, 9-12) (8). Lastly, one intracranial example arose in choroid plexus (7a). More tumors occur

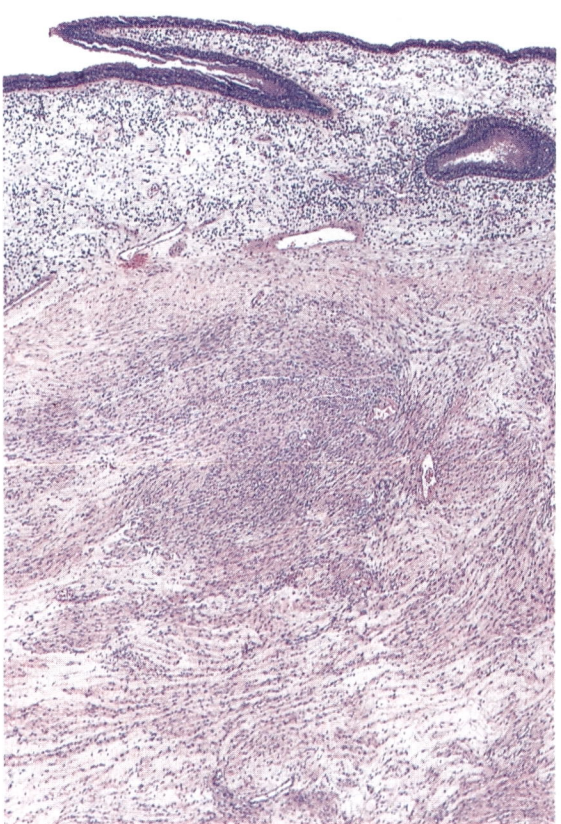

Figure 9-11
SOFT TISSUE PERINEURIOMA

This globular, gray-tan, 6-cm tumor (top) arose in the maxillary sinus of a 61-year-old woman and is seen as a demarcated lesion beneath the respiratory mucosa (bottom). For clinical details, see reference 8.

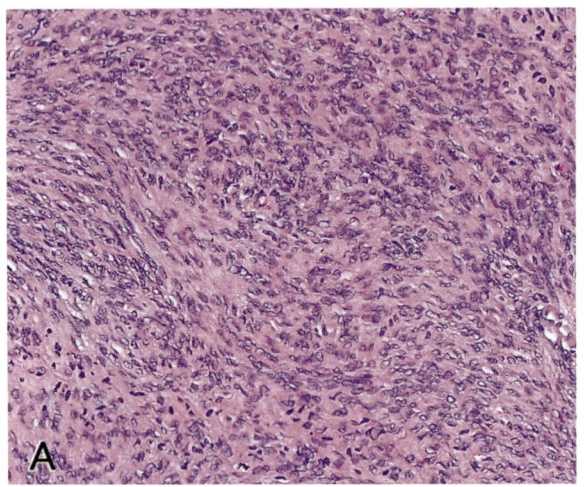
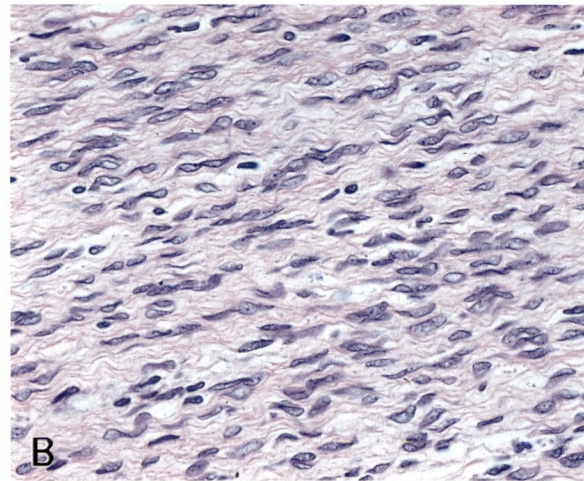
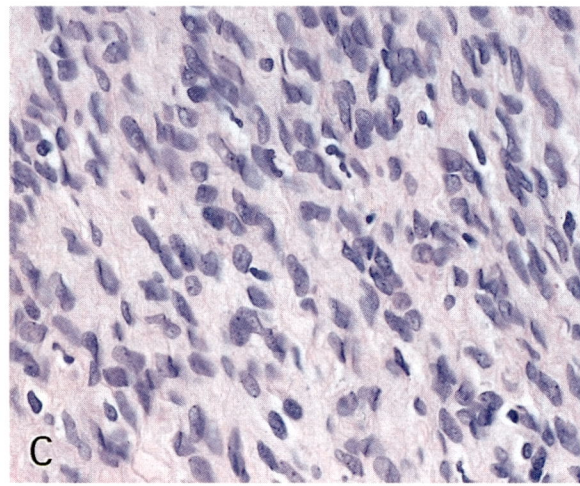

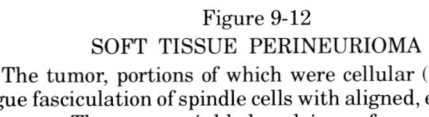

Figure 9-12
SOFT TISSUE PERINEURIOMA
The tumor, portions of which were cellular (A), features vague fasciculation of spindle cells with aligned, elongate cell processes. The wavy, wrinkled nuclei vary from narrow (B) to plumper than those of most schwannomas (C).

in women than in men, in a ratio of 4 to 1. Although both adolescents and the elderly may be affected, most patients with soft tissue perineuriomas are middle aged. No examples have been reported in association with neurofibromatosis type 1 (NF1).

Gross Findings. At surgery, soft tissue perineuriomas are generally unassociated with an identifiable nerve (figs. 9-11, 9-14). One exception is an example occurring in association with a mandibular nerve (14a). Although initially considered a meningioma, retrospective study confirmed its perineurial nature. Discrete but unencapsulated, they are nodular or ovoid, range in size from 1.5 to 20 cm, and are white-tan, rubbery to firm, or gritty. Perineuriomas do not exhibit the "bag of worms" appearance so characteristic of plexiform neurofibroma. One very large example showed similar degenerative changes to so-called ancient

schwannoma, including necrosis, cyst formation, collagenization, and histiocytic infiltrates (1). Osseous metaplasia is rare (20).

Microscopic Findings. Histologically, the soft tissue perineurioma is a well-circumscribed tumor encased by a thin or only moderately thick fibrous capsule and unassociated with a nerve. The histologic pattern is variable, ranging from alignment of tumor cells in elongate bundles, to interweaving fascicles, loose whorls, and vague storiform arrangements (figs. 9-12, 9-13). A typical "cracking" artifact is commonly see (fig. 9-13C). A distinctive feature of the collagenous zones of some tumors is dissection of collagen by tumor cells with resultant encirclement of collagen bundles and nodules (figs. 9-13, 9-19). In most cases, the stroma is collagen rich. Although sclerosis is a dominant feature in lesions arising in the hands (fig. 9-14) (7), we have

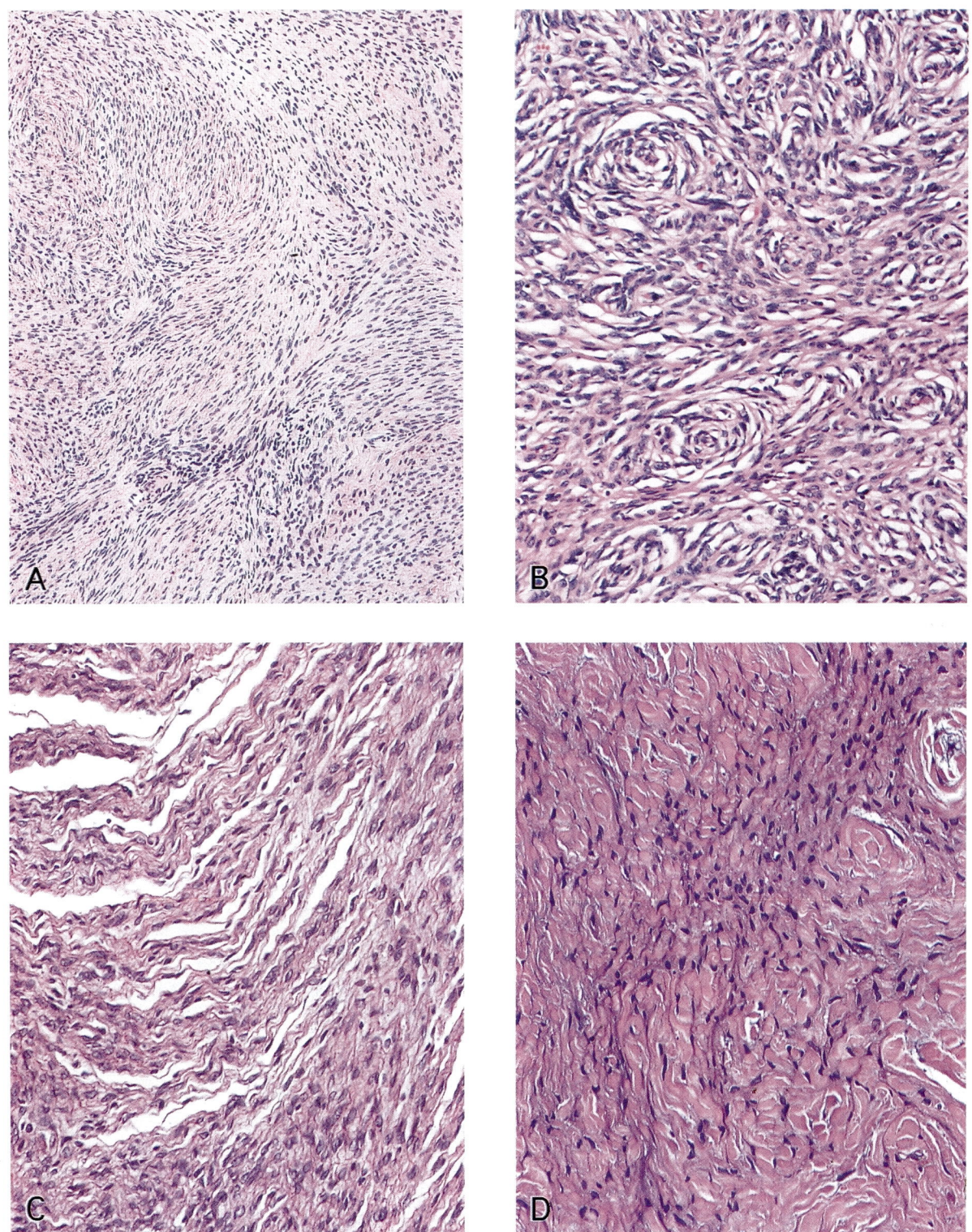

Figure 9-13
SOFT TISSUE PERINEURIOMA
Pattern variations include sinuous bundles (A), whorls (B), a commonly seen cracking artifact (C), and dissection of collagen into bundles and nodules (D).

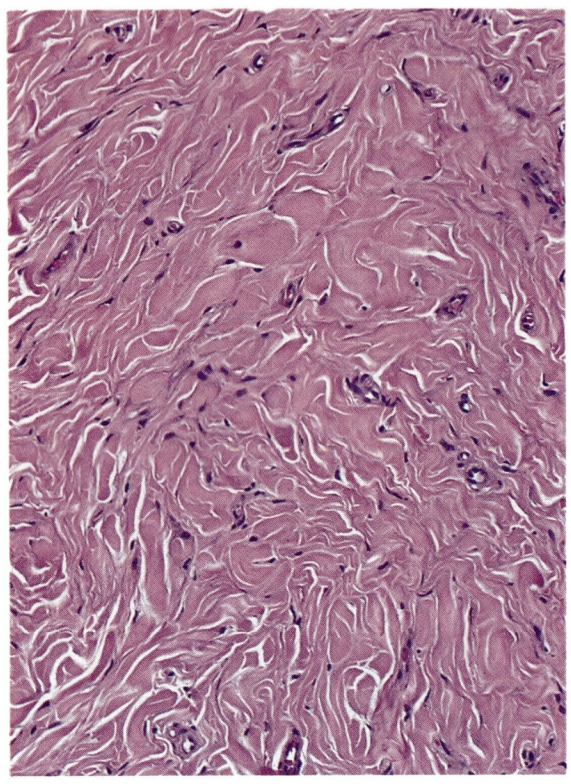 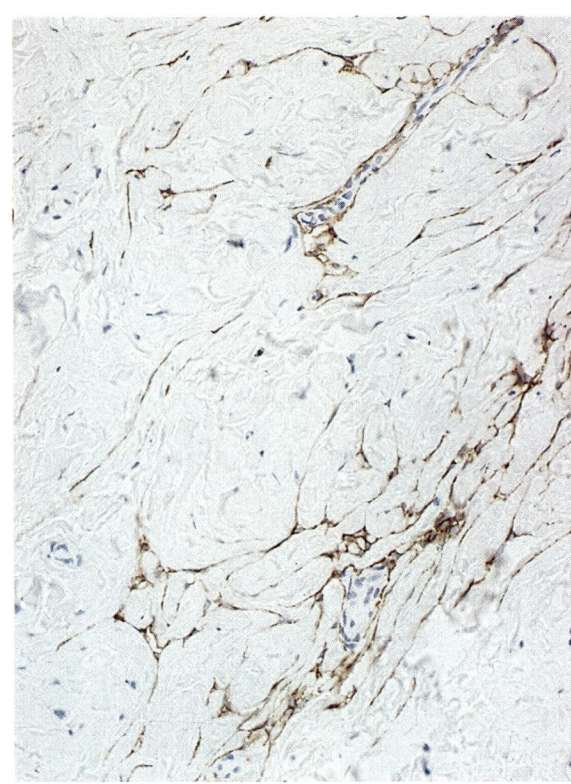

Figure 9-14
SCLEROSING SOFT TISSUE PERINEURIOMA
Left: Advanced sclerosis is often seen in tumors of the hand.
Right: Staining for EMA confirms the diagnosis. (Courtesy of Dr. J. Fetch, Washington, D.C.)

seen it in longstanding perineuriomas occurring at other sites (8a). Myxoid changes are infrequent and have been seen in only three tumors: the intercellular matrix in two cases was slightly myxoid, while in one case there was a loose reticular arrangement of tumor cells due to the presence of abundant myxoid material (26).

The cells of soft tissue perineurioma possess elongated to often disc-shaped nuclei as evident by their appearing variously thin or coin-shaped in different planes of section, as well as long, very thin, eosinophilic processes. Both the nuclei and cell processes may be curved or wavy in configuration. In most cases, the overall appearance is that of a fibroma-like lesion with curved or wrinkled cells. Although mild nuclear hyperchromasia may be noted, pleomorphism or degenerative change of the sort seen in ancient schwannoma and atypical neurofibroma is rarely encountered (1); we have seen only an occasional example, usually a large tumor of long standing (fig. 9-15)

(8a). Mitoses are absent or very infrequent. Blood vessels, although inconspicuous, are often numerous. Psammoma body formation is very uncommon (25). Necrosis is lacking. Special stains such as silver impregnations for axons are negative, as are myelin stains.

Immunohistochemical Findings. By definition, in order to be classified as a perineurioma, a tumor should exhibit membranous immunoreactivity for EMA (figs. 9-14–9-16). Since tumor cell processes are often thin and widely separated, prolonged incubation or a higher antibody titer than is used to label carcinomas may be required to obtain a positive reaction. Lack of S-100 protein staining further distinguishes perineuriomas from Schwann cell neoplasms. Immunoreactivity for laminin and collagen type 4 is also seen and is attributed to the presence of pericellular basement membrane, albeit incomplete (see below). CD34 staining is evident in a minority of cases. Pertinent negative reactions include desmoplakin, desmin, and

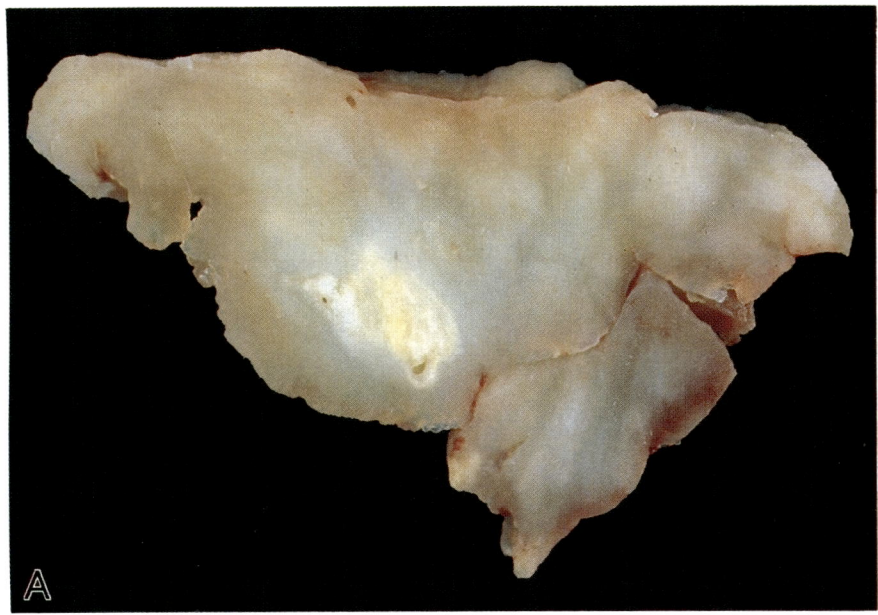

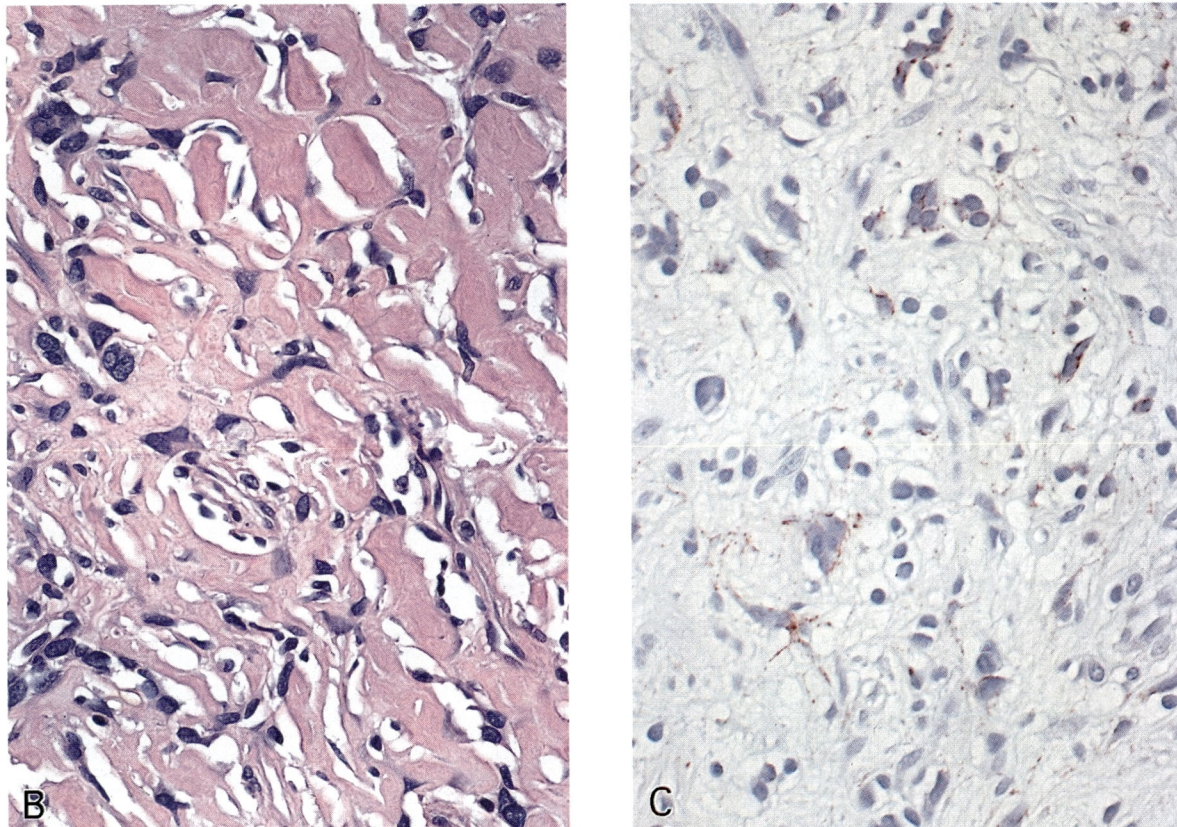

Figure 9-15

SOFT TISSUE PERINEURIOMA

Degenerative changes analogous to those of schwannoma and neurofibroma are rarely seen. These include dystrophic calcification (A), and dense collagenization as well as nuclear abnormalities (B). Note EMA immunoreactivity (C). (From Hirose T, Scheithauer BW. Sclerosing perineurioma: a distinct entity? Int J Surg Pathol (in press).

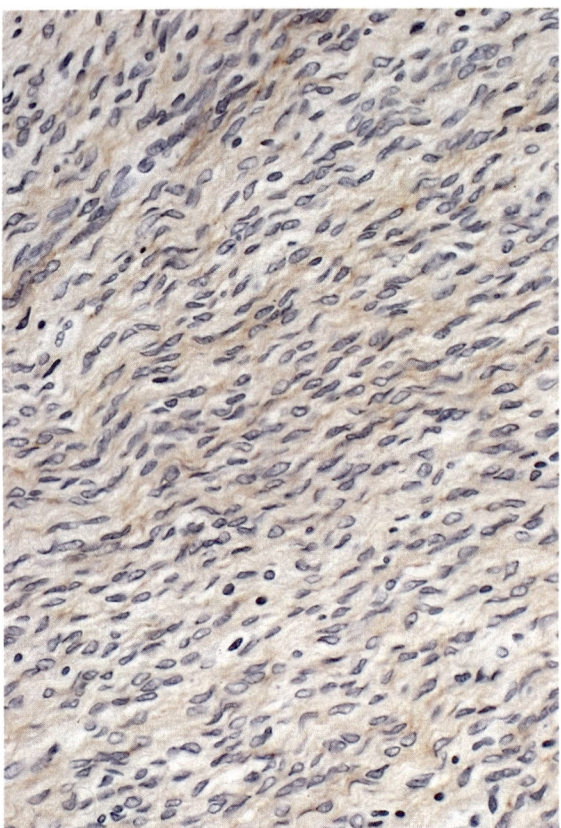 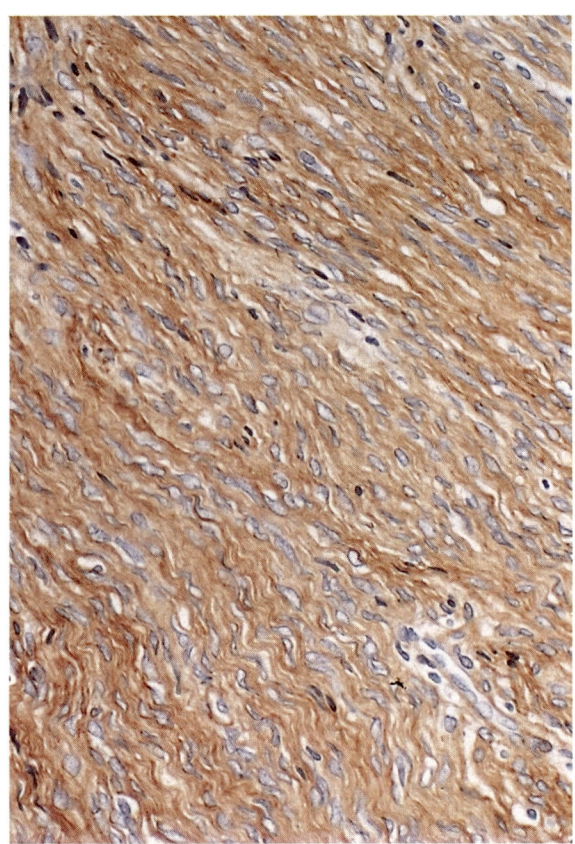

Figure 9-16
SOFT TISSUE PERINEURIOMA

Left: Reactivity for EMA is requisite to the diagnosis.
Right: Diffuse laminin immunostaining is attributed to the presence of pericellular basement membranes.

smooth muscle actin. As in virtually all soft tissue neoplasms, vimentin stains uniformly.

Ultrastructural Findings. Given the variation in the sensitivity of EMA immunoreactivity among various laboratories, electron microscopy continues to play an important role in the diagnosis of soft tissue perineurioma. Such tumors are composed of normal-appearing perineurial cells that are usually loosely organized in a collagenous or myxocollagenous stroma (fig. 9-16). Seen in cross section, stromal collagen fibrils may appear as circular aggregates surrounded by perineurial cell processes (fig. 9-17). Diagnostic attributes of neoplastic perineurial cells include an elongate nucleus with variably clumped, marginated chromatin, an inconspicuous nucleolus, long thin cytoplasmic processes, cytoplasm containing few organelles and scant filaments, prominent pinocytotic vesicles distributed along the cell membrane and occasionally in the cytoplasm, an often discon-

tinuous basement membrane thinner than that lining normal perineurial cells, and scattered rudimentary intercellular junctions (figs. 9-16, 9-18) (4,6,8,13,15,19,24,25,27). Dissection and encirclement of collagen bundles is also a common feature (fig. 9-19). Ribosome-lamella complexes were a prominent feature of one tumor (4a).

Differential Diagnosis. The differential diagnosis of extraneural perineurioma includes a number of benign and low-grade malignant spindle cell tumors with a collagenous or myxocollagenous stroma. Immunohistochemistry is instrumental in excluding most lesions. Neurofibroma (S-100 protein positive), extracranial meningioma (S-100 protein or keratin positive, lacking basement membranes as well as pinocytotic vesicles), *dermatofibrosarcoma protuberans* and extrapleural *solitary fibrous tumor,* which are not confined to the pleura (both CD34 positive), and *myoepithelioma* (cytokeratin and actin positive),

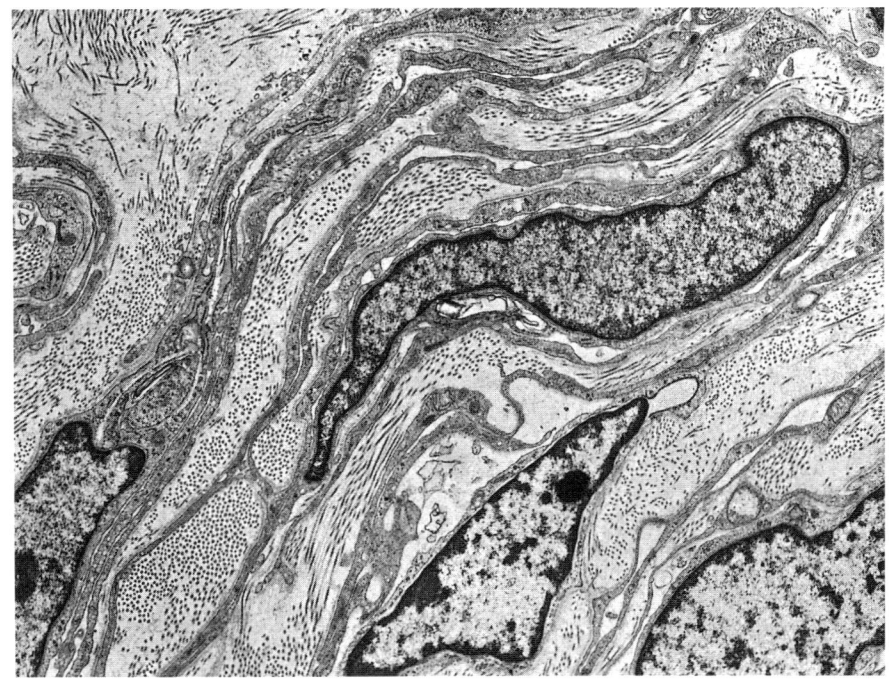

Figure 9-17
SOFT TISSUE
PERINEURIOMA
OF THE
MAXILLARY SINUS
The spindle-shaped tumor cells closely resemble normal perineurial cells in a collagenous stroma. Note the long thin processes (X10,600).

Figure 9-18
SOFT TISSUE
PERINEURIOMA: DETAIL
OF PERINEURIAL
CELL PROCESSES
Note the pinocytotic vesicles (arrow), remnants of basement membrane (arrowhead), and cross-sectioned collagen fibrils (asterisk). A portion of a nucleus is also seen (X48,300).

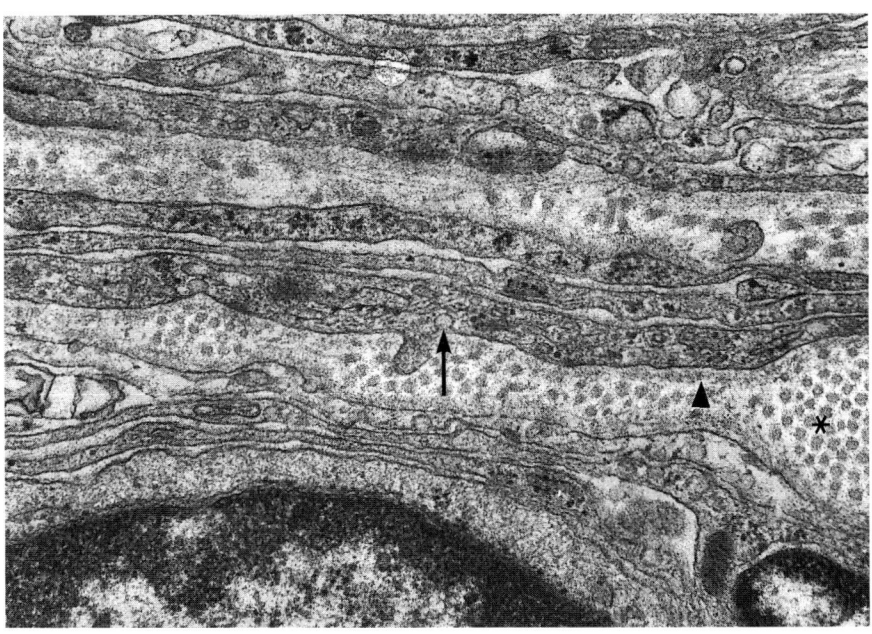

when occurring in such myoepithelium-containing organs as the breast, may all be confused with soft tissue perineurioma. Also in the differential are circumscribed soft tissue *fibroma, low-grade fibrosarcoma,* and *fibromyxoid sarcoma* (8). As mentioned, the definitive ways to confirm a diagnosis of perineurioma are electron microscopy, "the gold standard," and immunostaining for EMA and collagen 4 or laminin.

Treatment and Prognosis. The best treatment of soft tissue perineurioma is complete excision. The prognosis is excellent. To date, no cases have recurred or metastasized following complete resection. Even in instances in which

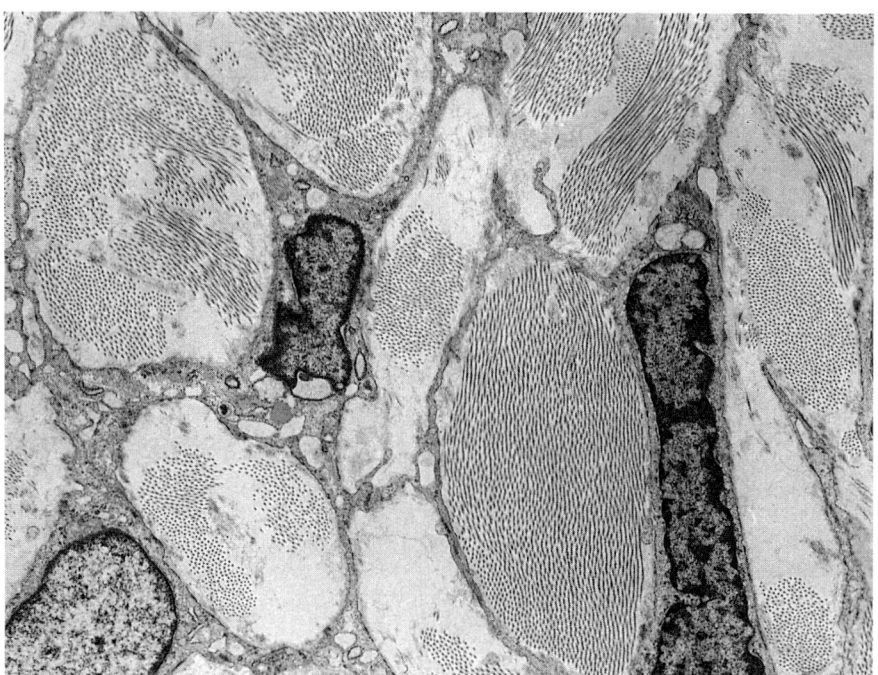

Figure 9-19
SOFT TISSUE
PERINEURIOMA
Encirclement of collagen bundles by the long processes of perineurial cells is a common feature of this tumor (X7,500).

total excision may be difficult, as in the nasal cavity-maxillary sinus example referred to above (8), we advocate careful observation rather than aggressive adjuvant therapy.

NERVE SHEATH MYXOMA
AND NEUROTHEKEOMA

Definition. Nerve sheath myxoma is a usually cutaneous, multilobulated, predominantly myxoid, spindle cell neoplasm exhibiting Schwann cell differentiation. Neurothekeoma is a cutaneous, multilobulated, variably myxoid and moderately to hypercellular neoplasm composed of clustered, spindled, and epithelioid cells lacking either Schwann or perineurial cell differentiation.

In the literature, nerve sheath myxoma has also been referred to as *cutaneous lobular neuromyxoma, perineurial myxoma,* and *pacinian neurofibroma.*

General Comments. Nerve sheath myxoma was originally illustrated by Harkin and Reed in their 1969 Fascicle (39) and was subsequently discussed in greater detail by Reed in 1985 (49). It has become nosologically linked with neurothekeoma, a cutaneous neoplasm described by Gallagher and Helwig in 1980 (37) and regarded by them as being of nerve sheath origin. The

reasons the two became linked were their common location in the skin; their nodular, lobular, or nested growth pattern; an entire or partial composition of spindle cells; and variable content of stromal mucin. Furthermore, both lesions occasionally show features suggesting an origin from cutaneous nerves. The conclusion that a link existed between these two tumors was flawed, in that it was based upon only two large published series (37,49), one consisting solely or mainly of neurothekeomas (37) and the other of a mix of both tumors (49). Until recently, therefore, the prevailing view was that nerve sheath myxoma and neurothekeoma were predominantly myxoid and cellular variants of the same tumor. However, recent ultrastructural and immunohistochemical studies have led to a contrary interpretation (30). Based upon the finding of S-100 protein immunoreactivity (28,48,56) as well as of ultrastructural features of Schwann cell differentiation (28,29,34,48,54), we consider the nerve sheath myxoma to be a form of Schwann cell tumor. To date, no similar features have been reported in neurothekeomas which, as a rule, do not stain for S-100 protein (32,33,35,41) and exhibit ultrastructural features resembling either those of fibroblasts (32) or of undifferentiated polygonal cells (29). It has also been suggested that some cellular neurothekeomas show evidence of smooth muscle differentiation (35). In our opinion, immunohistochemistry, particularly staining for S-100 protein, and electron microscopy, play a role in the evaluation of that minority of lesions not readily classified by routine histochemical methods.

Clinical Features. The *nerve sheath myxoma* typically occurs in adults during the third through the fifth decades and preferentially affects females at a ratio of 2 to 1. Although widely distributed, its site of predilection is the skin of the hands (28,34,40,54), less frequently that of the back (28,38), arm (36), and face or neck (36, 38). Similar lesions have also occurred in the intraspinal space (48) and oral mucosa (44,47,51, 53,55,56). Typical examples present as mobile, flesh-colored to translucent nodules undergoing slow, painless growth. No association with neurofibromatosis has been reported.

The *neurothekeoma* is also a cutaneous tumor. It occurs primarily in children and young adults, the mean patient age being 22 years in one large series (37). The cellular variant (see below) shows no sex predilection. The female to male ratio is approximately 2 to 1. Most neurothekeomas involve skin of the face, arms, and shoulders. Facial lesions often arise in the nasomalar, nasolabial, and lower forehead regions. The thumb and lower extremities are uncommon, albeit reported sites (37). We have observed two examples arising in skin and subcutaneous tissue of the breast.

Gross Findings. In general, the clinical appearance of neurothekeoma is indistinguishable from that of nerve sheath myxoma. Both are solitary, circumscribed, firm, sometimes multilobular, and variably myxoid lesions. Both tumors range in size from 0.5 to 3.0 cm. Aside from one nerve sheath myxoma found to extend into the neurovascular bundle of a digit (34), neither tumor shows a gross association with nerve. One purported example appears to represent a myxoid schwannoma (45). On sectioning, nerve sheath myxomas are characteristically gray-white, whereas neurothekeomas tend to be gray-tan, a difference related to the greater content of mucin in myxomas. Ulceration of the overlying epidermis is rare and hyperpigmentation is lacking.

Microscopic Findings. Typically, both nerve sheath myxoma and neurothekeoma are multinodular tumors with a variably myxoid stroma. They are nonencapsulated, infiltrate collagen bundles of the dermis, and extend with a pushing margin into subcutaneous tissue (figs. 9-20, 9-21). Round to ovoid and of varying size, the constituent lobules are demarcated by usually thin collagen bands containing delicate blood vessels (figs. 9-20– 9-23). Lobule configuration is most variable in neurothekeoma (fig. 9-24). Secondary involvement of a small cutaneous nerve is rarely seen.

The lobules of *nerve sheath myxoma* contain stellate, spindle, and occasional epithelioid cells disposed in a loose network within an abundant myxoid matrix (figs. 9-20, 9-25). Cellularity may vary. The cells often possess lightly eosinophilic, thin cytoplasmic processes that extend in bipolar or multipolar fashion from small round or ovoid nuclei (fig. 9-25). The overall appearance is that of compartmentalized bags of mucin filled with thin "stringy" cells. Nuclei contain faintly granular chromatin and frequently exhibit several vacuoles. The cytoplasm can be vacuolated as well. Occasional multinucleate giant cells may also be seen. Mitotic figures are rare (fig. 9-25) (28,38,40). Supporting the view that such tumors are possibly myxoid variants of schwannoma is the occasional finding of an example with focal Verocay bodies. Histochemically, the mucin within this tumor is strongly Alcian blue reactive (fig. 9-20D) and consists of hyaluronic acid and perhaps chondroitin sulfates 4 and 6 (28,34).

Unlike nerve sheath myxoma, *neurothekeoma* is a moderately to markedly cellular lesion with less of a myxoid matrix than is seen in nerve sheath myxoma (figs. 9-21, 9-22). Constituent cells are both spindle and, to a varying extent, epithelioid in shape (fig. 9-23). The plump epithelioid cells possess abundant eosinophilic cytoplasm. Multinucleate cells are commonly seen (fig. 9-27). At low magnification, cell processes are inconspicuous. The cells of neurothekeoma often are closely aggregated and in some cases form whorls (fig. 9-23). Myxoid matrix, when present, often varies in quantity from lobule to lobule (37,49). Only on occasion does myxoid change focally approach that seen in nerve sheath myxoma (fig. 9-24C). The same is true of lobule cellularity (figs. 9-23, 9-27). Hyperchromatic nuclei are frequent, and mitotic counts as high as 10 per 10 high-power fields have been reported (fig. 9-27) (49). As in nerve sheath myxoma, the Alcian blue–positive mucin within neurothekeoma is hyaluronic acid rich (fig. 9-22, right). Necrosis is lacking (fig. 9-22, right).

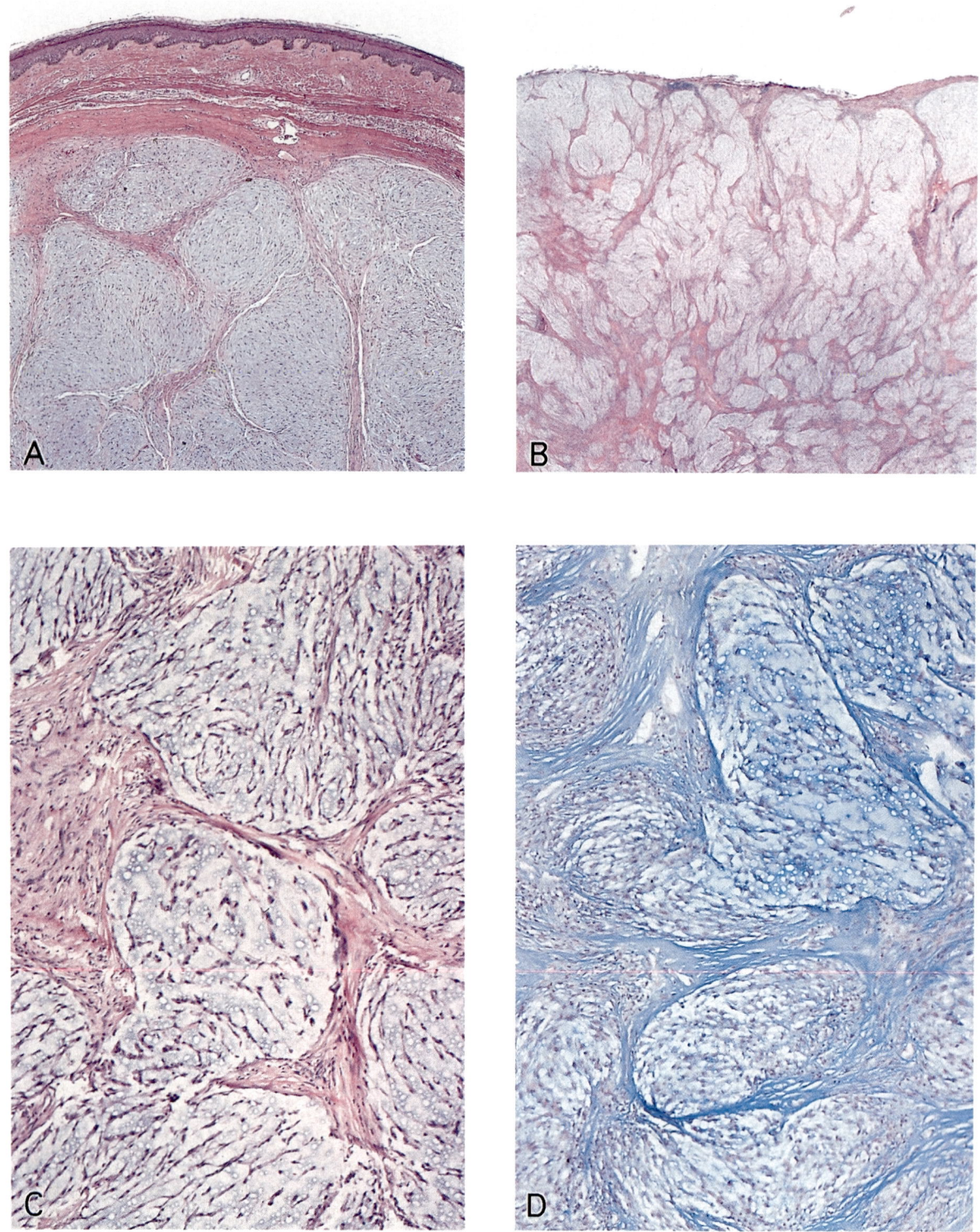

Figure 9-20
NERVE SHEATH MYXOMA

These micrographs of two different tumors show compressive demarcation relative to surrounding tissue (A) and varying degrees of interstitial collagen as well as scant hemosiderin deposition (B). Note their distinct lobularity, septation, and high mucin content (C). The latter is highlighted on Alcian blue stain (D).

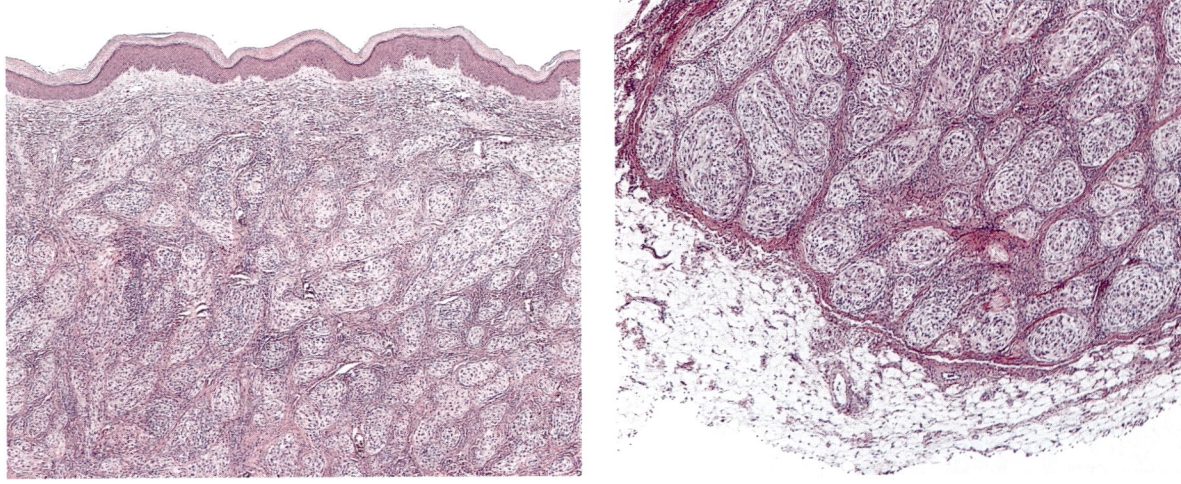

Figure 9-21
NEUROTHEKEOMA
This discrete lesion occupies the dermis, exhibits a narrow grenz zone relative to overlying epidermis (left), and is demarcated relative to underlying subcutaneous adipose tissue (right).

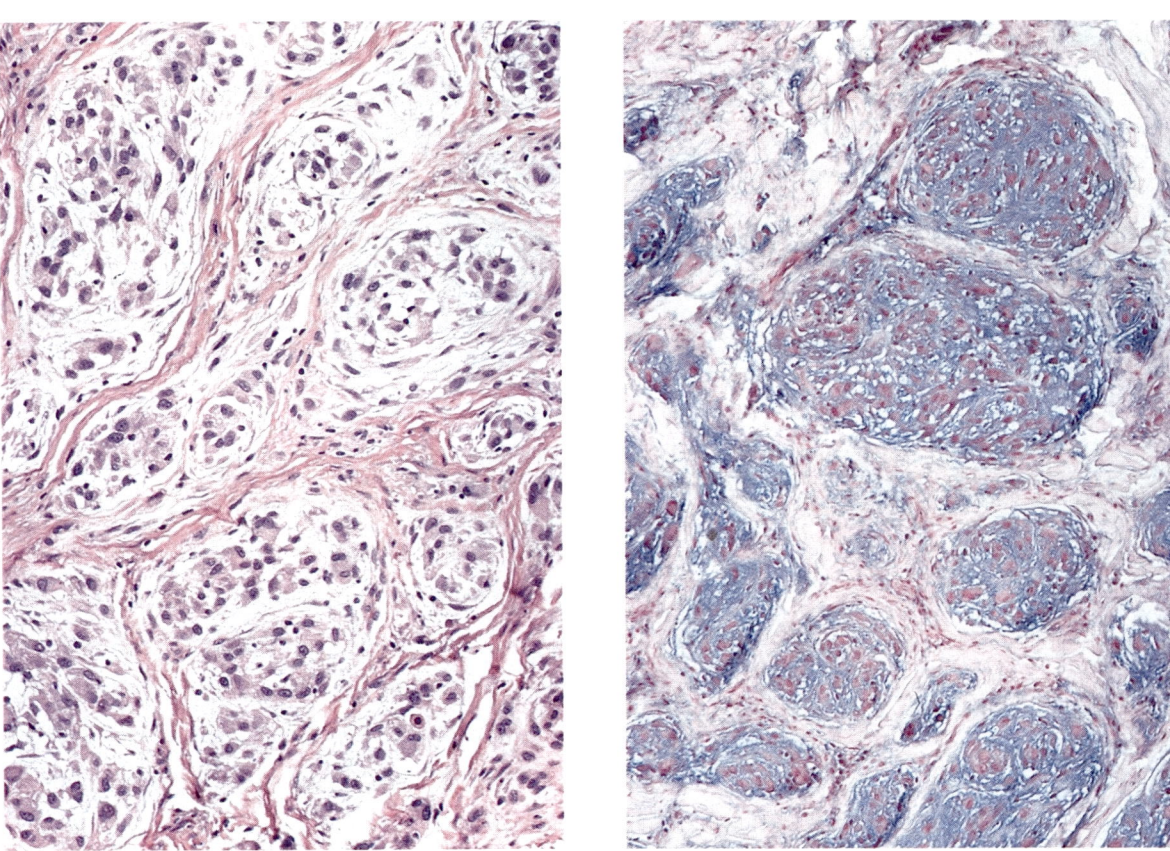

Figure 9-22
NEUROTHEKEOMA
Left: The formation of cellular nests, usually round to ovoid in configuration, is a conspicuous feature of neurothekeoma.
Right: Stromal mucin, here seen on Alcian blue stain, may be abundant in loose textured nodules.

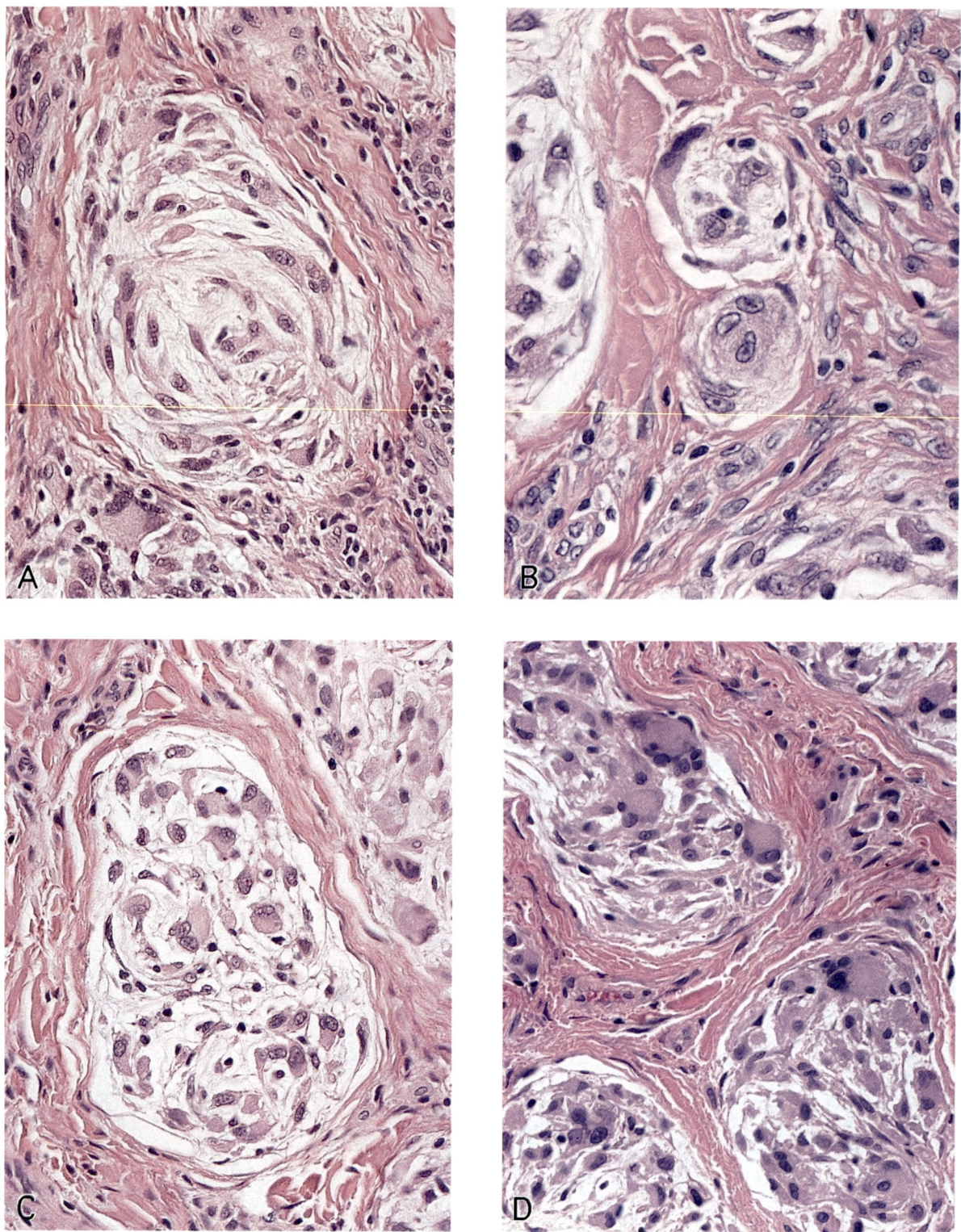

Figure 9-23

NEUROTHEKEOMA

Cytologic features vary from spindle cells arranged in loose to compact whorls (A,B) to epithelioid (C) and occasionally multinucleate cells (D).

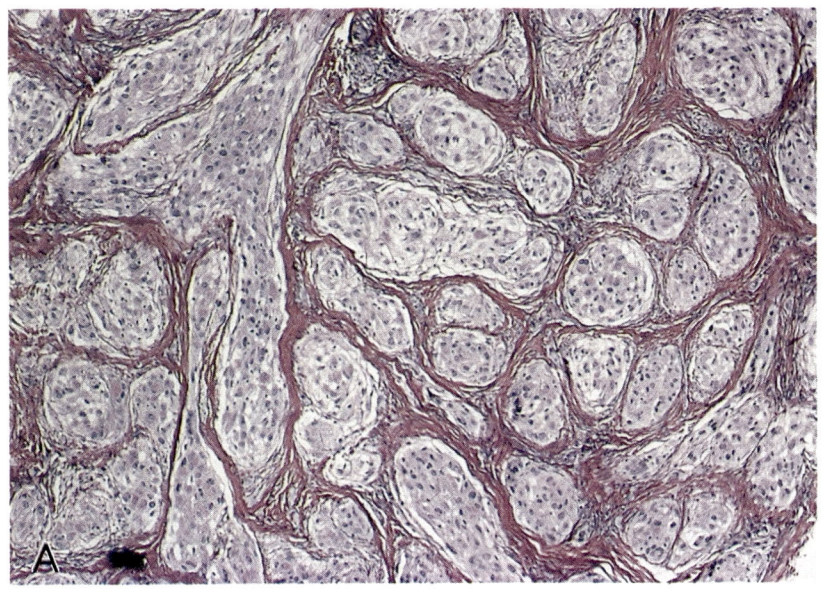

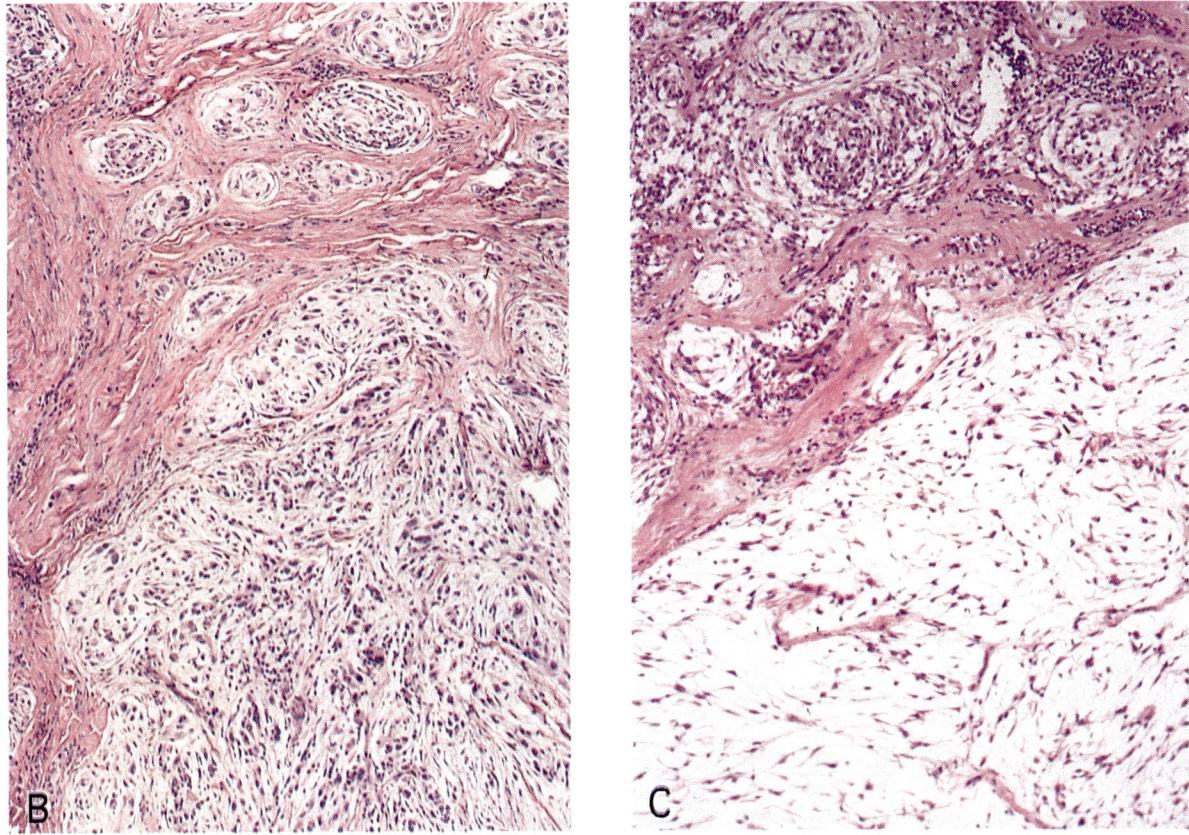

Figure 9-24
NEUROTHEKEOMA

Nodule configuration is often variable. A reticulin preparation (A) shows some nodules to be elongate. Apparent coalescence of nodules is less commonly seen (B). Neurothekeomas only infrequently exhibit loose textured, mucoid elements resembling nerve sheath myxoma (C).

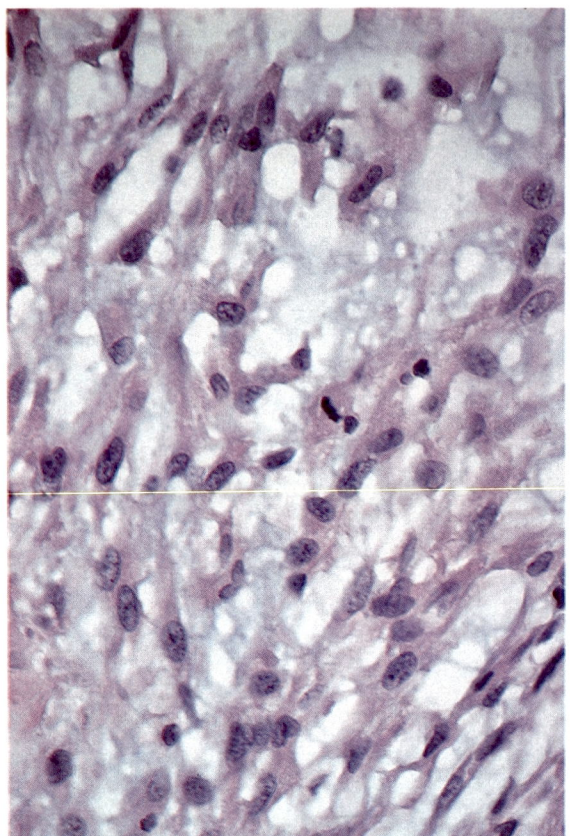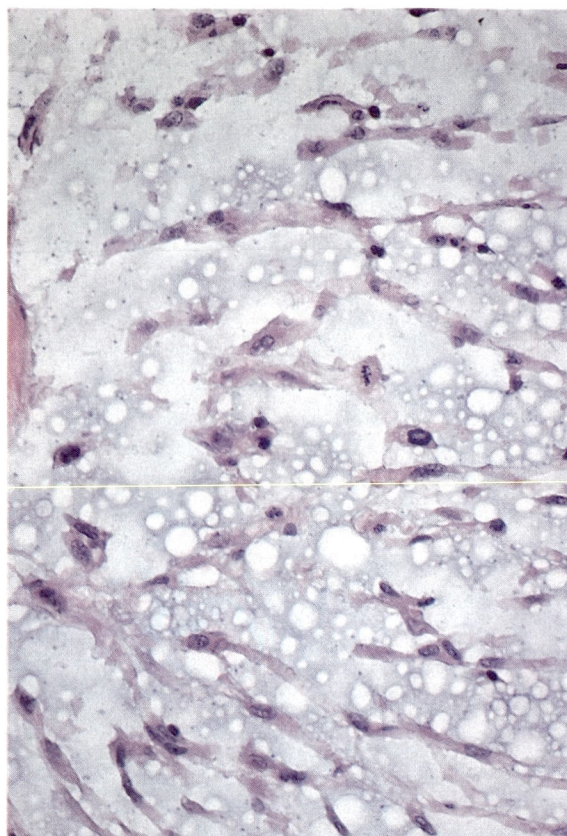

Figure 9-25
NERVE SHEATH MYXOMA
Both figures show variation in nuclear appearance and cytoplasmic volume. Mitotic activity is infrequent (left) and is of no significance. Note the abundance of often bubbly mucin (right).

Figure 9-26
MYXOID SCHWANNOMA
MIMICKING NERVE
SHEATH MYXOMA

Although uncommon, occasional schwannomas show abundant stromal mucin accumulation. This example showed not only a collagenous capsule, a feature alien to nerve sheath myxoma, but the presence of compact islands of Antoni A tissue typical of schwannoma.

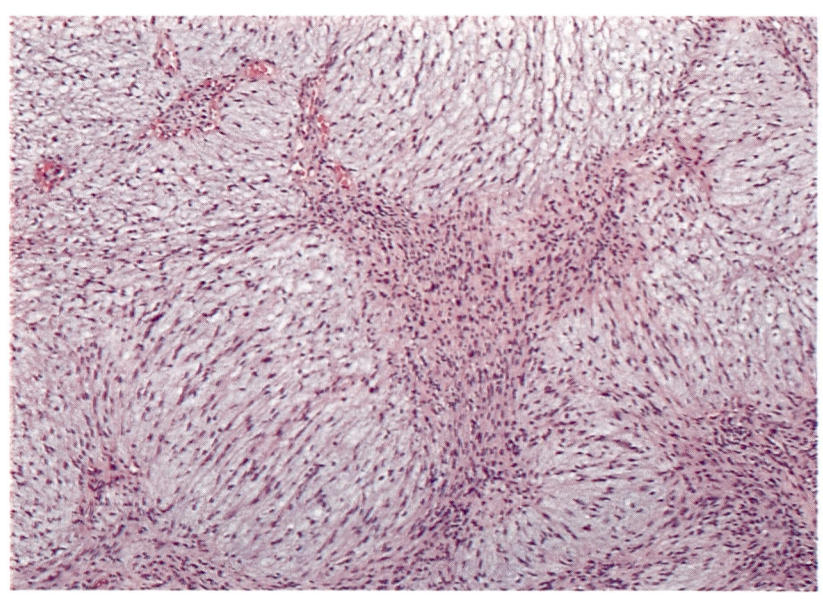

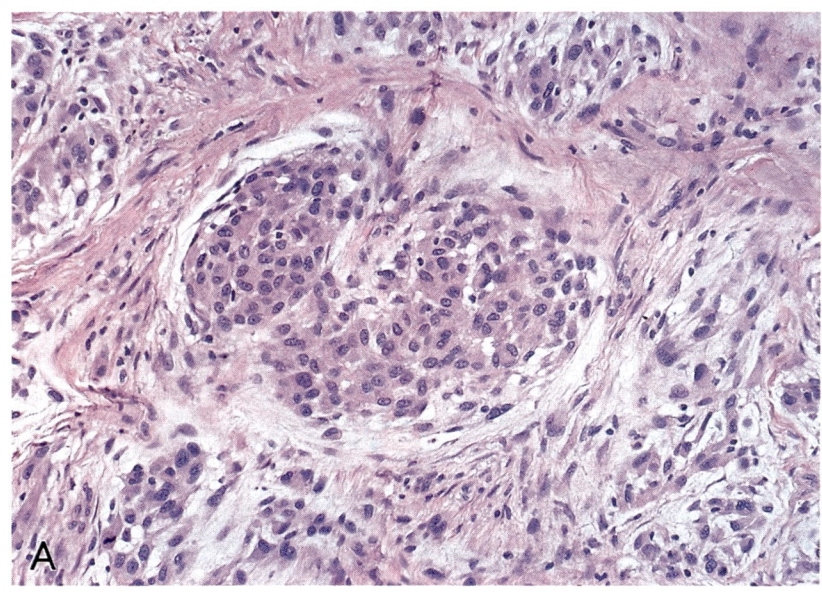

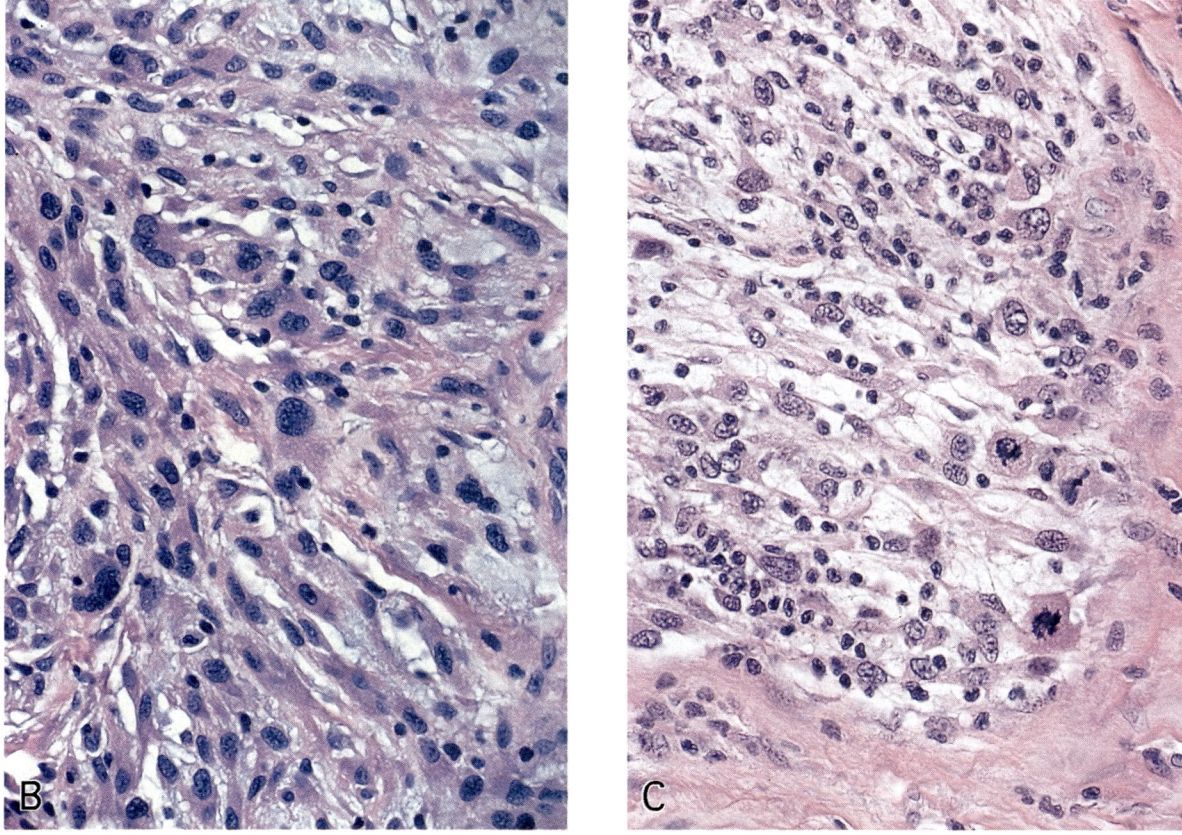

Figure 9-27
NEUROTHEKEOMA

Crowded nodules of cells with higher nuclear-cytoplasmic ratios may be seen in otherwise ordinary tumors (A), but marked atypia (B) is uncommon. Mitoses are seen, but are only rarely frequent or abnormal (C).

A hypercellular variant of neurothekeoma termed *cellular neurothekeoma,* which possesses little or no myxoid stroma, has also been described (figs. 9-28, 9-29) (32,33,50). This tumor features fairly discrete lobules and fascicles of primarily epithelioid cells which, unlike those of conventional neurothekeoma, show a more clearly infiltrative pattern of growth. Although occasional examples superficially invade muscle or vessels, complete resection appears to be curative (34a). The cells of cellular neurothekeoma have abundant eosinophilic or pale-staining cytoplasm and vesicular nuclei with evenly dispersed chromatin. Nuclear pleomorphism, hyperchromasia, and a mitotic index as high as 10 or even 15 mitoses per 10 high-power fields (33,34a) may be observed. Melanin pigmentation has not been reported.

Immunohistochemical Findings. Nerve sheath myxomas usually are reactive for S-100 protein (fig. 9-30, left) (28,34,36,52), whereas neurothekeomas are not (30,31,33). The same is true of basement membrane staining for collagen type 4 or laminin (fig. 9-30, right). The delicate EMA-immunoreactive layer of spindle cells often surrounding some lobules of nerve sheath myxoma appears to represent residual perineurium (52). In contrast, neurothekeomas lack EMA staining entirely (43). Vimentin preparations are strongly positive in both nerve sheath myxoma and neurothekeoma (fig. 9-31). In addition to lack of S-100 protein and EMA reactivity in both conventional and cellular neurothekeomas, the latter are also negative for Leu 7, protein gene product (PGP) 9.5, myelin basic protein, and desmin (32,33,34a,35,42). NK1/C3 staining is characteristic of neurothekeomas as a whole (fig. 9-31, right) (34a); nerve sheath myxomas react more sparingly or not at all. Inexplicably, one study of cellular neurothekeomas reported focal staining for smooth muscle actin in a minority of cases (35).

Ultrastructural Findings. Nerve sheath differentiation of one type or another has been reported to occur in light microscopically typical nerve sheath myxoma (28,34,38,48,54,56). Although the findings were variously interpreted as evidence of Schwann cell or perineurial differentiation, a critical review of published illustrations and reported immunoreactivities indicates that the constituent cells are schwannian. Argenyi et al. (29) also recently reported that

Schwann cells surrounded by a continuous basement membrane is the main constituent of classic nerve sheath myxoma.

In contrast to nerve sheath myxoma, schwannian or perineurial cell differentiation usually is lacking in neurothekeoma (29,30). Ultrastructural studies performed by us upon one conventional and one cellular neurothekeoma (fig. 9-32) revealed neoplastic cells with well-developed, often dilated rough endoplasmic reticulum and lack of basement membranes, features indicative of fibroblastic differentiation. The same features were noted in a cellular neurothekeoma by Barnhill et al. (32). Yet another view was expressed by Argenyi et al. (29), who in a study of 11 neurothekeomas found an undifferentiated polygonal cell to predominate. Interestingly, the authors also found evidence suggesting partial divergent differentiation to Schwann, smooth muscle, fibroblastic, and myofibroblastic cells.

Differential Diagnosis. Several processes, not all neoplastic, enter into the differential diagnosis of nerve sheath myxoma and neurothekeoma. These include focal mucinosis, myxoid schwannoma and neurofibroma, and low-grade myxofibrosarcoma (low-grade myxoid malignant fibrous histiocytoma). With regard to cellular neurothekeoma, both spindle and epithelioid cell (Spitz) nevus and desmoplastic (neurotrophic) melanoma enter into the differential.

A non-neoplastic process occasionally associated with hyperthyroidism, *focal mucinosis* lacks not only the circumscription and lobulation so typical of nerve sheath myxoma and neurothekeoma, but their cellularity as well (53).

Occasional myxoid schwannomas mimic nerve sheath myxoma in showing remarkable mucin accumulation (9-26). Unlike nerve sheath myxoma, *myxoid schwannomas* exhibit a collagenous capsule and often islands of Antoni A tissue. The distinction of nerve sheath myxoma from *neurofibroma* of the diffuse dermal type poses no problem in that nerve sheath myxomas are demarcated proliferations. At the light microscopic level, the distinction from plexiform neurofibroma is more difficult; however, unlike nerve sheath myxoma, clusters of stellate and epithelioid cells as well as a syncytial arrangement of the cells are uncommon and there are at least small numbers of neurofilament protein–reactive axons.

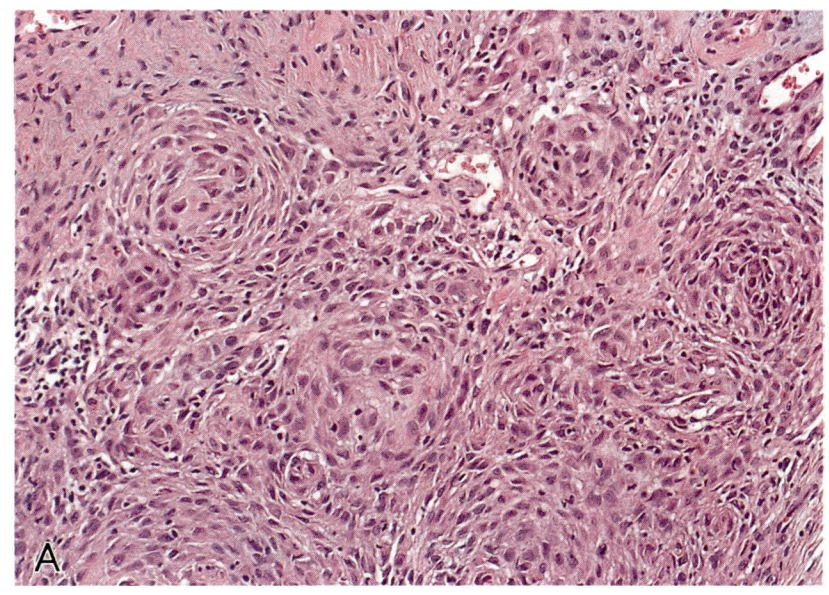

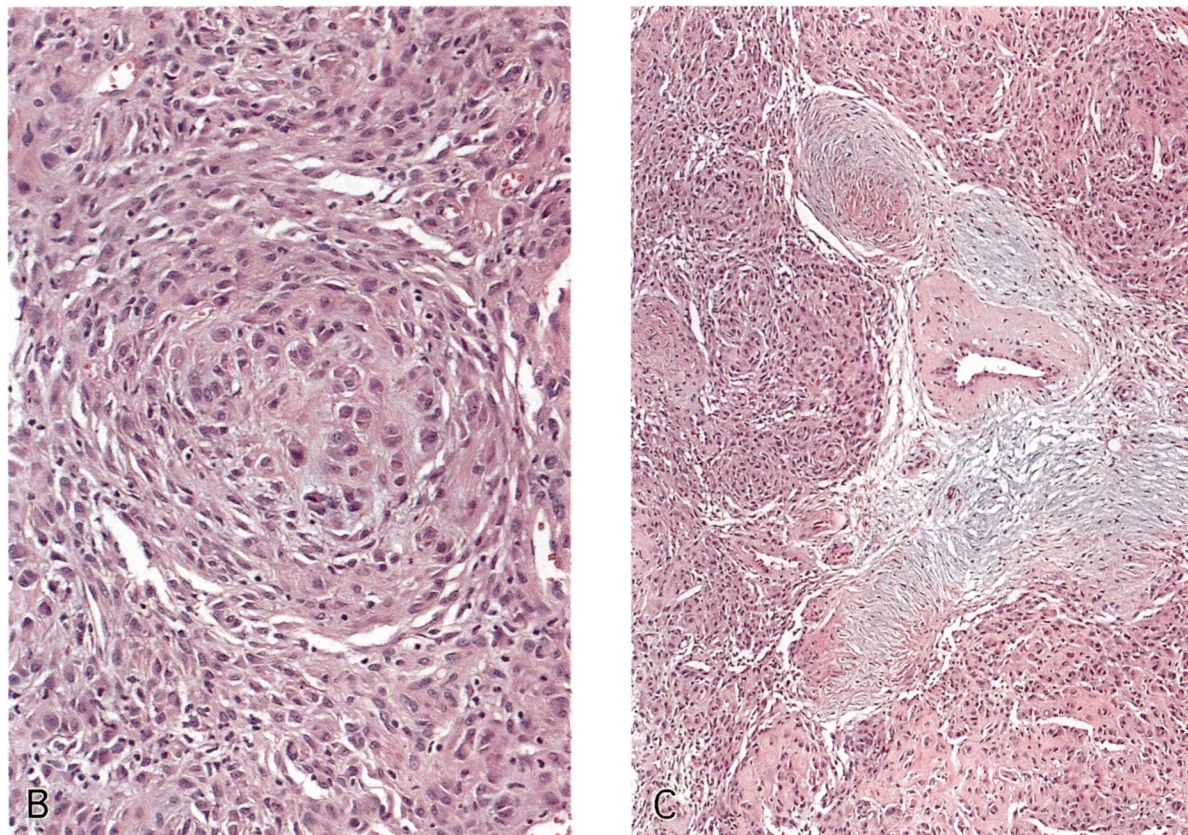

Figure 9-28
CELLULAR NEUROTHEKEOMA

Such tumors feature cellular nodules and relatively little mucoid matrix (A,B). Stromal mucin in this example is concentrated about vessels where it separates lamellae of tumor cells (C).

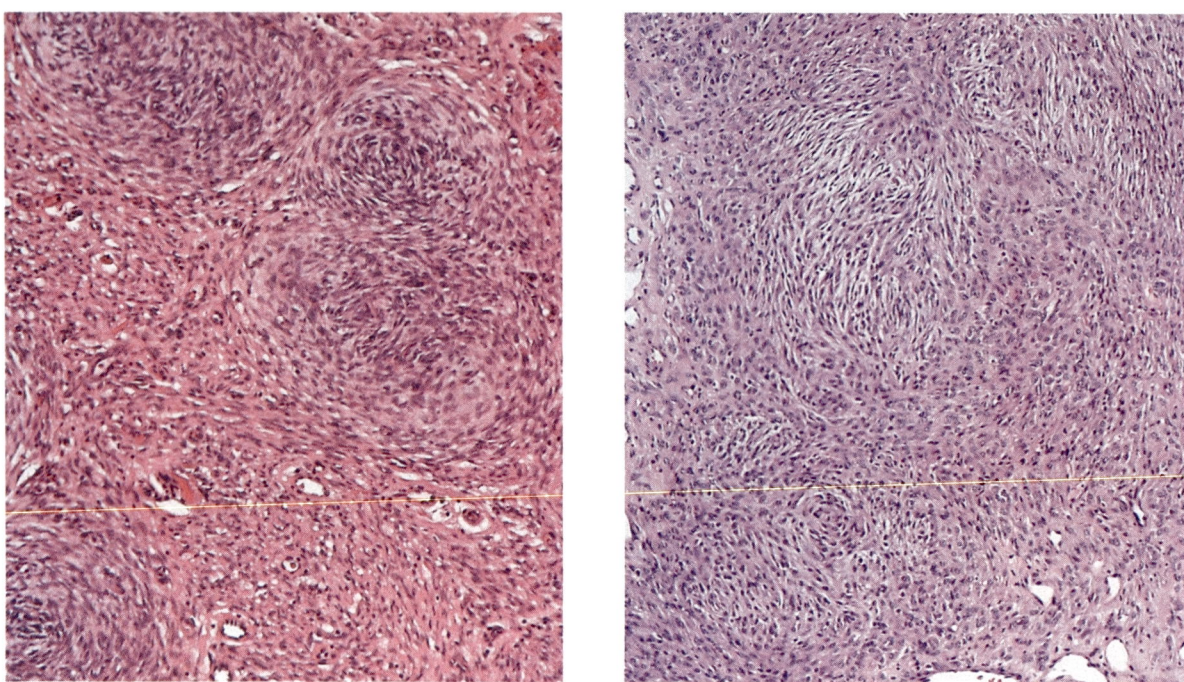

Figure 9-29
CELLULAR NEUROTHEKEOMA
This even more cellular example shows less sharply delineated (left) as well as vague nodules (right), all lacking mucin.

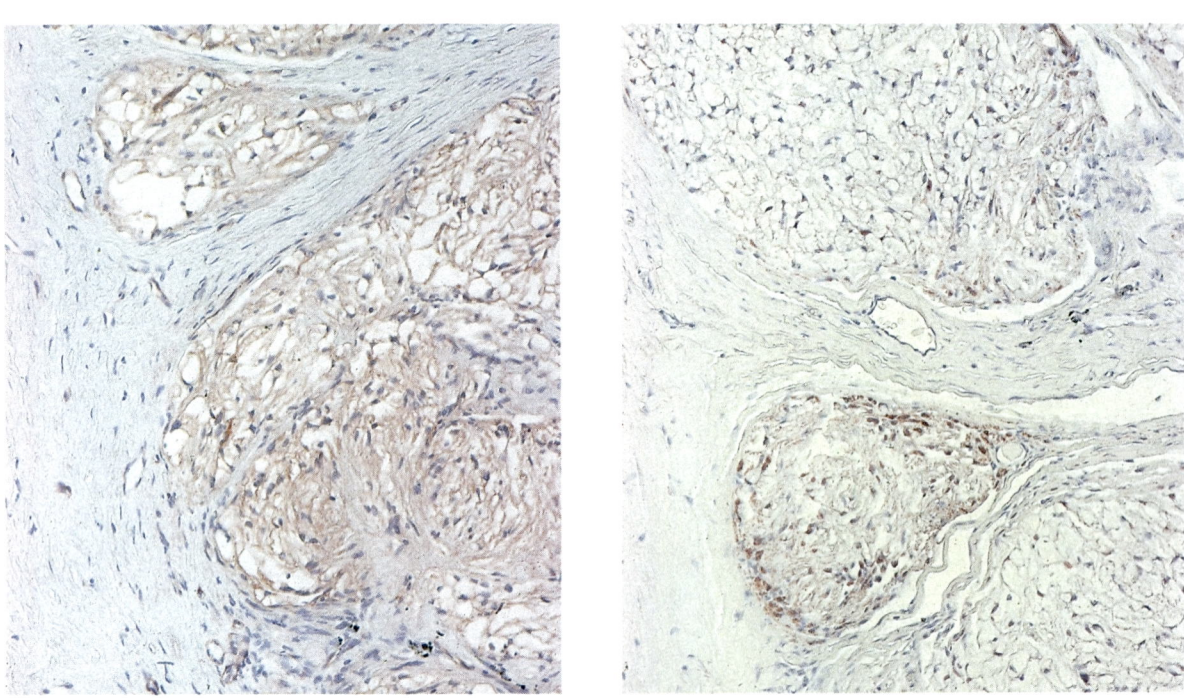

Figure 9-30
NERVE SHEATH MYXOMA
Immunoreactivity for S-100 protein (left) and collagen 4 (right) further supports the concept that these lesions are schwannian in nature. Note considerable variation in S-100 protein staining (left).

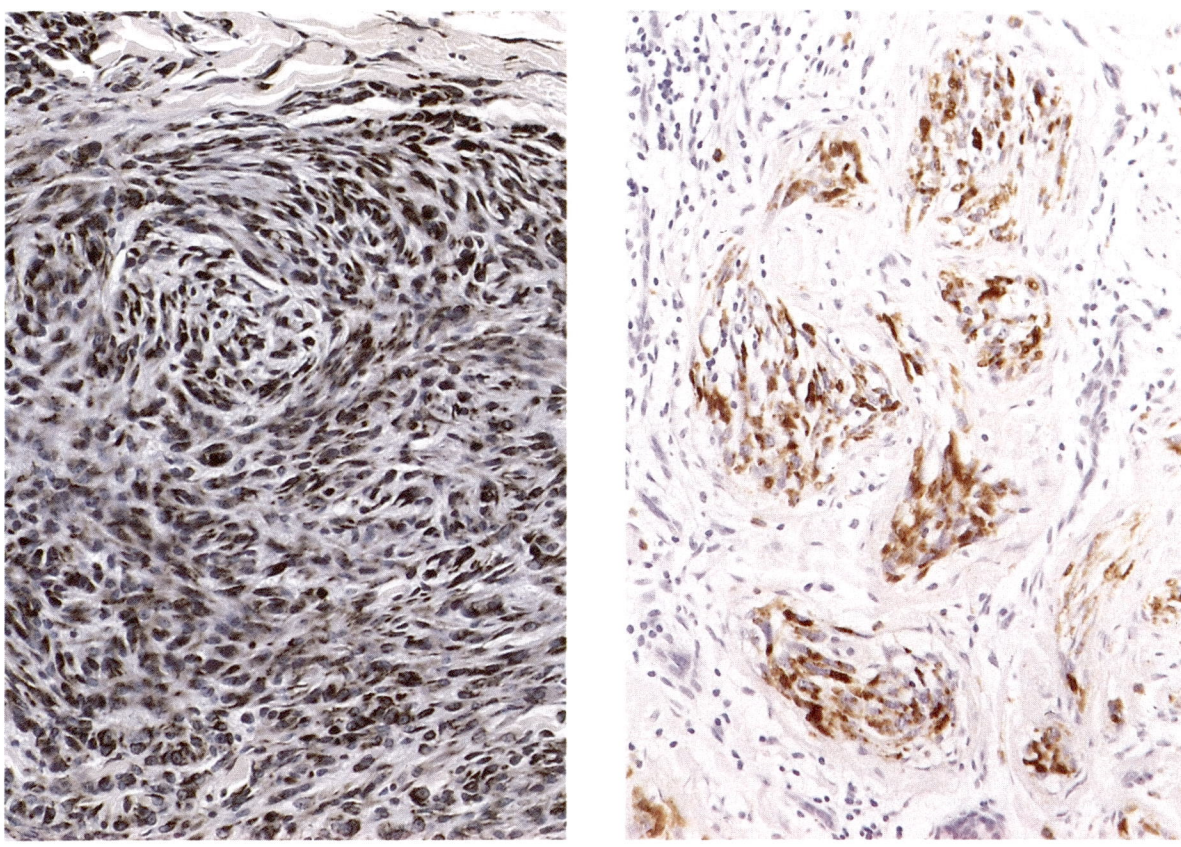

Figure 9-31
CELLULAR NEUROTHEKEOMA
Whether conventional or cellular, as in this example, the cells of neurothekeoma are vimentin immunoreactive (left). Staining for NK1/C3 is also typical (right). Unlike nerve sheath myxoma, neurothekeomas do not stain for S-100 protein and collagen 4.

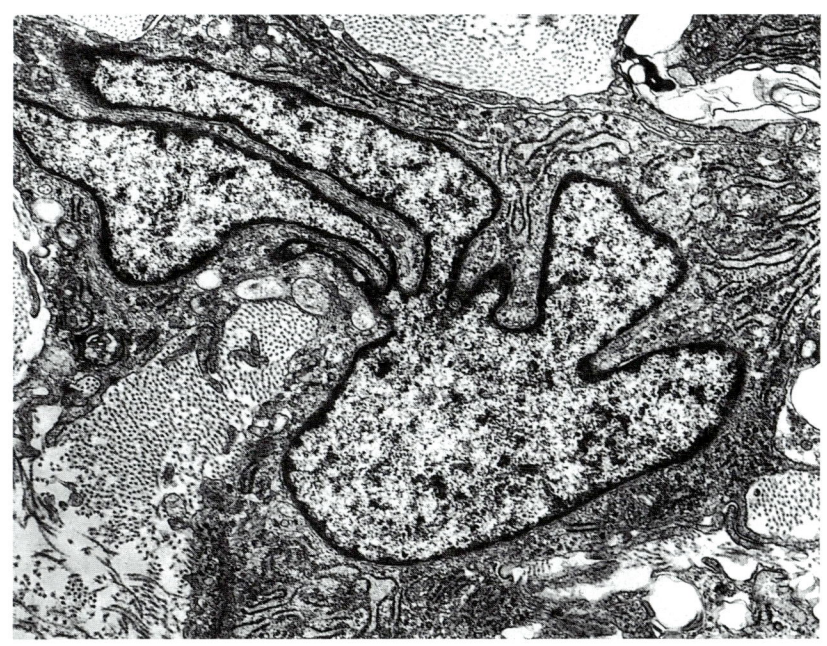

Figure 9-32
CELLULAR NEUROTHEKEOMA
The tumor shows fibroblastic features including prominent rough endoplasmic reticulum and lack of basement membrane (X16,700).

Although *low-grade myxofibrosarcoma* may be mistaken for nerve sheath myxoma, the former occurs in older patients, is generally larger, and often involves deeper soft tissues of the thigh and arm (46). In addition, myxofibrosarcoma generally exhibits a more prominent vasculature, a prominent fibrous component, greater degrees of cellularity and nuclear atypia, and often some pleomorphism.

The distinction of cellular neurothekeoma from *Spitz nevus* rests upon the usual presence in the latter of a junctional component, melanin pigment, and individual cell infiltration of the dermis (33). The *desmoplastic melanoma* is richer in collagen than neurothekeoma and often shows epidermal lentiginous melanocytic hyperplasia, larger nuclei, and, at least focally, marked hyperchromasia (33). Mild chronic inflammation is also a common feature of desmoplastic melanoma. The finding of melanosomes at the ultrastructural level distinguishes both these melanocytic lesions from nerve sheath myxoma and neurothekeoma. Inasmuch as desmoplastic melanoma often is nonreactive for HMB-45, this stain will not serve as a diagnostic determinant.

Treatment and Prognosis. Both nerve sheath myxoma and neurothekeoma are benign neoplasms. In the two largest series of these tumors, those of Gallagher and Helwig (37) and Pulitzer and Reed (49), consisting of 123 cases, only 3 recurrences were noted. Not a single example of either tumor has been reported to metastasize. Conservative, complete excision is curative. Cellular neurothekeomas behave in a similar benign fashion; resection is curative (33).

BENIGN GRANULAR CELL TUMOR

Definition. This is a tumor composed of eosinophilic granular cells which often are PAS positive, immunoreactive for S-100 protein, and ultrastructurally contain large numbers of secondary lysosomes. Synonyms include *granular cell schwannoma, granular cell neurofibroma,* and *granular neurogenic tumor.*

General Comments. Granular cell tumor (GCT) is an uncommon lesion which at one time was considered to be myogenic in nature, hence the now antiquated term "granular cell myoblastoma" (58,59). The current concept that it is a neural tumor originated with Feyrter (80–82), and was later promoted by Fust and Custer (87,88) and Fisher and Wechsler (84). Several lines of evidence support the neural derivation of GCT, including their close association with small to medium-sized nerves (88). These include cranial nerves, either within the cranium (70,71,103,123) or in their extracranial course (64,68), as well as spinal nerves (65,79,99,141). The neurogenic nature of most GCTs is also suggested by their immunoreactivity for S-100 protein (62,104,118,124, 130,131,142), Leu-7 (57,103), and the distinctive proteins of peripheral nerve myelin P0 and P2 (114); the occurrence of GCTs with ultrastructural features of schwannian differentiation (57); and the rare finding of granular change in ordinary schwannoma (see fig. 7-18D,E). Immunoreactivity for markers of muscle differentiation is lacking. Numerous electron microscopic studies, including early reports (84,89), also support the concept that most GCTs are neural in nature (see below).

Malignant GCT, some which are histologically indistinguishable from benign GCT, are discussed in chapter 11.

Clinical Features. GCTs affect all age groups, but their incidence peaks in the fourth through the sixth decades (132). Pediatric examples are uncommon and must not be confused with congenital gingival granular cell tumor or "epulis," a histologically similar lesion presenting in neonates and typically arising in the mucosa of the alveolar ridge (see differential diagnosis) (135,137). The majority of GCTs occur in females (104,122), and in at least three large series, blacks were preferentially affected (122,139). Most present as solitary masses, but up to 10 percent are multiple (95,102, 113,124). With the possible exception of a single example, no association exists between this unusual tumor and neurofibromatosis (102). Only rarely is a diagnosis of GCT clinically suspected (98).

GCTs occur at numerous anatomic sites. Most frequently affected are the skin and subcutaneous tissue (fig. 9-33), particularly that of the head, neck, trunk, and extremities (122). The single most common site, however, the location of one fourth of all lesions, is the tongue (fig. 9-34A) (98,122), especially its lateral borders, tip, and dorsum (60, 110). Breast lesions represent 5 to 15 percent of all GCTs (76,122); the lower figure corresponds to involvement of breast parenchyma alone, while the higher figure includes examples affecting overlying skin and subcutaneous tissue (132,135).

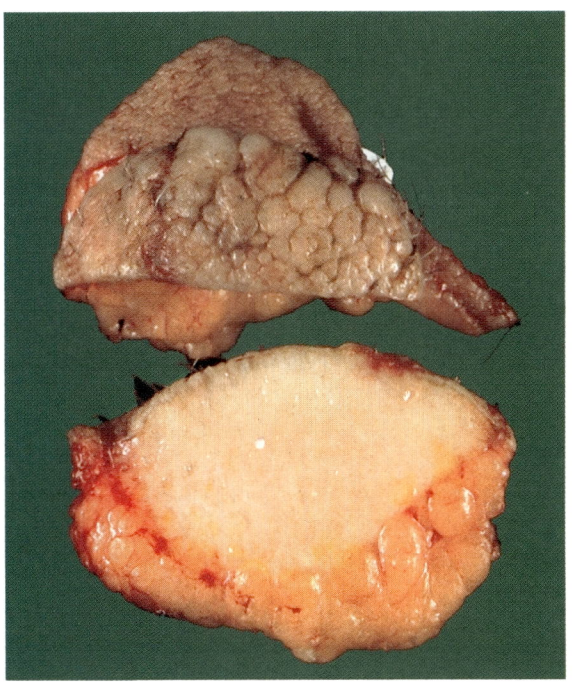
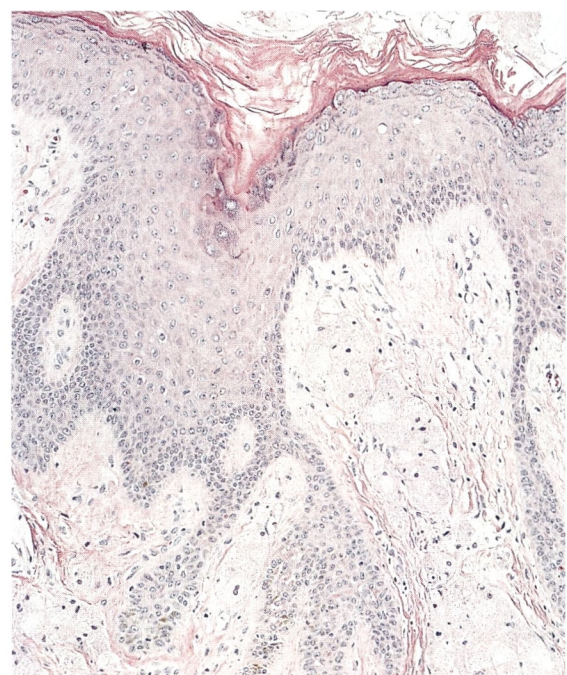

Figure 9-33
GRANULAR CELL TUMOR

Left: The squamous mucosa overlying this vulvar lesion is markedly hypertrophic, lending a cobblestone appearance (top). On cut section the pale, white, nonencapsulated nodule lies within submucosal adipose tissue (bottom).

Right: Microscopically, the squamous mucosa shows marked pseudoepitheliomatous hyperplasia (right). (Courtesy of Dr. J. Goellner, Rochester, Minnesota.)

Viscera are only infrequently involved by GCT. In the respiratory tract, the larynx is most often affected; in Peterson's series (122) 7 percent of cases occurred in this location. The majority of laryngeal GCTs are confined to the posterior aspect of a true vocal cord. Subglottic examples are rare and occur primarily in children (67,74,90,135). Interestingly, the frequency of bronchial lesions is about half that of laryngeal tumors, but the trachea is rarely involved.

Approximately 5 percent of GCTs present in the gastrointestinal tract (122). While the esophagus, large bowel, and perianal region account for the majority of cases (92,94), examples have occurred at all levels, including stomach and small bowel. Most esophageal tumors arise in the distal portion, while tumors involving the large bowel are distributed throughout its length (94). Although most gastrointestinal tumors are solitary, and involve the lamina propria or submucosa (figs. 9-34B,C), multiplicity is not uncommon. The greatest number of multiple GCTs reported to date were two cases of 26 and 52

lesions per case; in both instances the colon was the affected site (66,107). GCTs also involve the gallbladder and biliary tract (94).

Gross Findings. GCTs usually present as solitary, nodular lesions seldom measuring greater than 3 cm in maximum dimension. Circumscribed lesions are more common than poorly demarcated or grossly infiltrative tumors (98,132). When present, surface irregularity of skin or involvement of squamous mucosa by tumor is often due to accompanying pseudoepitheliomatous hyperplasia (fig. 9-33). On cross section the generally firm tumors appear gray-white to yellow (fig. 9-33, left). In one reported example, as well as a case of our own (fig. 9-35), cutaneous plaques or multinodularity was a reflection of an unusual, plexiform pattern of growth (99).

Microscopic Findings. The cells of GCT are disposed in sheets, nests, lobules, or ribbons (figs. 9-36A,B, 9-37A, 9-38A) accompanied by variable amounts of connective tissue. Occasional examples are extensively collagenized (fig. 9-36B). Limited infiltration of surrounding

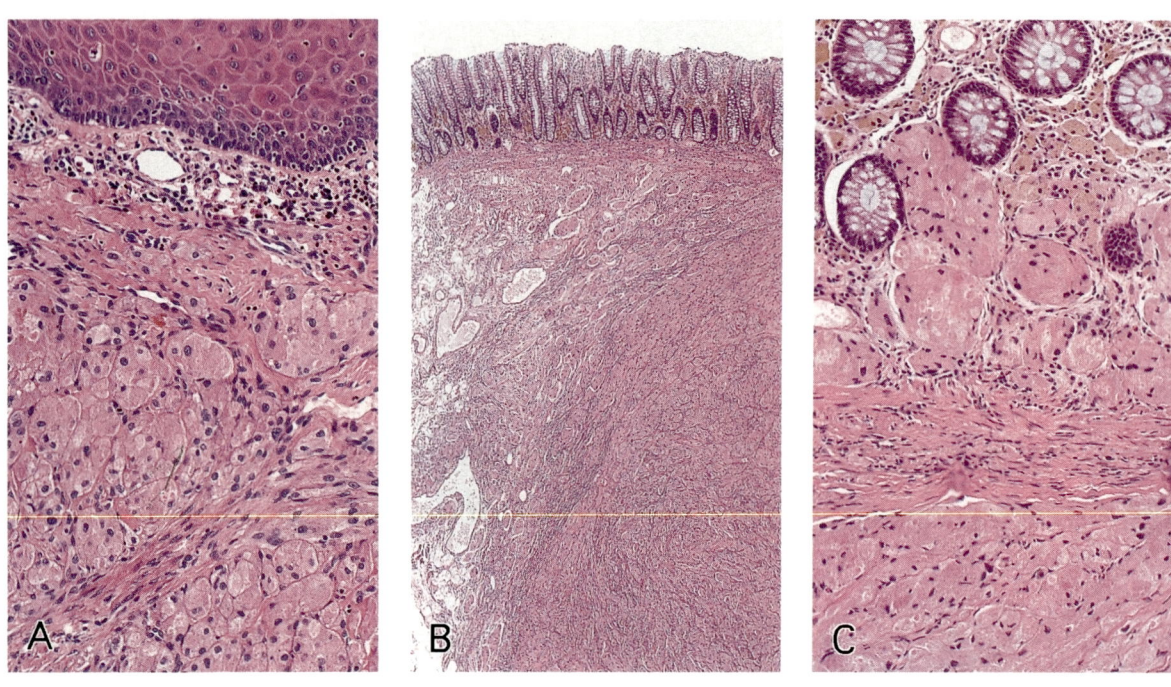

Figure 9-34
GRANULAR CELL TUMOR
Examples arising in the tongue (A) and the colon (B,C) show the tendency of GCT to involve lamina propria and submucosa.

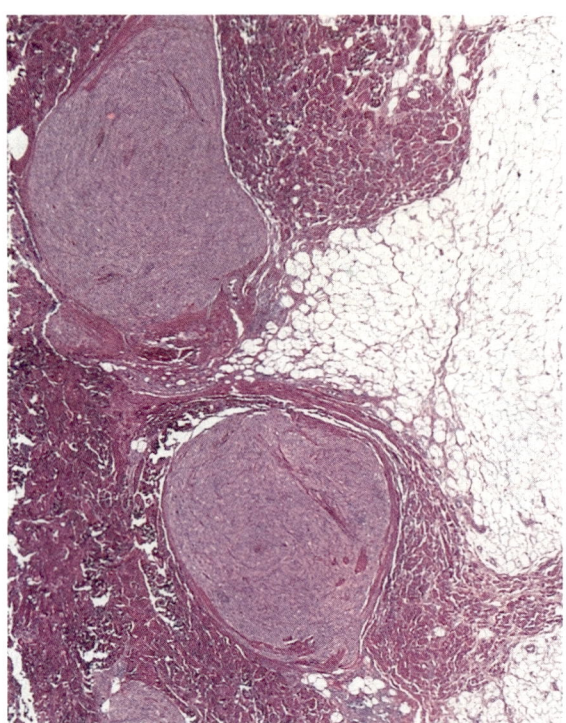

Figure 9-35
GRANULAR CELL TUMOR
Rare dermal examples show a plexiform pattern of growth.

adipose tissue may be seen (fig. 9-36D). Aggregates of lymphoid cells are found at the periphery of most lesions (fig. 9-36D). GCTs are composed of monotonous, plump, polyhedral to elongate cells with distinct cell borders. Their abundant eosinophilic cytoplasm is granular in appearance due to the high content of lysosomes (figs. 9-34A,C, 9-37A). Nuclei are small and regular, somewhat hyperchromatic, and generally contain inconspicuous nucleoli. Occasional tumors show degenerative nuclear changes (fig. 9-37C). In addition to granularity, a near constant feature of GCT is the presence in occasional cells of one or several eosinophilic cytoplasmic globules, some encompassed by a halo (fig. 9-38A). A typical but less obvious feature is refractile eosinophilic lysosomes, termed "angulate bodies," seen within stromal histiocytes (fig. 9-38C) (78,125,126). The cytoplasmic granules of tumor cells are moderately PAS positive (figs. 9-37B, 9-38B) and diastase resistant. The same is true of globules and angulate bodies (fig. 9-38B,D). In addition, the tumor cells stain with Sudan black B and are magenta in trichrome preparations. These various cellular features of

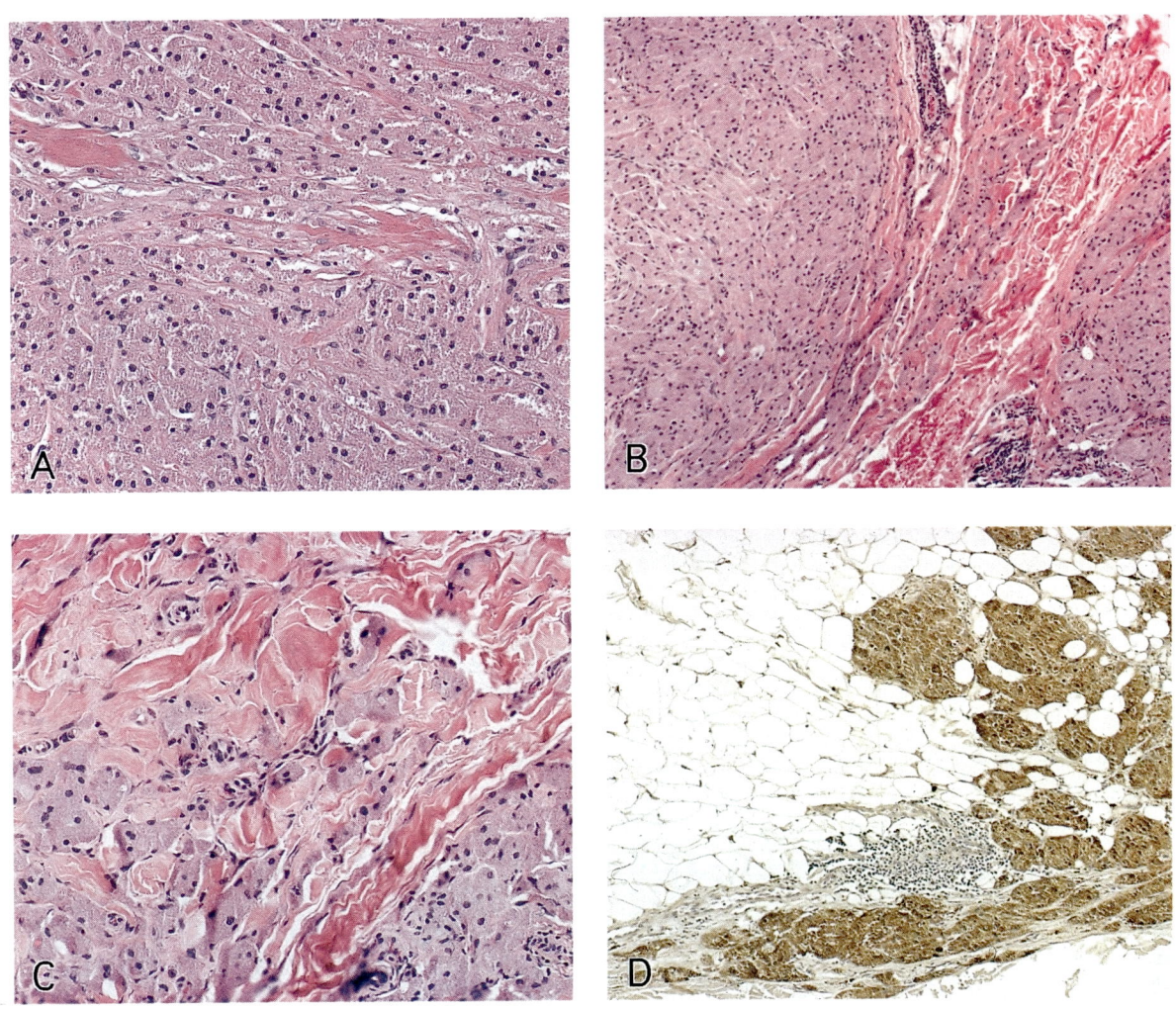

Figure 9-36
GRANULAR CELL TUMOR

Although often disposed in sheets (A), with uniform, polyhedral cells grouped between delicate fibrovascular septa (A), multinodularity is common (B). Occasional tumors are fibrotic (C). Local infiltration of surrounding or adipose tissue is often seen (D, S-100 protein immunostain). Note focal chronic inflammation in the tumor periphery (D).

GCT are constant and are readily appreciated in cytologic preparations (fig. 9-39) (85,86,101, 144). Multinucleation, nuclear pleomorphism, readily identifiable nucleoli, and mitotic figures are uncommon features. The pattern of reticulin staining varies considerably, surrounding either individual or clustered granular cells. Cytoplasmic striations are absent.

Most GCTs are superficial and involve dermis and subcutaneous tissue, although some involve deep soft tissues, including muscle. As previously noted, gastrointestinal GCTs affect primarily the lamina propria and submucosa (fig. 9-34). A notable feature, given its bearing upon the assumed differentiation of GCTs, is the not uncommon involvement of small nerves in or around the tumor (fig. 9-40). Larger nerves are less often affected (fig. 9-41). In other instances the neural derivation of GCT is suggested simply by the finding of residual axons within a tumor. Also, rare dermal examples exhibit a decidedly plexiform pattern of nerve involvement (fig. 9-34) (99). Lastly, the pseudoepitheliomatous hyperplasia of squamous epithelium overlying some GCTs can closely mimic well-differentiated squamous cell carcinoma.

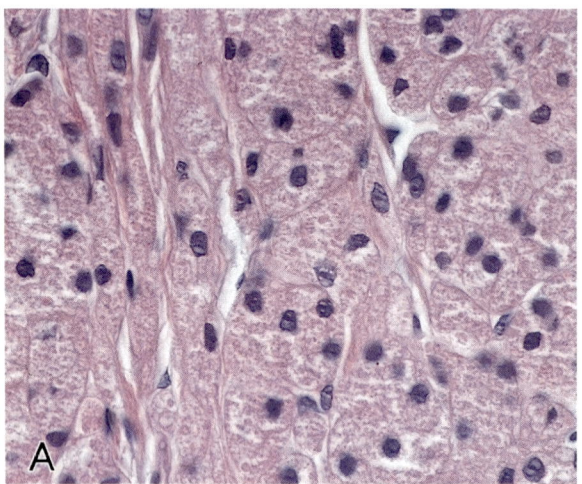

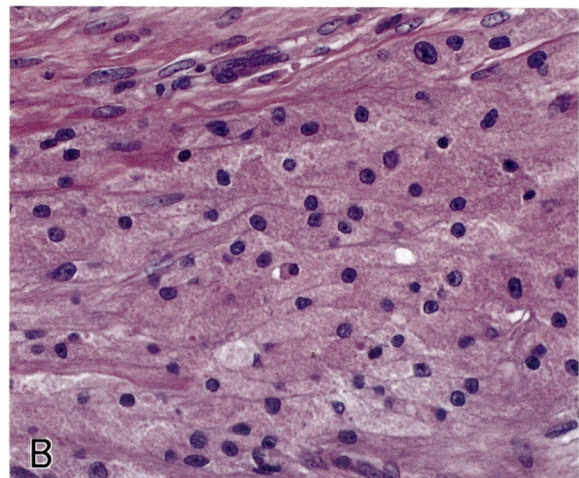

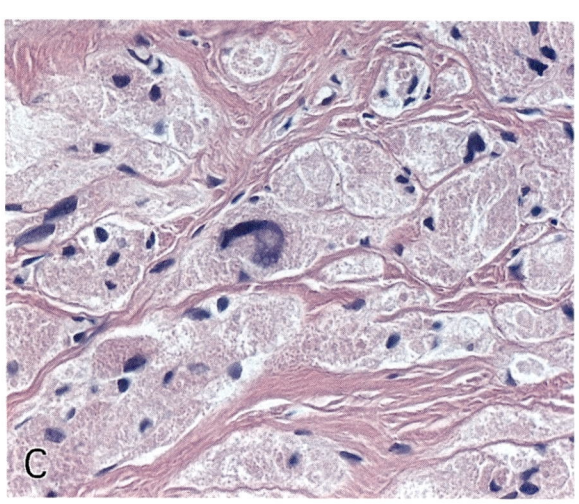

Figure 9-37
GRANULAR CELL TUMOR
Due to the accumulation of often large lysosomes, the cells appear coarsely granular (A), a feature highlighted on PAS stain (B). Note the variation in nuclear features, ranging from more open chromatin and discernible nucleoli (A), to rather dense chromatin (B). Degenerative nuclear atypia is occasionally seen (C).

Immunohistochemical Findings. A number of markers, none specific, are consistently exhibited by GCTs. These include variable degrees of immunoreactivity for S-100 protein (figs. 9-41C, 9-42) (62,77,104,109,112,116,120,130,142), the macrophage markers alpha-1-antichymotrypsin (120,129) and CD68 (fig. 9-42C) (83,97), neuron-specific enolase (83), and vimentin. Leu-7 reactivity is present in about one third of GCTs (104). Staining has also been reported for two myelin-associated proteins, the integral myelin protein P0 and the peripheral myelin protein P2 (114). Immunoreactivity for myelin basic protein (MBP) is less consistently observed (69,73,104,121). Whereas one investigator found MBP reactivity in 13 of 21 granular cell tumors (104), another study of six cases reported none (73). A number of series have reported lack of both neurofilament protein and

glial fibrillary acidic protein (GFAP) in GCT (69, 109,114,118,138). Stains for collagen 4 typically show perilobular staining around small or sizable clusters (fig. 9-42D). Angulate body–containing histiocytes are CD68 immunoreactive and do not stain for S-100 protein (126).

Ultrastructural Findings. The fine structural features of GCTs are highly characteristic. The light microscopic granularity of the polygonal to spindle-shaped tumor cells is due to the presence of large numbers of pleomorphic secondary lysosomes within their cytoplasm. These vary in type and include autophagosomes, residual bodies, multivesicular bodies, and material resembling ceroid lipofuscin (figs. 9-43, 9-44) (57, 61,65,69,71,75,84,109,111,113,124,125,143). Ultrastructurally, these lysosomes consist of membrane-bound aggregates of microgranules and

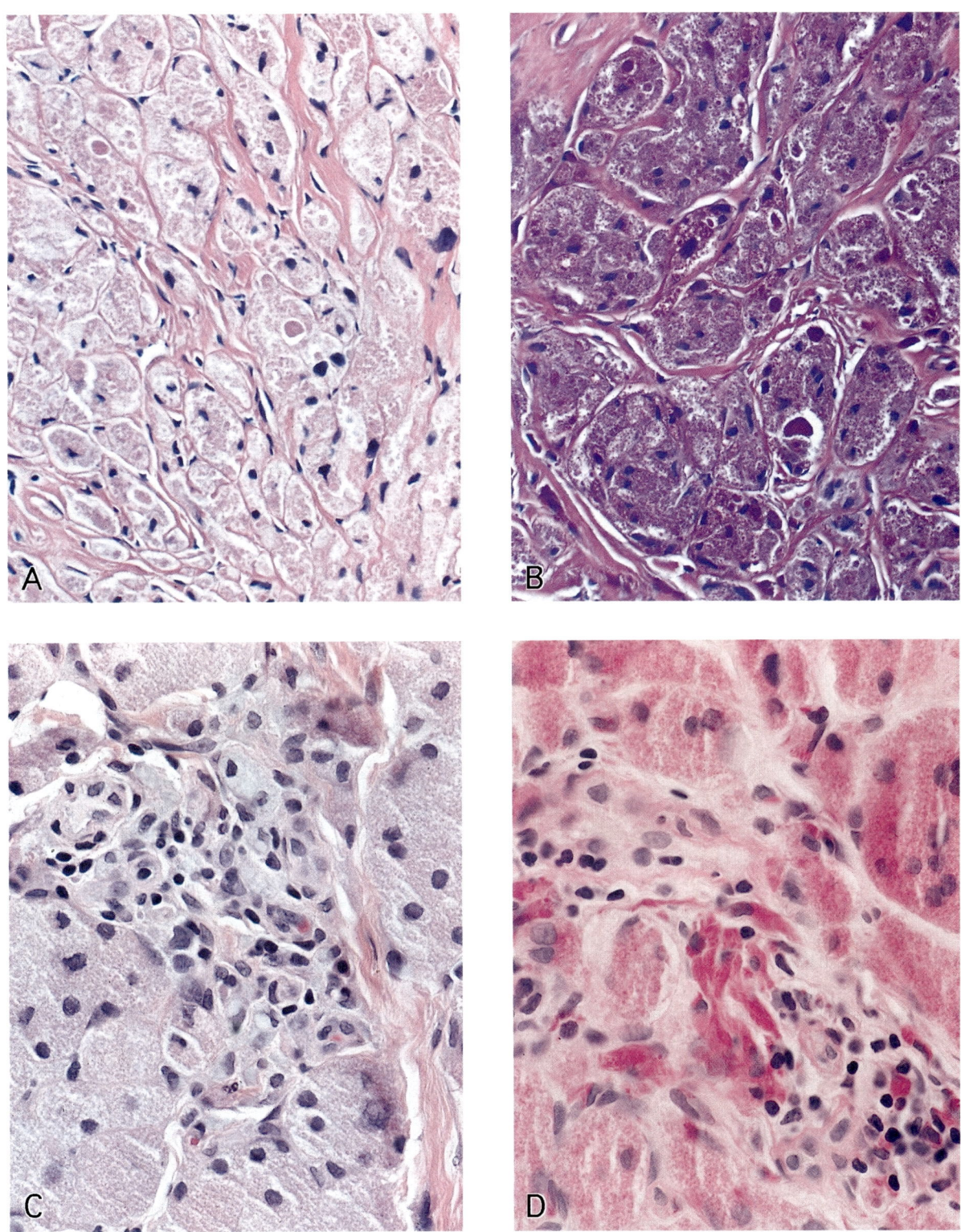

Figure 9-38
GRANULAR CELL TUMOR
Two cytologic features characteristic of GCT include the formation of globules corresponding to giant lysosomes (A, center) and the presence of angulate bodies (C). Both are accentuated on PAS stain (B and D).

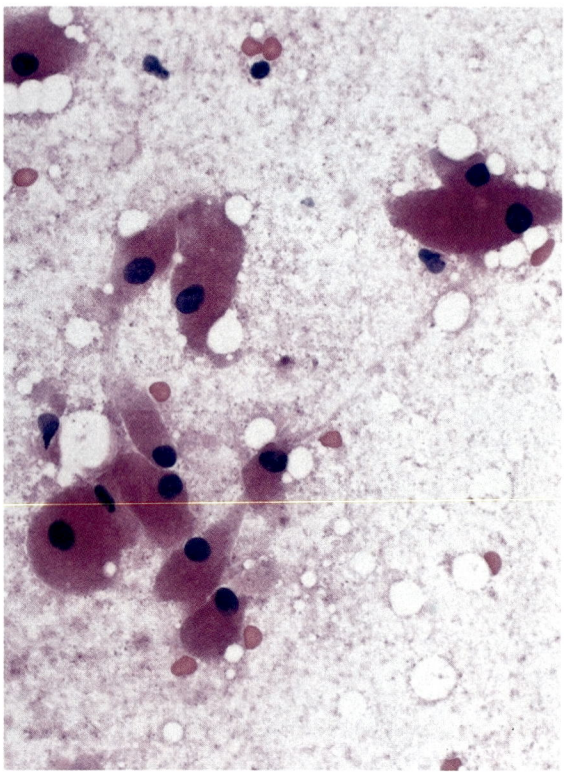

Figure 9-39
GRANULAR CELL TUMOR: CYTOLOGY
On smear preparations the cells appear epithelioid, often
angular in configuration, and possess dense granular cytoplasm.

irregularly shaped, variably electron-dense masses containing assorted inclusions, among them remnants of organelles and concentric lamellae (figs. 9-43, 9-44). The latter have been likened to myelin debris. Stromal fibrohistiocytic cells intimately associated with the granular tumor cells frequently contain numerous membrane-bound structures featuring parallel arrays of "microtubules" and scattered dense lipid bodies variously termed angulate bodies (126), angulate lysosomes (78), or Gaucher-like bodies (fig. 9-45) (91). These unusual secondary lysosomes are only rarely found within the cytoplasm of the granular tumor cells. The peripheral nerve origin of most GCTs is supported by varying degrees of granular transformation of recognizable Schwann cells, a distinct basement membrane often surrounding granular cell clusters (fig. 9-44), the occasional presence of long-spacing collagen, and the presence among tumor cells of arrays of neuritic processes (57,65,71,75,84,124,127,128,140).

As will be further discussed below, ultrastructural studies also are useful for excluding mimics of GCT, such as granular cell leiomyoma (57,72), leiomyosarcoma (133), angiosarcoma (105), ameloblastoma (119,134), and glioblastoma (96).

Differential Diagnosis. With the exception of examples involving breast parenchyma, GCTs seldom present a diagnostic problem. Due to their induration and infiltrative margins, GCTs of the breast are notoriously difficult to distinguish from mammary *carcinoma*. This is true both grossly and microscopically, particularly at frozen section (63,93,115,136). The distinction from carcinoma is most easily achieved by immunohistochemistry; unlike carcinoma, GCTs are KP-1 (CD68) positive (97) and lack keratin and epithelial membrane antigen staining. Since carcinomas may be S-100 protein reactive, this determinant cannot be relied upon.

Although granular cells may occasionally be encountered in schwannoma and neurofibroma, the differing basic nature of these tumors is readily apparent. For example, we have not encountered a schwannoma with widespread granular change, despite their frequent expression of CD68 immunoreactivity (see fig. 7-25D) (97). The three tumors bearing the closest histologic resemblance to GCT are congenital GCT or "epulis" (135,137), granular cell leiomyoma, and malignant GCT (57,72). Although *congenital GCT* or *epulis* shares many histologic similarities with benign GCT, important differences exist. The former arises exclusively on the alveolar ridge of newborns and histologically demonstrates a plexiform capillary pattern, not present in GCT. Unlike GCT, the cells of congenital gingival tumors lack globular cytoplasmic inclusions, S-100 protein (100,135,137) and neuron-specific enolase immunoreactivity (83), and an association with angulate body–containing histiocytes and pseudoepithelial hyperplasia. Furthermore, congenital GCT of the gingiva does not recur. Even if incompletely excised, the majority undergo spontaneous regression. Gingival GCT has no malignant counterpart (137). The distinction of GCT from *granular cell leiomyoma* may require either immunohistochemical staining for muscle markers such as HHF-35 and smooth muscle actin, or recourse to electron microscopy (57,72). Interestingly, granular cell change in smooth muscle tumors may be associated with immunoreactivity for neuron-specific enolase

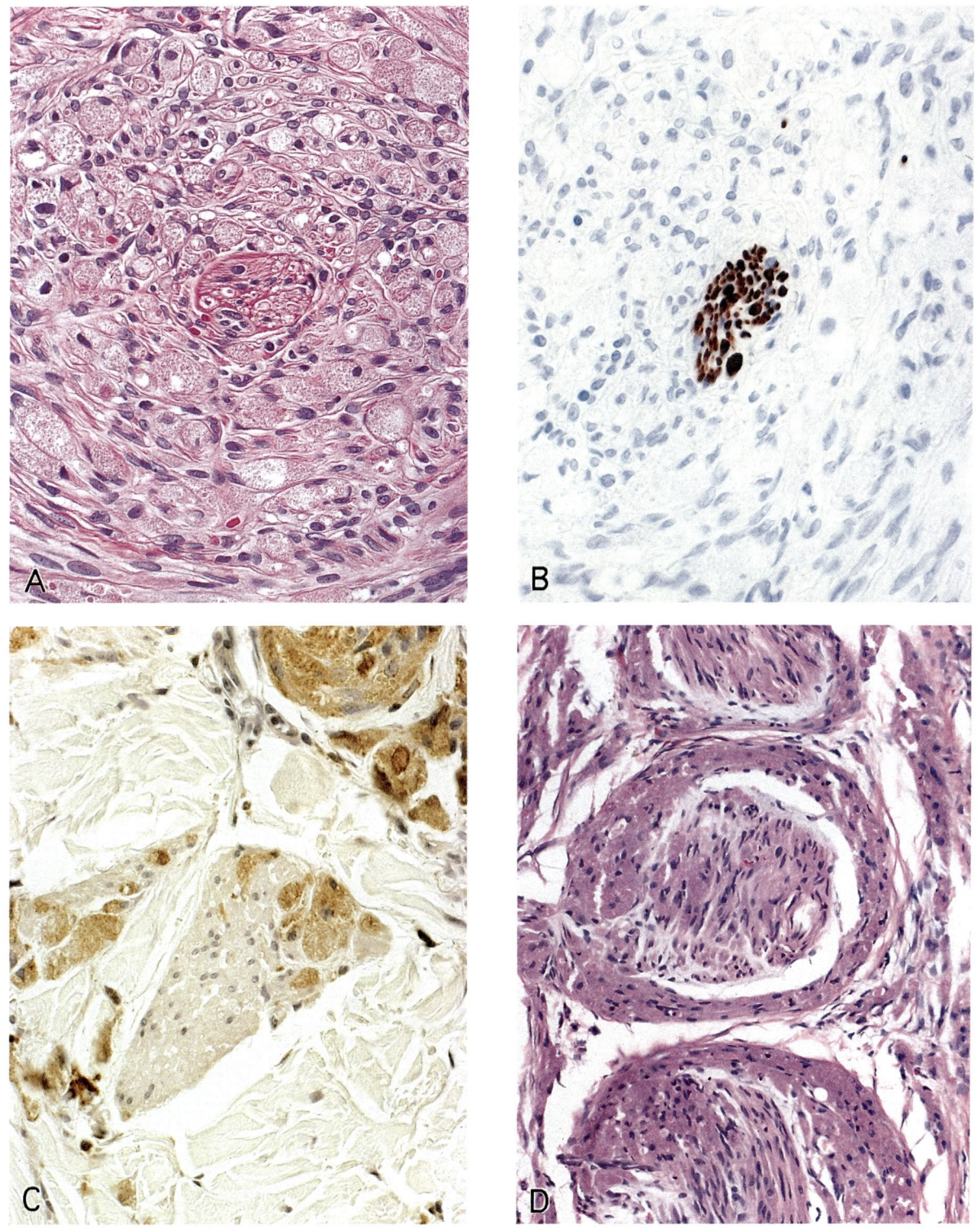

Figure 9-40
GRANULAR CELL TUMOR

Careful sampling sometimes shows GCTs to be associated with minute nerves (A), a feature highlighted by neurofilament protein immunostaining (B; same case as fig. 9-35). Although perineural growth is the rule, in some cases granular cells actually lie within the nerve (C, S-100 protein immunostain). On occasion, perineural involvement is conspicuous (D).

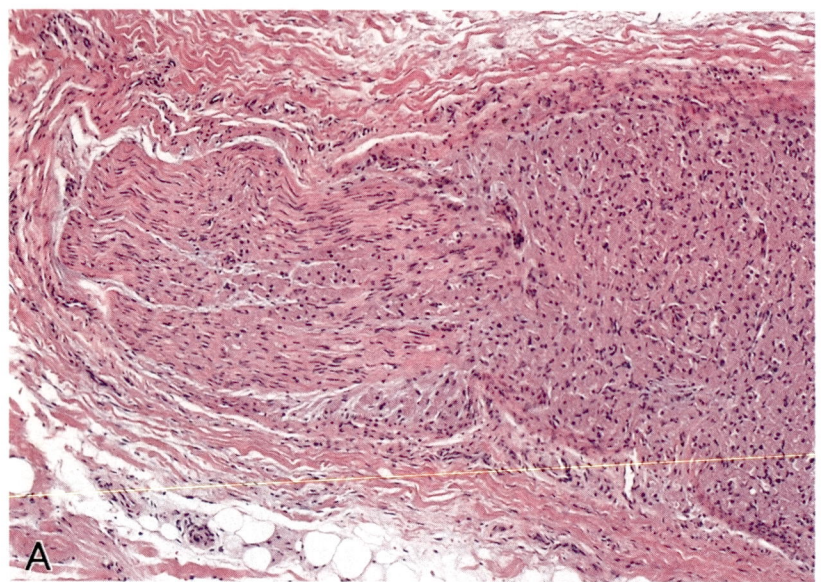

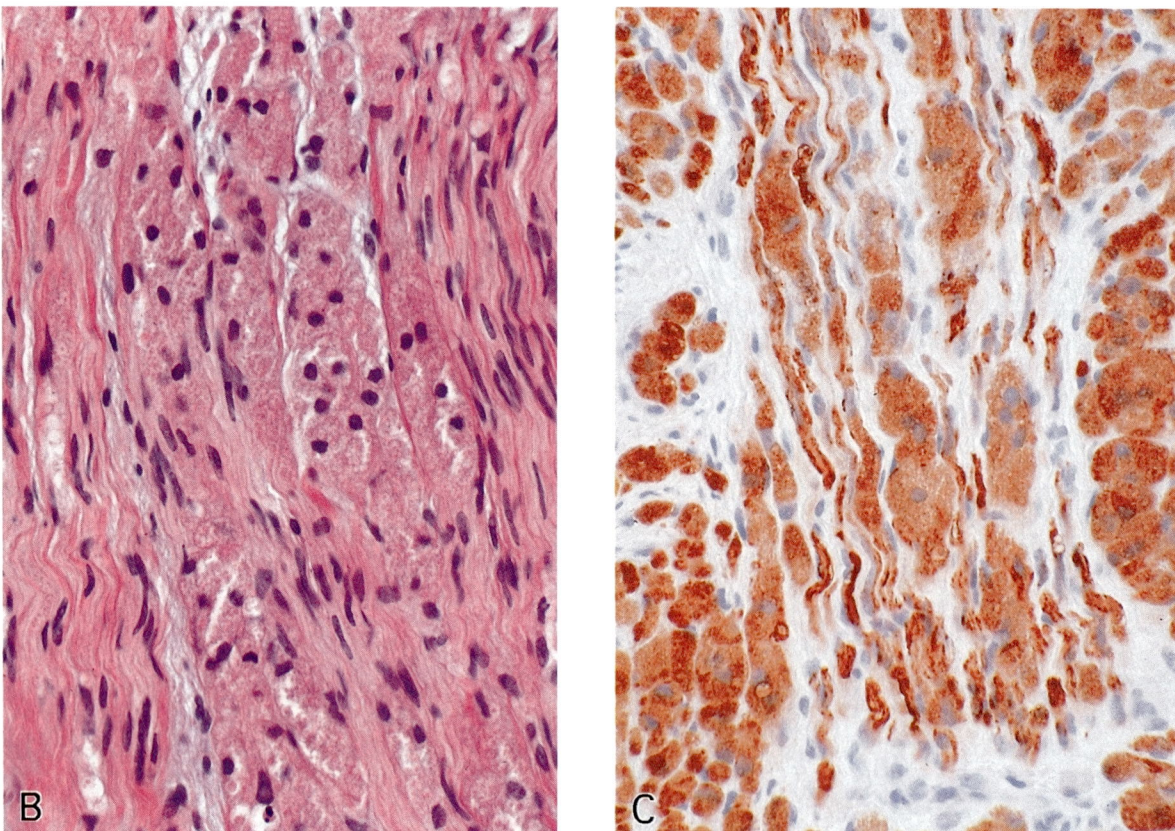

Figure 9-41

GRANULAR CELL TUMOR

This lesion arose in a grossly recognizable nerve. At low power (A), the contours of the affected nerve are still apparent (left). In addition to a solid growth phase (A, right), permeation of the nerve is readily seen at higher power (B). The granular cells are most apparent on S-100 protein immunostain (C). The latter permits comparison of the neoplastic cells to aligned Schwann cells of the underlying nerve.

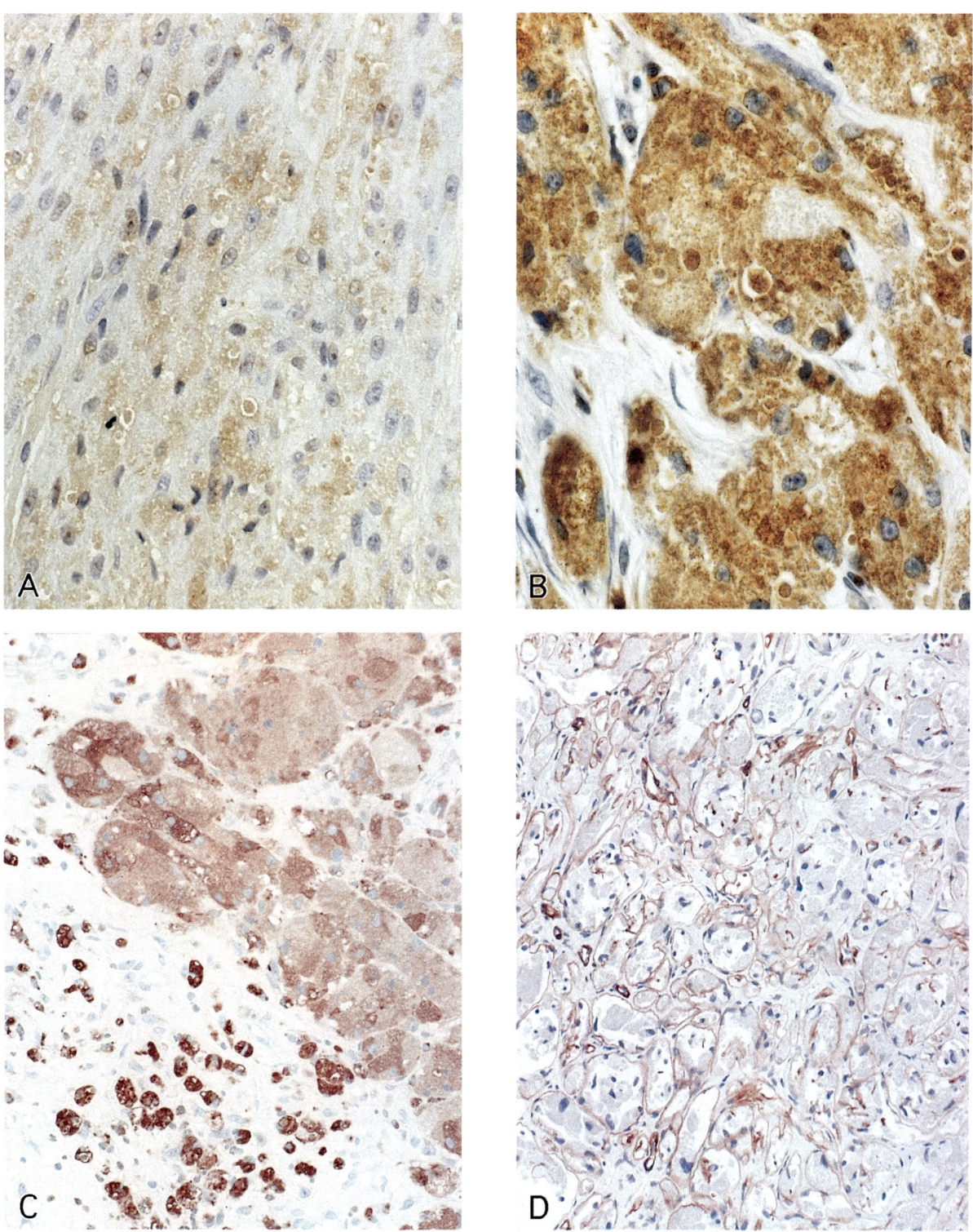

Figure 9-42
GRANULAR CELL TUMOR

Immunoreactivity for S-100 protein varies considerably from one tumor to the next (A,B). Staining for CD68 is also a typical feature of GCT (C); note stronger staining of the small stromal histiocytes than of tumor cells. Collagen 4 staining highlights basement membranes around cell clusters of varying size (D).

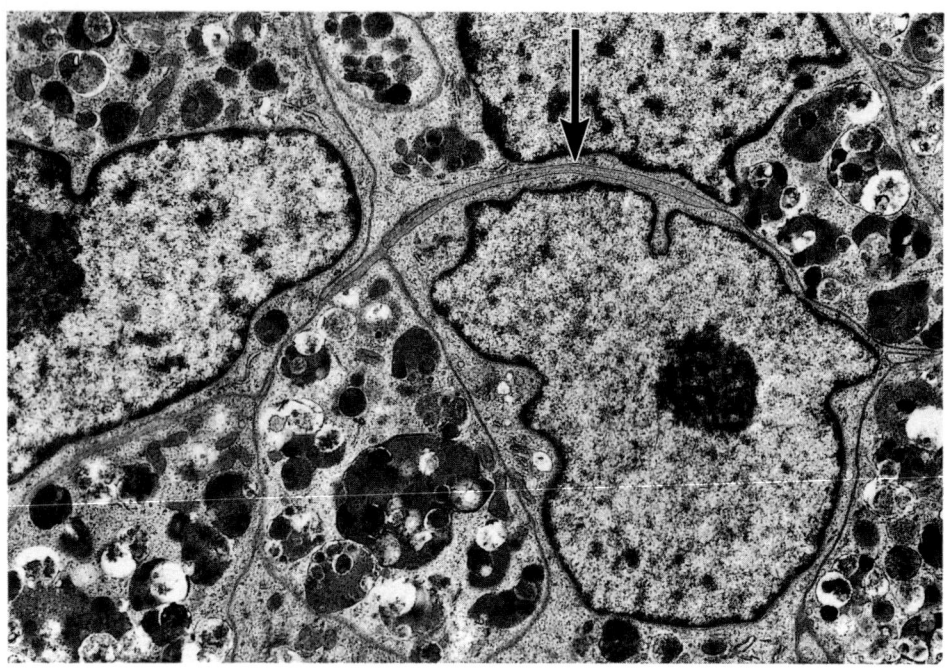

Figure 9-43
GRANULAR CELL TUMOR

Portions of clusters of Schwann cells contain numerous pleomorphic secondary lysosomes. Note the basement membrane (arrow) separating cell clusters (X10,100).

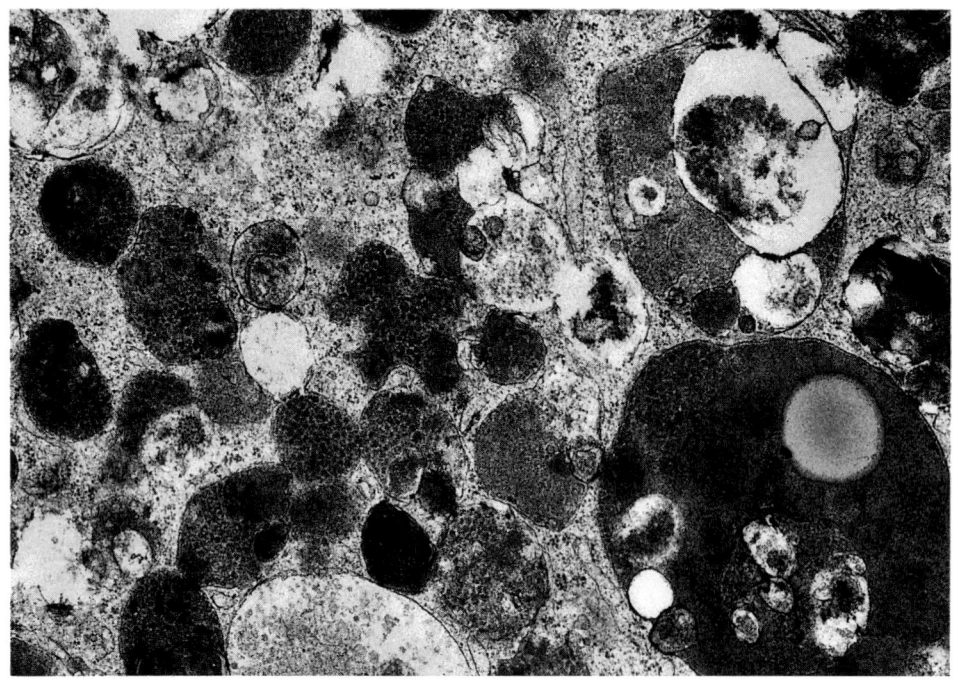

Figure 9-44
GRANULAR CELL TUMOR

Detail of the cytoplasm of a granular cell. Numerous pleomorphic secondary lysosomes are illustrated, as described in the text (X26,000).

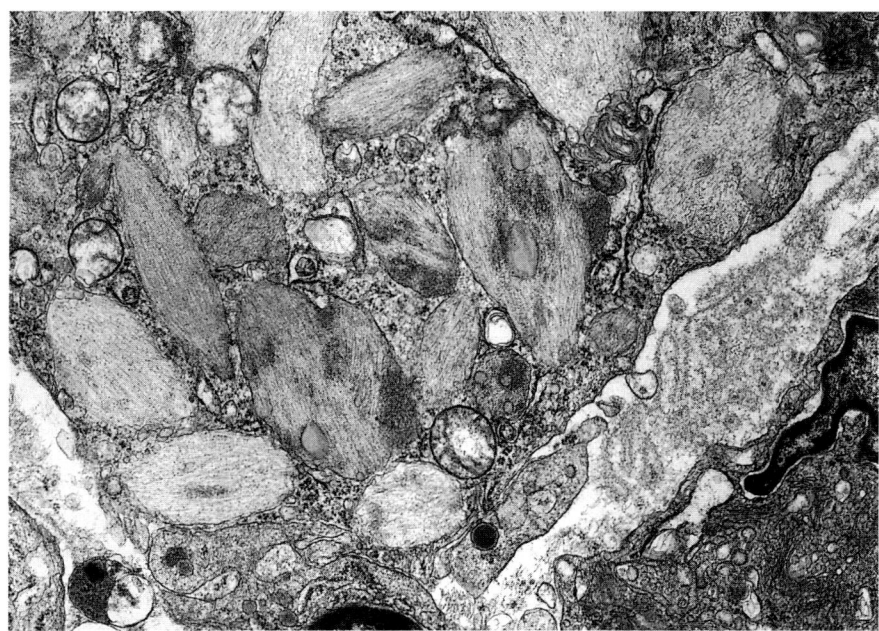

Figure 9-45
GRANULAR CELL TUMOR
Membrane limited angulate bodies (angulate lysosomes) containing numerous aligned microtubules are a common feature of the histiocytes associated with GCTs (X20,000).

and NKI/C3, a melanoma-associated antigen (108). Most clinically *malignant GCTs* are histologically indistinguishable from benign GCT. The remainder show cellular pleomorphism, marked hyperchromasia, mitotic activity, and focal necrosis, features lacking in benign examples. Unlike *rhabdomyoma,* GCTs lack cytoplasmic cross striations as well as immunohistochemical and ultrastructural features of myogenic differentiation. Unlike *hibernomas,* the cells of GCTs do not have vacuolated cytoplasm. Finally, intracerebral *astrocytic tumors* with granular cell features can be distinguished from benign GCT by the lack of GFAP staining in the latter (106,117,118).

Treatment and Prognosis. The recommended treatment of benign GCT is local excision, preferably with negative margins. The recurrence rate is estimated at 2 to 8 percent when margins of resection are deemed free of involvement, and 21 to 50 percent after incomplete excision (60).

GANGLIONEUROMA

Definition. This benign neoplasm is composed of mature autonomic ganglion cells, satellite cells, and an abundance of unmyelinated as well as occasional myelinated axons with their accompanying Schwann cells, all in a fibrous stroma.

General Comments. Although originally described by Loritz in 1870 (169), it was Stout (188)

who first summarized the clinicopathologic features of ganglioneuromatous tumors. In doing so, he found that a minority of cases were composite tumors containing either a diffuse admixture or localized collections of neuroblastoma cells; such lesions metastasized at rates of 18 and 65 percent, respectively. In contrast, tumors lacking neuroblastoma cells did not metastasize. Such "fully differentiated" examples he referred to as ganglioneuromas. Although they had a benign clinical outcome, a postoperative mortality rate of 10 percent was noted in instances in which resection was aggressive. As a result, Stout emphasized the need to distinguish histologically between pure ganglioneuroma and similar tumors which in addition contained less differentiated components.

The origin of ganglioneuroma, particularly its relationship to neuroblastic neoplasms, remains unsettled. There is little doubt that the ganglion cells present in all ganglioneuromas at one time had their origin in neuroblasts. However, whether most ganglioneuromas are distinct from neuroblastoma in having uniformly matured at a pace approximating that of normal development is unclear. Maturation to ganglioneuroma by neuroblastoma or ganglioneuroblastoma is also known to occur, both at primary sites, either spontaneously or after therapy, and in metastases (153,155,156,160,170,186). The occurrence of such maturation suggests that a proportion of ganglioneuromas may represent fully differentiated neuroblastomas, despite differences in patient age and tumor distribution (see below).

Ganglioneuromas may occur in association with or transition from other neuroectodermal tumors. Examples of the former include concurrent ganglioneuroma and schwannoma of the vagus nerve (162), and the association of an adrenal ganglioneuroma in neurofibromatosis type 1 (NF1) (161). Examples of the latter are referred to as "composite tumors" and include ganglioneuroma arising from pheochromocytoma (175), to be discussed below, and the occurrence of ganglioneuromatous components in extra-adrenal paragangliomas, such as of the cauda equina region (183,187) and duodenum (182).

Ganglioneuroma is a tumor of older children and young adults. At presentation the majority of patients are between 10 and 20 years of age. The lesion also shows a distinct female predilection. Most patients come to attention due to the tumor's mass effect or its incidental finding at physical examination or imaging studies. Occasional examples are first noted at autopsy.

Ganglioneuromas rarely occur in animals, but have been reported to arise in association with C cell hyperplasia in the rat thyroid (152).

Clinical Features. Ganglioneuromas most commonly arise at sites in which sympathetic ganglia are found, specifically the mediastinum, retroperitoneum, and pelvis. They represent 5 percent of all tumors of the mediastinum, a site at which most are paraspinal. Also frequently affected are retroperitoneal sympathetic ganglia and the adrenal medulla. Most pelvic examples are presacral or coccygeal. Less common are skull base, parapharyngeal region, and cranial nerve ganglia lesions (162). Aware of examples involving such odd sites as the uterus, ovary, kidney, breast, and vulva, Stout (188) anticipated the finding of ganglioneuromas at further unusual sites. Their reported occurrence in viscera (see below), choroid of the eye (191), posterior cranial fossa (165), spinal intradural space (168), and mandible (194) have proven him right. Although ganglioneuromatous tumors occur in skin (159), the architecture of some (167,179) differs significantly from that of classic ganglioneuroma.

Although most ganglioneuromas arise in sympathetic ganglia, a minority originate in viscera.

Whether they represent parasympathetic counterparts to the ganglioneuromas noted above remains to be determined, but it is convenient to view them as such.

Visceral involvement by ganglioneuromatous proliferations as a whole is broadly divided into diffuse and localized varieties. Diffuse examples, such as occur in the alimentary tract in the setting of multiple endocrine neoplasia type IIb (MEN IIb), are discussed in chapter 5. Localized visceral ganglioneuromas unassociated with a heritable syndrome are rare. Unlike neurofibromas occurring in the setting of NF1, most of which arise in stomach and small bowel, localized visceral ganglioneuromas affect primarily the colon and rectum (148). Appendiceal lesions have also been reported (195) as have localized ganglioneuromas of lung (171), urinary bladder (192), and prostate (178); the latter tumor occurred in a patient with NF1. Visceral ganglioneuromas are generally smaller than their soft tissue counterparts and lack a neuroblastoma association.

A minority of ganglioneuromas are endocrinologically functional: best known is their association with the "watery diarrhea syndrome" (Verner-Morrison syndrome), a condition mediated by tumoral production of vasoactive intestinal polypeptide (VIP). This hormone may be elaborated by differentiating and mature ganglion cells in ganglioneuroma and ganglioneuroblastoma, as well as in composite ganglioneuroma-pheochromocytoma (173,190). Not surprisingly, such composite tumors may also be associated with hypertension (175). Virilization is rarely observed (145). One ganglioneuroma was reportedly associated with myasthenia gravis (177). Elevation of urinary catecholamine metabolites, including vanylmandelic acid and homovanillic acid, may be seen in association with pure ganglioneuromas. Levels appear to be related to tumor size (169a). Significant elevations (more than three times normal) should prompt a careful search for a neuroblastoma component.

Although uncommon, the association of ganglioneuroma with NF1 is well established. In addition, ganglioneuromas are occasionally familial but unassociated with a specific syndrome (180). Whether heritable or sporadic in occurrence, ganglioneuromas are far less common than are schwannoma and neurofibroma.

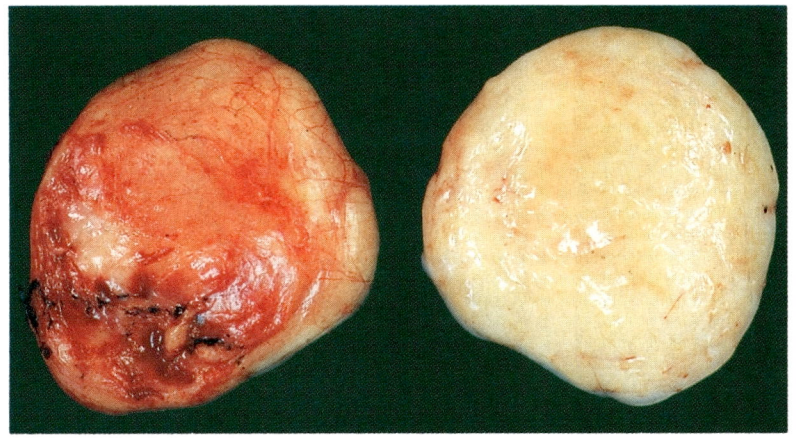

Figure 9-46
GANGLIONEUROMA
Grossly (top) most ganglioneuromas are ovoid in shape, but unlike schwannomas are often flattened rather than globoid. A thick pancake shape is common. Occasional examples are multilobate. Microsections show them to be enveloped by a thin fibrous pseudocapsule (bottom).

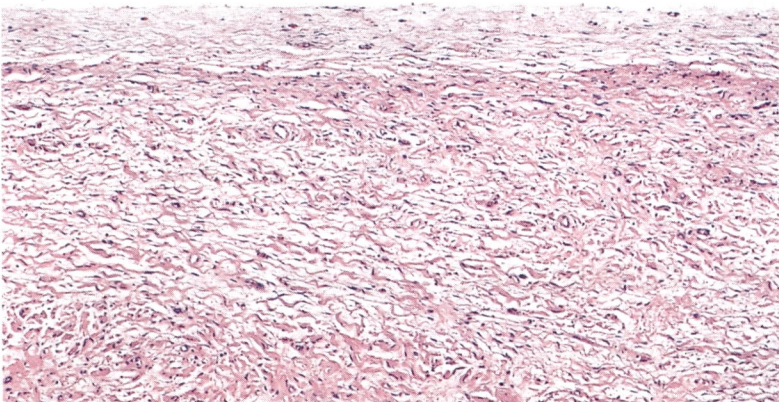

Radiographic Findings. Radiographically, ganglioneuromas appear as solitary, smooth-contoured masses. Paraspinous tumors are often associated with expansion of a spinal foramen and occasionally with intraspinal extension. On computerized tomography (CT) ganglioneuromas are sharply defined masses that show soft tissue attenuation. Delicate or amorphous calcification is occasionally seen, but is far less frequent than in neuroblastoma. Contrast enhancement is most pronounced on magnetic resonance imaging (MRI) scans which also show cyst formation the best. On ultrasound, ganglioneuromas are hypoechoic and hypovascular.

Gross Findings. Ganglioneuromas are large, circumscribed, smooth-contoured masses of varied ovoid shapes (figs. 9-46–9-49). Most are smaller than 15 cm, but rare tumors attain a size of 50 cm and weigh up to 6 kg. Although they appear grossly encapsulated, ganglioneuromas often possess only

a thin pseudocapsule (fig. 9-46). Focally, some tumors exhibit a direct, irregular interface with adjacent soft tissue (fig. 9-49, right). In such instances, adherence to surrounding tissue may complicate resection. The same is true of tumors with an irregular contour that encompasses vital anatomic structures (fig. 9-49). In all but their shape, which is globular to lobulate rather than fusiform, ganglioneuromas grossly resemble neurofibroma. Nearly all ganglioneuromas are solitary; only rare examples have been multiple, as in one instance in which several tumors involved an entire segment of the sympathetic chain (185). The majority are solid, but cyst formation may be seen (fig. 9-48). Only a minority of ganglioneuromas show gross calcification. On cut surface most are firm, homogeneous or patchy light tan, and often somewhat translucent (figs. 9-46, 9-47).

Ganglioneuromatous maturation is known to occur in pheochromocytoma. On occasion the two

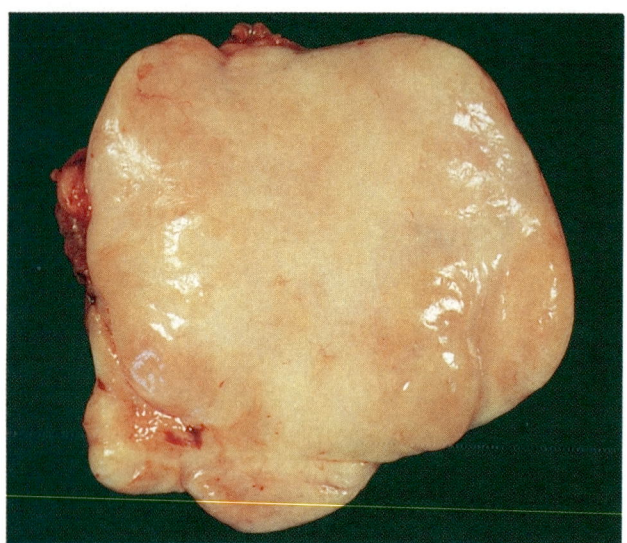
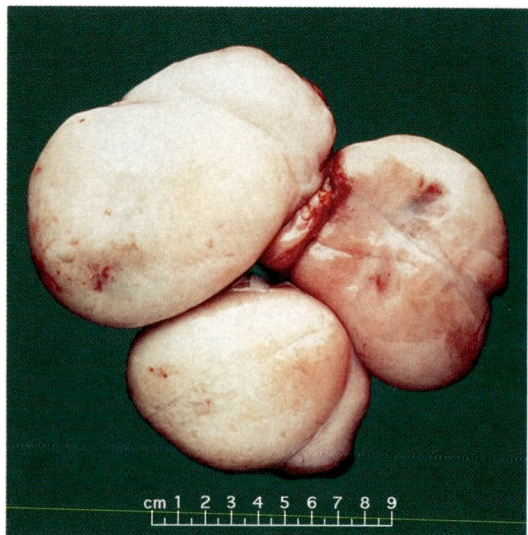

Figure 9-47
GANGLIONEUROMA
The cut surfaces of these posterior mediastinal examples vary from soft, pale, translucent, and mucin-rich (left) to firm and somewhat fibrous (right). The range closely resembles that exhibited by neurofibroma, and is a reflection of the uniform cellularity of the lesion.

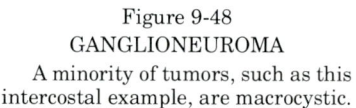

Figure 9-48
GANGLIONEUROMA
A minority of tumors, such as this intercostal example, are macrocystic.

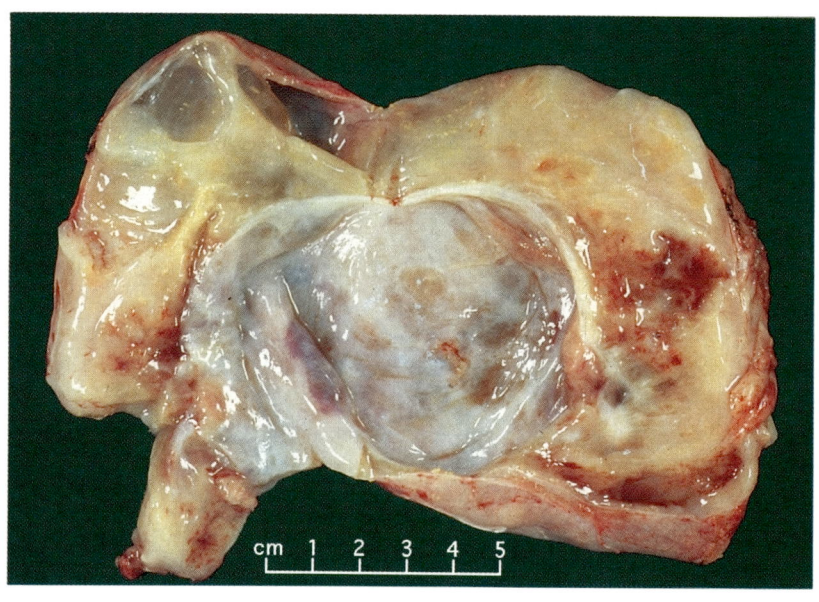

elements are grossly evident, the tan ganglioneuroma component being distinct from the red-brown pheochromocytoma (figs. 9-50A,B). The two components may also be dramatically highlighted by fixation in Zenker's solution which shows the pheochromocytoma to be strongly chromaffin positive (dark brown). Microsections usually show the two tumor elements to be spatially distinct (fig. 9-50C). With the exception of a single example occurring in the region of the organs of Zuckerkandl (193), composite tumors reported to date have all arisen in the adrenal gland. In one instance, the process was bilateral (151).

Microscopic Findings. The essential features of ganglioneuroma include ganglion cells, their long axonal processes with accompanying

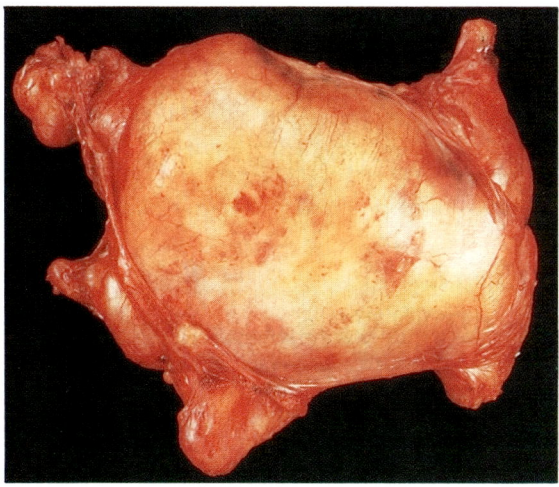

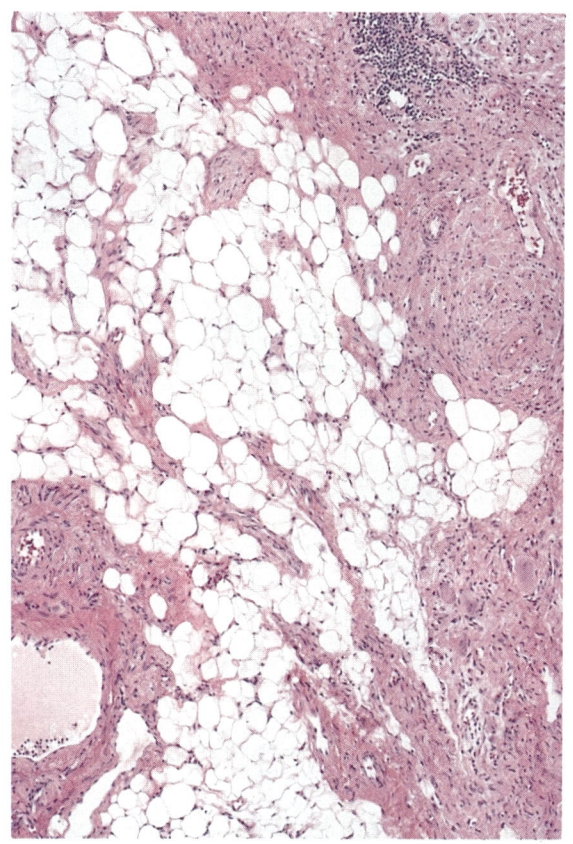

Figure 9-49
GANGLIONEUROMA

Above: Irregular in contour, with peripheral lobulation, this posterior mediastinal lesion was adherent to surrounding structures.

Right: Occasional tumors lack complete encapsulation and focally infiltrate surrounding soft tissue.

Schwann sheaths, and satellite cells which encompass the ganglion cells (fig. 9-51). By thorough sampling, the presence of neuroblasts and a diagnosis of ganglioneuroblastoma must be excluded. Ganglion cells within ganglioneuromas may be either localized (fig. 9-51B) or widely scattered (fig. 9-51C). As a result, individual histologic sections may lack ganglion cells almost entirely, and consist only of fields of neuritic processes with ensheathing Schwann cells (fig. 9-52C). Indeed, the shear number of neuritic processes in ganglioneuromas often appears out of all proportion to the number of parent ganglion cells. Compactly arrayed or loose textured, the processes typically form aligned, entangled bundles (fig. 9-52A,B). The microscopic appearance of the bundles varies with their orientation (fig. 9-53). Despite considerable morphologic variation (fig. 9-54), ganglion cells are well differentiated and readily recognized by: 1) their size which, due to varying amounts of often abundant eosinophilic to amphophilic cytoplasm, is generally greater than 20 μm; 2) the

presence of single or multiple vesicular nuclei which are often eccentrically placed and feature prominent single nucleoli; and 3) the finding of Nissl substance, which varies from scant to relatively abundant (fig. 9-55A). Cytologic abnormalities include pleomorphism, multinucleation, vacuolation, and the presence of large, often pale, spherical cytoplasmic inclusions (fig. 9-54C,D), some resembling Lewy bodies. Secretory granules may be evident on argyrophil (Grimelius) stain, but this is not a uniform feature (fig. 9-55B). Surrounding the ganglion cells are varying numbers of satellite cells, modified Schwann cells with often flattened nuclei. As a rule, their number and uniformity of distribution falls short of that seen in normal ganglia. As previously noted, axons are abundant. Although silver stains, such as Bodian or Bielschowsky preparations, stain the axons, their small diameter makes them difficult to see (fig. 9-55C). Binding of peanut agglutinin, a marker of advanced neuronal differentiation, also labels ganglion cells and their processes

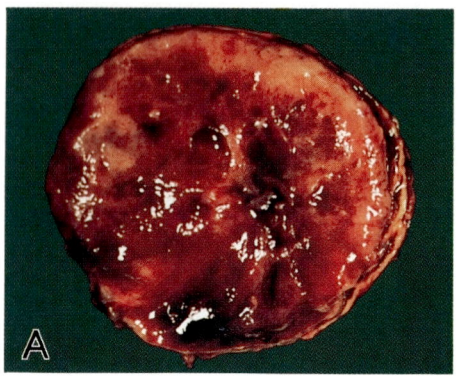

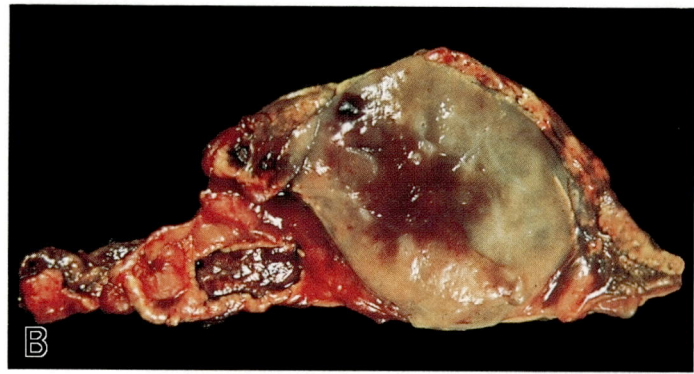

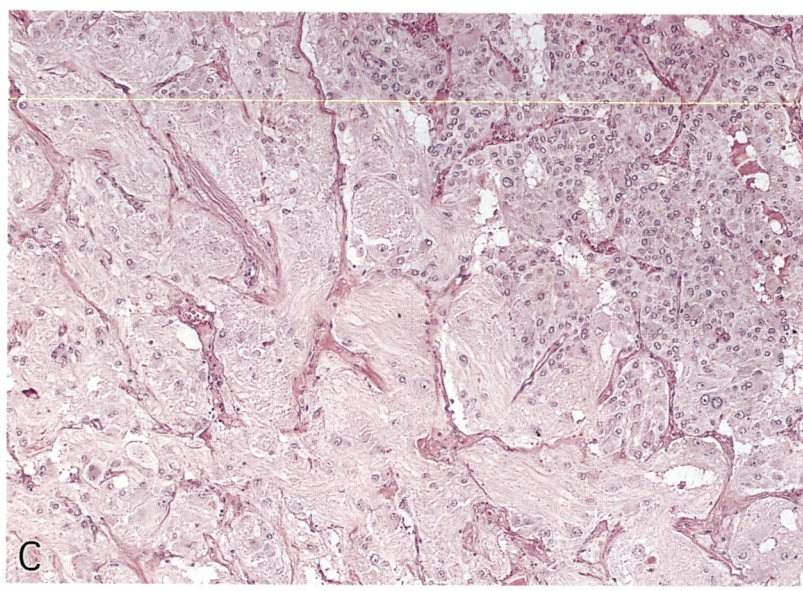

Figure 9-50
GANGLIONEUROMATOUS
MATURATION OF
PHEOCHROMOCYTOMA
(COMPOSITE
PHEOCHROMOCYTOMA—
GANGLIONEUROMA)
The process may be grossly evident and varies in extent. Firm and cream colored, such foci may be limited, as beneath the capsule (A), or may comprise the majority of the tumor (B). Microscopically, the two components are typically distinct (C). (A and B, courtesy of Dr. J. A. Carney, Rochester, MN.)

(163). Although Schwann cell cytoplasm surrounds axons, myelination is usually limited to entrapped normal nerve fibers (fig. 9-56). For this reason, myelin stains, such as the Luxol-fast blue, are generally negative (fig. 9-55D). If present, residual normal sympathetic ganglion tissue is recognized by its characteristic anatomic distribution of ganglion cells and by the traversing, aligned nerve fiber bundles (see fig. 2-17).

Ganglioneuromas often undergo degenerative changes. For instance, ganglion cells come to contain brown cytoplasmic pigment (fig. 9-57A), consisting not of true melanin but of pigmented lysosomes or "neuromelanin" (158). Both argyrophil and argentaffin positive, it differs from lipofuscin in that it lacks PAS and acid-fast reactivity, and does not autofluoresce (176). Stromal degenerative changes are also common, particularly in large tumors. These include mainly

fibrosis or some degree of mucin accumulation as occurs in neurofibroma (fig. 9-57B). As a result, Alcian blue positivity may be evident and trichrome stains may show impressive collagen deposition. The presence of adipose tissue in occasional ganglioneuromas usually takes the form of ill-defined lobules at the periphery of a tumor (fig. 9-49, right). Vascular hyalinization may be the basis of focal hemorrhage and of resultant cystic change. When present, lymphocytic infiltrates are usually centered upon vessels (fig. 9-57C); they should not be mistaken for neuroblasts. The distinction is readily made on leukocyte common antigen (LCA) immunostain. Mast cells may also be present in small number. Whereas coarse, patchy calcification is common, psammoma bodies are only rarely found (151).

Although in most cases of composite ganglioneuroma-pheochromocytoma the two components

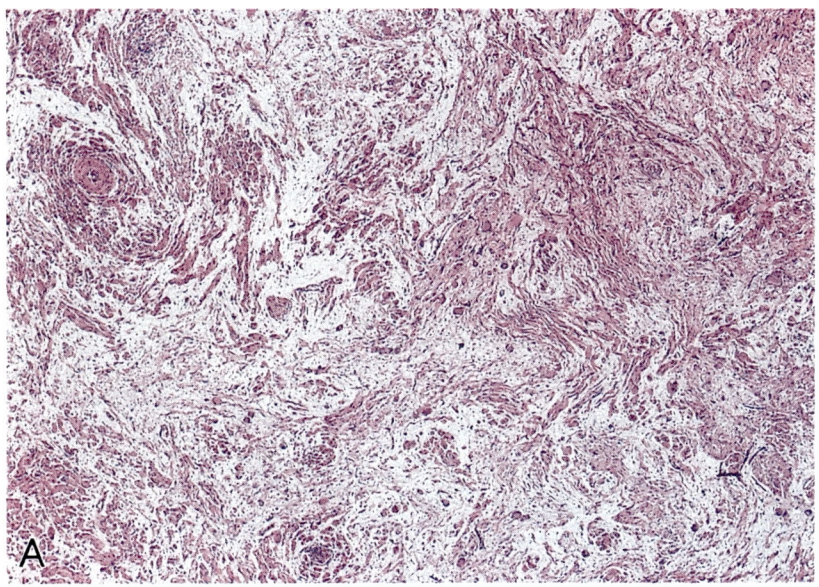

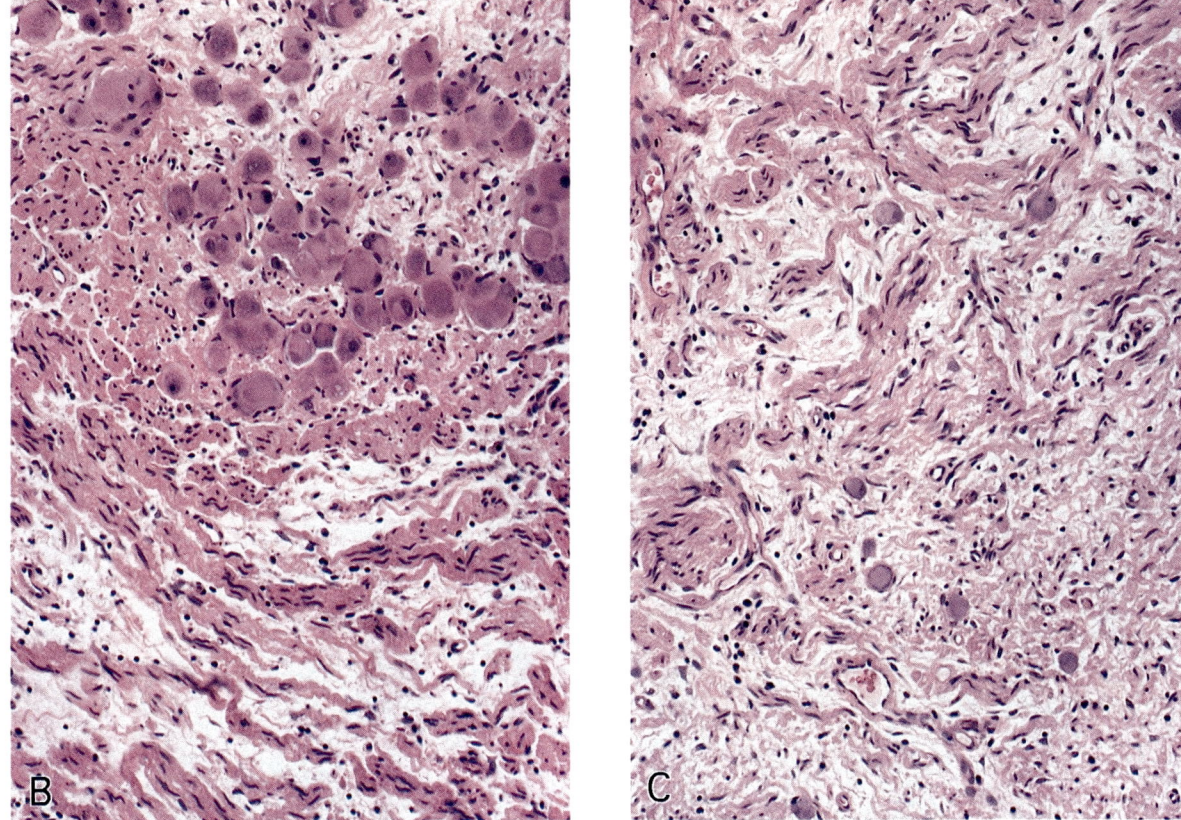

Figure 9-51
GANGLIONEUROMA

The essential components of this tumor include ganglion cells, their processes, and ensheathing Schwann cells (A). These vary in proportion and in their distribution. This example exhibited areas with numerous, concentrated ganglion cells (B) and other areas in which they were dispersed (C).

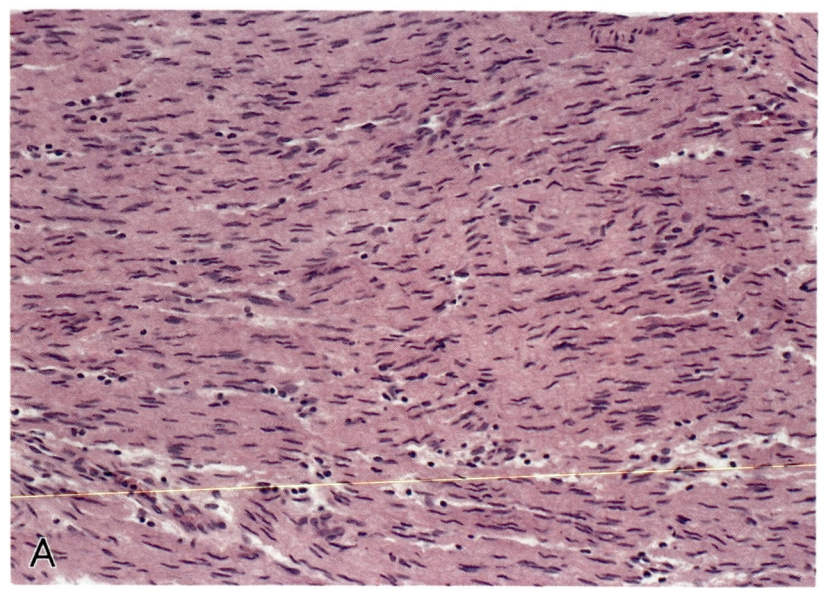

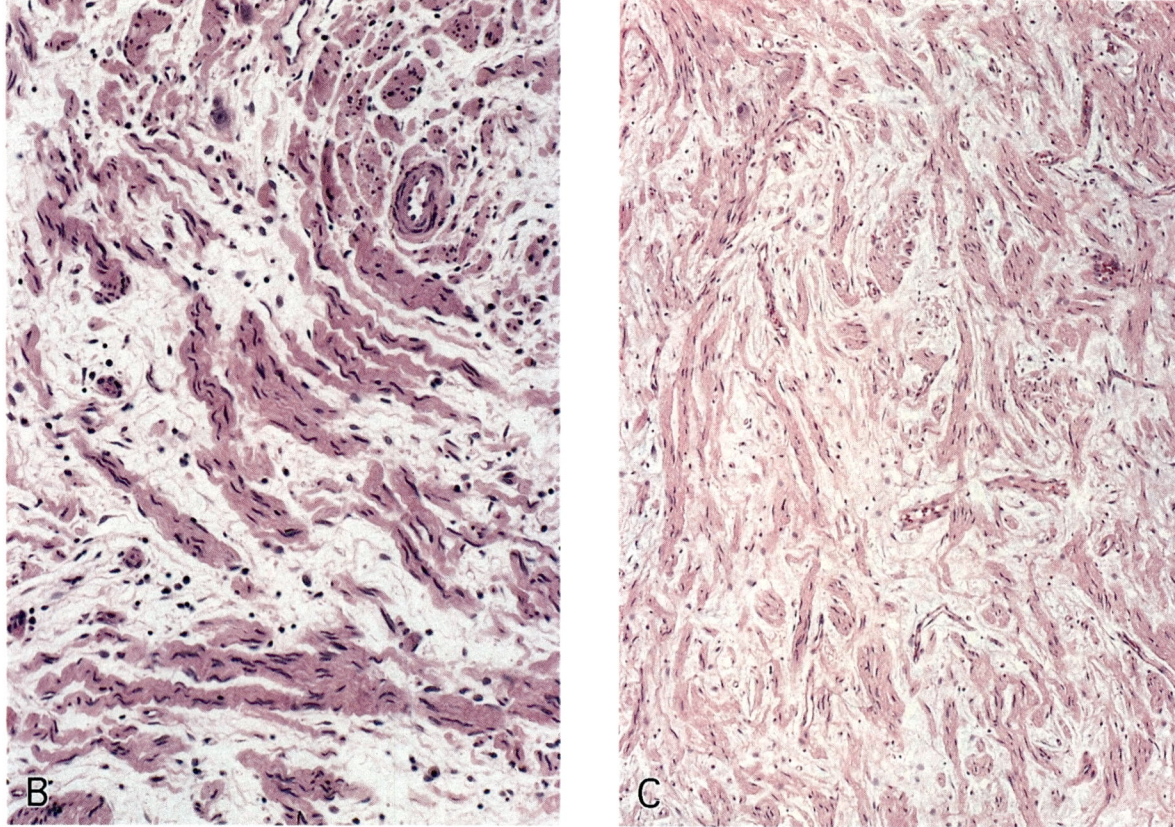

Figure 9-52
GANGLIONEUROMA

The arrangement of nerve fibers varies from compact, aligned bundles, the appearance of which mimics that of schwannoma (A), to fields wherein nerve fiber bundles of varying size are dispersed (B). Short of the finding of scattered ganglion cells, the jumbled bundles may mimic the pattern of a neurofibroma (C).

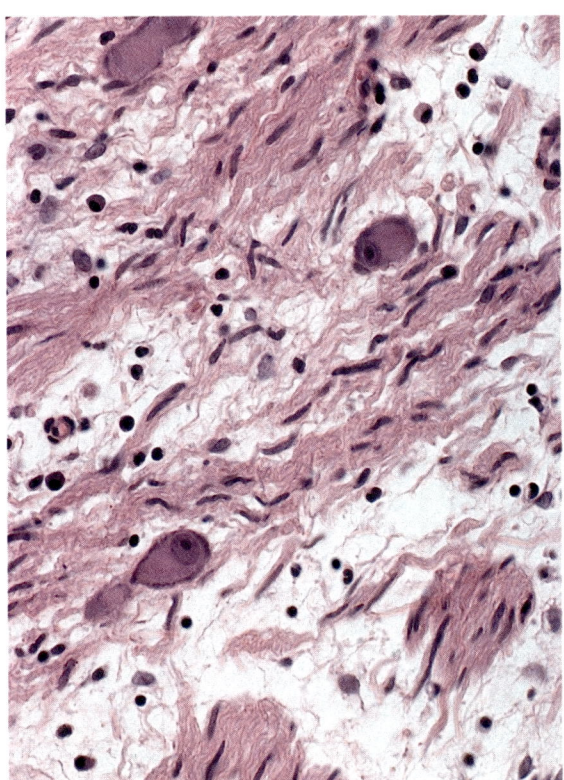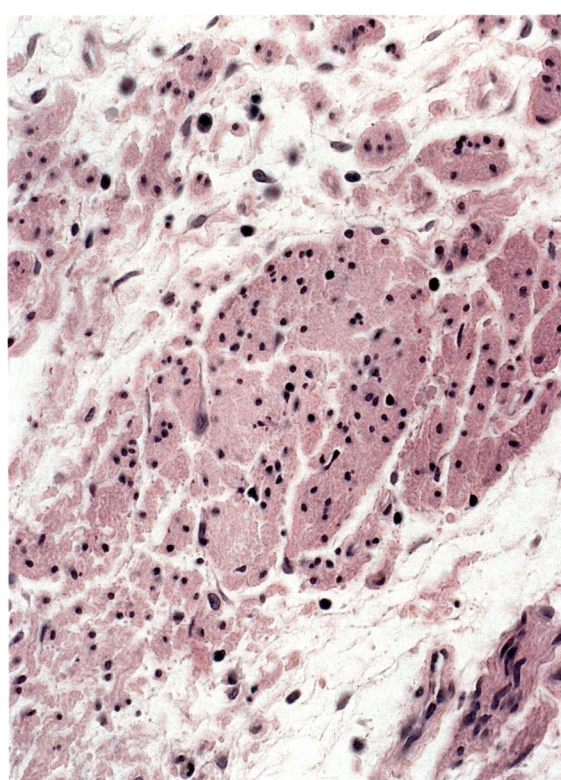

Figure 9-53
GANGLIONEUROMA
Whether longitudinally (left) or cross cut (right), nerve fiber bundles vary markedly in appearance.

are minimally admixed (fig. 9-50C) (146,151, 173,190,193), one example arising in nodular and diffuse adrenal medullary hyperplasia of MEN IIb (150) showed a clear transition of pheochromocytes to intermediate cells and ganglion cells. Although cells of all three types exhibited tyrosine hydroxylase activity, the process of transition was accompanied by loss of phenylethanolamine-N-methyltransferase, the enzyme that synthesizes epinephrine. One morphologically unique, testosterone-secreting adrenal ganglioneuroma consisted in part of nodules of Leydig cells containing lipochrome pigment and Reinke crystalloids (145).

Immunohistochemical Findings. Ganglion cells and their axonal processes stain for synaptophysin (fig. 9-58A), neurofilament protein (fig. 9-58B), and tubulin, as well as for neuron-specific enolase, a rather nonspecific marker of neuronal differentiation (147,181). Staining for neurofilament protein includes reactivity for the high molecular weight phosphorylated epitope

(174,189). The Schwann cell element of ganglioneuroma exhibits strong staining for S-100 protein (fig. 9-58C) and may also show myelin basic protein (189) as well as GFAP expression. In addition, collagen 4 reactivity highlights the basal lamina surrounding Schwann cells. Although chromogranin A staining within the cytoplasm of ganglion cells is said to be a regular finding (189), we have found it to vary (fig. 9-59, left). Of hormones elaborated by ganglioneuroma, VIP is the best known (fig. 9-59, right) (173,190). This substance is frequently demonstrable in differentiating and mature ganglion cells, even in lesions unassociated with the watery diarrhea syndrome (fig. 9-59, right). Calcitonin immunoreactivity has also been reported (173).

Ultrastructural Findings. The fine structural features of ganglioneuroma are similar to those of mature sympathetic ganglia. The ganglion cells are characterized by 1) large, round to oval, electron-lucent nuclei with prominent nucleoli; 2) abundant cytoplasm containing well-developed,

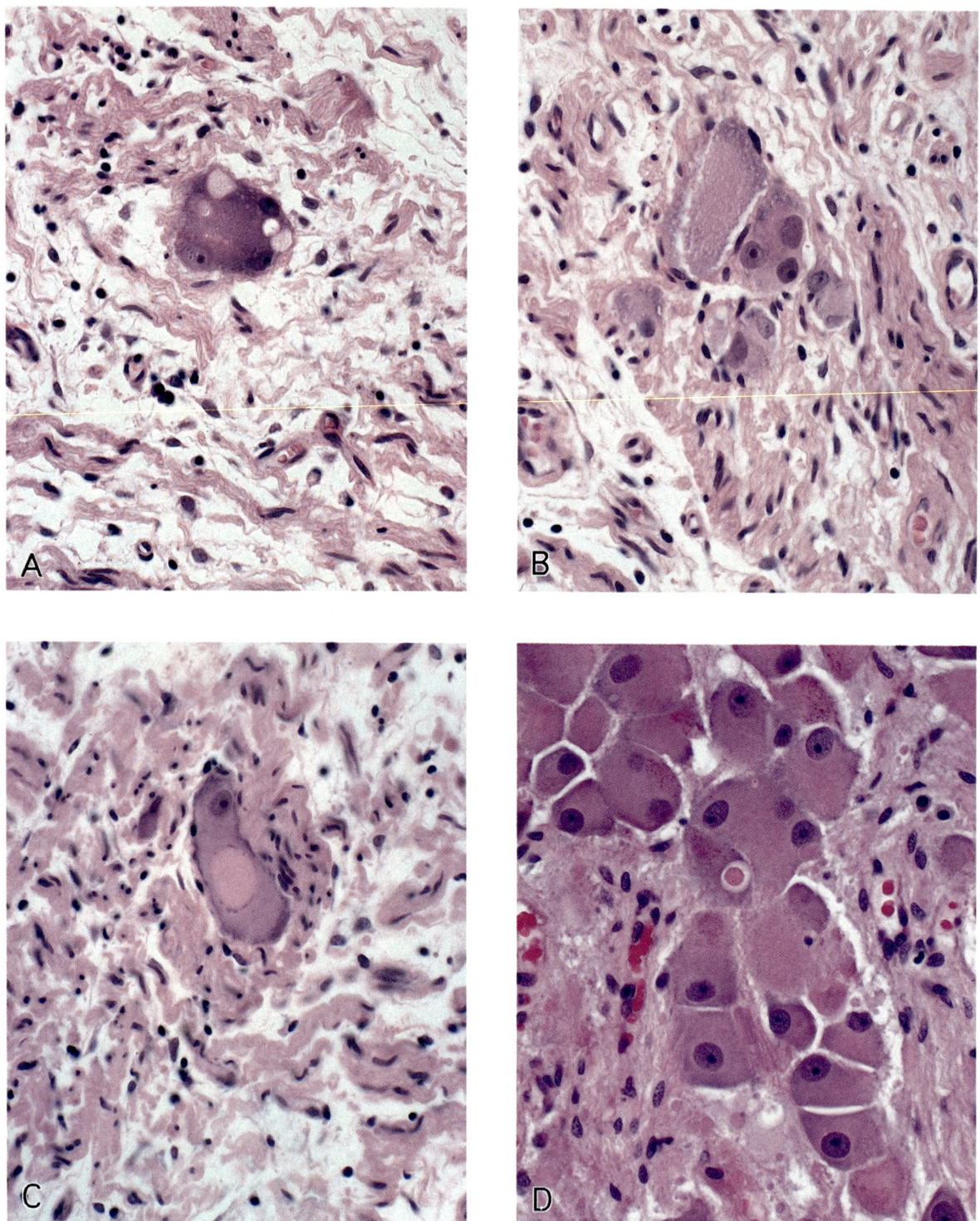

Figure 9-54
GANGLIONEUROMA

Even at high power the distribution of ganglion cells varies, some being isolated (A), others clustered (B). Many but not all contain abundant Nissl substance. Note large vesicular nuclei and prominent nucleoli, hallmarks of ganglion cells. Cytologic abnormalities are common and include multinucleation (A,B), vacuolation (A), and spherical, eosinophilic cytoplasmic masses (C,D), some closely resembling Lewy bodies (D; see also fig. 9-58). (D courtesy of Dr. Jon Wilson, New York, NY.)

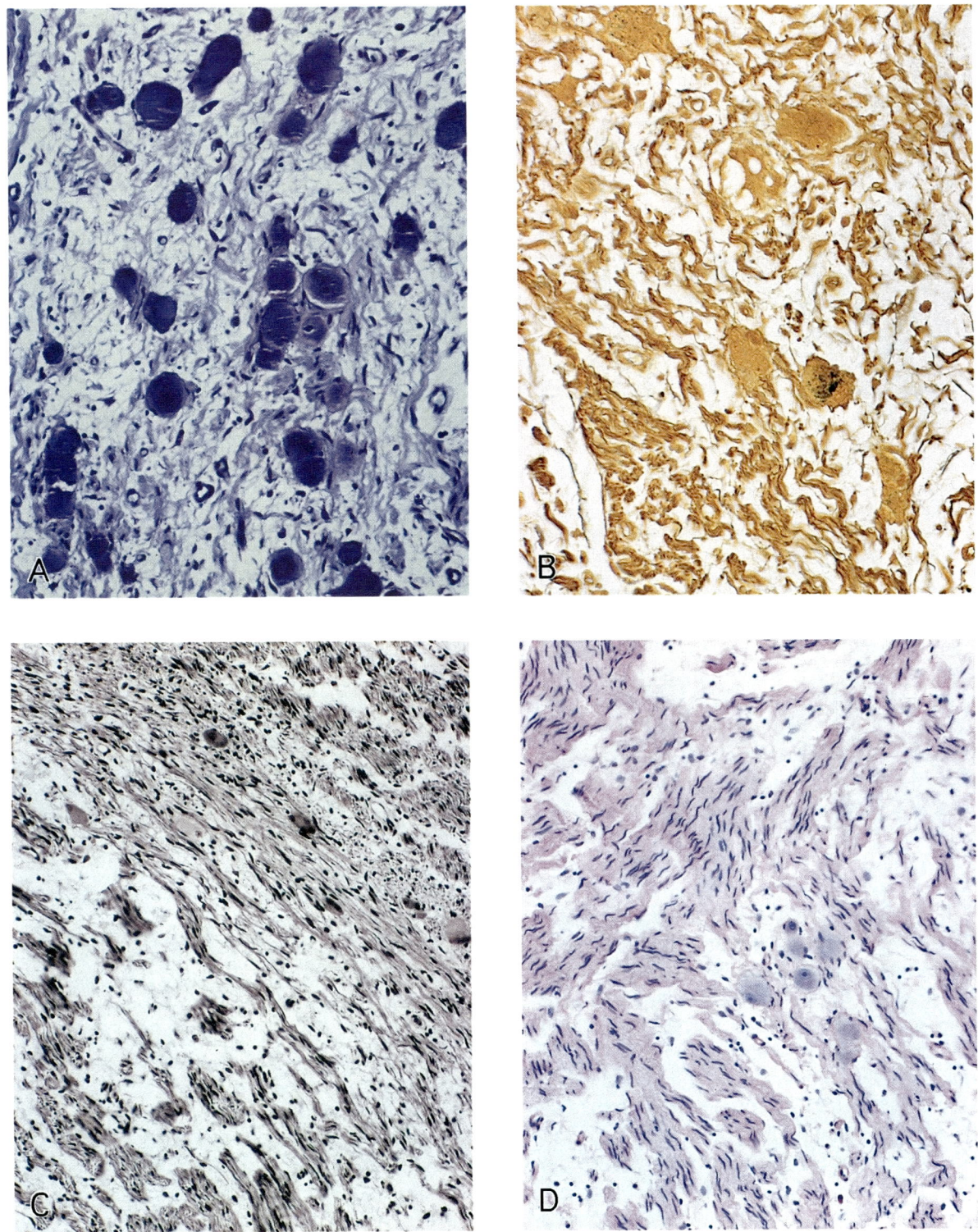

Figure 9-55
GANGLIONEUROMA

Ganglion cells vary in their content of Nissl substance (A) and argyrophilic granules (B). Their processes are readily visualized on silver impregnations (C), but myelin stains are typically negative (D). (A, cresyl violet; B, Grimelius; C, Bielschowsky; D, Luxol-fast blue–periodic acid–Schiff stains.)

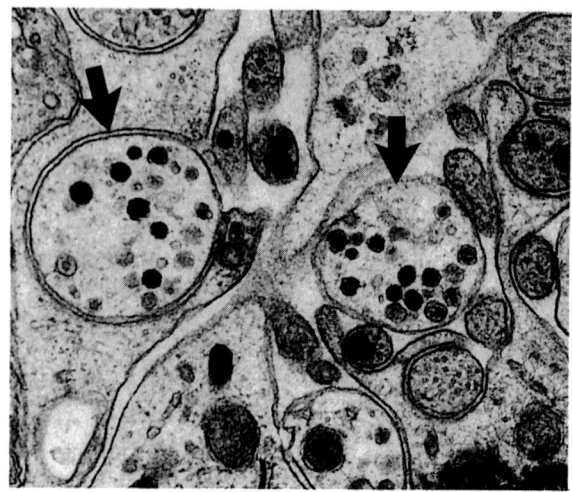

Figure 9-56
GANGLIONEUROMA

Two cross-sectioned axons (arrows) contain dense-core neurosecretory granules with an average diameter of 100 nm (X27,000).

often dilated rough endoplasmic reticulum; 3) a prominent Golgi apparatus and numerous pleomorphic secondary lysosomes; 4) bundles of intermediate filaments (neurofilaments) which extend into proximal processes; 5) scattered microtubules; and 6) dense core neurosecretory granules ranging in diameter from 90 to 130 nm (figs. 9-56, 9-60). In one case, 125-nm granules were thought to correlate with the presence of calcitonin, and coexisting 350-nm granules with VIP (173). Rarely seen presynaptic terminations of axons reportedly contain 40- to 60-nm vesicles. Tubular inclusions (172) and Pick-like bodies (149) also have been reported to occur within the cytoplasm of ganglion cells. While most axons are unmyelinated, scattered myelinated examples, presumably overrun normal nerve fibers, are found in many tumors (fig. 9-61). The flattened satellite cells encompassing ganglion cells are surrounded by basal lamina on their external surface (fig. 9-60). The interstitium of ganglioneuroma contains varying quantities of collagen fibrils and scattered Luse bodies (long-spacing collagen). Ultrastructural studies, while useful in delineating architecture and cellular makeup of ganglioneuroma, are generally not required for diagnosis.

Differential Diagnosis. Ganglioneuroma is readily distinguished from *neurofibroma* and

schwannoma, both of which lack both a ganglion cell component and abundant unmyelinated nerve fibers. Confusion only arises at surgery, on gross examination, and at microscopy in cases in which these *nerve sheath tumors* overrun *dorsal root* or *sympathetic ganglia* (fig. 9-62). The residua of normal ganglia are characterized by orderly arrangement and uniform cytology of clustered ganglion cells as well as by separation of such clusters by organized bundles of myelinated or unmyelinated nerve fibers. Intraneural neurofibromas lack the high density of nerve fibers that characterize ganglioneuroma; instead, nerve fibers in neurofibromas are few in number, are often myelinated, and are either widely separated by intervening neurofibroma tissue or lie bundled at the center of affected nerve fascicles. Another distinguishing feature is the presence of more extensive stromal mucin (mucopolysaccharide) in neurofibromas. Elements of schwannoma not seen in ganglioneuroma include a thick capsule, an often peripherally displaced or partly intracapsular myelinated nerve, hyalinized blood vessels, Antoni A and B patterns, palisading of cells, and Verocay bodies. Localized mucosal neuromas, such as of the pharynx (154), may feature overrun ganglion cells and thereby enter into the differential diagnosis of ganglioneuroma.

As previously noted, ganglioneuromatous maturation is known to occur in both pheochromocytoma (fig. 9-50) and in the spectrum of neuroblastic tumors. *Composite ganglioneuroma-pheochromocytoma* was discussed in detail above. Adequate tissue sampling is key to the correct diagnosis of such neoplasms. With regard to neuroblastoma, its primary sites differ from those of ganglioneuroma. In the majority of cases, the former are infradiaphragmatic and the latter supradiaphragmatic. Neuronal neoplasms often mistaken for ganglioneuroma include "immature ganglioneuroma" and ganglioneuroblastoma. *Immature ganglioneuroma* is characterized by a broad range of ganglion cell maturation, absence of or only rare neuroblasts, and often abundant axonal processes unassociated with Schwann cells (fig. 9-63). *Ganglioneuroblastoma* (fig. 9-64), particularly of the stroma-rich type (184), enters into the differential diagnosis since a nonrepresentative biopsy of the latter may contain only the mature ganglionic element. Adequate sampling is always a necessity. The finding of immature

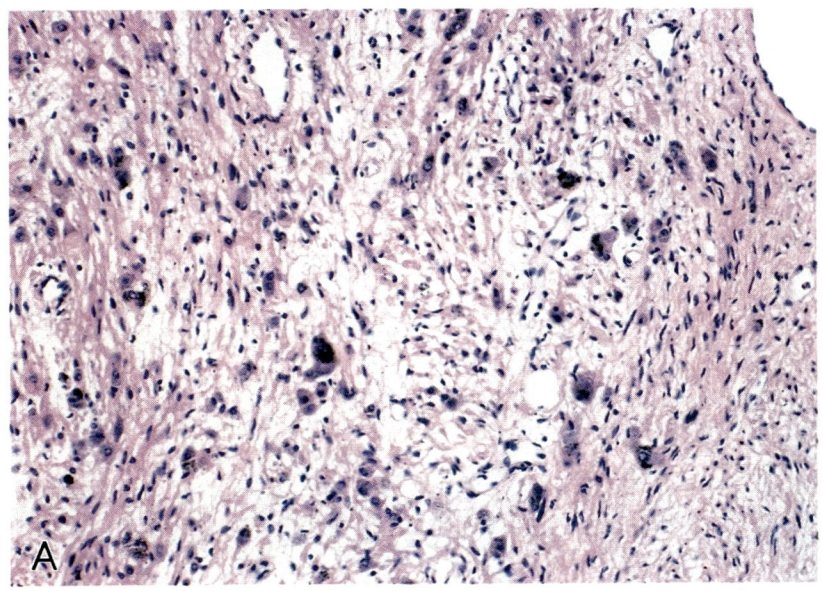

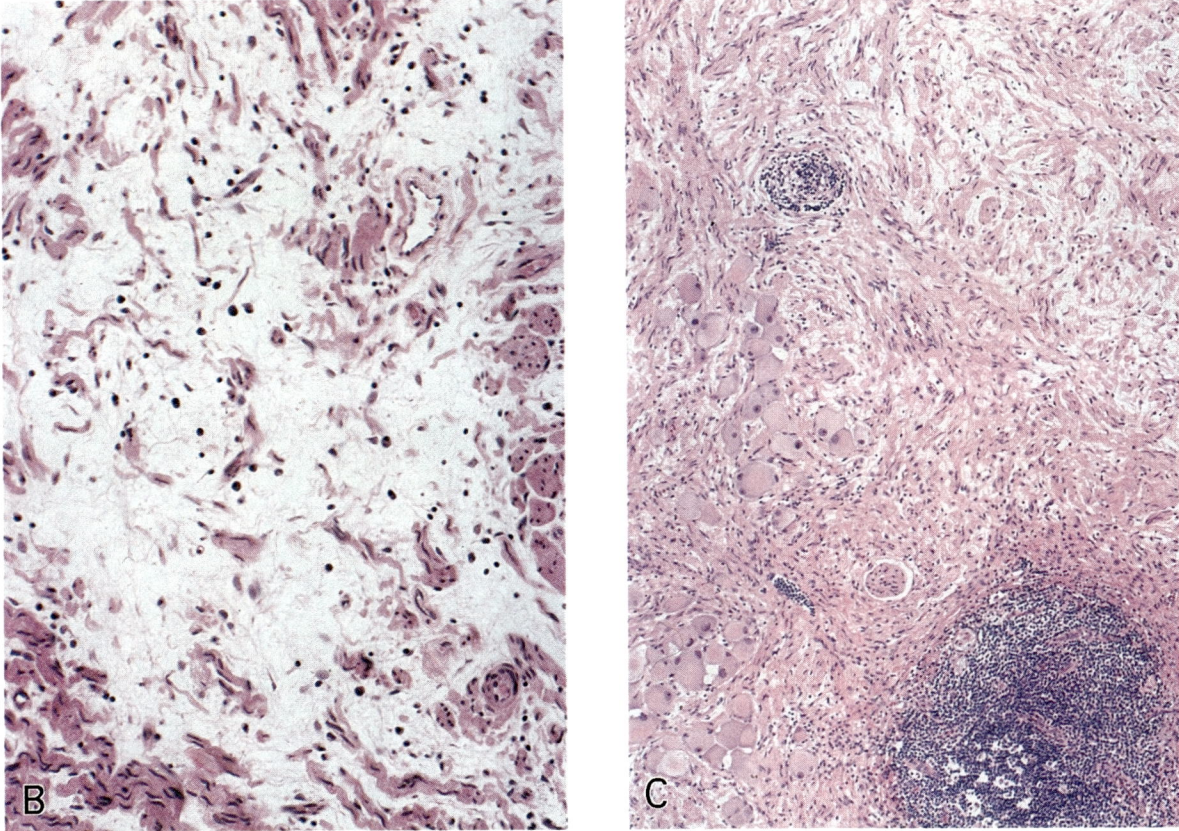

Figure 9-57
GANGLIONEUROMA

Neuromelanin deposition (A) is commonly seen and is considered a degenerative feature. The same is true of stromal mucin accumulation (B) and fibrosis or chronic inflammation (C).

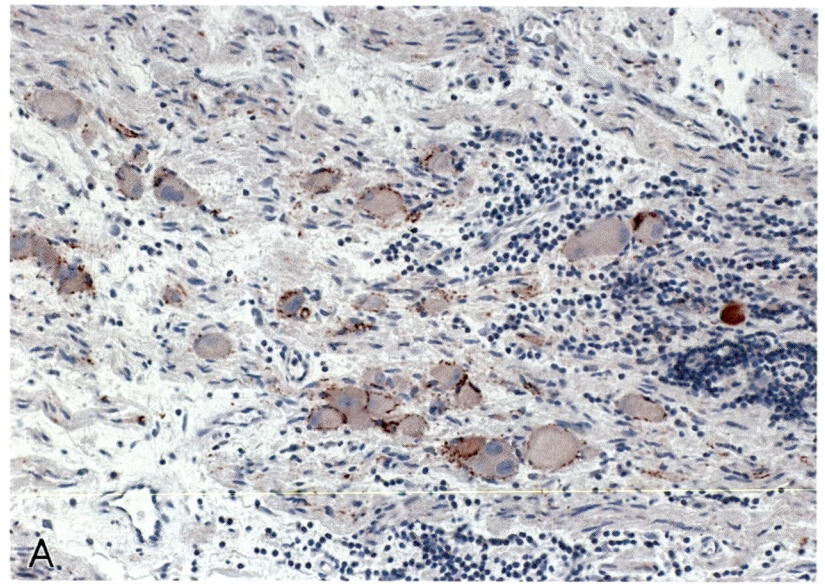

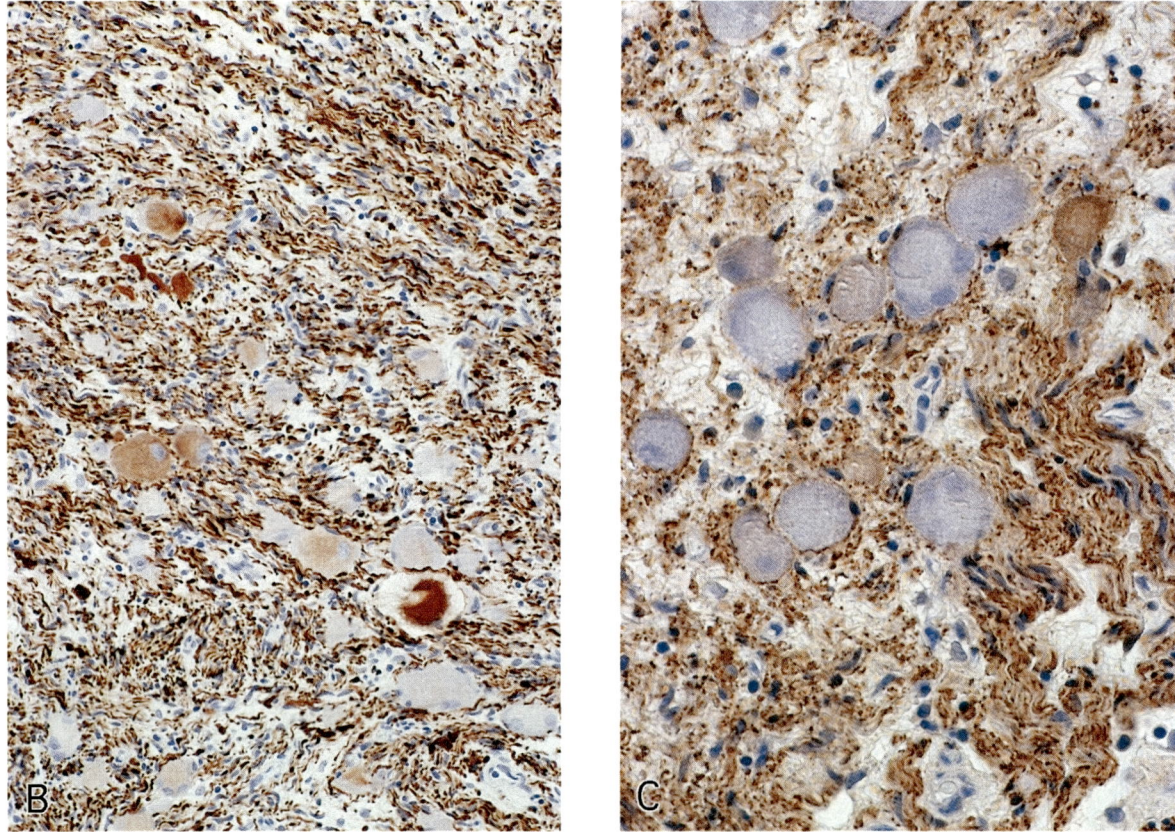

Figure 9-58
GANGLIONEUROMA

Ganglion cells show reactivity for synaptophysin (A) and neurofilament protein (B). Note that the latter also stains spherical cytoplasmic neurofilament accumulations and ganglion cell processes. The ensheathing Schwann cells are S-100 protein reactive (C).

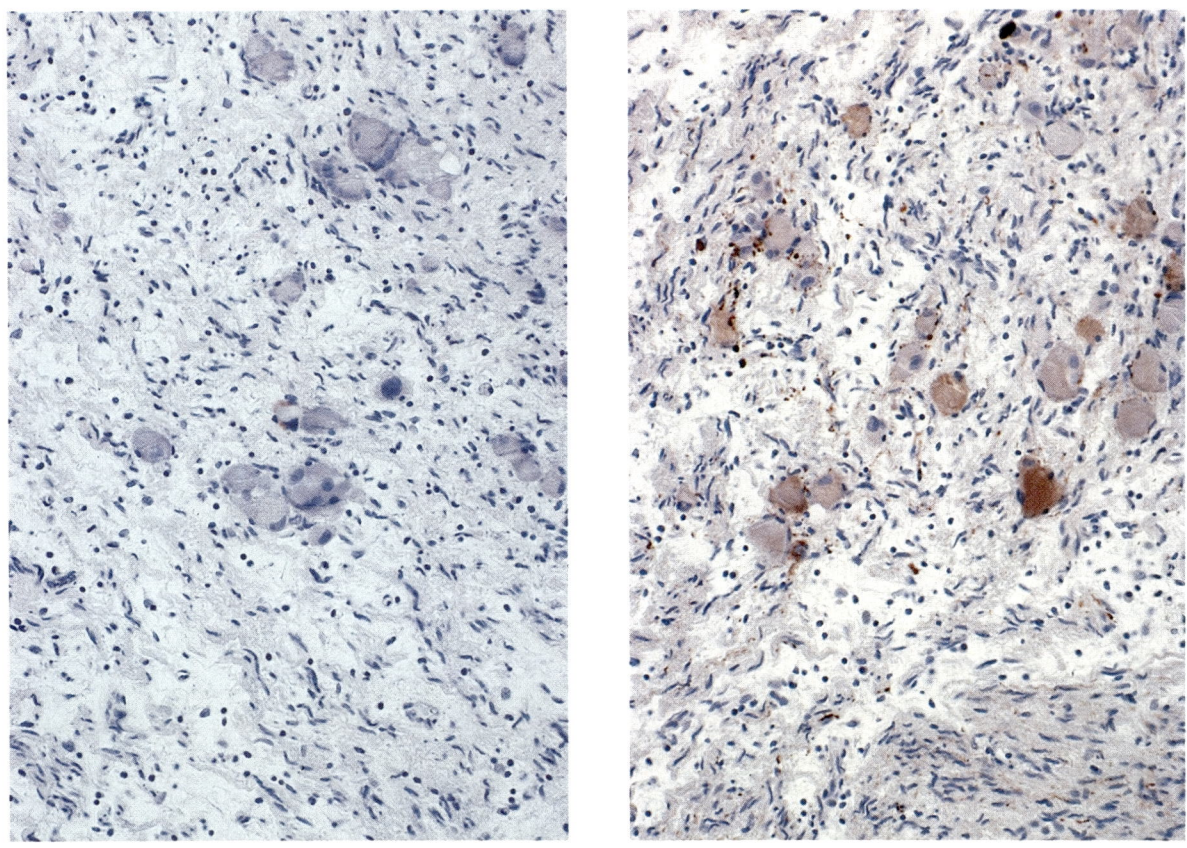

Figure 9-59
GANGLIONEUROMA
Chromogranin staining of ganglion cells (left) reflects their content of hormones and neurotransmitter substances, in this case vasoactive intestinal polypeptide (VIP) (right).

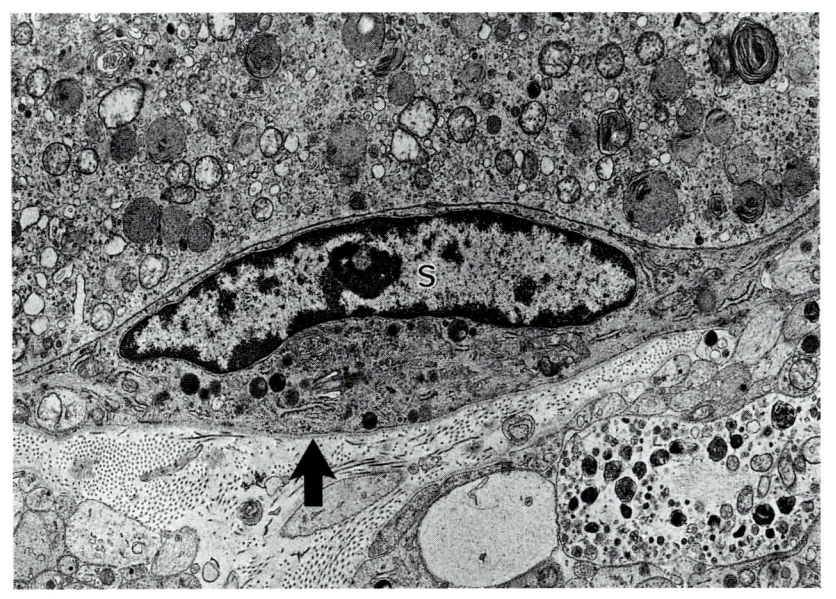

Figure 9-60
GANGLIONEUROMA
A portion of a ganglion cell (top) is intimately surrounded by an elongate satellite cell (center). Note that numerous lysosomal inclusions are found in the cytoplasm of the ganglion cell and that the outer cell membrane of the satellite cell is separated from the stroma by a thin basement membrane (arrow) (X9,700).

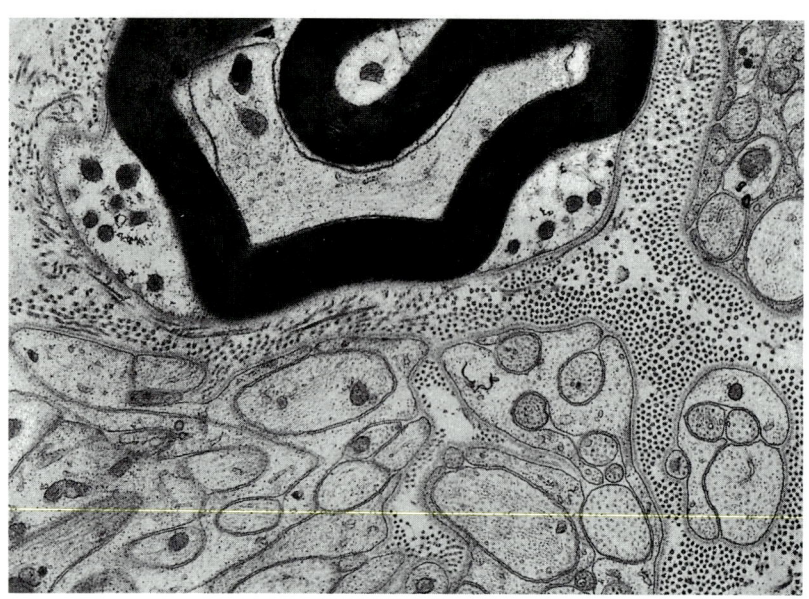

Figure 9-61
GANGLIONEUROMA
Prominent unmyelinated axons (bottom) are much smaller than a normal, apparently entrapped myelinated axon (top). The stroma consists of numerous collagen fibrils, here seen in cross section (X12,100).

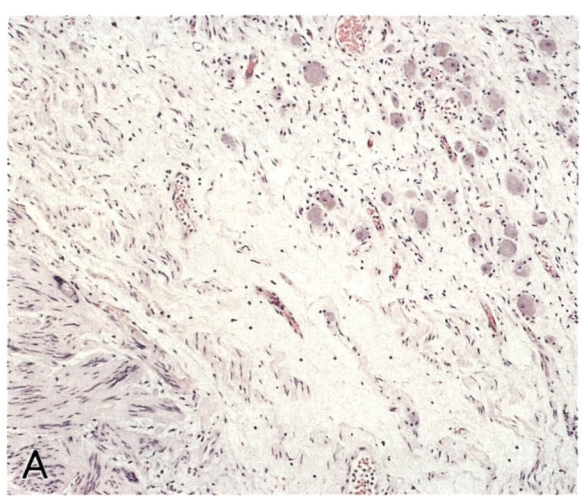

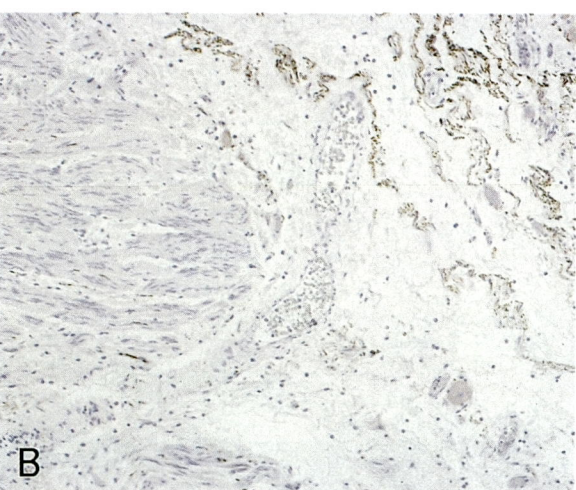

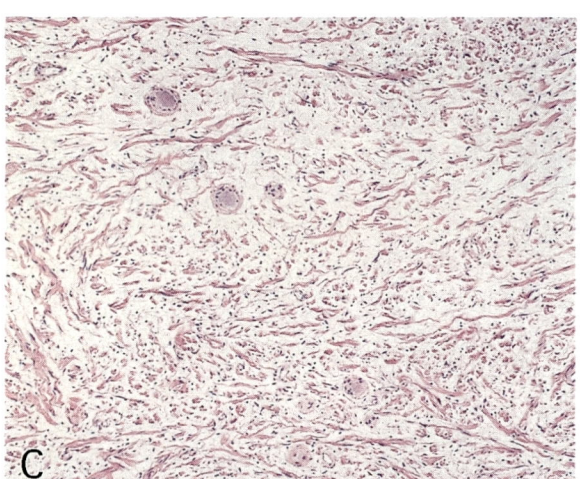

Figure 9-62
GANGLIONEUROMA
Mimicry of ganglioneuroma may result when schwannomas involve dorsal root ganglia (A). Unlike ganglioneuroma, the schwannoma component is devoid of nerve fibers and well-formed Schwann sheaths (B, neurofilament protein immunostain). In a similar manner, neurofibromas may also mimic ganglioneuromas (C).

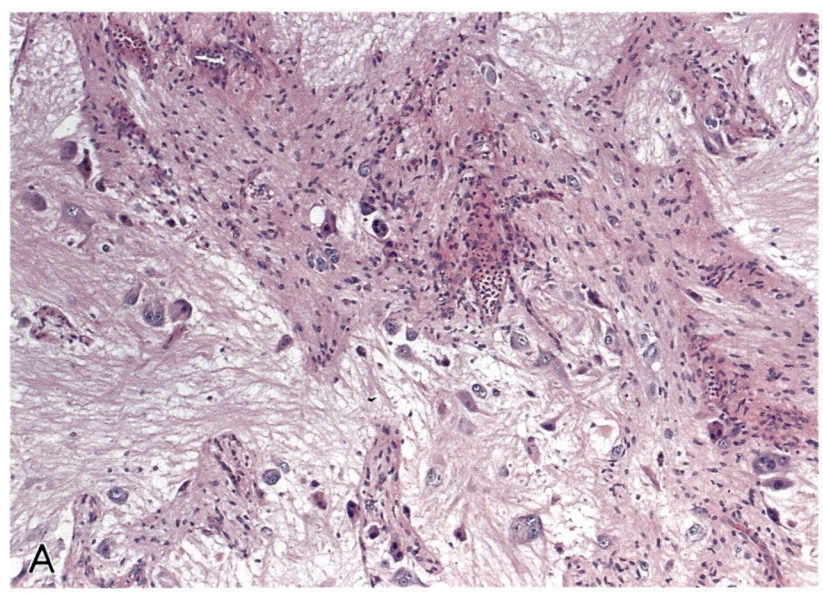

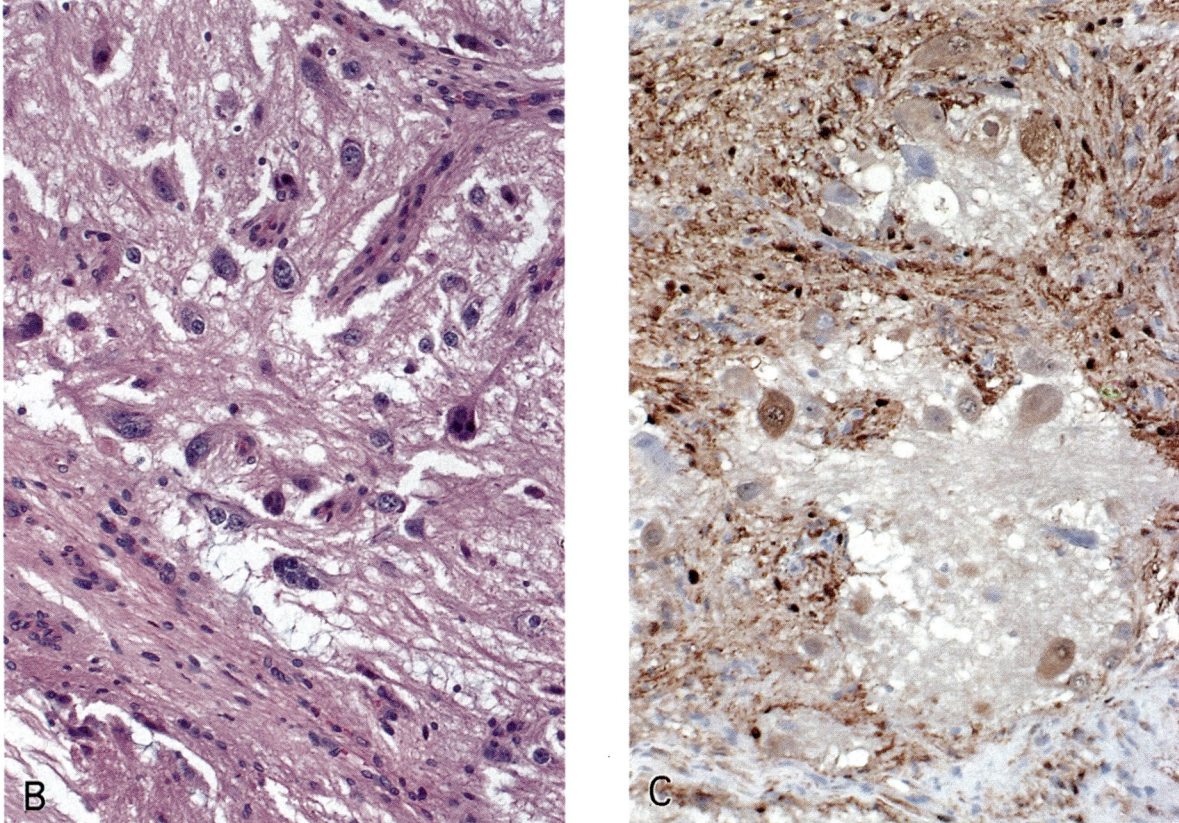

Figure 9-63
"IMMATURE" GANGLIONEUROMA

This neuronal neoplasm mimics mature ganglioneuroma and consists of both mature ganglion cells and smaller forms with less cytoplasm and smaller nucleoli (A,B). Atypia as well as rare neuroblasts may be seen (B). Neuronal processes unassociated with Schwann cells are a common feature (A,B) and readily evident on H&E (A,B) and S-100 protein stains (C).

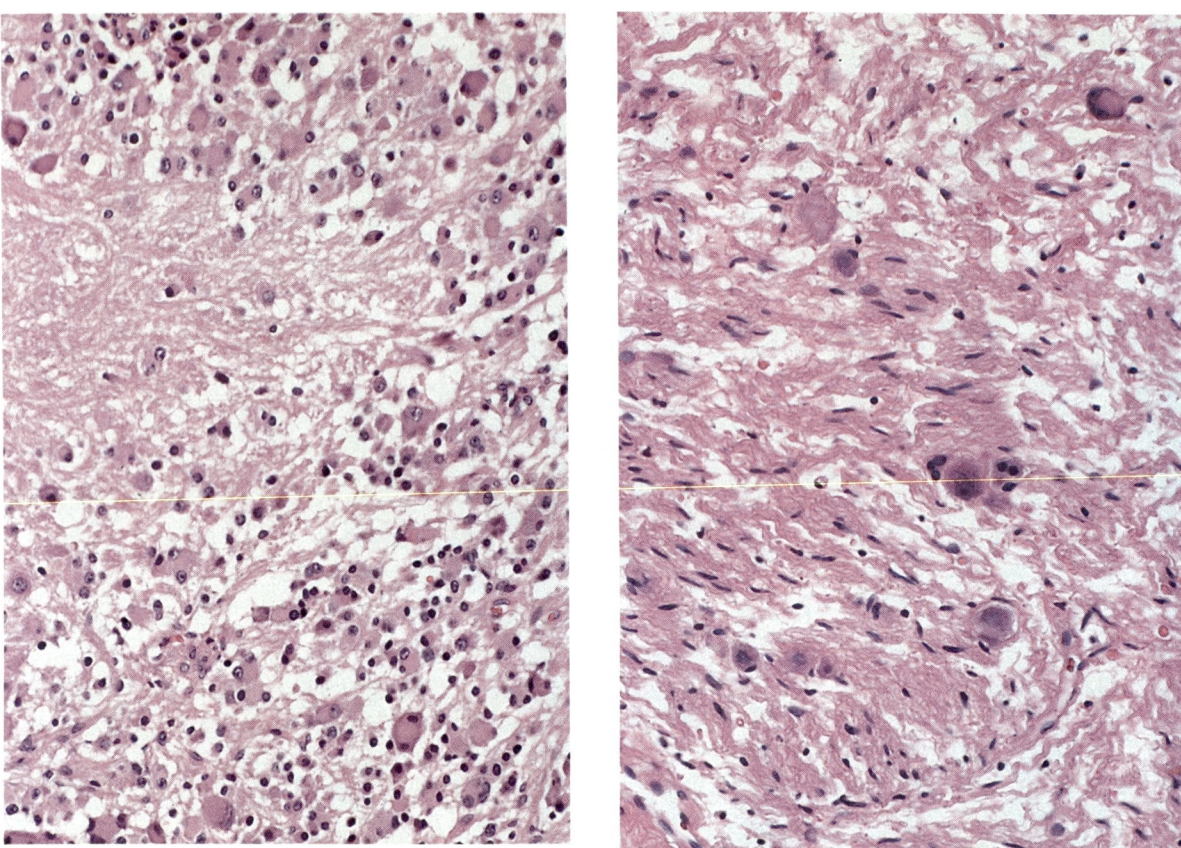

Figure 9-64
GANGLIONEUROBLASTOMA
This neuronal neoplasm consists of both neuroblastic (left) and variably mature ganglioneuromatous components (right). Careful sampling of such tumors is required to avoid an erroneous diagnosis of ganglioneuroma.

neurons with little cytoplasm and ones lacking vesicular nuclei as well as prominent nucleoli should prompt a search for neuroblasts. In expressing neuron-specific enolase and synaptophysin reactivity, neuroblasts are usually readily distinguished from the scattered, leukocyte common antigen–positive lymphocytes often seen in ganglioneuroma. As previously noted, maturation of neuroblastoma or ganglioneuroblastoma metastases may also mimic ganglioneuroma (fig. 9-65).

Ganglioneuroma is a common component of the histologically malignant heterogenous tumor variously referred to as ectomesenchymoma (164) and "gangliorabdomyosarcoma" (166), a lesion discussed in more detail under MPNST ex ganglioneuroma in chapter 11.

Treatment and Prognosis. Ganglioneuromas are benign tumors that cause symptoms due to mass effects or, far less often, to endocrine activity. Resection is curative, even in instances in which intimate adherence to or growth around nearby structures complicates resection. The occasional finding of ganglioneuroma in regional lymph nodes or at remote sites indicates that maturation of a metastatic neuroblastoma has taken place. The prognosis in such instances is also excellent. Nonetheless, at least one example of recurrence of neuroblastoma 15 years after conversion to ganglioneuroma has been reported (157). On rare occasion, ganglioneuroma may give rise to malignant peripheral nerve sheath tumor (MPNST) (see chapter 11).

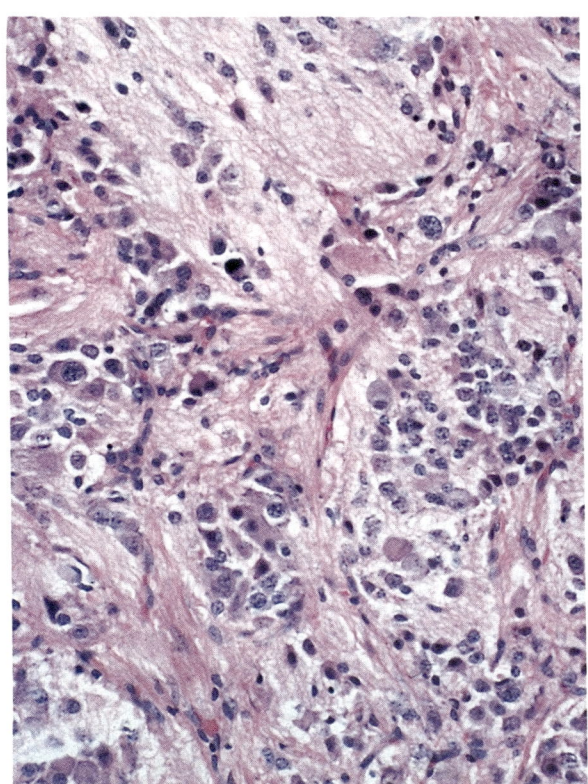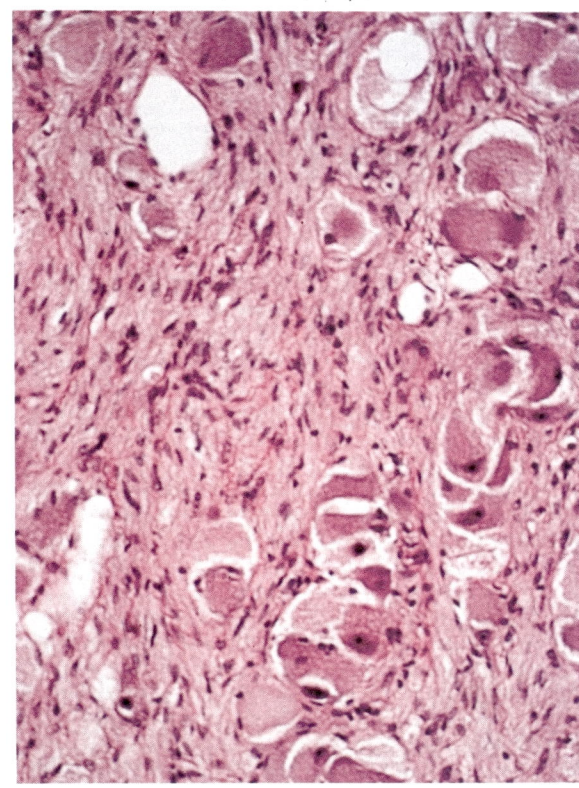

Figure 9-65
NEUROBLASTOMA WITH GANGLIONEUROMATOUS MATURATION OF METASTASIS
This adrenal primary (left) showed remarkable maturation in its orbital metastasis (right).

REFERENCES

Perineurioma

1. Aoki T, Hisaoka M, Hashimoto H, Nakata H, Sakai A, Okabe S. Giant degenerative perineurial cell tumor. Skeletal Radiol 1996;25:757–61.

2. Appenzeller O, Kornfeld M. Macrodactyly and localized neuropathy. Neurology 1974;24:767–71.

2a. Bégin LR. Perineurioma of the finger: case report of a rare peripheral nerve sheath neoplasm of pure perineurial cell lineage. J Hand Surg 1998;23A:342–47.

3. Bilbao JM, Khoury NJ, Hudson AR, Briggs SJ. Perineurioma (localized hypertrophic neuropathy). Arch Pathol Lab Med 1984;108:557–60.

4. Carneiro F, Brandão O, Correia AC, Sobrinho-Simões M. Spindle cell tumor of the breast. Ultrastruct Pathol 1989;13:593–8.

4a. Dhimes P, Martinez-Gonzalez MA, Carabias E, Perez-Espejo G. Ultrastructural study of a perineurioma with ribosome-lamella complexes. Ultrastruct Pathol 1996;20:167–72.

4b. Donnellan R, Rughubar K, Govender D, Chetty R. Perineurioma: an unusual cause of an external auditory canal polyp. ORL J Otorhinolaryngol Relat Spec 1997;59:336–8.

5. Emory TS, Scheithauer BW, Hirose T, Wood M, Onofrio BM, Jenkins RB. Intraneural perineurioma: a clonal neoplasm associated with abnormalities of chromosome 22. Am J Clin Pathol 1995;103:696–704.

6. Erlandson RA. The enigmatic perineurial cell and its participation in tumors and in tumor-like entities. Ultrastruct Pathol 1991;15:335–51.

7. Fetch JF, Miettinen M. Sclerosing perineurioma. Am J Surg Pathol 1997;21:1433–42.

7a. Giannini C, Scheithauer BW, Cosgrove T, et al. Intracranial perineurioma. Neurosurgery (in press).

8. Giannini C, Scheithauer BW, Jenkins RB, et al. Soft tissue perineurioma. Evidence for an abnormality of chromosome 22, criteria for diagnosis, and review of the literature. Am J Surg Pathol 1997;21:164–73.

8a. Hirose T, Scheithauer BW. Sclerosing perineuroma: a distinct entity? Int J Surg Pathol (in press).

9. Hirose T, Scheithauer BW, Sano T. Malignant perineurioma: a study of 8 cases [Abstract]. Mod Pathol 1997;10:10A.

10. Hirose T, Sumitomo M, Kudo E, et al. Malignant peripheral nerve sheath tumor (MPNST) showing perineurial cell differentiation. Am J Surg Pathol 1989;13:613–20.

11. Inaba H, Hizawa K, Ii K, Iwasa S. Perineurioma. A distinctive form of the peripheral nerve tumor. Tokushima J Exp Med 1980;27:37–43.
12. Johnson PC, Kline DG. Localized hypertrophic neuropathy: possible focal perineurial barrier defect. Acta Neuropathol 1989;77:514–8.
13. Kahn DG, Duckett T, Bhuta SM. Perineurioma of the kidney. Report of a case with histologic, immunohistochemical, and ultrastructural studies. Arch Pathol Lab Med 1993;117:654–7.
14. Korthals JK, Gieron MA, Wisniewski HM. Nerve regeneration patterns after acute ischemic injury. Neurology 1989;39:932–7.
14a. Landini G, Kitano M. Meningioma of the mandible. Cancer 1992;69:2917–20.
15. Lazarus SS, Trombetta LD. Ultrastructural identification of a benign perineurial cell tumor. Cancer 1978;41:1823–9.
16. Li D, Schauble B, Moll C, Fisch U. Intratemporal facial nerve perineurioma. Laryngoscope 1996;106:328–33.
17. Mentzel T, Dei Tos AP, Fletcher CD. Perineurioma (storiform perineurial fibroma): clinicopathological analysis of four cases. Histopathology 1994;25:261–7.
18. Merck C, Angervall L, Kindblom LG, Odén A. Myxofibrosarcoma. A malignant soft tissue tumor of fibroblastic-histiocytic origin. A clinicopathologic and prognostic study of 110 cases using multivariate analysis. Acta Pathol Microbiol Immunol Scand [A] 1983;282(Suppl):1–40.
19. Ohno T, Park P, Akai M, et al. Ultrastructural study of perineurioma. Ultrastruct Pathol 1988;12:495–504.
20. Peckham NH, O'Boynick PL, Meneses A, Kepes JJ. Hypertrophic mononeuropathy. A report of two cases and review of the literature. Arch Pathol Lab Med 1982;106:534–7.
20a. Rank JP, Rostad SW. Perineurioma with ossification. A case report with immunohistochemical and ultrastructural studies. Arch Pathol Lab Med 1998;122:366–70.
21. Reed RJ, Harkin JC. Supplement to tumors of the peripheral nervous system. 2nd Series, Fascicle 3 [Supplement]. Armed Forces Institute of Pathology, 1983:S15–6.
22. Simpson DA, Fowler M. Two cases of localized hypertrophic neurofibrosis. J Neurol Neurosurg 1966;29:80–4.
22a. Smith K, Skelton H. Cutaneous fibrous perineurioma. J Cutan Pathol 1998;25:333–7.
23. Thomas PK, Bhagat S. The effect of extraction of the intrafascicular contents of peripheral nerve trunks on perineurial structure. Acta Neuropathol 1978;43:135–41.
24. Tranmer BI, Bilbao JM, Hudson AR. Perineurioma: a benign peripheral nerve tumor. Neurosurgery 1986;19(1):134–8.
25. Tsang WY, Chan JK, Chow LT, Tse CC. Perineurioma: an uncommon soft tissue neoplasm distinct from localized hypertrophic neuropathy and neurofibroma. Am J Surg Pathol 1992;16:756–63.
26. Ushigome S, Takakuwa T, Kyuga M, Tadokoro M, Shinagawa T. Perineurial cell tumor and the significance of the perineurial cells in neurofibroma. Acta Pathol Jpn 1986;36:973–87.
26a. Val-Bernal JF, Hernando M, Garijo MF, Villa P. Renal perineurioma in childhood. Gen Diagn Pathol 1997;143:75–81.
27. Weidenheim KM, Campbell WG Jr. Perineurial cell tumor. Immunocytochemical and ultrastructural characterization. Relationship to other peripheral nerve tumors with a review of the literature. Virchows Arch [A] 1986;408:375–83.

Neurothekeoma

28. Angervall L, Kindblom LG, Haglid K. Dermal nerve sheath myxoma. A light and electron microscopic, histochemical and immunohistochemical study. Cancer 1984;53:1752–9.
29. Argenyi ZB, Kutzner H, Seaba MM. Ultrastructural spectrum of cutaneous nerve sheath myxoma/cellular neurothekeoma. J Cutan Pathol 1995;22:137–45.
30. Argenyi ZB, LeBoit PE, Santa Cruz D, Swanson PE, Kutzner H. Nerve sheath myxoma (neurothekeoma) of the skin: light microscopic and immunohistochemical reappraisal of the cellular variant. J Cutan Pathol 1993;20:294–303.
31. Aronson PJ, Fretzin DF, Potter BS. Neurothekeoma of Gallagher and Helwig (dermal nerve sheath myxoma variant): report of a case with electron microscopic and immunohistochemical studies. J Cutan Pathol 1985;12:506–19.
32. Barnhill RL, Dickersin GR, Nickeleit V, et al. Studies on the cellular origin of neurothekeoma: clinical, light microscopic, immunohistochemical and ultrastructural observations. J Am Acad Dermatol 1991;25:80–8.
33. Barnhill RL, Mihm MC Jr. Cellular neurothekeoma. A distinctive variant of neurothekeoma mimicking nevomelanocytic tumors. Am J Surg Pathol 1990;14:113–20.
34. Blumberg AK, Kay S, Adelaar RS. Nerve sheath myxoma of digital nerve. Cancer 1989;63:1215–8.
34a. Busam KJ, Mentzel T, Colpaert C, Barnhill RL, Fletcher CD. Atypical or worrisome features in cellular neurothekeoma. A study of 10 cases. Am J Surg Pathol 1998;22:1067–72.
35. Calonje E, Wilson-Jones E, Smith NP, Fletcher CD. Cellular neurothekeoma: an epithelioid variant of pilar leiomyoma? Morphological and immunohistochemical analysis of a series. Histopathology 1992;20:397–404.
36. Fletcher CD, Chan JK, McKee PH. Dermal nerve sheath myxoma: a study of three cases. Histopathology 1986;10:135–45.
37. Gallager RL, Helwig EB. Neurothekeoma—a benign cutaneous tumor of neural origin. Am J Clin Pathol 1980;74:759–64.
38. Goldstein J, Lifshitz T. Myxoma of the nerve sheath. Report of three cases, observations by light and electron microscopy and histochemical analysis. Am J Dermatopathol 1985;7:423–9.
39. Harkin JC, Reed RJ. Myxoma of nerve sheath. Tumors of the peripheral nervous system. Atlas of Tumor Pathology, 2nd Series, Fascicle 3. Washington, D.C.: Armed Forces Institute of Pathology, 1969:60–5.
40. Holden CA, Wilson-Jones E, MacDonald DM. Cutaneous lobular neuromyxoma. Br J Dermatol 1982;106:211–5.
41. Husain S, Silvers DN, Halpern AJ, McNutt SN. Histologic spectrum of neurothekeoma and the value of immunoperoxidase staining for S-100 protein in distinguishing it from melanoma. Am J Dermatopathol 1994;16:496–503.

42. Jones TJ, Hammerton W, Shrank AB, Nicholls PE. Cellular neurothekeoma—the Shropshire experience [Abstract]. J Pathol 1991;163:161A.

43. Kao GF, Penneys NS. Immunohistochemical findings of 34 neurothekeomas (benign peripheral nerve sheath tumor) [Abstract]. J Cutan Pathol 1990;17:304.

44. Katsourakis M, Kapranos N, Papanicolaou SI, Patrikiou A. Nerve-sheath myxoma (neurothekeoma) of the oral cavity: a case report and review of the literature. J Oral Maxillofac Surg 1996;54:904–6.

45. Kleinschmidt-DeMasters BK, Lillehei KO. Intraneural neurothekeoma: case report. Neurosurgery 1995;37:333–5.

46. Mentzel T, Calorje E, Wadden C, et al. Myxofibrosarcoma. Clinicopathologic analysis of 75 cases with Eupharis on the low grade variant. Am J Surg Pathol 1996;20:391–405.

47. Mincer HH, Spears KD. Nerve sheath myxoma in the tongue. Oral Surg Oral Med Oral Pathol 1974;37:428–30.

48. Paulus W, Jellinger K, Perneczky G. Intraspinal neurothekeoma (nerve sheath myxoma). A report of two cases. Am J Clin Pathol 1991;95:511–6.

49. Pulitzer DR, Reed RJ. Nerve sheath myxoma (perineurial myxoma). Am J Dermatopathol 1985;7:409–21.

50. Rosati LA, Fratamico CM, Eusebi V. Cellular neurothekeoma. Appl Pathol 1986;4:186–91.

51. Sist TC, Green GW. Benign nerve sheath myxoma: light and electron microscopic features of two cases. Oral Surg Oral Med Oral Pathol 1979;47:441–4.

52. Theaker JM, Fletcher CD. Epithelial membrane antigen expression by the perineurial cell: further studies of peripheral nerve lesions. Histopathology 1989;14:581–92.

53. Tomich CE. Oral focal mucinosis. Oral Surg Oral Med Oral Pathol 1974;38:714–24.

54. Webb JN. The histogenesis of nerve sheath myxoma: report of a case with electron microscopy. J Pathol 1979;127:35–7.

55. Wright BA, Jackson D. Neural tumors of the oral cavity, a review of the spectrum of benign and malignant oral tumors of the oral cavity and jaw. Oral Surg Oral Med Oral Pathol 1980;49:509–22.

56. Yamamoto H, Kawana T. Oral nerve sheath myxoma. Report of a case with findings of ultrastructural and immunohistochemical studies. Acta Pathol Jpn 1988;38:121–7.

Benign Granular Cell Tumor

57. Abenoza P, Sibley RK. Granular cell myoma and schwannoma: fine structural and immunohistochemical study. Ultrastruct Pathol 1987;11:19–28.

58. Abrikossoff A. Myomas originating from transversely striated voluntary musculature. Virchow Arch [A] 1926;260:215–33.

59. Abrikossoff AI. Weitere Untersuchungen (ber myoblastenmyome. Virchows Arch Path Anat 1931; 280:723–40.

60. Alessi DM, Zimmerman MC. Granular cell tumors of the head and neck. Laryngoscope 1988;98:810–4.

61. Alvarez-Fernandez E, Carretero-Albinana L. Bronchial granular cell tumor. Presentation of three cases with tissue culture and ultrastructural study. Arch Pathol Lab Med 1987;111:1065–9.

62. Armin A, Connelly EM, Rowden G. An immunoperoxidase investigation of S-100 protein in granular cell myoblastomas: evidence for Schwann cell derivation. Am J Clin Pathol 1983;79:37–44.

63. Baeten CG, Weidema WF, Willebrand D, De Jong R. Granular cell tumor of the breast. Neth J Surg 1989;41–5:111–3.

64. Bangle R Jr. An early granular cell myoblastoma confined within a small peripheral myelinated nerve. Cancer 1953;6:790–3.

65. Bedetti CD, Martinez AJ, Beckford NS, May M. Granular cell tumor arising in myelinated peripheral nerves. Light and electron microscopy and immunoperoxidase study. Virchows Arch [A] 1983;402:175–83.

66. Bodic O, Couderc JP, Guilliere P. Tumeur à cellules granulluses colique plurifocale. Ann Pathol 1992; 12:130–4.

67. Booth JB, Osborn DA. Granular cell myoblastoma of the larynx. Acta Otolaryngol 1970;70:279–93.

68. Budzilovich GN. Granular cell "myoblastoma" of vagus nerve. Acta Neuropathol 1968;10:162–5.

69. Buley ID, Gatter KC, Kelly PM, Heryet A, Millard PR. Granular cell tumours revisited. An immunohisto-chemical and ultrastructural study. Histopathology 1988;12:263–74.

70. Carvalho GA, Lindeke A, Tatagiba M, Ostertag H, Samii M. Cranial granular-cell tumor of the trigeminal nerve. Case report. J Neurosurg 1994;81:795–8.

71. Chimelli L, Symon L, Scaravilli F. Granular cell tumor of the fifth cranial nerve: further evidence for Schwann cell origin. J Neuropathol Exp Neurol 1984;43:634–42.

72. Christ ML, Ozzello L. Myogenous origin of granular cell tumor of the urinary bladder. Am J Clin Pathol 1971;56:736–49.

73. Clark HB, Minesky JJ, Agrawal D, Agrawal HC. Myelin basic protein and P2 protein are not immunohistochemical markers for Schwann cell neoplasms. A comparative study using antisera to S-100, P2, and myelin basic proteins. Am J Pathol 1985;121:96–101.

74. Compagno J, Hyams VJ, Ste-Marie P. Benign granular cell tumors of the larynx: a review of 36 cases with clinicopathologic data. Ann Otol Rhinol Laryngol 1975;84:1–7.

75. Damiani S, Koerner FC, Dickersin GR, Cook MG, Eusebi V. Granular cell tumor of the breast. Virchows Arch [A] 1992;420:219–26.

76. DeMay RM, Kay S. Granular cell tumor of the breast. Pathol Annu 1984;19:121–48.

77. Dhillon AP, Rode J. Immunohistochemical studies of S-100 protein and other neural characteristics expressed by granular cell tumor. Diagn Histopathol 1983;6:23–8.

78. Dingemans KP, Mooi WJ, van den Bergh Weeman MA. Angulate lysosomes. Ultrastruct Pathol 1983;5:113–22.

79. Enghardt MH, Jordan SE. Granular cell tumor of a digital nerve. Cancer 1991;68:1764–9.

80. Feyrter F. Uber die granularen Neurome (sog. Myoblastenmyome). Virchows Arch [A] 1952;322:66–72.

81. Feyrter F. Uber die granularen neurogenen Gewachse. Beitr Pathol Anat 1949;110:181–208.

82. Feyrter F. Uber eine eigenartige Geschwulstform des Nervengewebes im menschlichen Verdauungsschlauch. Virchows Arch [A] 1935;295:480–501.

83. Filie AC, Lage JM, Azumi N. Immunoreactivity of S-100 protein, alpha-1-antitrypsin, and CD68 in adult and congenital granular cell tumors. Mod Pathol 1996;9:888–92.

84. Fisher ER, Wechsler H. Granular cell myoblastoma—a misnomer. Electron microscopic and histochemical evidence concerning its Schwann cell derivation and nature (granular cell schwannoma). Cancer 1962;15:936–54.

85. Frable MA, Fischer RA. Granular cell myoblastomas. Laryngoscope 1976;86:36–42.

86. Franzen S, Stenkvist B. Diagnosis of granular cell myoblastoma by fine-needle aspiration biopsy. Acta Pathol Microbiol Scand 1968;72:391–5.

87. Fust JA, Custer RP. Granular cell "myoblastoma" and granular cell neurofibromas: separation of the neurogenous tumors from the myoblastoma group. Am J Pathol 1948;24:674.

88. Fust JA, Custer RP. On neurogenesis of so-called granular cell myoblastoma. Am J Clin Path 1949;19:522–35.

89. Garancis JC, Komorowski RA, Kuzman JF. Granular cell myoblastoma. Cancer 1970;25:542–50.

90. Garud O, Bostad L, Elverland HH, Mair IW. Granular cell tumor of the larynx in a 5-year-old child. Ann Otol Rhinol Laryngol 1984;93:45–7.

91. Ghadially FN. Ultrastructural pathology of the cell and matrix. 3rd ed. London: Butterworths, 1988:589–765.

92. Goldblum JR, Rice TW, Zuccaro G, Richter JE. Granular cell tumors of the esophagus: a clinical and pathologic study of 13 cases. Ann Thorac Surg 1996;62:860–5.

93. Gordon AB, Fisher C, Palmer B, Greening WP. Granular cell tumor of the breast. Europ J Surg Oncol 1985;11:269–73.

94. Johnston J, Helwig EB. Granular cell tumors of the gastrointestinal tract and perianal region: a study of 74 cases. Dig Dis Sci 1981;26:807–16.

95. Kanabe S, Watanabe I, Lotuaca L. Multiple granular cell tumors of the ascending colon: microscopic study. Dis Colon Rectum 1978;21:322–8.

96. Kornfeld M. Granular cell glioblastoma: a malignant granular cell neoplasm of astrocytic origin. J Neuropathol Exp Neurol 1986;45:447–62.

97. Kurtin PJ, Bonin DM. Immunohistochemical demonstration of the lysosome associated glycoprotein CD 68 (KP-1) in granular cell tumors and schwannomas. Hum Pathol 1994;25:1172–8.

98. Lack EE, Worsham GF, Callihan MD, et al. Granular cell tumor: a clinicopathologic study of 110 patients. J Surg Oncol 1980;13:301–16.

99. Lee J, Bhawan J, Wax F, Farber J. Plexiform granular cell tumor. A report of two cases. Am J Dermatopathol 1994;16:537–41.

100. Lifshitz MS, Flotte TJ, Greco A. Congenital granular cell epulis. Immunohistochemical and ultrastructural observations. Cancer 1984;53:1845–8.

101. Lowhagen T, Rubio CA. The cytology of the granular cell myoblastoma of the breast. Report of a case. Acta Cytol 1977;21:314–5.

102. Martin RW, Nelder KH, Boyd AS, Coates PW. Multiple cutaneous granular cell tumors and neurofibromatosis in childhood. Arch Dermatol 1990;126:1051–6.

103. May M, Beckford NS, Bedetti CD. Granular cell tumor of facial nerve diagnosed at surgery for idiopathic facial nerve paralysis. Otorhinolaryngol Head Neck Surg 1985;93:122–6.

104. Mazur MT, Shultz JJ, Myers JL. Granular cell tumor. Immunohistochemical analysis of 21 benign tumors and one malignant tumor. Arch Pathol Lab Med 1990;114:692–6.

105. McWilliam LJ, Harris M. Granular cell angiosarcoma of the skin: histology, electron microscopy and immunohistochemistry of a newly recognized tumor. Histopathology 1985;9:1205–16.

106. Melaragno MJ, Prayson RA, Murphy MA, Hassenbusch SJ, Estes ML. Anaplastic astrocytoma with granular cell differentiation: case report and review of the literature. Hum Pathol 1993;24:805–8.

107. Melo CR, Melo IS, Schmitt FC, Fagundes R, Amendola D. Multicentric granular cell tumor of the colon: report of a patient with 52 tumors. Am J Gastroenterol 1993;88:1785–7.

108. Mentzel T, Wadden C, Fletcher CD. Granular cell change in smooth muscle tumours of skin and soft tissue. Histopathology 1994;24:223–31.

109. Miettinen M, Lehtonen E, Lehtola H, Ekblom P, Lehto VP, Virtanen I. Histogenesis of granular cell tumour—an immunohistochemical and ultrastructural study. J Pathol 1984;142:221–9.

110. Miller AS, Liefer C, Chen SY, Harwick RD. Oral granular cell tumors. Report of 25 cases with electron microscopy. Oral Surg Oral Med Oral Pathol 1977;44:227–37.

111. Mittal KR, True LD. Origin of granules in granular cell tumor. Intracellular myelin formation with autodigestion. Arch Pathol Lab Med 1988;112:302–3.

112. Mori O, Hachisuka H, Sakamoto F, Nomura H, Sasai Y. Immunohistochemical observation of S-100 protein and neuron specific enolase in the tumour cells of granular cell tumour. Acta Histochem 1988;83:33–8.

113. Moscovic EA, Azar HA. Multiple granular cell tumors ("myoblastomas"). Case report with electron microscopic observations and review of the literature. Cancer 1967;20:2032–47.

114. Mukai M. Immunohistochemical localization of S-100 protein and peripheral nerve myelin proteins (P2 protein, P0 protein) in granular cell tumors. Am J Pathol 1983;112:139–46.

115. Mulcare R. Granular cell myoblastoma of the breast. Ann Surg 1968;168:262–8.

116. Nakajima T, Watanabe S, Sato Y. An immunoperoxidase study of S-100 protein distribution in normal and neoplastic tissues. Am J Surg Pathol 1982;6:715–27.

117. Nakamura T, Hirato J, Hotchi M, Kyoshima K, Nakamura Y. Astrocytoma with granular cell tumor-like changes. Report of a case with histochemical and ultrastructural characterization of granular cells. Acta Pathol Jpn 1990;40:206–11.

118. Nakazato Y, Ishizeki J, Takahashi K, Yamaguchi H. Immunohistochemical localization of S-100 protein in granular cell myoblastoma. Cancer 1982;49:1624–8.

119. Nasu M, Takagi M, Yamamoto H. Ultrastructural and histochemical studies of granular cell ameloblastoma. J Oral Pathol 1984;13:448–56.

120. Nathrath WB, Remberger K. Immunohistochemical study of granular cell tumours. Demonstration of neuron specific enolase, S-100 protein, laminin, and alpha-1-antichymotrypsin. Virchows Arch [A] 1986;408:421–34.

121. Penneys NS, Adachi K, Ziegels-Weissman J, Nadji M. Granular cell tumors of the skin contain myelin basic protein. Arch Pathol Lab Med 1983;107:302–3.

122. Peterson LJ. Granular cell tumor. Review of the literature and report of a case. Oral Surg Oral Med Oral Pathol 1974;37:728–35.

123. Rao TV, Puri R, Reddy GN. Intracranial trigeminal nerve granular cell myoblastoma. Case report. J Neurosurg 1983;59:706–9.

124. Seo IS, Azarelli B, Warner TF, Goheen MP, Senteney GE. Multiple visceral and cutaneous granular cell tumors. Ultrastructural and immunocytochemical evidence of Schwann cell origin. Cancer 1984;53:2104–10.

125. Shintaku M, Sasaki M. Angulate body cell: an immunohistochemical and ultrastructural study. Brain Tumor Pathol 1992;9:41–7.

126. Sobel HJ, Marquet E. Granular cells and granular cell lesions. Pathol Ann 1974;9:43–79.

127. Sobel HJ, Marquet E, Schwarz R. Is schwannoma related to granular cell myoblastoma? Arch Pathol 1973;95:396–401.

128. Sobel HJ, Marquet E, Avrin TA, Schwarz R. Granular cell myoblastoma. An electron microscopic and cytochemical study illustrating the genesis of granules and aging of myoblastoma cells. Am J Pathol 1971;65:59–78.

129. Soini Y, Miettinen M. Widespread immunoreactivity for alpha-1-antichymotrypsin in different types of tumors. Am J Clin Pathol 1988;90:131–6.

130. Stefansson K, Wollmann RL. S-100 protein in granular cell tumors. Cancer 1982;49:1834–8.

131. Stefansson K, Wollmann RL, Jerkovic M. S-100 protein in soft tissue tumors derived from Schwann cells and melanocytes. Am J Pathol 1982;106:261–8.

132. Strong EW, McDivitt RW, Brasfield RD. Granular cell myoblastoma. Cancer 1970;25:415–22.

133. Suster S, Rosen LB, Sanchez JL. Granular cell leiomyosarcoma of the skin. Am J Dermatopathol 1988;10:234–9.

134. Tandler B, Rossi EP. Granular cell ameloblastoma: electron microscopic observation. J Oral Pathol 1977;6:401–12.

135. Torsiglieri AJ, Handler SD, Uri AK. Granular cell tumors of the head and neck in children: the experience at the Children's Hospital of Philadelphia. Int J Ped Otorhinolaryngol 1991;21:249–58.

136. Townsend MC, Stellato TA. Granular cell myoblastoma of the breast: a report of five cases and a review. Breast 1985;11:12–5.

137. Tucker MC, Rusnock EJ, Azumi N, Hoy GR, Lack EE. Gingival granular cell tumors of the newborn. An ultrastructural and immunohistochemical study. Arch Pathol Lab Med 1990;114:895–8.

138. Ulrich J, Heitz PU, Fischer T, Obrist E, Gullotta F. Granular cell tumors: evidence for heterogenous tumor cell differentiation: an immunocytochemical study. Virchows Arch [Cell Pathol] 1987;53:52–7.

139. Vance SF III, Hudson RP Jr. Granular cell myoblastoma. Clinicopathologic study of forty-two patients. Am J Clin Path 1969;33:208–11.

140. Weiser G. Granular cell tumor (Granuläres Neurom Feyrter) und Schwannsche Phagen. Elektronenoptische Untersuchung von 3 Fällen. Virchows Arch [A] 1978;380:49–57.

141. Weisman RA, Konrad HR, Canalis RF. Granular cell myoblastoma involving the recurrent laryngeal nerve. Arch Otolaryngol 1980;106:294–7.

142. Weiss SW, Langloss JM, Enzinger FM. The role of S-100 protein in the diagnosis of soft tissue tumors with particular reference to benign and malignant Schwann cell tumors. Lab Invest 1983;49:299–308.

143. Willén R, Willén H, Baldin G, Albrechtsson U. Granular cell tumour of the mammary gland simulating malignancy. A report of two cases with light microscopy, transmission electron microscopy and immunohistochemical investigation. Virchows Arch [A] 1984;403:391–400.

144. Zajdela A, Laurent M, Durand JC. Cytologic de quelques tumeurs benignes rares due sein. Bull Cancer 1975;62:401–10.

Ganglioneuroma

145. Aguirre P, Scully RE. Testosterone-secreting adrenal ganglioneuroma containing Leydig cells. Am J Surg Pathol 1983;7:699–705.

146. Balázs M. Mixed pheochromocytoma-ganglioneuroma producing catecholamines and various neuropeptides. Acta Med Scand 1988;224:403–8.

147. Becker H, Wirnsberger G, Ziervogel K, Hofler H. Immunohistochemical markers in ganglioneuroblastomas. Acta Histochem [Suppl] 1990;38:107–14.

148. Beer TW. Solitary ganglioneuroma of the rectum: report of two cases. J Clin Pathol 1992;45:353–5.

149. Bender BL, Ghatak NR. Light and electron microscopic observations on a ganglioneuroma. Acta Neuropathol (Berl) 1978;42:7–10.

150. Brady S, Lechan RM, Schwaitzberg SD, Dayal Y, Ziar J, Tischler AS. Composite pheochromocytoma/ganglioneuroma of the adrenal gland associated with multiple endocrine neoplasia 2A: case report with immunohistochemical analysis. Am J Surg Pathol 1997;21:102–8.

151. Chetty R, Duhig JD. Bilateral pheochromocytoma-ganglioneuroma of the adrenal in type 1 neurofibromatosis. Am J Surg Pathol 1993;17:837–41.

152. Crissman JW, Valerio MG, Asiedu SA, Evangelista-Sobel I. Ganglioneuromas of the thyroid gland in a colony of Sprague-Dawley rats. Vet Pathol 1991;28:354–62.

153. Cushing H, Wolbach SB. Transformation of malignant paravertebral sympathicoblastoma into benign ganglioneuroma. Am J Pathol 1927;3:203–16.

154. Daneshvar A. Pharyngeal traumatic neuromas and traumatic neuromas with mature ganglion cells (pseudoganglioneuromas). Am J Surg Pathol 1990;14:565–70.

155. Fox F, Davidson J, Thomas LB. Maturation of sympathicoblastoma into ganglioneuroma: report of 2 patients with 20- and 46-year survivals, respectively. Cancer 1959;12:108–16.

156. Garvin JH Jr, Lack EE, Berenberg W, Frantz CN. Ganglioneuroma presenting with differentiated skeletal metastases. Report of a case. Cancer 1984;54:357–60.

157. Goldman R, Winterling A, Winterling C. Maturation of tumors of the sympathetic nervous system. Cancer 1965;18:1510–6.

158. Graham DG. On the origin and significance of neuromelanin. Arch Pathol Lab Med 1979;103:359–62.

159. Hammond RR, Walton JC. Cutaneous ganglioneuromas: a case report and review of the literature. Hum Pathol 1996;27:735–8.

160. Hayes FA, Green AA, Rao BN. Clinical manifestations of ganglioneuroma. Cancer 1989;63:1211–4.

161. Jansson S, Dahlström A, Hansson G, Tisell LE, Ahlman H. Concomitant occurrence of an adrenal ganglioneuroma and a contralateral pheochromocytoma in a patient with von Recklinghausen's neurofibromatosis. An immunocytochemical study. Cancer 1989;63:324–9.

162. Johnson DC, Teleg M, Eberle RC. Simultaneous occurrence of a ganglioneuroma and a neurilemmoma of the vagus nerve: a case report. Otolaryngol Head Neck Surg 1981;89:75–6.

163. Kahn HJ, Baumal R, Thorner PS, Chan H. Binding of peanut agglutinin to neuroblastomas and ganglioneuromas: a marker for differentiation of neuroblasts into ganglion cells. Pediatr Pathol 1988;8:83–93.

164. Karcioglu Z, Someren A, Mathes SJ. Ectomesenchymoma. A malignant tumor of migratory neural crest (ectomesenchyme) remnants showing ganglionic, schwannian, melanocytic, and rhabdomyoblastic differentiation. Cancer 1977;39:2486–96.

165. Keefe JF, Kobrine AI, Kempe LG. Primary ganglioneuroma of the posterior cranial fossa: case report. Mil Med 1976;141:115–6.

166. Kodet R, Kasthuri N, Marsden HB, Coad NA, Raafat F. Gangliorhabdomyosarcoma: a histopathologic and immunohistochemical study of three cases. Histopathology 1986;10:181–93.

167. Lee JY, Martinez AJ, Abell E. Ganglioneuromatous tumor of the skin: a combined heterotopia of ganglion cells and hamartomatous neuroma: report of a case. J Cutan Pathol 1988;15:58–61.

168. Levy DI, Bucci MN, Weatherbee L, Chandler WF. Intradural extramedullary ganglioneuroma: case report and review of the literature. Surg Neurol 1992;37:216–8.

169. Loritz W. Ein Fall von gangliosen Neurom (Ganglion). Virchows Arch [Pathol Anat] 1870;49:435–41.

169a. Lucas K, Gula MJ, Knisely AS, Virgi MA, Wollman M, Blatt J. Catecholamine metabolites in ganglioneuroma. Med Pediatr Oncol 1994;22:240–3.

170. MacMillan R, Blanc WB, Santulli TV. Maturation of neuroblastoma to ganglioneuroma in lymph nodes. J Pediatr Surg 1976;11:461–2.

171. Markaki S, Edwards C. Intrapulmonary ganglioneuroma. A case report. Arch Anat Cytol Pathol 1987;35:183–4.

172. Matsuda M, Nagashima K. Cytoplasmic tubular inclusion in ganglioneuroma. Acta Neuropathol (Berl) 1984;64:81–4.

173. Mendelsohn G, Eggleston JC, Olson JL, Said SI, Baylin SB. Vasoactive intestinal peptide and its relationship to ganglion cell differentiation in neuroblastic tumors. Lab Invest 1979;41:144–9.

174. Molenaar WM, Baker DL, Pleasure D, Lee VM, Trojanowski JQ. The neuroendocrine and neural profiles of neuroblastomas, ganglioneuroblastomas and ganglioneuromas. Am J Pathol 1990;136:375–82.

175. Moore PJ, Biggs PJ. Compound adrenal medullary tumor. South Med J 1995;88:475–8.

176. Mullins JD. A pigmented differentiating neuroblastoma: a light and ultrastructural study. Cancer 1980;46:522–8.

177. Nagashima F, Hayashi J, Araki Y, et al. Silent mixed ganglioneuroma/pheochromocytoma which produces a vasoactive intestinal polypeptide. Int Med 1993;32:63–6.

178. Nassiri M, Ghazi C, Stivers JR, Nadji M. Ganglioneuroma of the prostate. A novel finding in neurofibromatosis. Arch Pathol Lab Med 1994;118:938–9.

179. Rios JJ, Diaz-Cano SJ, Rivera-Hueto F, Villar JL. Cutaneous ganglion cell choristoma. Report of a case. J Cutan Pathol 1991;18:469–73.

180. Robertson CM, Tyrrell JC, Pritchard J. Familial neural crest tumours. Eur J Pediatr 1991;150:789–92.

181. Sasaki A, Ogawa A, Nakazato Y, et al. Distribution of neurofilament protein and neuron-specific enolase in peripheral neuronal tumors. Virchows Arch [Pathol Anat] 1985;407:33–41.

182. Scheithauer BW, Nora FE, Lechago J, et al. Duodenal gangliocytic paraganglioma: clinicopathologic and immunocytochemical study of 11 cases. Am J Pathol 1986;86:559–65.

183. Schmitt HP, Wurster K, Bauer M, et al. Mixed chemodectoma—ganglioneuroma of the conus medullaris region. Acta Neuropathol 1982;57:275–81.

184. Shimada H, Chatten J, Newton WA Jr, et al. Histologic prognostic factors in neuroblastic tumors: definition of subtypes of ganglioneuroblastoma and an age-linked classification of neuroblastomas. JNCI 1984;73:405–16.

185. Shotton JC, Milton CM, Allen JP. Multiple ganglioneuroma of the neck. J Laryngol Otol 1992;106:277–8.

186. Sitarz AL, Santulli TV, Wigger HJ, Berdon WE. Complete maturation of neuroblastoma with bone metastases in documented stages. J Pediatr Surg 1975;10:533–6.

187. Sonneland PR, Scheithauer BW, Lechago J, Crawford BG, Onofrio BM. Paraganglioma of the cauda equina region: clinicopathologic study of 31 cases with special reference to immunocytology. Cancer 1986;58:1720–35.

188. Stout AP. Ganglioneuroma of the sympathetic nervous system. Surg Gynecol Obstet 1947;84:101–10.

189. Trojanowski JQ, Molenaar WM, Baker DL, Pleasure D, Lee VM. Neural and neuroendocrine phenotype of neuroblastomas, ganglioneuroblastomas, ganglioneuromas and mature versus embryonic human adrenal medullary cells. Prog Clin Biol Res 1991;366:335–41.

190. Trump DL, Livingston JN, Baylin SB. Watery diarrhea syndrome in an adult with ganglioneuroma-pheochromocytoma: identification of vasoactive intestinal peptide, calcitonin, and catecholamines and assessment of their biologic activity. Cancer 1977;40:1526–32.

191. Woog JJ, Albert DM, Craft J, Silberman N, Horns D. Choroidal ganglioneuroma in neurofibromatosis. Graefe's Arch Clin Exp Ophthalmol 1983;220:25–31.

192. Wyman HE, Chappell BS, Jones WR Jr. Ganglioneuroma of bladder: report of case. J Urol 1950;63:526–32.

193. Yoshimi N, Tanaka T, Hara A, Bunai Y, Kato K, Mori H. Extra-adrenal pheochromocytoma-ganglioneuroma. A case report. Pathol Res Pract 1992;188:1098–100.

194. Young WG. Histopathologic study of ganglioneuroma in the mandible. J Oral Surg 1967;25:327–35.

195. Zarabi M, LaBach JP. Ganglioneuroma causing acute appendicitis. Hum Pathol 1982;13:1143–6.

10

BENIGN AND MALIGNANT NON-NEUROGENIC TUMORS

PERIPHERAL NERVE AND ECTOPIC MENINGIOMA

Definition. This meningioma is one without a meningeal association and involves soft tissue, including peripheral nerve, skin, or viscera.

General Comments. In most instances, the finding of a meningioma outside the central nervous system (CNS) is due to direct extension of intracranial or intraspinal meningiomas via osseous foramina. This is expected given the intimate association of the arachnoid membrane with proximal, intradural segments of cranial and spinal peripheral nerves. In one large study of meningiomas (7), 90 percent of which arose from the cranial dura, extension outside the CNS was noted in 20 percent. In decreasing order of frequency, secondarily affected sites included the orbit, skull and scalp, paranasal sinuses and nose, and parotid and parapharyngeal regions. There were only three primary extracranial soft tissue meningiomas in this series, one involving the orbit and two the neck; none affected peripheral nerve.

Meningiomas are rarely primary in peripheral nerves. A review (4) found that of approximately 75 meningiomas reported to arise outside the CNS, only 2 arose in a major peripheral nerve (4,9). One additional case has recently been described (15). It is of note that several other examples, variously quoted as originating in nerve, did not in fact do so (1,5).

The spectrum of meningothelial lesions affecting subcutaneous tissue and skin extends beyond cutaneous meningiomas, some of which are nerve-associated, to include "rudimentary meningocele of the skin" (19,27), a presumably malformative lesion related to meningocele, and the closely related "hamartoma of scalp with ectopic meningothelial elements" (31). On occasion, the latter may be familial (12). Meningothelial cells may also contribute to "hairy polyp of the palate" (23).

Pathogenesis. Proposed mechanisms underlying the occurrence of meningiomas outside the CNS include: 1) extradural trapping of arachnoidal cells during development; 2) migration of arachnoidal cells along developing peripheral nerves; and 3) metaplasia of soft tissue or peripheral nerve sheath cells (17,30).

The distinction between lesions resulting from entrapment as opposed to migration is often difficult, since a parent nerve may not be found. Presumed examples of trapping include meningiomas involving calvarial diploe (11,14) and skin overlying the skull or spine (26,33). Rare examples of post-traumatic extracranial meningioma may also be viewed as a form of arachnoidal cell entrapment (35).

Peripheral meningiomas, perhaps arising by migration of arachnoidal cells along nerve, include those affecting soft tissues of the head and neck (13), parotid and parapharyngeal region (21), maxilla and oral cavity (28,32), nasopharynx (36), orbit, and temporal bone (13). Meningiomas of proximal nerve plexuses may also fall into this group (4,9,15). The simple fact that the leptomeninges are continuous with the perineurium (20) may explain the occurrence of proximal examples, but the occasional finding of arachnoidal cell nests around otherwise normal peripheral nerves (9) suggests that migration of these cells may also play a role.

The metaplasia concept perhaps better explains the finding of meningiomas at sites truly remote from the CNS. Experiments showing not only nerve sheath but a portion of the leptomeninges to be neuroectodermal in derivation (10) make this a plausible mechanism. A likely candidate to undergo arachnoidal metaplasia is the perineurial cell. Arachnoidal and perineurial cells share some similarities, both being vimentin and epithelial membrane antigen (EMA) reactive (34). There are differences, however. Electron microscopic studies show that meningothelial cells contain intermediate filaments and are interconnected by well-formed desmosomes, whereas perineurial cells are joined by tight junctions. Furthermore, perineurial cells possess a discontinuous pericellular basement membrane as well as pinocytotic vesicles, features alien to arachnoidal cells, and lack S-100 protein immunoreactivity, a feature evident in 18 percent of meningothelial meningiomas and 80 percent of fibrous meningiomas (3,37). Nonetheless, since an intimate association with nerve is noted in some heterotopic meningiomas, particularly cutaneous examples (33), arachnoidal metaplasia of nerve sheath or mesenchymal cells may well explain the occurrence of meningiomas at such remote sites as a finger (5), muscle of the thigh (29), and in viscera such as the lung (6,24).

Clinical Features. Peripheral meningiomas represent 1 percent of all meningiomas. Nearly all are sporadic in occurrence.

The two peripheral nerve tumors reported to date arose in adult females, both in the brachial plexus (4,9). A possible third example, a psammomatous meningioma, arose in the left neck of a 15-year-old male; firmly attached to the left accessory nerve, it also featured a fibrous string-like attachment to the vertebral column (8). One mandibular nerve tumor considered a meningioma (15) has since been found to be a perineurioma.

Of meningiomas arising outside the CNS, 45 percent are cutaneous meningiomas. Rare examples, due either to multifocality (38) or to an association with pheochromocytoma (25), are thought to be a manifestation of a phakomatosis. Lopez (17) divided cutaneous meningothelial lesions into three distinct clinicopathologic types. Probably congenital, those of type I occur in children and young adults and involve primarily the scalp, forehead, and paravertebral area. Some are presumed to originate in arachnoidal rests entrapped during development, and have been conceptually linked to "rudimentary meningocele of skin" (19,27) or to "hamartoma of scalp with ectopic meningothelial elements" (31). Type II lesions often arise along the distribution of cranial or spinal nerves, particularly in the orbital, nasal, aural, and buccal regions. Their genesis may be in arachnoidal cells accompanying nerves as they penetrate the skull. Such tumors occur primarily in adults. Type III lesions result from direct extension of intracranial meningiomas into skin, and affect primarily adults; spinal examples are rare (26).

Gross and Histologic Findings. The three peripheral nerve meningiomas reported to date were all centered upon or accompanied by medium-sized or large nerves, and were located in the epineurium (fig. 10-1A,B). As in the CNS, their morphologic spectrum includes a meningothelial (4) and a transitional example (9). Psammoma bodies were present in one instance (9). Atypical features indicative of aggressive behavior, such as brisk mitotic activity, hypercellularity, and necrosis were not noted. Immunohistochemistry, performed in one case, showed reactivity for EMA (fig. 10-1C) (4). Stains for S-100 protein were negative (fig. 10-1B) as were those for glial fibrillary acidic protein (GFAP), Leu-7, and keratin preparations. These results are consistent with the immunophenotype of meningioma (3,37). Typical ultrastructural features of meningioma were apparent in the two cases (4,9) and included intracytoplasmic intermediate filaments, interdigitating cell membranes, and well-formed desmosomes. Basement membrane was lacking.

Cutaneous meningiomas generally show histologic, immunohistochemical, and ultrastructural features typical of meningioma. Unencapsulated and invasive of connective tissue, some type I lesions are nerve-associated (33). The same is true of a significant proportion of type II tumors occurring in cranial nerve distributions. In the series of Lopez et al. (17), approximately 30 percent of type I lesions corresponded to what is termed "rudimentary meningocele" or "acoelic meningeal hamartoma" (19,27). Both these and the closely related "meningeal hamartoma of the scalp" (12,31) occur in newborns or young children and tend to be associated with underlying osseous defects or other congenital anomalies. Solid or partly cystic, they are relatively hypocellular and consist in large part of meningothelial cells dissecting between collagen bundles, a pattern which may mimic vascular neoplasms, particularly angiosarcoma (31).

Differential Diagnosis. In view of the frequency with which intracranial and spinal meningiomas extend peripherally through a dural root sleeve, confirmation of an ectopic origin requires careful attention to neuroimaging and operative findings. Rare soft tissue *meningiomas unassociated with nerve* (29) must also be excluded. The ease with which perineurioma may be confused with meningioma is illustrated by one mandibular tumor mimicking meningioma (15). Lastly, given the wide morphologic spectrum of meningiomas, the differential diagnosis is broad. In the context of a nerve-associated neoplasm, principal lesions include *schwannoma* and *soft tissue perineurioma*. Their salient morphologic and immunohistochemical differences from meningioma are summarized in Table

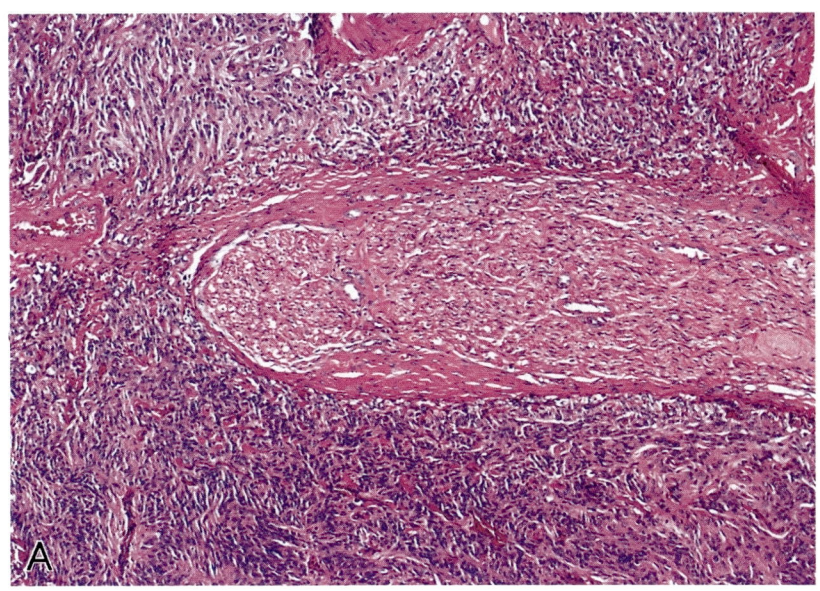

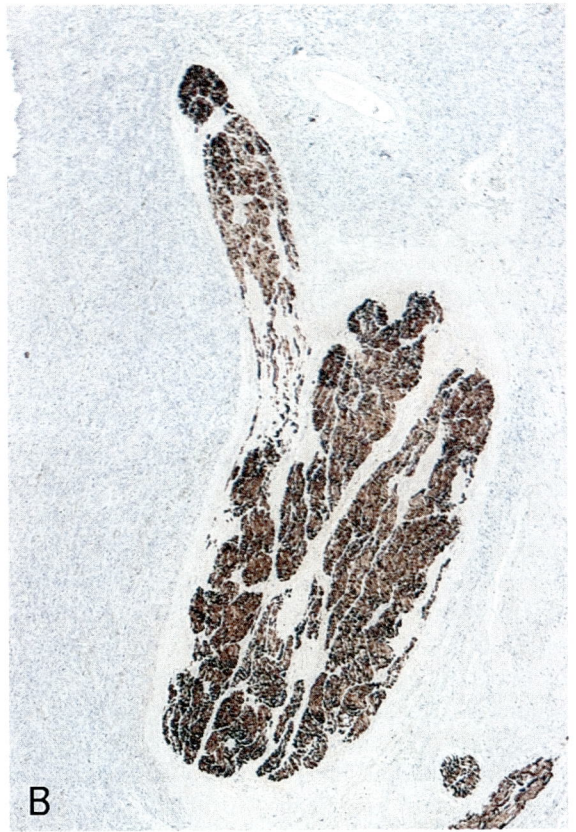

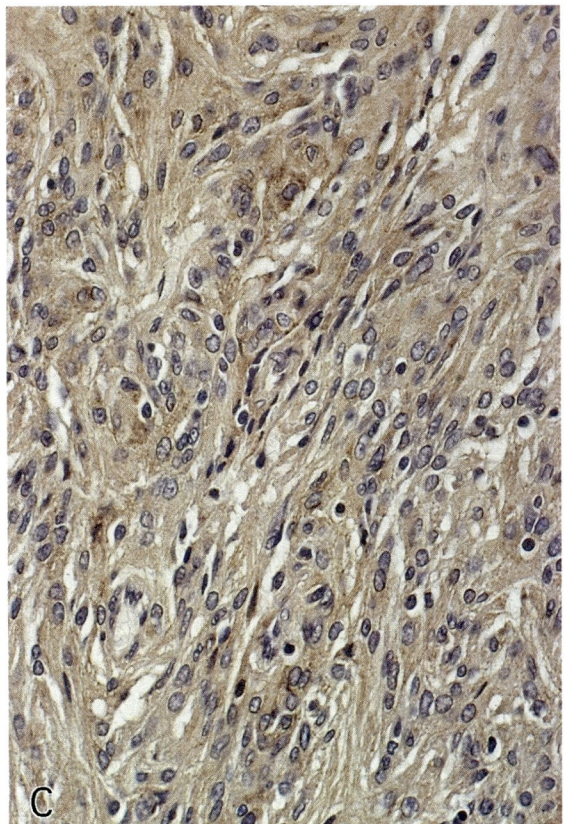

Figure 10-1
MENINGIOMA OF NERVE

This multiple recurrent, rather cellular meningothelial meningioma arose in the brachial plexus of a 50-year-old female with a long history of pain. It encased nerve fascicles (A), here accentuated on S-100 protein stain (B), and was EMA immunoreactive (C). (Courtesy of Drs. S. Coons, Phoenix, AZ and P.C. Johnson, Tuscon, AZ.)

Table 10-1
DIFFERENTIAL DIAGNOSIS

Features	Meningioma	Schwannoma	Soft Tissue Perineurioma
Antoni A and/or B pattern	(-)	Frequent	(-)
Verocay bodies	(-)	Frequent	(-)
Whorls	Frequent, tight	Rare, vague	Occasional, loose
Psammoma bodies	20%	Rare	(-)
Reticulin pattern	Variable	Intercellular	Intercellular
S-100 protein	18-80%	100%	(-)
EMA	70-95%	(-)	100%
Cytokeratin	5%	(-)	(-)
Interdigitating cell membranes	Yes	No	No
Entangled cell processes	No	Yes	No
Junctions	Well-formed desmosomes	Rudimentary	Rudimentary and tight
Basement membranes	Absent	Continuous	Discontinuous

10-1. A full discussion of the differential diagnosis of meningioma may be found in the Alas of Tumor Pathology, Tumors of the Central Nervous System (2).

Meningiomas secondarily involving nerve are far more common than ones arising primarily in nerve. Actual invasion of nerve by nearby meningiomas may have implications for their recurrence (16).

Treatment and Prognosis. Too few meningiomas of peripheral nerve have been described to draw conclusions regarding prognosis. The subtotally excised brachial plexus tumor of Coons and Johnson (4) was associated with multiple recurrences despite absence of atypia. After multiple partial resections and two courses of radiotherapy, the patient is alive at 17 years with persistent disease. None have metastasized, a rare occurrence in meningiomas at any site. The patient that Hallgrimsson et al. (8) treated by resection with sparing of the nerve was tumor-free at 3 years. Depending upon the nerve involved, gross total removal or simple debulking of tumor may be the treatment of choice. As at other sites, radiation therapy may be required when complete resection is not possible (4).

Although cutaneous meningiomas are benign, the prognosis varies with their location (35). Ones limited to skin (type I) are only locally infiltrative and are amenable to resection. Meningiomas of skin, particularly scalp lesions, may communicate with the underlying meninges; cautious resection is required in order to avoid a cerebrospinal fluid leak (22). Type II tumors have a guarded prognosis, due to their location and capacity for recurrence. Given the association of type III tumors with central disease, many are inoperable. Malignant primary cutaneous meningiomas undergoing distant metastasis are rare (18).

MISCELLANEOUS TUMORS AND TUMOR-LIKE LESIONS

Paraganglioma of Nerve Root

On occasion, extra-adrenal paragangliomas arise at sites in which paraganglia do not normally occur. These include the duodenum (64, 85), filum terminale (92), and pituitary (86). Rarely, large nerves are affected, particularly spinal nerve roots of the cauda equina (88,92,99) or other spinal levels (40). Of these, paraganglioma of cauda equina are by far the most common. With rare exception, they occur in adults, showing a 2 to 1 male predilection. Symptoms include low back pain, sensorimotor deficits, and bowel and bladder dysfunction. On computerized tomography (CT) and magnetic resonance imaging (MRI) scans, paragangliomas present as contrast-enhancing, sausage-shaped masses. Most measure several centimeters in size, but one massive, 13-cm example has been reported (99). Enveloped by a delicate fibrous

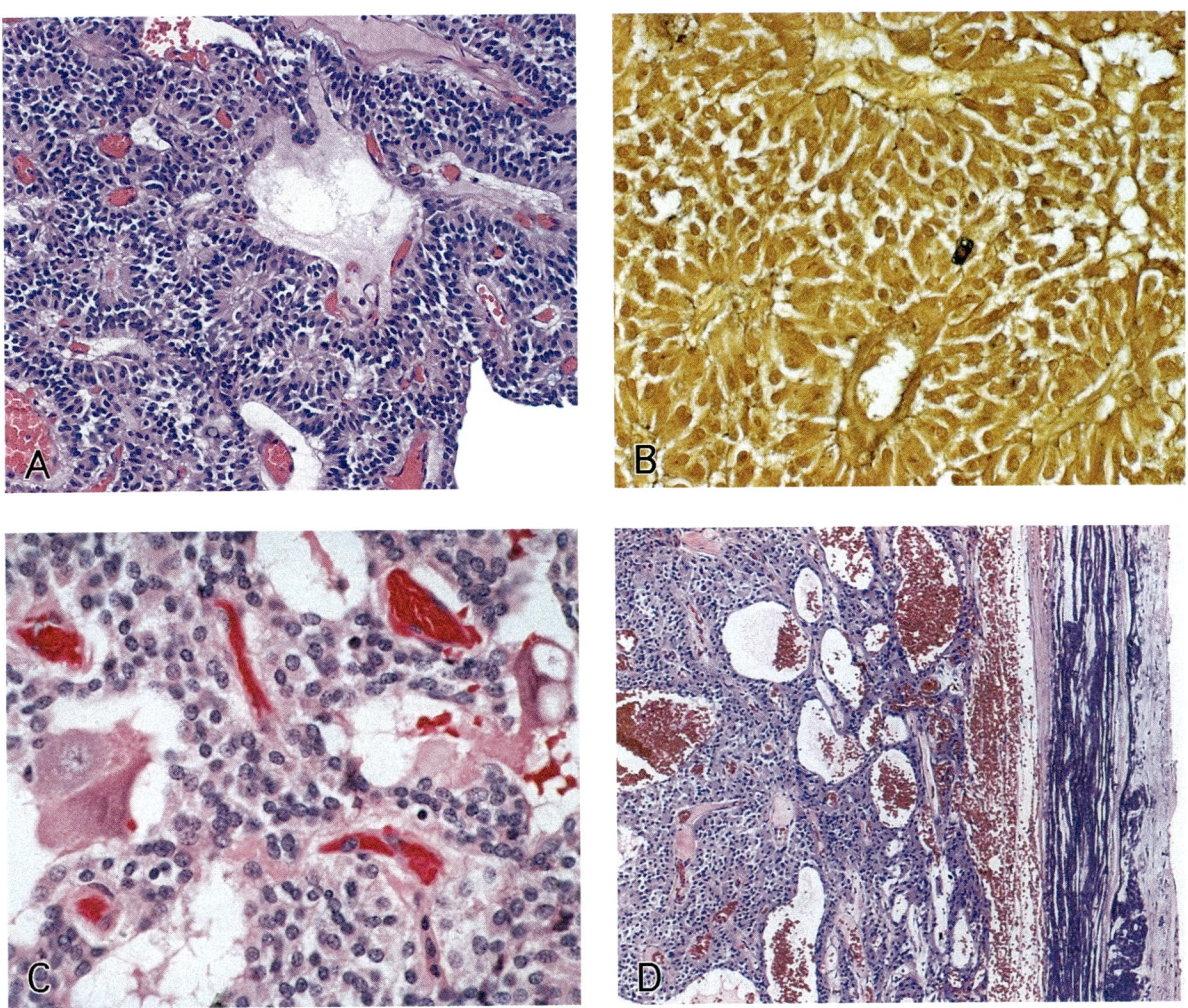

Figure 10-2
PARAGANGLIOMA OF NERVE ROOT
Although the occurrence of perivascular pseudorosettes and mucin accumulation may simulate myxopapillary ependymoma (A), argyrophilia (Grimelius stain) readily permits the correct diagnosis (B). Half of cauda equina lesions show ganglionic differentiation (C). Occasional examples have capsular calcifications (D). (D, courtesy of Dr. N. Karpinski, San Diego, CA.)

capsule, occasionally with microcalcification (fig. 10-2), their histologic patterns vary considerably. Most tumors show the typical zellballen pattern exhibited by paragangliomas at other sites. Yet others feature a ribbon or pseudorosette pattern resembling that of carcinoid tumor (fig. 10-2A). Ganglionic differentiation (fig. 10-2C) is seen in up to half of paragangliomas of the cauda equina region (92). The neuroendocrine nature of their chief cells is confirmed by the findings of argyrophilia (fig. 10-2B) and occasionally by argentaffin staining, as well as by immunoreactivity for neuron-specific enolase, synapto-

physin, chromogranin, and such neuropeptides as somatostatin, serotonin, or metenkephalin (59,65,92). Cytokeratin expression by chief cells is reportedly a feature of paragangliomas occurring in the cauda equina region (75). Clusters of chief cells are encircled by modified Schwann cells. Termed sustentacular cells, they demonstrate immunoreactivity for S-100 protein and GFAP. The ultrastructural findings are those of paragangliomas occurring at other sites (52). These include the presence within chief cells of 100- to 400-nm secretory granules, occasionally numerous or atypical mitochondria, moderately

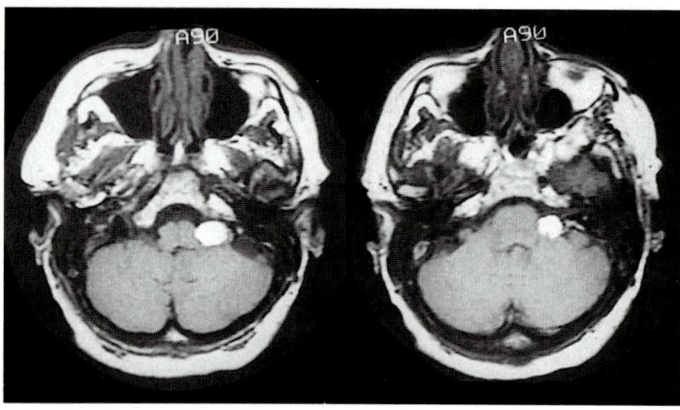

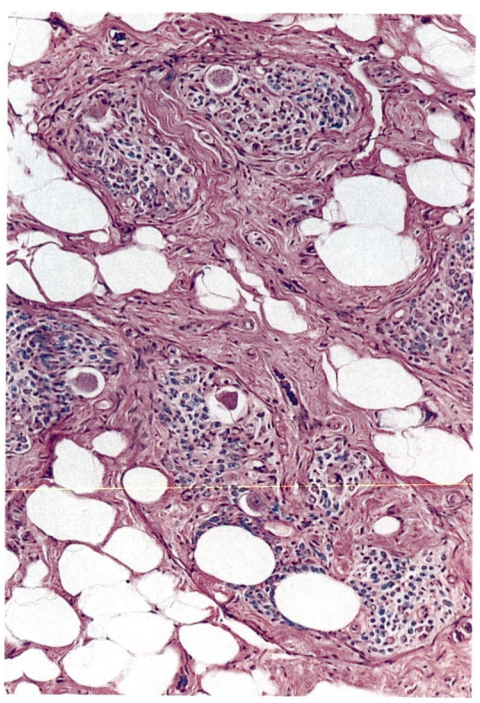

Figure 10-3
LIPOMA OF 8TH NERVE

Above: The MRI appearance of this lesion, here seen as a bright signal on T1-weighted sequence, is diagnostic. (Courtesy of Dr. G.M. Miller, Rochester, MN.)

Right: Note the entrapment of nerve fascicles and accompanying ganglion cells by benign adipose tissue. (Courtesy of Dr. P.C. Burger, Baltimore, MD.)

developed Golgi complexes, small stacks of rough endoplasmic reticulum, smooth endoplasmic reticulum, lysosomes in small number, and occasional arrays of intermediate filaments. Process formation and rudimentary junctions are also seen. Sustentacular cells vary in number and may be absent, particularly in malignant examples.

While the majority of nerve root paragangliomas lend themselves to gross total resection, a minority are locally invasive. Invasiveness is more often a feature of recurrent tumors. Of subtotally resected lesions, approximately 10 percent recur at 1 year (88). Paragangliomas of nerve are rarely malignant; only one example, a lesion occurring at the cervical level, has been reported (40). The aggressive potential of both adrenal and extra-adrenal paragangliomas is related to anaplastic changes reflected by a diminution of or lack of neuropeptide immunoreactivity (65,70) and sustentacular cells (65).

Spinal intradural paragangliomas must be distinguished from *myxopapillary ependymoma.* In contrast to paraganglioma, ependymomas far more often break through their capsules to involve surrounding leptomeninges and nerve roots, exhibit widespread GFAP positivity, and lack both neuronal differentiation and immunoreactivity for neuroendocrine markers (93).

Lipoma

Soft tissue lipomas secondarily compressing peripheral nerve are uncommon (76,94). They are well circumscribed by a delicate capsule, arise in subfacial tissue or in intermuscular planes, and are composed entirely of adipose tissue. In the upper extremity, the posterior interosseous nerve is most often affected (58). *Lipoma of nerve sheath,* defined as a discrete, delicately encapsulated epineurial lesion, is rare (see chapter 6, fig. 6-5, upper right) (83,93). Excision of both soft tissue and nerve sheath lipomas is curative and unassociated with neurologic deficits. Neither is accompanied by macrodactyly. For a discussion of lipofibromatous hamartoma of nerve, the reader is referred to chapter 6.

Cranial nerve lipomas are rare and present in adulthood. Most arise in the cerebellopontine angle where they affect the 8th or occasionally, other nerves (46,62,89). Although clinically confused with acoustic schwannoma, the neuroimaging characteristics of fat permit a preoperative diagnosis in nearly all instances. Microscopically, they consist of mature adipose tissue intimately associated with nerve fascicles, fibers, and ganglion cells (fig. 10-3, above). As is the case in lipomas affecting other CNS sites, the occasional presence of heterologous elements, such as muscle (see figs. 6-7, 6-8) (39), suggests that lipomas of the 8th nerve may be malformative rather than neoplastic in nature. The relation of such muscle-containing CNS lesions to intracranial neuromuscular choristoma (55), or rhabdomyomatous lesions with scant adipose tissue content (95) or none at all (100), remains unsettled (see Neuromuscular Choristoma, page 101).

Spinal epidural lipomatosis, a rare disorder often associated with the administration of exogenous steroids or with endogenous steroid excess, may produce radiculopathy (80). It affects primarily the thoracolumbar region and occurs mainly in obese males. Surgical decompression is the treatment of choice.

Vascular Tumors of Nerve

Benign vascular lesions rarely affect nerve. The clinicopathologic features of the approximately 15 reported *hemangiomas* were recently summarized (51a,82a,96). Fully half of patients are of pediatric age, but no sex predilection is apparent. There is also no association with prior trauma. In order of decreasing frequency, involved nerves include the median, ulnar, digital, peroneal, and tibial. Cranial nerves are rarely affected (70b). Pain is the most common symptom, although early lesions may present as asymptomatic lumps. Most are solitary globular lesions grossly mistaken for nerve sheath tumor. Multiple tumors are rare, as is extensive "hemangiomatosis" of a nerve (93a). Affecting primarily epineurium, the hemangiomas may be of cavernous or capillary type (fig. 10-4) (70a). We have encountered one example of spindle cell hemangioendothelioma. Hemangiomas showing a compact pattern of growth, particularly ones featuring mitotic activity, should not be mistaken for angiosarcoma (see below) (fig. 10-4D). An occasional feature of capillary hemangiomas is extramedullary hemopoiesis. Treatment has varied from intraneural dissection with gross total or partial tumor resection to excision of the affected nerve. With the exception of one case in which two partial resections failed to alleviate pain, thus necessitating amputation (93a), all patients have experienced symptomatic improvement without tumor recurrence. A conservative, nerve-sparing approach is therefore recommended.

Of particular note is a report of a case of *angiomatosis of nerve* (fig. 10-5) associated with multiple soft tissue tumors (fig. 10-6) in the setting of progressive peripheral neuropathy (57). It featured a massive proliferation of small vessels with abnormally thick walls, extensively replacing both the endoneurium and perineurium of multiple peripheral nerves (fig. 10-5A,B). That the constituent cells were either pericytes or smooth muscle cells was suggested by intense immunoreactivity for actin and smooth muscle actin (fig. 10-5C), as well as by the ultrastructural features. The patient also exhibited multiple, often partially calcified soft tissue tumors. Histologically these resembled infantile myofibromatosis (fig. 10-5D) and showed immunohistochemical and ultrastructural features of either smooth muscle or myofibroblastic differentiation. At surgery, a peripheral nerve branch appeared to course directly into one such tumor. This association of a diffuse polyneuropathy with widespread angiomatosis and multifocal soft tissue tumors (fig. 10-6) may well be a manifestation of a previously unrecognized syndrome. Soft tissue angiomatosis with involvement of small peripheral nerve fascicles has also been described (79).

Primary *angiosarcoma of nerve* is rare; only two cases have been reported (43,49). A detailed discussion of this and malignant vascular tumors secondarily affecting nerve are found in chapter 12.

The *glomus tumor,* an uncommon benign vascular tumor, rarely affects nerve. Only three cases have been reported; affected nerves included the radial nerve in the axillary region (fig. 10-7) (91), a digital nerve (66), and a dermal nerve in the shoulder (48). All occurred in adults and two involved grossly apparent nerves. In the dermal example, a nerve association was evident only at the histologic level where nerve fiber bundles traversed the lesion and a surrounding epineurium was observed (48). Tumors ranged from several millimeters to 2.5 cm in size. The lesions appeared discrete, the largest having the appearance of a schwannoma which shelled out with preservation of adjacent nerve fascicles (fig. 10-7, above) (91). A nerve-sparing surgical approach is therefore recommended. The occurrence of glomus tumors within nerve remains to be explained since glomus bodies are not normally encountered in nerve.

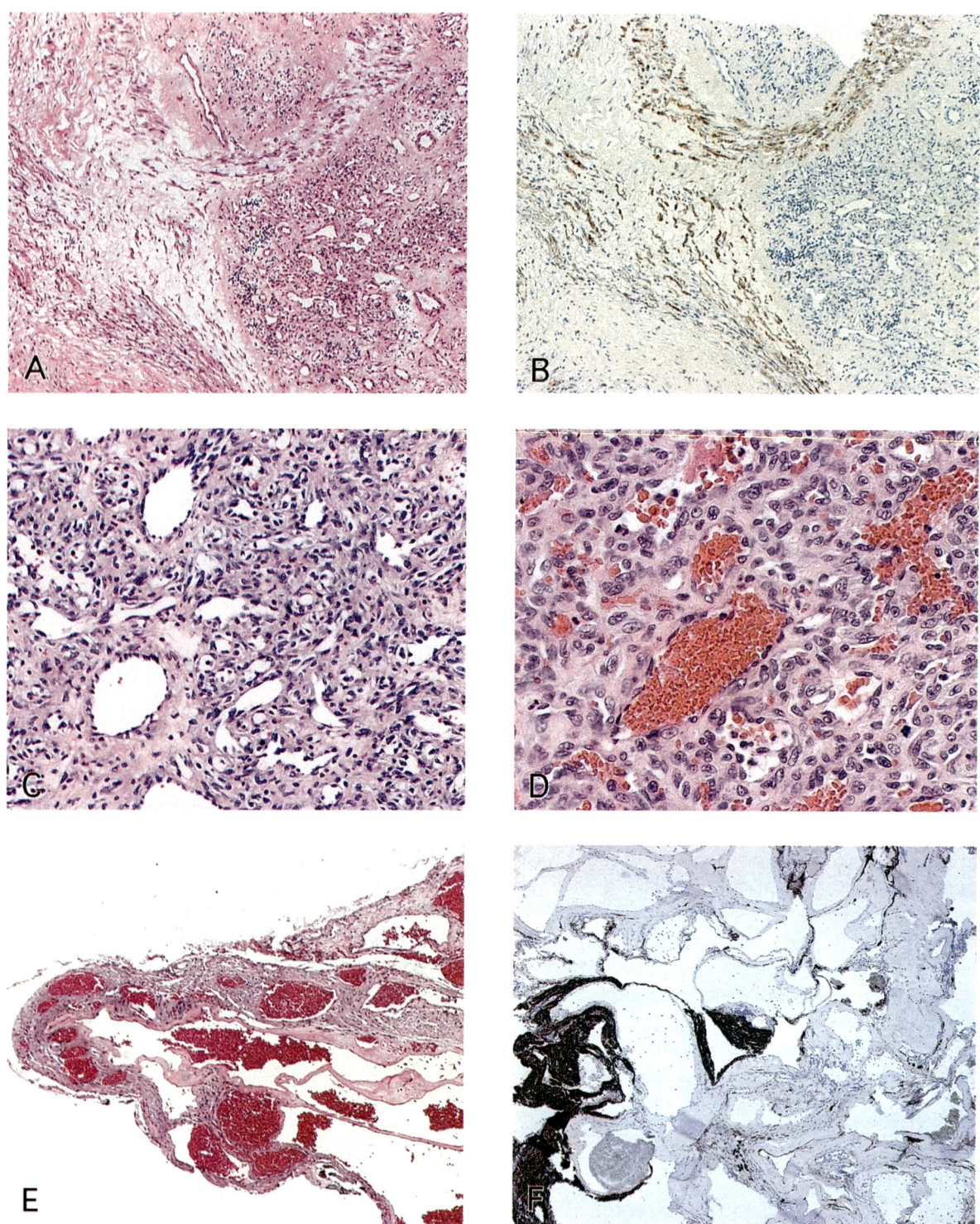

Figure 10-4
VASCULAR TUMORS OF NERVE

Capillary hemangiomas show lobular architecture (A) and lie in epineurium between nerve fascicles (B). Whereas most feature obvious lumen formation (C), occasional examples are cellular and mitotically active (D). Cavernous angiomas, such as this facial nerve lesion (E), consist of large vascular spaces composed of hyaline vessels (E). They too are epineurial in location (F, neurofilament protein immunostain). (E: Courtesy of Dr. D. Horoupian, Stanford, CA.)

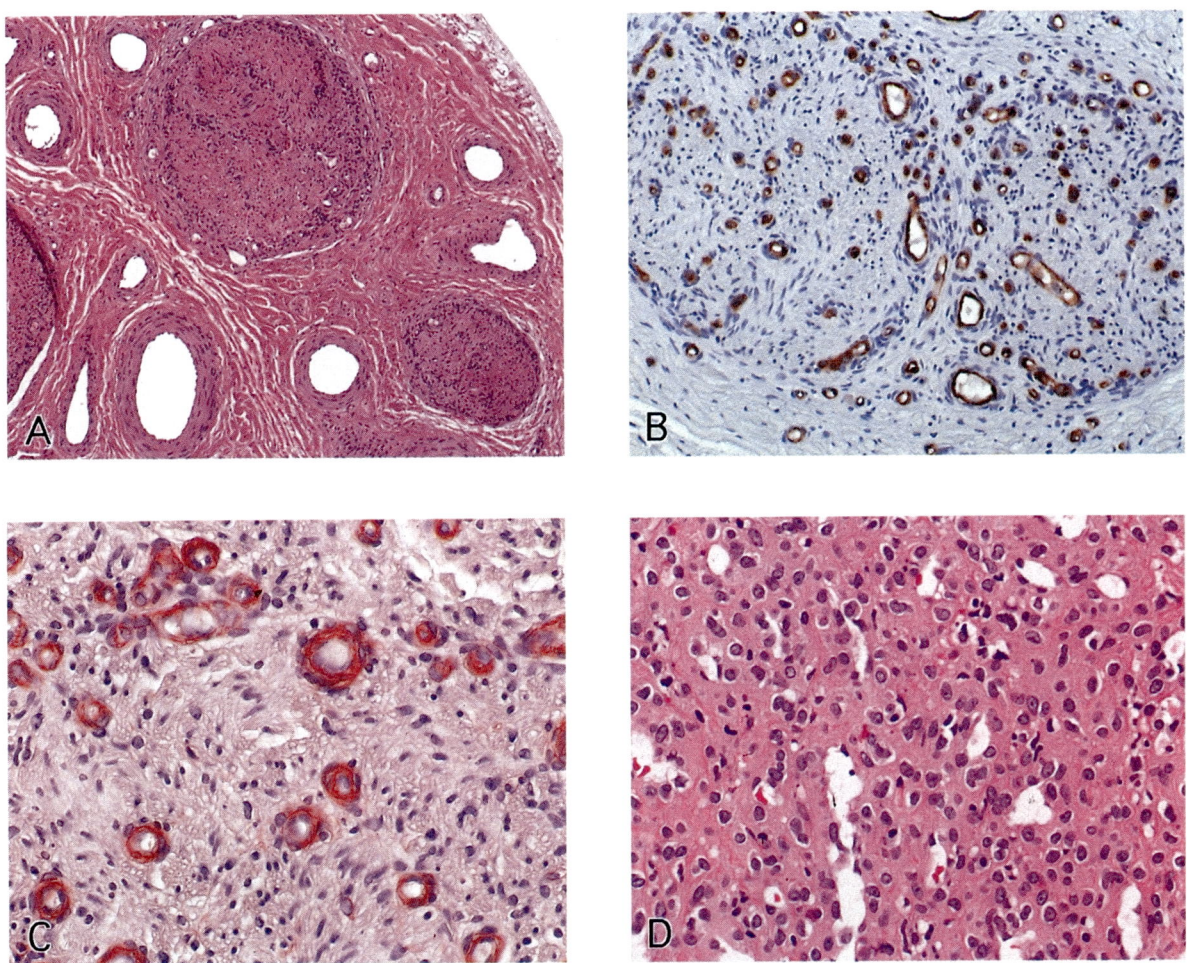

Figure 10-5
ANGIOMATOSIS OF PERIPHERAL NERVE

Sections of the sural nerve (A), show architecture of the perineurium and endoneurium to be retained. Myelinated fibers are severely and diffusely decreased. A striking proliferation of small vessels with thickened walls is present in the perineurium and extends into the endoneurium, partially replacing it. These vessels are accentuated on immunostains for factor VIII-related antigen (B). The cells present in the wall of the numerous, thickened perineurial and endoneurial vessels show intense immunoreactivity for alpha smooth muscle actin (C). The soft tissue nodules, this one from the lateral neck, show infantile myofibromatosis or hemangiopericytoma-like features (D). (All figures courtesy of Drs. C. Giannini and P.J. Dyck, Treviso, Italy and Rochester, MN, respectively.)

Only a single bona fide *hemangiopericytoma* of nerve has been described (99a). Involving the sciatic nerve of an adult, it was entirely limited to epineurium. On occasion, a rare MPNST shows a hemangiopericytoma-like pattern (see fig. 11-13D).

Hemangioblastoma of Nerve

Virtually limited to the CNS, this tumor of adulthood typically arises in the cerebellum. Depending upon their site in the brain or spinal cord, one third to nearly all are associated with von Hippel-Lindau disease, an inherited, autosomal dominant disorder characterized by retinal, cerebellar, and spinal hemangioblastomas; renal cell carcinoma; cysts or cystic neoplasms of the pancreas, liver, or epididymis; and pheochromocytoma (87). The 5 percent that arise in the spinal cord, often from its dorsal aspect, lie in close proximity to spinal nerve roots which may occasionally be directly involved (45,98). On the other hand, hemangioblastomas limited to

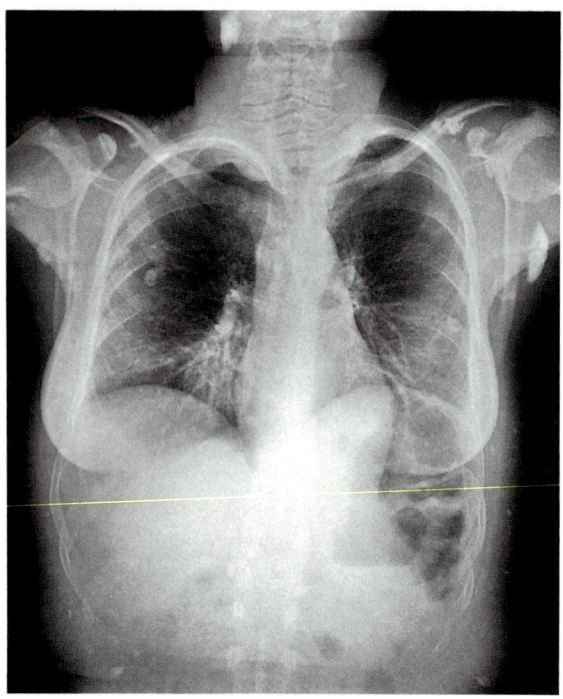
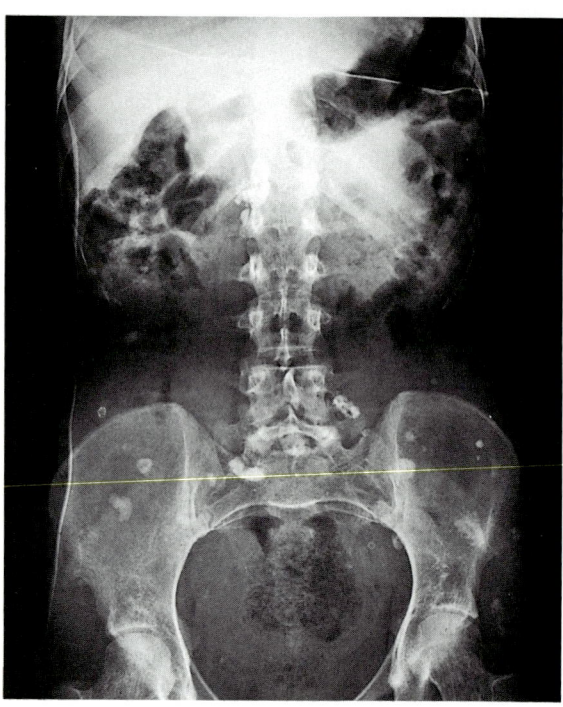

Figure 10-6

ANGIOMATOSIS OF PERIPHERAL NERVE WITH SOFT TISSUE TUMOR ASSOCIATION

Multiple, calcified, subcutaneous and deep soft tissue nodules ranging in size from 0.5 to 3 cm are present in the lateral neck, axilla, chest (left), and abdomen (right). (Fig. 1 from Giannini C, Wright A, Dyck PJ. Polyneuropathy associated with nerve angiomatosis and multiple soft tissue tumors. A newly recognized syndrome. Am J Surg Pathol 1995;19:1325–32.)

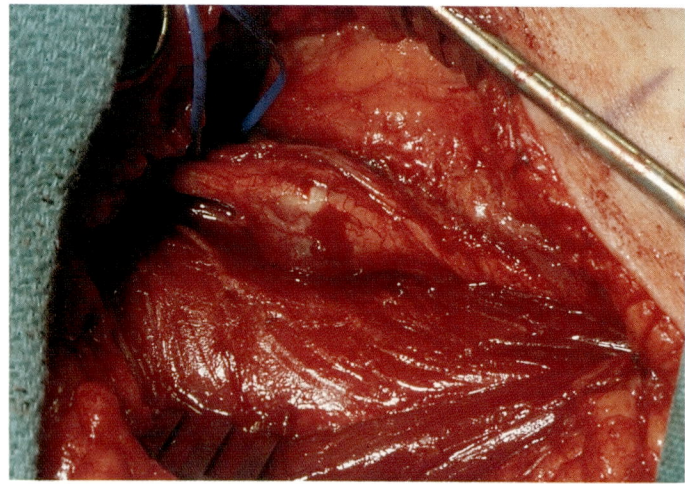
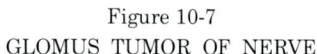
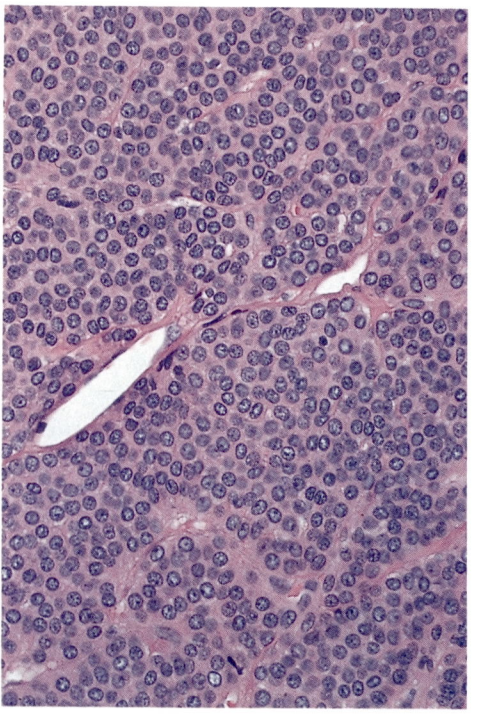

Figure 10-7

GLOMUS TUMOR OF NERVE

This well-demarcated brachial plexus example (above) arose in the epineurium of the radial nerve, displaced fascicles, and showed the typical histologic features of glomus tumor (right). For clinical details, see ref. 52. (Courtesy of Dr. S. E. MacKennan, St. Louis, MO.)

nerve are rare. With the exception of two reported examples (44,56), all have been intradural, arising either from a sensory nerve root (44,45,56, 60,98) or from a ganglion (67). Dumbbell-shaped tumors with intradural and extradural-extraspinal components are rare (81). In one instance (45), multiple cervical, thoracic, and lumbar hemangioblastomas of microscopic dimension were an incidental autopsy finding.

Approximately half of patients with hemangioblastoma of nerve have von Hippel-Lindau disease. Patient ages range from 17 to 79 years with no sex predilection. Sensory symptoms predominate, a reflection of the high frequency of posterior root involvement in intradural tumors. Several lesions measured 3.5 cm. With increase in tumor size, spinal cord or anterior root compression results in associated motor signs. Although invasion of nerve fascicles may necessitate sacrifice of the parent nerve, its sparing by microsurgical resection of the lesion appears to be the treatment of choice (56). Grossly, the tumors are demarcated, yellow-red, and associated with prominent feeder vessels. Microscopically, they are often multinodular and show microcystic degeneration. The cells are concentrated in the epineurium, frequently about feeder vessels of varying size (fig. 10-8A), but fascicular invasion is commonly seen. At higher magnification the stromal cells of hemangioblastoma, with their round nuclei and vacuolated, lipid-rich cytoplasm, fill the interstices between innumerable capillaries (fig. 10-8B). In areas in which fascicles are involved, the tumor cells lie among nerve fibers (fig. 10-8C). Termed "stromal cells," they are S-100 protein positive. Unlike some hemangioblastomas involving brain or spinal cord which on occasion exhibit unexplained GFAP reactivity, reported peripheral nerve examples are nonreactive for this antigen (44,56).

The differential diagnosis is primarily with *renal cell carcinoma,* a lesion often associated with von Hippel-Lindau disease. Renal cell carcinomas stain for keratin and EMA. It is of note, however, that 15 to 20 percent of primary and 50 percent of metastatic renal cell carcinomas are S-100 protein positive. The prognosis of hemangioblastoma is excellent. No reported examples have recurred. Whereas radiotherapy plays a limited role in the treatment of cerebellar and spinal hemangio-

blastomas (90), adjuvant treatment has not been employed in peripheral nerve lesions.

Adrenal Adenoma of Spinal Nerve Root

To date, four examples of heterotopic adrenal tissue within the nervous system have been described, including one intracranial "rest" composed of adrenal cortex and medulla (72), as well as three adrenal cortical adenomas of spinal nerve root (63,73). The clinicopathologic features of the latter were recently summarized (73). All were discrete tumors of the spinal region (fig. 10-9A) and involved either anterior or posterior roots. Unlike the adrenal rest, which was an incidental autopsy finding, the three adenomas of nerve root were symptomatic due to pressure effects. Their microscopic features were typical of adrenal adenoma (fig. 10-9B). In one case, biochemical measurement of adrenal steroid hormones showed high tumoral levels (63). In two other cases, immunohistochemistry demonstrated the presence of adrenal enzymes (fig. 10-9C) (73). Despite these findings, none of the lesions were endocrinologically active. Given their relatively discrete nature, gross total resection with sparing of the involved root was possible in all cases. No recurrences have been reported.

Hemopoietic Neoplasms

Primary Lymphoma of Nerve. Involvement of peripheral nerve usually occurs in the setting of disseminated lymphoma or is due to direct extension from contiguous disease (47,84). The subject is discussed in detail in chapter 12.

Primary non-Hodgkin lymphomas of peripheral nerve are rare. Of reported, well-characterized examples, all but one (97) have arisen in the sciatic nerve (fig. 10-10) (53,61,77,78,82). Adults ranged in age from 34 to 72 years (mean, 55 years). None had evidence of systemic lymphoma or immunodeficiency. Men were predominantly affected (5 to 1). Symptoms included progressive paresthesia, numbness, weakness, and pain. Involvement was unilateral but varied in terms of the level at which the nerve was involved; three affected the mid-portion of the nerve, one arose at the level of the femoral head, and another extended within nerve from the level of the ischium to the ankle; a lumbar root lesion was both intradural and extradural (97). Tumors formed fusiform enlargements of the

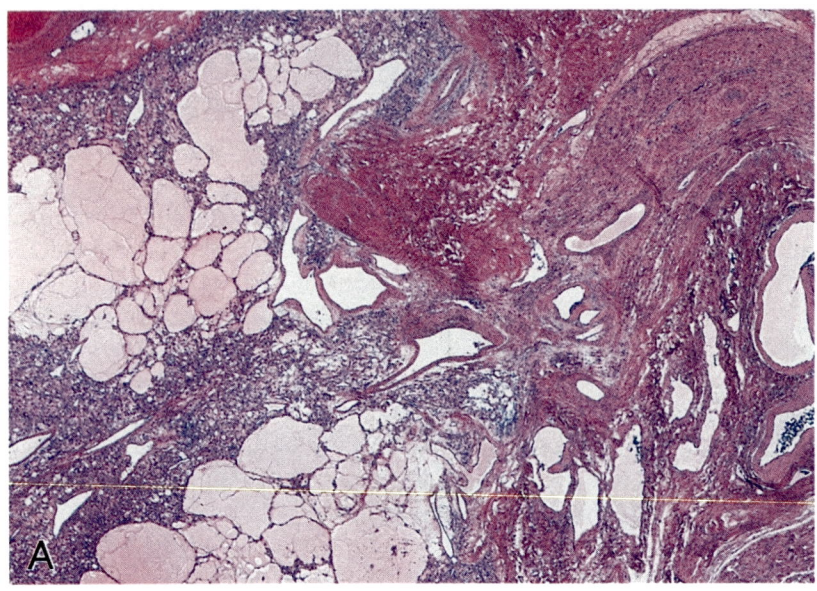

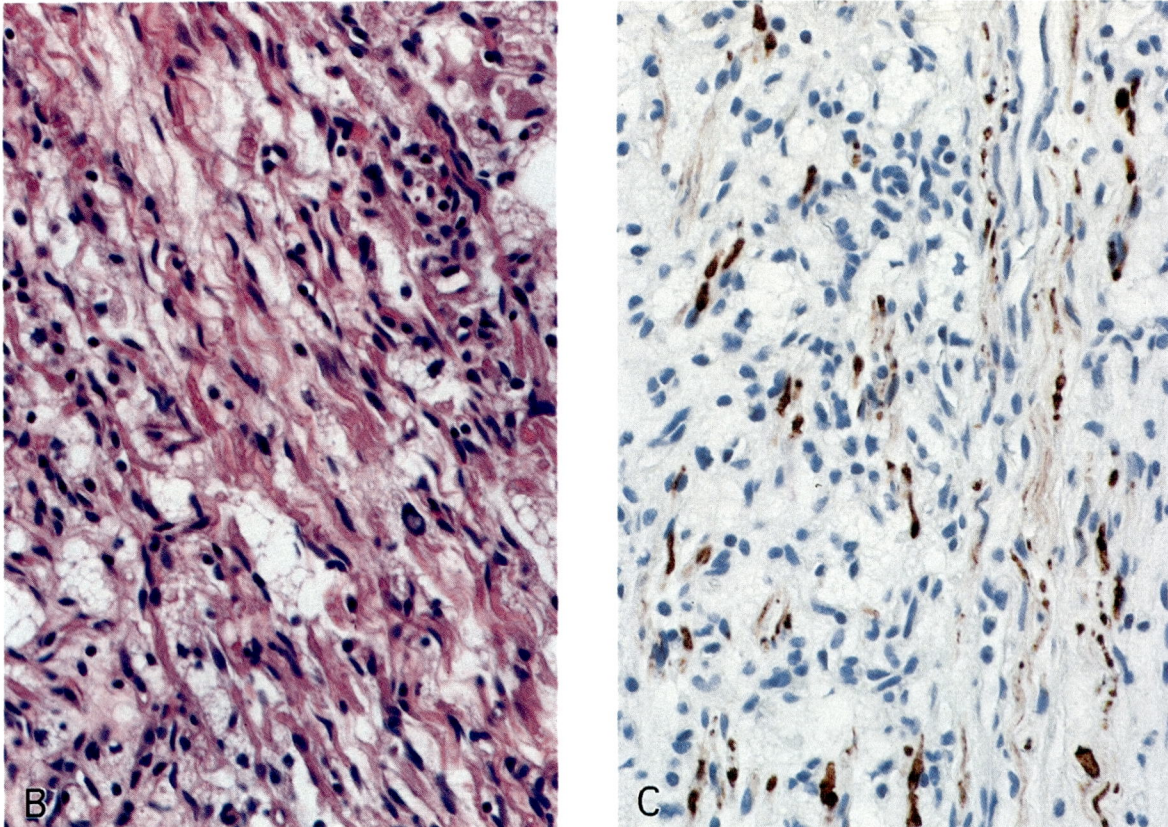

Figure 10-8
HEMANGIOBLASTOMA OF NERVE

The cellular, nodular, and multicystic tumor involves primarily the epineurium. Note a nerve fascicle traversing the lesion (A, upper right), and lipid-rich stromal cells within the interstices of the capillary network (B). Some degree of fascicular involvement was evident on neurofilament protein stain (C).

Figure 10-9
ADRENAL CORTICAL ADENOMA OF NERVE ROOT
The nodular tumor was delicately encapsulated (A) and readily separated from the parent nerve. Microscopically, it resembled adrenal cortex (B) and was seen on immunohistochemistry to contain cytochrome P 450-11b, a steroidogenic adrenal cortical enzyme (C).

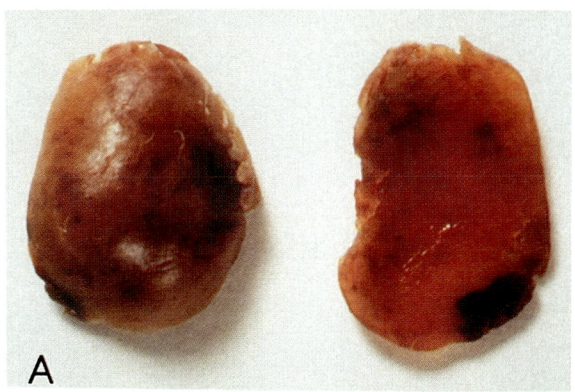

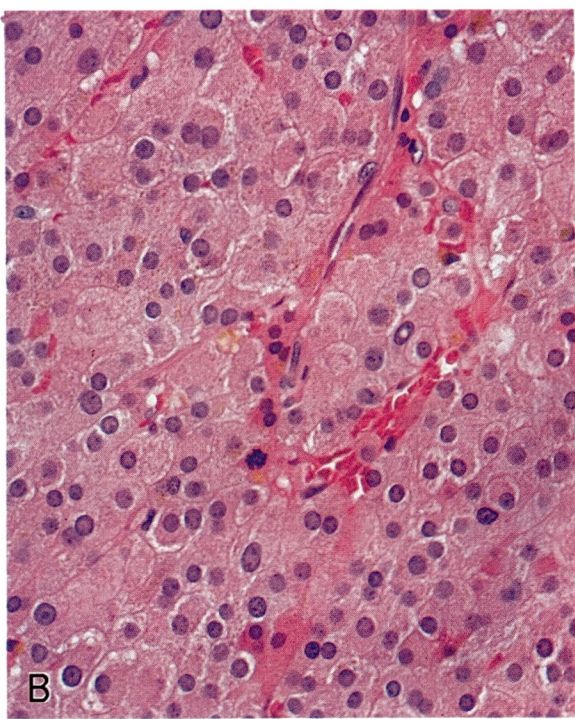

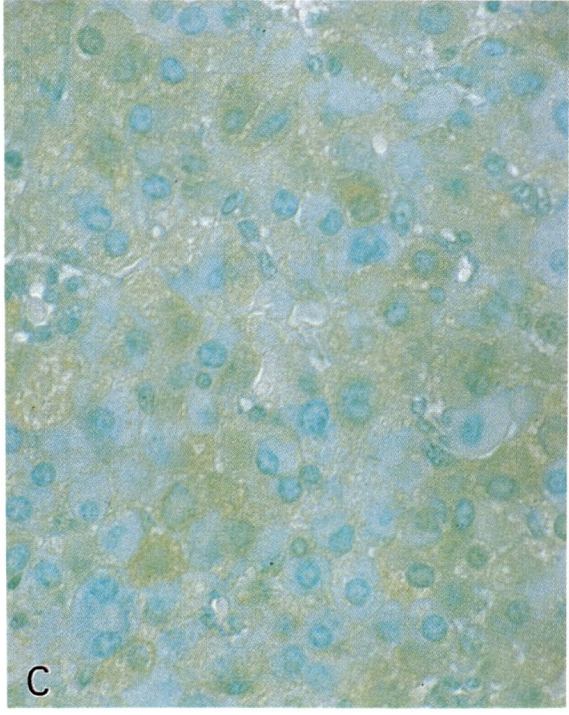

nerve, an appearance indistinguishable from nerve sheath tumors. All but two T-cell examples were B-cell lymphomas. Four were diffuse in histologic pattern and one was nodular. Three tumors were intermediate and two were high-grade types. Despite various combinations of resection, radiation, and chemotherapy, three tumors disseminated between 16 and 50 months of clinical onset. Details regarding the clinicopathologic findings in five of the six reported cases are summarized in a recent article on the subject (82). We have examined a diffuse, large

cell lymphoma of B-cell type arising in an intra-dural lumbar nerve root. Unassociated with systemic disease, it exhibited both an epineurial and intrafascicular pattern of growth (fig. 10-11).

Amyloidoma of Nerve. Once termed "tumefactive amyloidosis of nerve," amyloidomas of the peripheral nervous system are extremely rare. They are localized plasma cell tumors composed primarily of amyloid and only scant plasma cells. Most have involved the trigeminal (Gasserian) ganglion (41,42,50,51,69,71,74); in one case involvement was bilateral (74). Peripheral

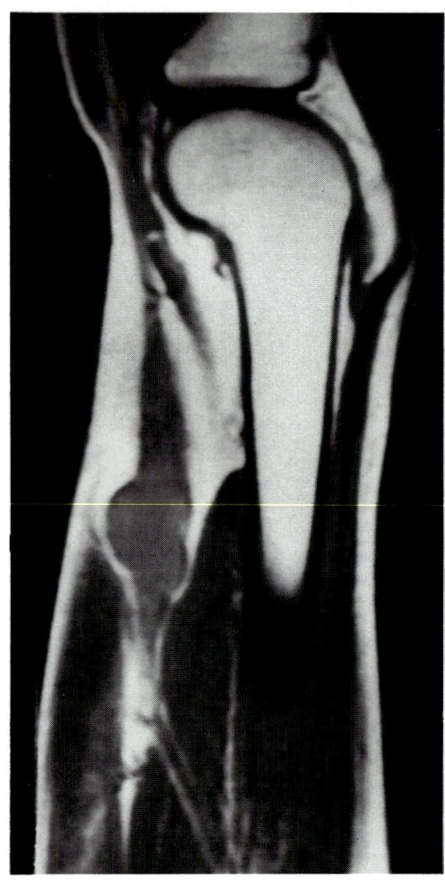

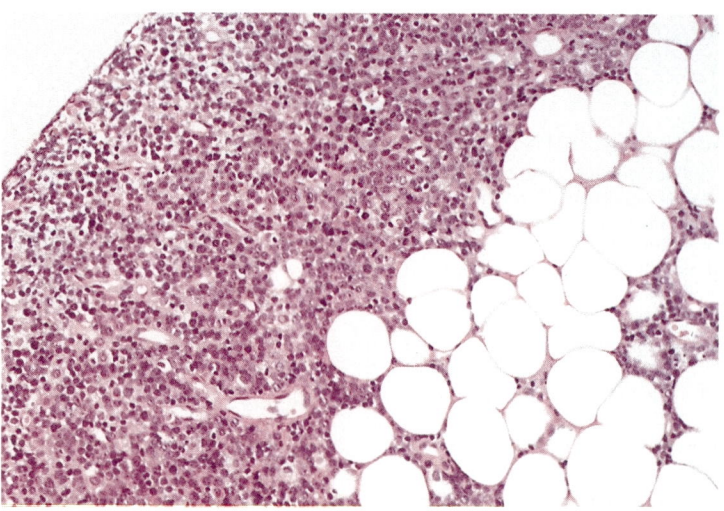

Figure 10-10
PRIMARY LYMPHOMA OF NERVE
An MRI scan clearly shows that the globular tumor arises in the sciatic nerve (left). Microsections of the sparing biopsy shows infiltration of epineurium (above); nerve-fascicles were not sampled. For clinical description, see ref. 82. (Courtesy of Dr. F Roncaroli, Bologna, Italy.)

nerves are less often involved; reported examples have included the infraorbital (68) and sciatic nerves (54). As in amyloidomas of the CNS, no association with systemic amyloidosis has been reported (69).

Although both central and peripheral amyloidomas are sparsely cellular, their localized occurrence and λ light chain immunoreactivity (69) suggest they are not simply pseudotumors. Supporting the concept that amyloidomas are neoplastic in nature and essentially represent "burned out plasmacytomas" are the findings of solely AL λ genome expression by in situ hybridization and immunoglobulin gene rearrangement (69).

Symptoms related to trigeminal nerve involvement include progressive numbness, dysesthesia, and neuralgia (41,42,50,51,54,68,69,74). In instances in which the lesion also extends into the cerebellopontine angle and jugular foramen, resultant hemifacial spasms, cerebellar signs, and hearing loss may be observed (71). On MRI, a hypodense mass is seen on T1-weighted im-

ages, one that enhances upon contrast administration. Edema is absent in surrounding brain.

The gross and histologic features of amyloidomas are typical. They are solitary, appear tan-brown, and are rubbery, waxy, or crumbly in consistency. Small foci of calcification may be observed.

In hematoxylin and eosin (H&E)–stained sections, amyloid appears as acellular, eosinophilic material. Unlike collagen, it is a homogeneous or delicately fibrillar rather than forming coarse bundles. Within ganglia and nerve, interstitial amyloid deposits extensively replace parenchyma (fig. 10-12A). Ganglion cells and nerve fibers are widely dispersed. Sparsely scattered lymphocytes and mature plasma cells vary in number but are generally scant. In addition to massive interstitial deposits, the walls of entrapped blood vessels typically also contain amyloid. The substance is Congo red positive and shows apple green birefringence under polarized light (fig. 10-12B) as well as bright yellow-green fluorescence in thioflavin T preparations.

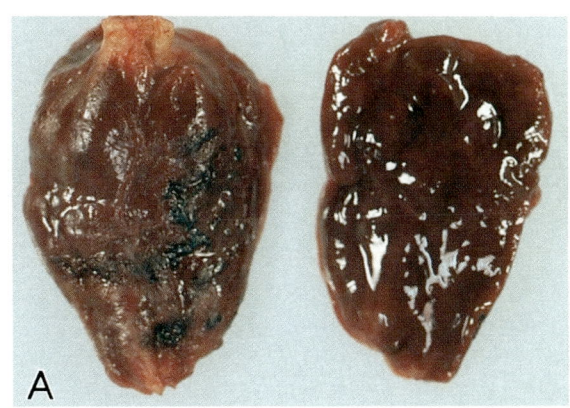

Figure 10-11
PRIMARY LYMPHOMA OF NERVE
This globular lumbar nerve root tumor of B-cell type was unassociated with disease elsewhere. It replaced the parent nerve (A, top) and infiltrated both epineurium and endoneurium (B). (C, neurofilament protein)

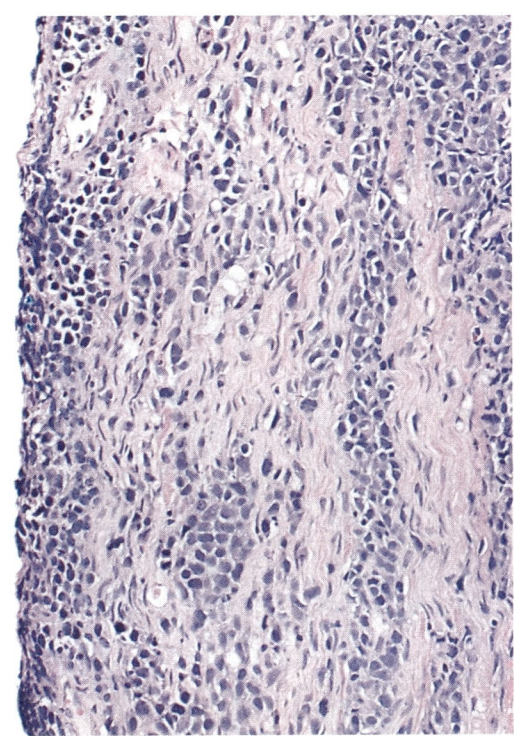

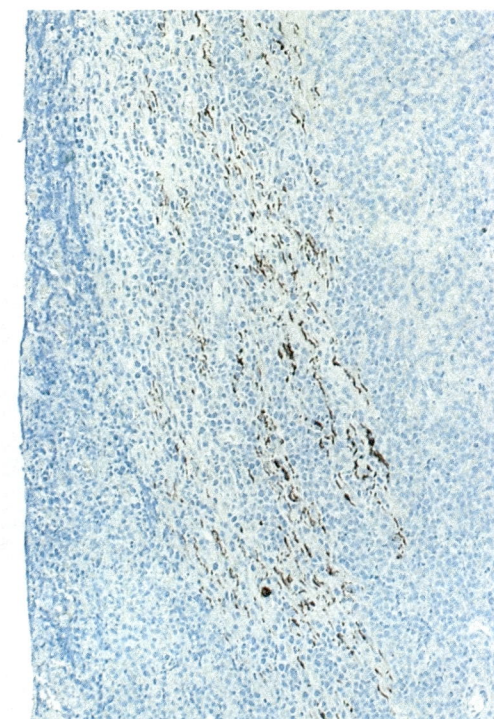

The amyloid in nerves affected by amyloidoma has been characterized both immunohistochemically and biochemically (42,69,74). Only AL λ expression has been observed (fig. 10-12C). With the exception of one case in which AA-protein immunoreactivity was focally observed in the absence of chronic inflammatory disease or circulating antinuclear antibodies, no other amyloid protein subunits, e.g., AA-protein, β-amyloid A4 protein, transthyretin, β2-microglobulin, cystatin C, or gelsolin, have been detected (74). Monotypic B lymphocytes and plasma cells are not found in peripheral blood. At the ultrastructural level, aggregates of amyloid are composed of non-branching fibrils with a diameter of 8 to 12 nm.

Since amyloidomas of peripheral nerves are well demarcated, unifocal lesions unassociated with systemic disease, surgical removal is curative.

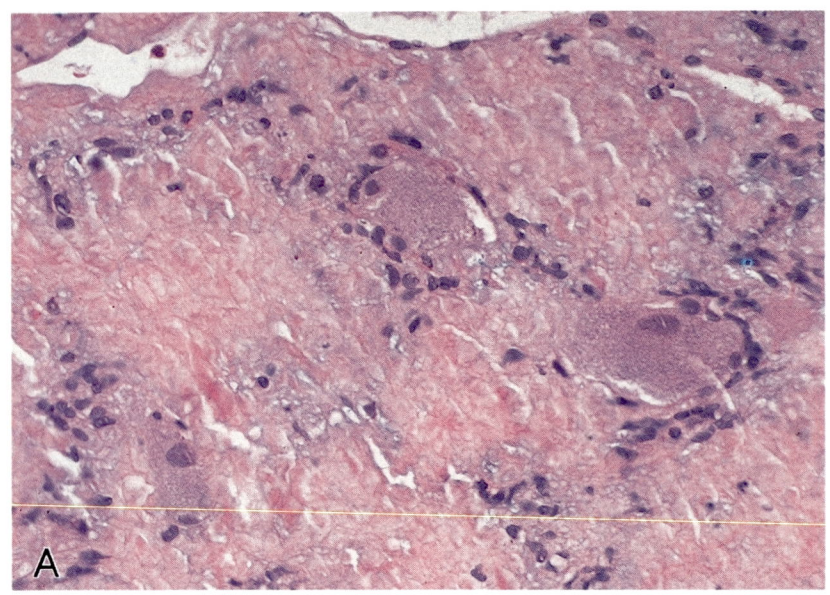

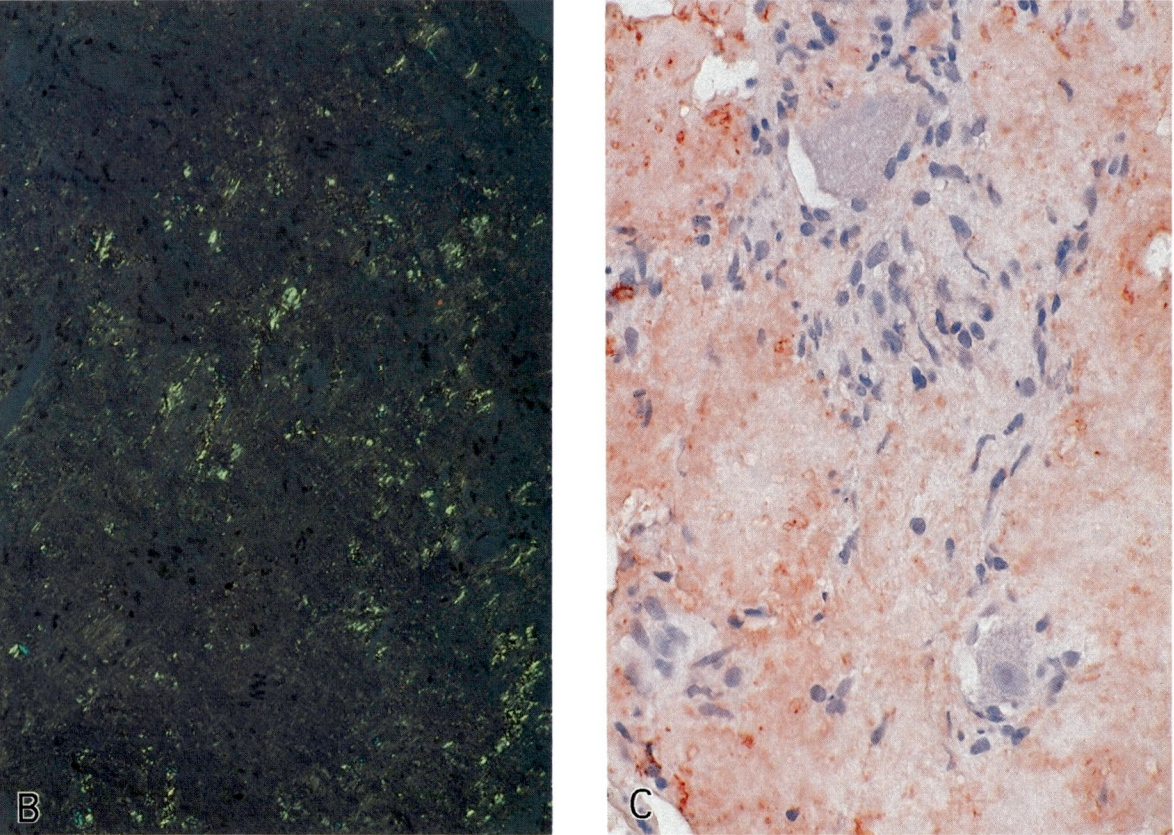

Figure 10-12
AMYLOIDOMA OF NERVE

This tumor-like deposit affected the trigeminal (Gasserian) ganglion. Note the residual ganglion cell (A), apple green birefringence on polarized light (B), and Ig λ immunoreactivity (C).

REFERENCES

Meningioma of the Peripheral Nervous System

1. Apatenko AK, Sementsov PN. Arachnoidendotheliomas (meningiomas, psammomas) of the skin. Arkh Patol 1974;36:34–42.
2. Burger PC, Scheithauer BW. Tumors of the central nervous system. Atlas of Tumor Pathology, 3rd Series, Fascicle 10. Washington, D.C.: Armed Forces Institute of Pathology, 1994:275–7.
3. Carneiro SS, Scheithauer BW, Nascimento AG, Hirose T, Davis DH. Solitary fibrous tumor of the meninges: a lesion distinct from fibrous meningioma: a clinicopathologic and immunohistochemical study. Am J Clin Pathol 1996;106:217–24.
4. Coons SW, Johnson PC. Brachial plexus meningioma, report of a case with immunohistochemical and ultrastructural examination. Acta Neuropathol 1988;77:445–8.
5. Daugaard S. Ectopic meningioma of a finger. Case report. J Neurosurg 1983;58:778–80.
6. Drlicek M, Grisold W, Lorber J, Hachl H, Wuketich S, Jellinger K. Pulmonary meningioma. Immunohistochemical and ultrastructural features. Am J Surg Pathol 1991;15:455–9.
7. Farr HW, Gray GF Jr, Vrana M, Panio M. Extracranial meningioma. J Surg Oncol 1973;5:411–20.
8. Hallgrimsson J, Bjornsson A, Gudmundsson G. Meningioma of the neck—case report. J Neurosurg 1970;32:695–9.
9. Harkin JC, Reed RJ. Tumors of the peripheral nervous system. Atlas of Tumor Pathology, 2nd Series, Fascicle 3. Washington, D.C.: Armed Forces Institute of Pathology, 1969:18.
10. Harvey SS, Burr HS, Van Canpenhout E. Development of the meninges: further experiments. Arch Neurol Psychiatry 1933;29:683–90.
11. Henderson JW. Meningioma. In: Orbital tumors. 3rd ed. Raven Press, 1994:377–90.
12. Hirakawa E, Kobayashi S, Terasaka K, Ogino T, Terai Y, Ohmori M. Meningeal hamartoma of the scalp. A variant of primary cutaneous meningioma. Acta Pathol Jpn 1992;42:353–7.
13. Kershisnik M, Callender DL, Batsakis JG. Pathology consultation. Extracranial, extraspinal meningiomas of the head and neck. Ann Otol Rhinol Laryngol 1993;102:967–70.
14. Kulali A, Ilcayto R, Rahmanli O. Primary calvarial ectopic meningiomas. Neurochirurgia 1991;34:174–7.
15. Landini G, Kitano M. Meningioma of the mandible. Cancer 1992;69:2917–20.
16. Larson JJ, van Loveren HR, Balko MG, Tew JM Jr. Evidence of meningioma infiltration into cranial nerves: clinical implications for cavernous sinus meningiomas. J Neurosurg 1995;83:596–9.
17. Lopez DA, Silvers DN, Helwig EB. Cutaneous meningiomas—a clinicopathologic study. Cancer 1974;34:728–44.
18. Mackay B, Bruner JM, Luna MA, Guillamondegui OM. Malignant meningioma of the scalp. Ultrastruct Pathol 1994;18:235–40.
19. Marrogi AJ, Swanson PE, Kyriakos M, Wick MR. Rudimentary meningocele of the skin. Clinicopathologic features and differential diagnosis. J Cutan Pathol 1991;18:178–88.
20. McCabe JS, Low FN. The subarachnoid angle: an area of transition in peripheral nerve. Anat Rec 1969;164:15–33.
21. Nichols RD, Knighton RS, Chason JL, Strong DD. Meningioma in the parotid region. Laryngoscope 1987;97:693–6.
22. Nochomovitz LE, Jannotta F, Orenstein JM. Meningioma of the scalp. Light and electron microscopic observations. Arch Pathol Lab Med 1985;109:92–5.
23. Olivares-Pakzad BA, Tazelaar HD, Dehner LP, Kasperbauer JL, Bite U. Oropharyngeal hairy polyp with meningothelial elements. Oral Surg Oral Med Oral Pathol Oral Radiol Endod 1995;79:462–8.
24. Robinson PG. Pulmonary meningioma. Report of a case with electron microscopic and immunohistochemical findings. Am J Clin Pathol 1992;97:814–7.
25. Shnitka TK, Bain GO. Cutaneous meningioma (psammoma). Autopsy findings in a previously reported case. Arch Dermatol 1959;80:410–2.
26. Shuangshoti S, Boonjunwetwat D, Kaoroptham S. Association of primary intraspinal meningiomas and subcutaneous meningioma of the cervical region: case report and review of literature. Surg Neurol 1992;38:129–34.
27. Sibley DA, Cooper PH. Rudimentary meningocele: a variant of "primary cutaneous meningioma." J Cutan Pathol 1989;16:72–80.
28. Simpson MT, Sneddon KJ. Extracranial meningioma of the oral cavity. Br J Oral Maxillofac Surg 1987;25:520–5.
29. Singh RV, Yeh JS, Broome JC, Campbell DA. Primary ectopic intramuscular meningioma of the thigh. Clin Neurol Neurosurg 1993;95:245–7.
30. Smith AT, Selecki BR, Stening WA. Ectopic meningioma. Med J Aust 1973;1:1100–4.
31. Suster S, Rosai J. Hamartoma of the scalp with ectopic meningothelial elements: a distinctive benign soft tissue lesion that may simulate angiosarcoma. Am J Surg Pathol 1990;14:1–11.
32. Susuki H, Gilbert EF, Zimmermann B. Primary extracranial meningioma. Arch Pathol 1967;84:202–6.
33. Theaker JM, Fletcher CD, Tudway AJ. Cutaneous heterotopic meningeal nodules. Histopathology 1990;16:475–9.
34. Theaker JM, Gatter KC, Esiri MN, Fleming KA. Epithelial membrane antigen and cytokeratin expression by meningiomas: an immunohistochemical study. J Clin Pathol 1986; 39:435–9.
35. Walters GA, Ragland RL, Knorr JR, Malhotra R, Gelber ND. Post-traumatic cutaneous meningioma of the face. AJNR Am J Neuroradiol 1994;15:393–5.
36. Weinberger JM, Birt BD, Lewis AJ, Nedzelski JM. Primary meningioma of the nasopharynx: case report and review of ectopic meningioma. J Otolaryngol 1985;14:317–22.
37. Winek RR, Scheithauer BW, Wick MR. Meningioma, meningeal hemangiopericytoma (angioblastic meningioma), peripheral hemangiopericytoma, and acoustic schwannoma. A comparative immunohistochemical study. Am J Surg Pathol 1989;13:251–61.
38. Winkler M. Über Psammone der Haut und des Unterhautgewebes. Virchows Arch 1904;178:323–50.

Miscellaneous Tumors

39. Apostiledes PJ, Spetzler RF, Johnson PC. Ectomesenchymal hamartoma (benign "ectomesenchymoma") of the VIIIth nerve. Case report. Neurosurgery 1995;37:1204–7.

40. Blades DA, Hardy RW, Cohen M. Cervical paraganglioma with subsequent intracranial and intraspinal metastases. Case report. J Neurosurg 1991;75:320–3.

41. Borghi G, Tagliabue G. Primary amyloidosis of the gasserian ganglion. Acta Neurol Scand 1961;37:105–10.

42. Bornemann A, Bohl J, Hey O, et al. Amyloidoma of the gasserian ganglion as a cause of symptomatic neuralgia of the trigeminal nerve: report of three cases. J Neurol 1993;241:10–4.

43. Bricklin AS, Rushton HW. Angiosarcoma of venous origin arising in the radial nerve. Cancer 1977; 39:1556–8.

44. Brodkey JA, Buchignani JA, O'Brien TF. Hemangioblastoma of the radial nerve: case report. Neurosurgery 1995;36:198–201.

45. Browne TR, Adams RD, Roberson GH. Hemangioblastomas of the spinal cord. Review and report of five cases. Arch Neurol 1976;33:435–41.

46. Burger PC, Scheithauer BW. Tumors of the central nervous system. Atlas of Tumor Pathology, 3rd Series, Fascicle 10. Armed Forces Institute of Pathology, 1994,301–2.

47. Burger PC, Scheithauer BW, Vogel FS. Surgical pathology of the central nervous system and its coverings. 3rd ed. New York: Churchill Livingstone, 1991:359–65.

48. Calonje E, Fletcher CD. Cutaneous intraneural glomus tumor. Am J Dermatopathol 1995;17:395–8.

49. Conway JD, Smith MB. Hemangio-endothelioma originating in a peripheral nerve. Report of a case. Ann Surg 1951;134:138–41.

50. Daly DD, Love JG, Dockerty MB. Amyloid tumor of the gasserian ganglion. J Neurosurg 1957;14:347–52.

51. DeCastro S, Sparks JR, Lapey JD, Freidberg SR. Amyloidoma of the gasserian ganglion. Surg Neurol 1976;6:357–9.

51a. Ergin MT, Druckmiller WH, Cohen P. Intrinsic hemangiomas of the peripheral nerves. Report of a case and review of the literature. Conn Med 1998;62:209–13.

52. Erlandson RA. Diagnostic transmission electron microscopy of tumors. Raven Press: New York, 1994:616–22.

53. Eusebi V, Bondi A, Cancellieri A, Canedi L, Frizzera G. Primary malignant lymphoma of sciatic nerve. Am J Surg Pathol 1990;14:881–5.

54. Gabet JY, Durand DV, Bady B, Kopp N, Sindou M, Levrat R. Pseudo-tumeur amyloïde du neerf sciatique. Rev Neurol 1989;145:872–6.

55. Gersdorff MC, Decat M, Duprez T. Neuromuscular hamartoma of the internal auditory canal. Eur Arch Oto-Rhino-Laryngol 1996;253:440–2.

56. Giannini C, Scheithauer BW. Hemangioblastoma of peripheral nerve. Mod Pathol 1998 (In press).

57. Giannini C, Wright A, Dyck PJ. Polyneuropathy associated with nerve angiomatosis and multiple soft tissue tumors. A newly recognized syndrome. Am J Surg Pathol 1995;19:1325–32.

58. Guthikonda M, Rengachary SS, Balko MG, van Loveren H. Lipofibromatous hamartoma of the median nerve: case report with magnetic resonance imaging correlation. Neurosurgery 1994;35:127–32.

59. Hirose T, Sano T, Mori K, et al. Paraganglioma of the cauda equina: an ultrastructural and immunohistochemical study of two cases. Ultrastruct Pathol 1988;12:235–43.

60. Ismail SM, Cole G. Von Hippel-Lindau syndrome with microscopic hemangioblastomas of the spinal nerve roots: case report. J Neurosurg 1984;60:1279–81.

61. Kanamori M, Matsui H, Yudoh K. Solitary T-cell lymphoma of sciatic nerve: case report. Neurosurgery 1995;36:1203–5.

62. Kato T, Sawamure Y, Abe H. Trigeminal neuralgia caused by a cerebellopontine-angle lipoma: case report. Surg Neurol 1995;44:33–5.

63. Kepes JJ, Boynick PO, Jones S, Baum D, McMillan J, Adams ME. Adrenal cortical adenoma in the spinal canal of an 8-year-old girl. Am J Surg Pathol 1990;5:481–4.

64. Kepes JJ, Zacharias DL. Gangliocytic paragangliomas of the duodenum. Report of two cases with light and electron microscopic examination. Cancer 1971;27:61–70.

65. Kliewer KE, Wen DR, Cancilla PA, Cochran AJ. Paraganglioma: assessment of prognosis by histologic, immunohistochemical, and ultrastructural techniques. Hum Pathol 1989;20:29–39.

66. Kline SC, Moore JR, deMente SH. Glomus tumor originating within a digital nerve. J Hand Surg 1990; 15A:98–101.

67. Krücke W. Pathologie der peripheren nerven. In: Olivecrona H, Tönnis W, Krenkel W, eds. Handbuch der Neurochirurgie. Berlin: Springer-Verlag, 1974:164–7.

68. Kyle RA, Bayrd ED. Amyloidosis: review of 236 cases. Medicine 1975;54:271–99.

69. Laeng RH, Altermatt HJ, Scheithauer BW, Zimmermann DR. Amyloidomas of the nervous system: a monoclonal B-cell disorder with monotypic amyloid and light chain lambda amyloid production. Cancer 1998;82:362–74.

70. Linnoila RI, Lack EE, Steinberg SM, Keiser HR. Decreased expression of neuropeptides in malignant paragangliomas: an immunohistochemical study. Hum Pathol 1988;19:41–50.

70a. Mastronaroli L, Guiducci A, Frondizi D, et al. Intraneural capillary hemangioma of the cauda equina. Eur Spine J 1997;6:278–80.

70b. Matius-Guice X, Alejo M, Sole T, et al. Cavernous angiomas of the cranial nerves. J Neurosurg 1990;73:620–2.

71. Matsumoto T, Tani E, Maeda Y, Natsume S. Amyloidomas in the cerebellopontine angle and jugular foramen. J Neurosurg 1985;62:592–6.

72. Meyer AW. A congenital intracranial intradural adrenal. Anat Rec 1917;12:43–94.

73. Mitchell A, Scheithauer BW, Sasano H, Hubbard EW, Ebersold MJ. Symptomatic intradural adrenal adenoma of the spinal nerve root: report of two cases. Neurosurgery 1993;32:658–62.

74. O'Brien TJ, McKelvie PA, Vrodos N. Bilateral trigeminal amyloidoma: an unusual case of trigeminal neuropathy with a review of the literature. Case report. J Neurosurg 1994;81:780–3.

75. Orrell JM, Hales SA. Paragangliomas of the cauda equina have a distinctive cytokeratin immunophenotype. Histopathology 1992;21:479–81.

76. Phalen GS, Kendrick JI, Rodriquez JM. Lipomas of the upper extremity. A series of fifteen tumors in the hand and wrist and six tumors causing nerve compression. Am J Surg 1971;121:298–306.

77. Pillay PK, Hardy RW, Wilbourn AJ, Tubbs RR, Lederman RJ. Solitary primary lymphoma of the sciatic nerve: case report. Neurosurgery 1988;23:370–1.

78. Purhoit DP, Dick DJ, Perry RH, Lyons PR, Schofield IS, Foster JB. Solitary extranodal lymphoma of sciatic nerve. J Neurol Sci 1986;74:23–34.

79. Rao VK, Weiss SW. Angiomatosis of soft tissue. An analysis of the histologic features and clinical outcome in 51 cases. Am J Surg Pathol 1992;16:764–71.

80. Robertson SC, Traynelis VC, Follett KA, Menezes AH. Idiopathic spinal epidural lipomatosis. Neurosurgery 1997;41:68–75.

81. Rohde V, Voigt K, Grote EH. Intra-extradural hemangioblastoma of the cauda equina. Zentralbl Neurochir 1995;56:78–82.

82. Roncaroli F, Poppi M, Riccioni L, Frank F. Primary non-Hodgkin's lymphoma of the sciatic nerve followed by localization in the central nervous system: case report and review of the literature. Neurosurgery 1997;40:618–22.

82a. Roncarolli F, Scheithauer BW, Kraus WE. Hemangioma of spinal nerve root. J Neurosurg 1999 (in press).

83. Rusko RA, Larsen RD. Intraneural lipoma of the median nerve—case report and literature review. J Hand Surg [Am] 1981;6:388–91.

84. Russell DS, Rubinstein LJ. Nervous system involvement by lymphomas, histiocytoses and leukemias. In: Russell DS, Rubinstein LJ, eds. Pathology of the nervous system. 5th ed. Baltimore: Williams & Wilkins, 1989:590–638.

85. Scheithauer BW, Nora FE, LeChago J, et al. Duodenal gangliocytic paraganglioma: clinicopathologic and immunocytochemical study of 11 cases. Am J Clin Pathol 1986;86:559–65.

86. Scheithauer BW, Parameswaran A, Burdick B. Intrasellar paraganglioma: report of a case in a sibship of von Hippel-Lindau disease. Neurosurgery 1996;38(2):396–9.

87. Seizinger BR. Toward the isolation of the primary genetic defect in von Hippel-Lindau disease. Ann N Y Acad Sci 1991;615:332–7.

88. Singh RV, Yeh JS, Broome JC. Paraganglioma of the cauda equina: a case report and review of the literature. Clin Neurol Neurosurg 1993;95:109–13.

89. Singh SP, Cottingham SL, Slone W, Boesel CP, Welling DB, Yates AJ. Lipomas of the internal auditory canal. Arch Pathol Lab Med 1996;120:681–3.

90. Smalley S, Schomberg PJ, Earle JD, Laws ER Jr, Scheithauer BW, O'Fallon JR. Radiotherapeutic considerations in the treatment of hemangioblastomas of the central nervous system. Int J Radiat Oncol Biol Phys 1990;18:1165–71.

91. Smith KA, Mackinnon SE, Macauley RJ, Mailis A. Glomus tumor originating in the radial nerve: a case report. J Hand Surg 1992;17A:665–7.

92. Sonneland PR, Scheithauer BW, LeChago J, Crawford BG, Onofrio BM. Paraganglioma of the cauda equina region. Clinicopathologic study of 31 cases with special reference to immunocytology and ultrastructure. Cancer 1986;58:1720–35.

93. Sonneland PR, Scheithauer BW, Onofrio BM. Myxopapillary ependymoma. A clinicopathologic and immunocytochemical study of 77 cases. Cancer 1985;56:883–93.

93a. Stewart SF, Bettin ME. The motor significance of hemangioma with report of a case of plexiform telangiectasis of the sciatic nerve and its branches. Surg Gynecol Obstet 1924;39:307–17.

94. Terzis JK, Daniel RK, Williams HB, Spencer PS. Benign fatty tumors of the peripheral nerves. Ann Plast Surg 1978;1:193–216.

95. Vandewalle G, Brucher JM, Michotte A. Intracranial facial nerve rhabdomyoma. Case report. J Neurosurg 1995;83:919–22.

96. Vigna PA, Kusior MF, Collins MB, Ross JS. Peripheral nerve hemangioma. Potential for clinical aggressiveness. Arch Pathol Lab Med 1994;118:1038–41.

97. Viswanathan R, Swamy NK, Vago J, Dunsker SB. Lymphoma of the lumbar nerve root: case report. Neurosurgery 1997;41:479–82

98. Wisoff HS, Suzuki Y, Llena JF, Fine DI. Extramedullary hemangioblastoma of the spinal cord: case report. J Neurosurg 1978;48:461–4.

99. Wolansky LJ, Stewart VA, Pramanik BK, et al. Giant paraganglioma of the cauda equina in adolescent: magnetic resonance imaging demonstration. J Neuroimaging 1996;6:54–6.

99a. Young JN, Friedman AH, Harrelson JM, Rossitch E Jr, Alston S, Rozear M. Hemangiopericytoma of the sciatic nerve. Case report. J Neurosurg 1991;74:512–5.

100. Zwick DL, Livingston K, Clapp L, Kosnik E, Yates A. Intracranial trigeminal nerve rhabdomyoma/choristoma in a child: a case report and discussion of possible histogenesis. Hum Pathol 1989;20:390–2.

11

PRIMARY MALIGNANT TUMORS OF PERIPHERAL NERVE

In addition to Schwann and perineurial cells, the normal nerve sheath contains an assortment of specialized but less site-specific mesenchymal cells, including fibroblasts, endothelial cells, pericytes, and epineurial lipocytes. While it is possible for any cell of the nerve sheath to give rise to a malignant tumor, most better differentiated malignant peripheral nerve sheath tumors (MPNSTs) exhibit Schwann cell characteristics. Thus, MPNSTs as a whole, even poorly differentiated examples, are generally regarded as being of Schwann cell origin (82). This includes MPNSTs developing de novo without genetic predisposition; unassociated with an obvious precursor lesion, but occurring within otherwise unremarkable peripheral nerve in the setting of neurofibromatosis 1 (NF1); arising in transition from a sporadic or NF1-associated neurofibroma; and rarely, arising from schwannoma, ganglioneuroma, ganglioneuroblastoma, or pheochromocytoma. In each instance the precursor Schwann cell assumes a different form: a non-neoplastic Schwann cell in normal nerve; a benign neoplastic Schwann cell in the schwannoma, ganglioneuroma, and ganglioneuroblastoma; a sustentacular cell (modified Schwann cell) in paraganglioma; and a benign, presumably neoplastic and genetically altered Schwann cell capable of multidirectional differentiation in neurofibroma (97). By virtue of their common spindle cell morphology and capacity for collagen production, malignant tumors of peripheral nerve derived from or growing as neoplastic Schwann cells, perineurial cells, or fibroblasts appear histologically similar. Therefore, although the terms "malignant schwannoma" and "neurofibrosarcoma" have been applied to primary malignant tumors of peripheral nerve, the use of such histologically specific terms is inappropriate. In an effort to be all inclusive, we use the noncommittal designation malignant peripheral nerve sheath tumor.

Given the complex structure of peripheral nerve, a meaningful discussion of MPNST must take into consideration the compartmental anatomy of nerve. Perineurium as well as endoneurium, with its high content of Schwann cells, are clearly indigenous to nerve. The same is not true of epineurium, the elements of which are common to all soft tissues. We therefore exclude from the category of MPNST any sarcoma involving only epineurium but sparing nerve fascicles. Since epineurial fibrous tissue is contiguous with surrounding connective tissue, malignant neoplasms involving only this portion of the nerve sheath may have arisen in extraneural soft tissue. Epineurial tumors are thus grouped among extrinsic, soft tissue tumors secondarily affecting peripheral nerve. Although, as a manifestation of metaplastic change, angiosarcoma has been described as a component of MPNST and of neurofibroma, we do not regard as MPNST those pure angiosarcomas arising in peripheral nerve vasculature.

MALIGNANT PERIPHERAL NERVE SHEATH TUMOR (MPNST)

Definition. This category includes any malignant tumor arising from or differentiating toward cells intrinsic to peripheral nerve sheath. These tumors are also termed *neurogenic sarcoma, neurofibrosarcoma,* and *malignant schwannoma.* Excluded are tumors of epineurial soft tissue and endothelial tumors originating from peripheral nerve vasculature.

General Comments. MPNSTs comprise approximately 5 percent of all malignant soft tissue tumors (56) and have a varied origin. Most are derived from neurofibromas or arise de novo in normal peripheral nerves (18,44). Extremely rare examples arise in schwannoma (97), ganglioneuroma/ganglioneuroblastoma (73), or pheochromocytoma (62,65,74). Although a majority of MPNSTs show some evidence of Schwann cell differentiation, a significant proportion are so anaplastic as to preclude the assessment of differentiation. Cells in a small minority of MPNSTs have the features of fibroblasts or perineurial cells (40,42). To be all inclusive, therefore, it is necessary to use the noncommittal designation MPNST as opposed to the more restrictive synonyms noted above.

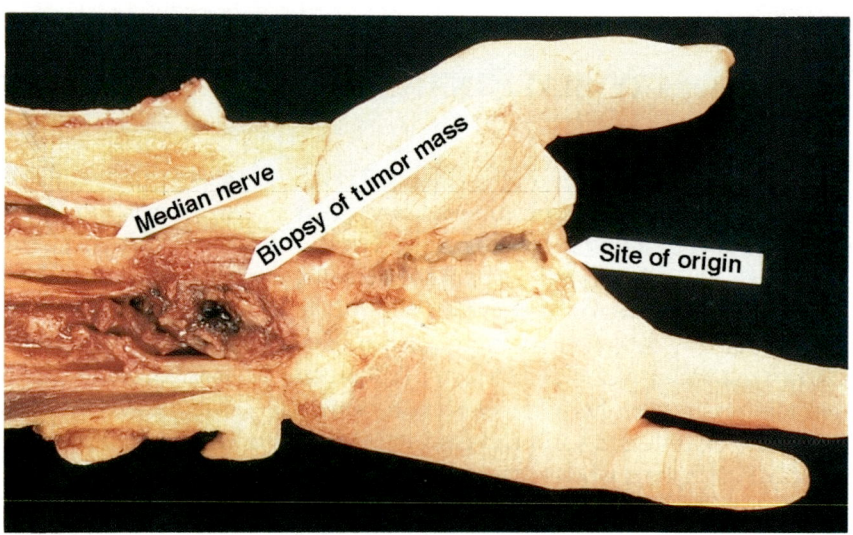

Figure 11-1
POSTRADIATION MPNST
Arising at the base of a finger, now amputated, this tumor underwent intraneural spread to form a mass at the wrist. Thereafter, continued extensive proximal growth within the median nerve required an amputation.

Since MPNSTs often closely resemble non-neural soft tissue tumors, morphologic features alone may not permit their recognition. As a result, several diagnostic guidelines have been formulated.

Widely accepted criteria for a diagnosis of MPNST require that the tumor conform to one of the following: 1) arises within a peripheral nerve; 2) arises in transition from a benign or other malignant peripheral nerve tumor (neurofibroma, schwannoma, ganglioneuroma/ganglioneuroblastoma, or pheochromocytoma); 3) develops in a patient with NF1 (von Recklinghausen's disease) and exhibits the same histologic features as do a majority of MPNSTs arising from nerves; or 4) develops in a patient without NF1, but exhibits the same histologic features as do most MPNSTs and shows either or both immunohistochemical and ultrastructural features of Schwann or perineurial cell differentiation. The clinical and pathologic characteristics of those few MPNSTs arising from schwannoma, ganglioneuroma, ganglioneuroblastoma, or pheochromocytoma differ significantly from the more conventional MPNSTs. As a result they will be separately discussed as MPNST variants.

Clinical Features. Most MPNSTs affect adults from 20 to 50 years of age and show a slight female predominance. The tumor may also present in childhood and adolescence (17,59); in one large series (17), this represented about 13 percent of the cases. Patients rarely present before the age of 6 years (1). Between 50 and 60 percent of MPNSTs occur in patients with NF1 (18, 44,50,78). In two large series, the mean age of MPNST patients with and without this inherited disorder was 28 and 36 years compared to 40 and 44 years, respectively (18,44). NF1 predisposes to the development of MPNST. Reports of the incidence with which this occurs vary from 2 percent (10–12) to as high as 16 (70) and 29 percent (43); the latter estimates appear heavily biased by selection factors. In the Mayo Clinic experience, the incidence was 4.6 percent (18), whereas in a study of a nationwide cohort of 212 Danish patients with NF1 followed for 39 years, Sorensen et al. (79) found a lower incidence of 1.9 percent. In contrast, the reported incidence of MPNST in the general population is 0.0001 percent (18). Although rare, examples of multiple MPNSTs have been described (50,51,54); all have occurred in the setting of NF1.

In addition to hereditary factors, ionizing radiation due to therapeutic or occupational exposure (fig. 11-1) may contribute to the development of up to 11 percent of all MPNSTs (16,28, 154) and 20 percent of paraspinous examples (50). Foley et al. (28) found the mean latency period between irradiation and clinical presentation of the MPNST to be 18.1 years (range, 4 to 41 years), while for Ducatman and Scheithauer (16) it was 15.6 years (range, 5 to 26 years). Exposure to chemical carcinogens, although a factor in experimental MPNST induction (9,25,49), has not been shown to play a role in human cases.

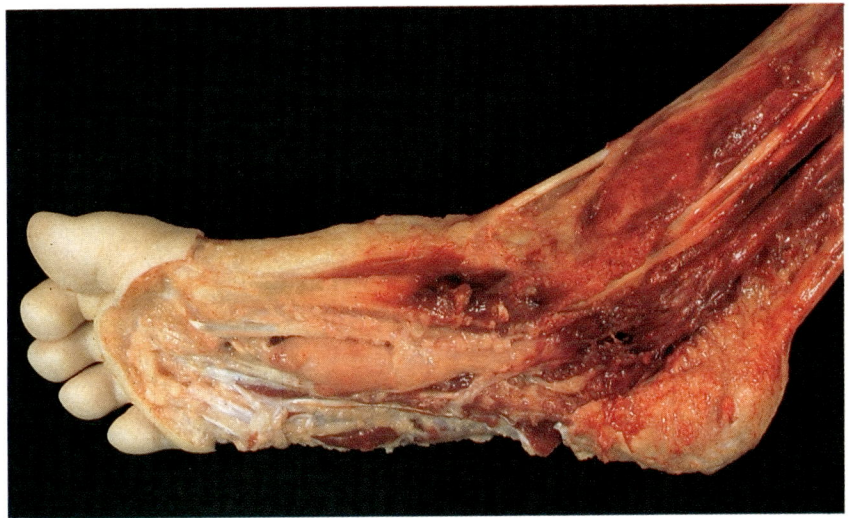

Figure 11-2
MPNST
This small example, arising in and limited to a plantar nerve, is fusiform in shape and displaces surrounding soft tissue.

Localization. Large and medium-sized nerves are distinctly more prone to involvement than small nerves. Common sites of origin include the buttock and thigh, brachial plexus and upper arm, and paraspinal nerves. The sciatic nerve is the most frequently affected. MPNSTs of cranial nerves are uncommon, the trigeminal being the most often involved (98), followed by the acoustic nerve (5,34,52,58,66). With the exception of one trigeminal nerve tumor showing unequivocal histologic evidence of origin from a schwannoma (29,97), MPNSTs of cranial nerves appear to arise de novo. A single example of intracerebral MPNST has also been reported (80). Visceral MPNSTs are rare, usually occurring in the setting of NF1, and often associated with multiple neurofibromas, from which they appear to arise by malignant transformation (55). Most reported examples either antedate immunohistochemistry or lack support of this method or ultrastructural evidence; this is a problem, given the occurrence of other spindle cell neoplasms in the gut (see Differential Diagnosis).

Gross Findings. The gross appearance of MPNST varies, depending upon whether the tumor involves a large nerve (figs. 11-2–11-4), evolves from a neurofibroma of solitary (fig. 11-5) or plexiform type (fig. 11-6), or presents with no grossly visible evidence of either origin (fig. 11-7). The frequency with which a coexisting neurofibroma is found varies among patients with and without NF1; in one large series the respective rates were 81 percent and 41 percent (18). In

practice, a coexisting neurofibroma is far more often microscopically than grossly apparent. Regardless of the setting in which they occur, the majority of MPNSTs exceed 5 cm in greatest dimension (18,44). Those arising from nerve roots or major nerves are often fusiform (figs. 11-2, 11-3) but some do grow eccentrically from the parent nerve to assume a globoid configuration (fig. 11-4). A globular growth pattern also characterizes the majority of MPNSTs unassociated with a neurofibroma or a visible nerve (fig. 11-7). MPNSTs that arise within plexiform neurofibromas may be grossly inapparent or multifocal. Thorough sectioning of all plexiform neurofibromas is therefore recommended.

Most MPNSTs are surrounded by a fibrous pseudocapsule of varying thickness formed by compaction and invasion of surrounding soft tissues as well as by accompanying reactive fibrosis (figs. 11-3, 11-4, 11-7). Unlike the soft, translucent character of neurofibromas, the cut surface of a MPNST is usually firm, gray-tan, and opaque (figs. 11-3–11-7). Areas of necrosis are grossly apparent in approximately 60 percent of cases (figs. 11-3, 11-4, 11-7) (44). Active bone destruction may be observed (fig. 11-8). Although irregular margins and lack of homogeneity on computerized tomography (CT) and magnetic resonance imaging (MRI) scans are features suggestive of malignancy (fig. 11-9, left), their occasional absence (fig. 11-9, right) makes a significant proportion of MPNSTs indistinguishable from benign nerve sheath tumors (see figs. 7-6,

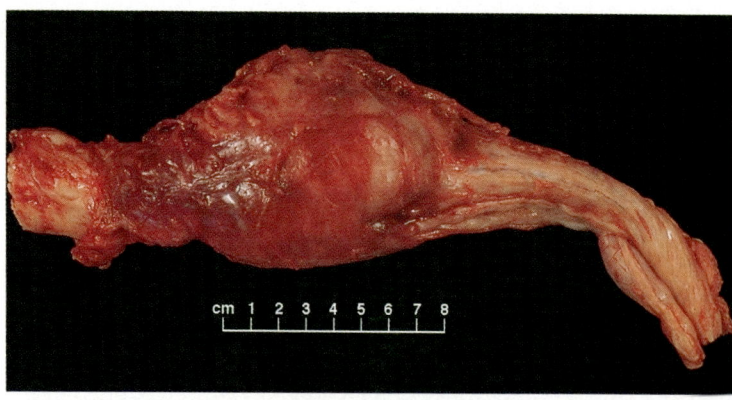

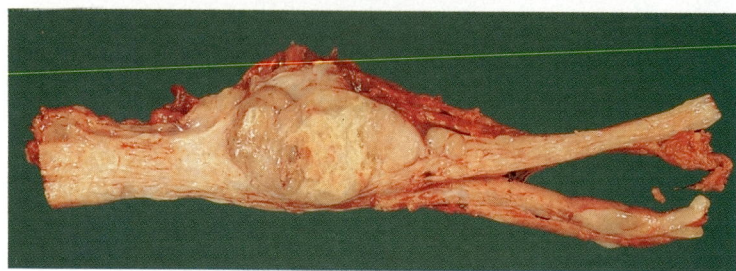

Figure 11-3
MPNST

This fusiform to globoid sciatic nerve tumor (top) arose in a plexiform neurofibroma just proximal to the bifurcation in the popliteal fossa. Invasion of perineural soft tissue, skeletal muscle in this case, contributes to the formation of a pseudocapsule. On cut section (bottom), the tumor shows extensive necrosis. This example arose in the setting of NF1.

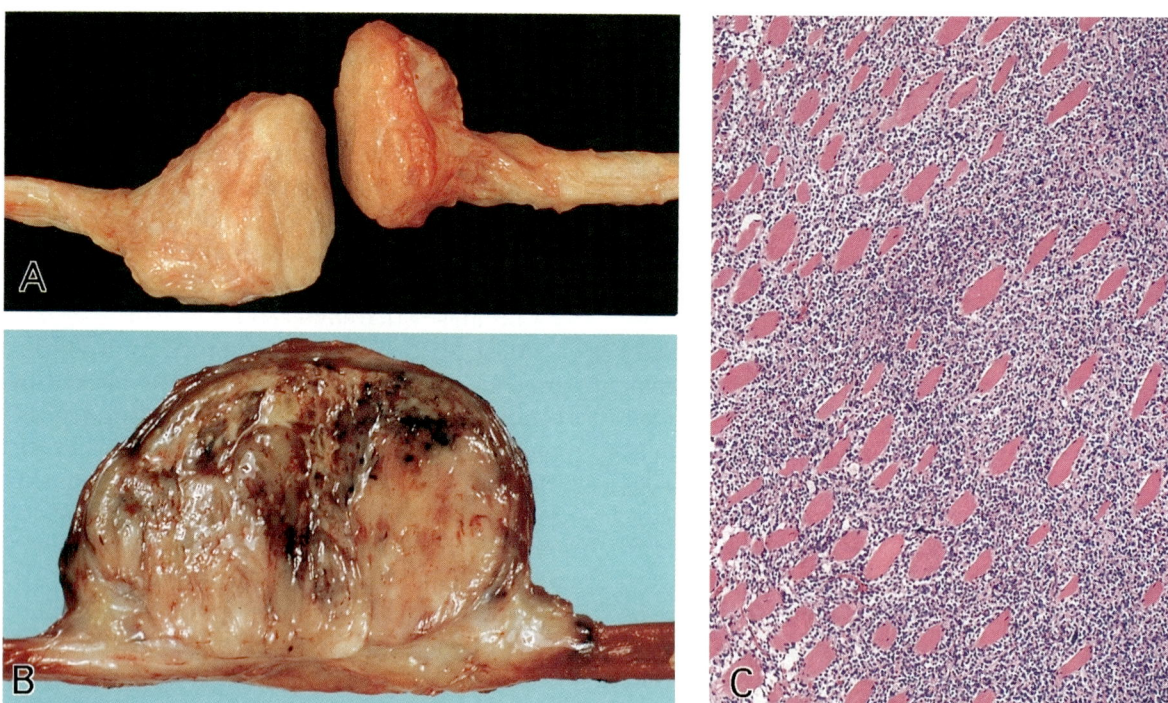

Figure 11-4
MPNST

This cross-sectioned sciatic nerve tumor is homogeneous and firm (A). The surrounding pseudocapsule consists of fibromuscular tissue in part infiltrated by tumor. Yet another example of a more globular MPNST (B) cut in longitudinal section shows it to be eccentric to the originating sciatic nerve. The fleshy partially necrotic lesion possesses a pseudocapsule which has been sharp-dissected from surrounding connective tissues. Note residual infiltrated skeletal muscle. Microsections of such a pseudocapsule (C) often show infiltration of skeletal muscle.

8-8, 8-9, 8-18). As a rule, MPNSTs lack the "target sign" so typical of localized intraneural neurofibroma (5a).

Sampling of soft tissue tumors suspected of being MPNSTs should be thorough in order to identify an associated nerve or neurofibroma, to determine the presence of heterologous elements, and to establish an accurate histologic grade. We suggest at least one section per centimeter of greatest tumor dimension. Given the tendency of MPNSTs arising in sizable nerves to undergo intraneural extension (figs. 11-1, 11-10, 11-16), it is imperative at the time of surgery to undertake frozen section assessment of proximal and distal nerve margins. Spread within nerves should particularly be sought in paraspinous tumors (50). Of the 25 cases of Kourea et al. (50), 10 tumors encroached upon the spinal column: 4 exhibited vertebral body involvement, 2 reached a vertebral foramen by proximal extension along nerve root, 2 had epidural involvement with or without spinal cord compression, and 2 extended intradurally. Intradural paraspinal extension by MPNST has also been described by others (76a,93).

Microscopic Findings. The histologic spectrum of MPNSTs is more varied than that of any other soft tissue tumor (figs. 11-11–11-14). Furthermore, their neural nature generally cannot be proven on conventionally stained material. The diagnosis thus rests on identifying one or more of the features listed in the general comment section above. Diagnostically helpful findings include an origin from nerve, intraneural (intrafascicular) spread within or beyond the main tumor mass, involvement of a ganglion, and identification of an associated solitary or plexiform neurofibroma.

Most MPNSTs are highly cellular, spindle cell proliferations (fig. 11-11A,B). Infrequently, bundles of such cells may show striking variation in cell density, imparting a "tapestry" appearance (44,50). The elongate tumor cells often feature hyperchromatic nuclei, are mitotically active, and possess moderate amounts of faintly eosinophilic cytoplasm. Nuclei generally have rounded or tapered ends, but are not blunt (fig. 11-15). In less cellular areas, they sometimes have a wavy contour. Although most MPNSTs closely resemble fibrosarcoma, large, pleomorphic, and often multinucleated tumor cells are found in about one third of the tumors (44), an appearance sometimes con-

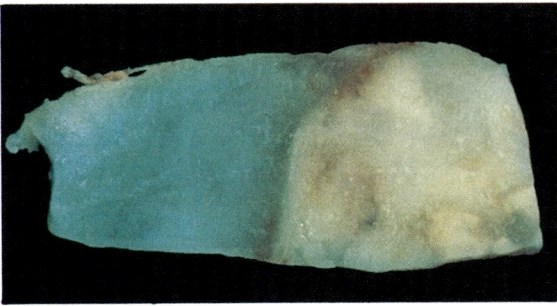

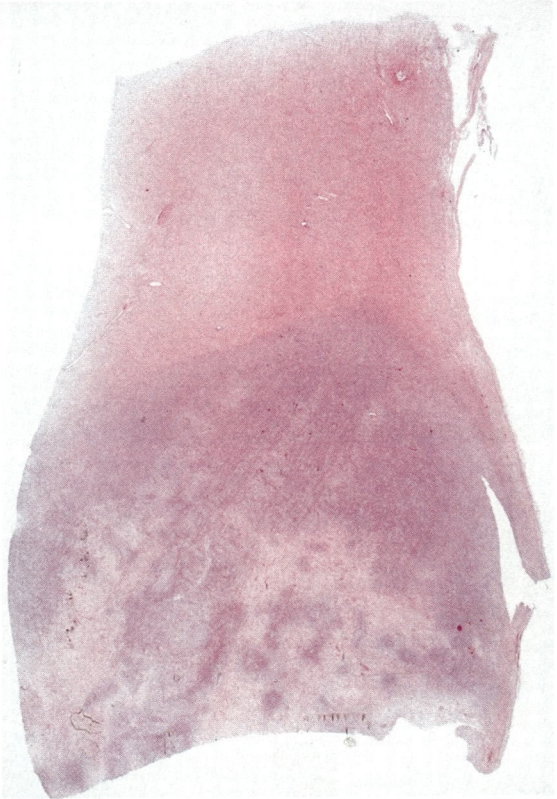

Figure 11-5
MPNST ARISING IN NEUROFIBROMA
These gross (top) and whole mount sections (bottom) show the transition from neurofibroma to sarcoma to be abrupt.

fused with that of pleomorphic malignant fibrous histiocytoma (fig. 11-11D). Tumors with only minor nuclear atypia, a small cell component, and epithelioid cells may also be seen (fig. 11-13). In addition to an often dominant, cellular, fibrosarcoma-like growth pattern, less cellular areas may feature a fibrous or myxoid stroma (fig. 11-13F). Infrequently, tumor cells are arranged in a storiform pattern (fig. 11-11E), as loose whorls mimicking "tactile differentiation" (fig. 11-14), or in curlicues.

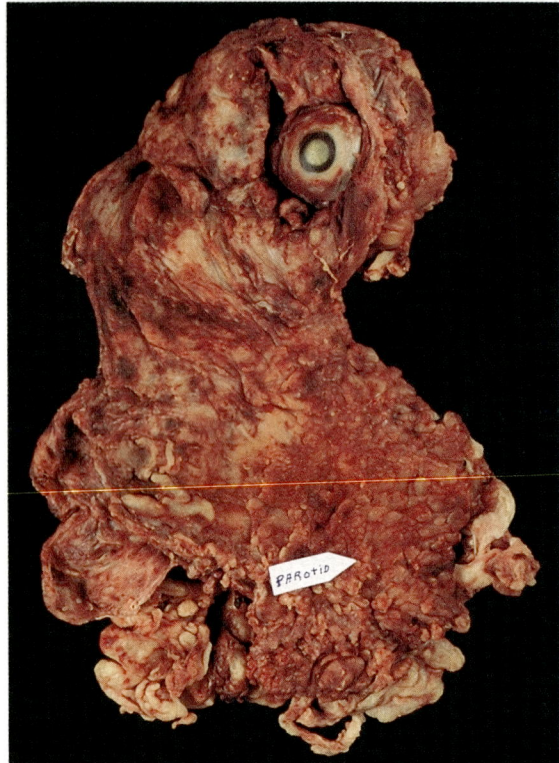

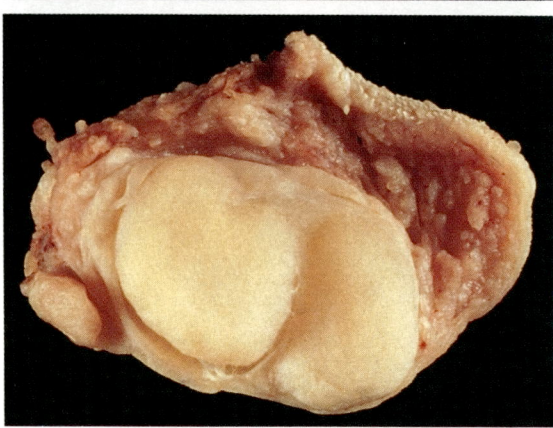

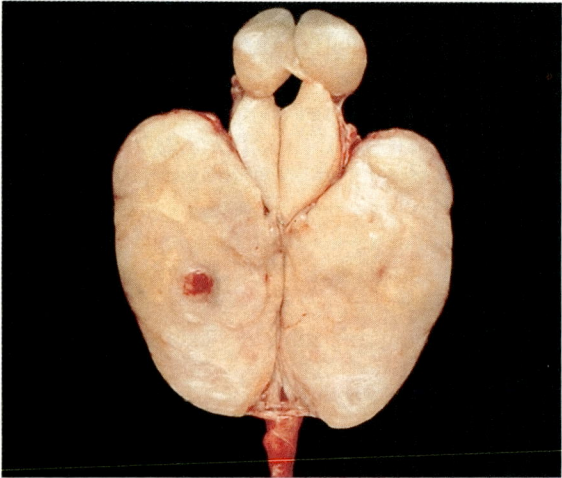

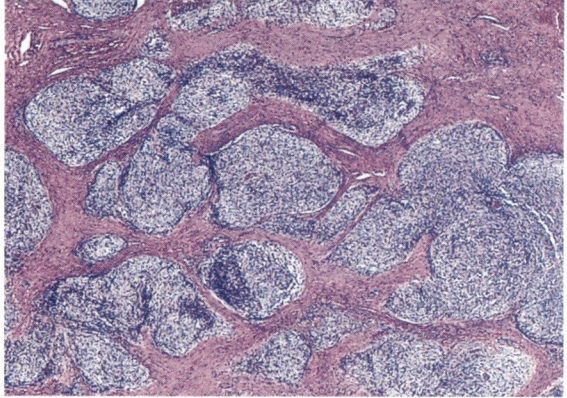

Figure 11-6

MPNST ARISING IN A PLEXIFORM NEUROFIBROMA

Left: This extensive NF1-associated facial lesion (top) showed a firm, lobular, and rather demarcated MPNST deep within its substance (bottom).

Right: This unusual example from a 17-year-old female with NF1 presented as one large nodule in a vagus nerve containing numerous smaller neurofibromas (top). The sympathetic chain (smaller specimen) also contained a neurofibroma. In yet another case (bottom), the MPNST involved numerous plexiform nerve branches.

Nuclear palisading is very uncommon (fig. 11-13C). Perivascular crowding of tumor cells is often seen in myxoid or edematous tumors (fig. 11-12D). Highly vascular lesions may focally resemble hemangiopericytoma (88), but the pattern is rarely extensive (fig. 11-13D). Approximately 5 percent of MPNSTs are epithelioid in nature. Yet another 15 percent (17) exhibit an array of heterologous mesenchymal rhabdomyoblasts, benign or malignant cartilage and bone, or epithelial glandular, squamous, or neuroendocrine elements. Such special variants are separately discussed later.

Most MPNSTs are high-grade tumors in which mitotic figures are usually readily identified (fig. 11-15) and may be abnormal. In the majority of cases a mitotic index of at least 4 per 10 high-power fields is seen. Areas of geographic necrosis with or without pseudopalisading are seen in approximately two thirds of cases (fig. 11-12A,B) (44). Geographic necrosis is found with equal frequency in tumors associated with NF1 (70 percent) and those occurring sporadically (65 percent) (44). Pattern variation typifies MPNST (fig. 11-12C,D). In addition to direct soft tissue spread,

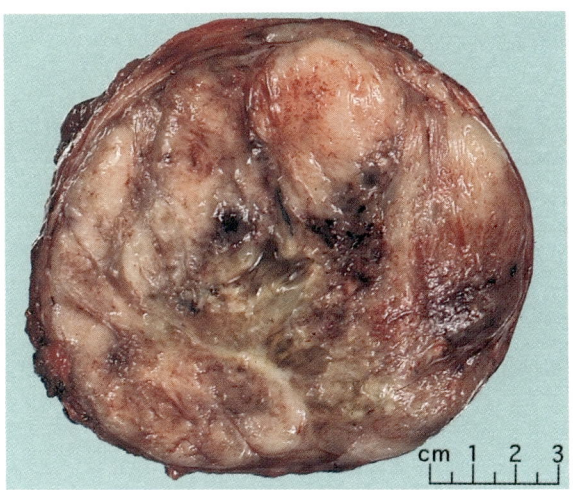

Figure 11-7
MPNST

Some tumors, such as this paraspinous example, are grossly unassociated with a recognizable nerve. Their recognition as MPNST is aided by knowledge of an association with neurofibromatosis, histologic evidence of an origin in neurofibroma, or by immunohistochemical or ultrastructural evidence of nerve sheath differentiation.

there may be intraneural extension (figs. 11-1, 11-10, 11-16A,B) and vascular (fig. 11-16C) or osseous invasion (fig. 11-16D).

Only a small proportion of MPNSTs, 15 percent in one large series (18), are low-grade tumors. These are less cellular than high-grade lesions, contain fewer hyperchromatic cells distributed in a variably collagenized stroma, and often show gradual transition to residual neurofibroma. Mitotic figures are infrequent or rare and tumor necrosis is lacking.

Low-Grade MPNST—Minimal Diagnostic Criteria. The distinction of neurofibromas with varying degrees of atypia from MPNST is often difficult (fig. 11-17). Authoritative textbooks (19,26) necessarily skirt the issue of what constitute minimal criteria of low-grade MPNST, be the tumors neurofibroma derived or de novo in occurrence. To date, no correlative morphologic-prognostic studies have specifically addressed the issue. The problem is compounded by the fact that transformation of neurofibroma to MPNST may be a focal finding in an otherwise benign, readily resected lesion, and inadequate sampling of ostensibly low-grade tumors may preclude identification of high-grade, prognostically significant elements. In the setting of a cellular or mildly

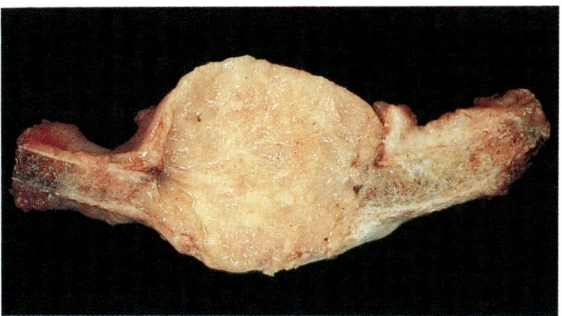

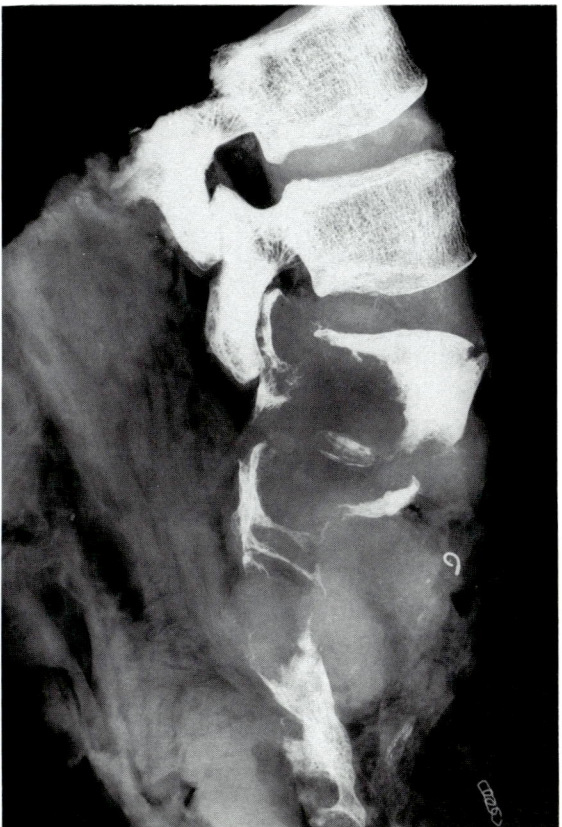

Figure 11-8
BONE INVOLVEMENT IN MPNST

Frank bone (rib) destruction, as seen in a gross specimen of a chest wall MPNST (top) and in a specimen X ray of a sacral example (bottom) may be a presenting feature. The same is also true of soft tissue sarcomas.

atypical neurofibroma, a distinction between benignancy and malignancy that rests entirely on the finding of any mitoses, however scarce (26), appears to us to be an overstatement. Those MPNSTs arising in transition from plexiform neurofibroma pose a particular problem, because anticipation of malignant change runs high in large examples,

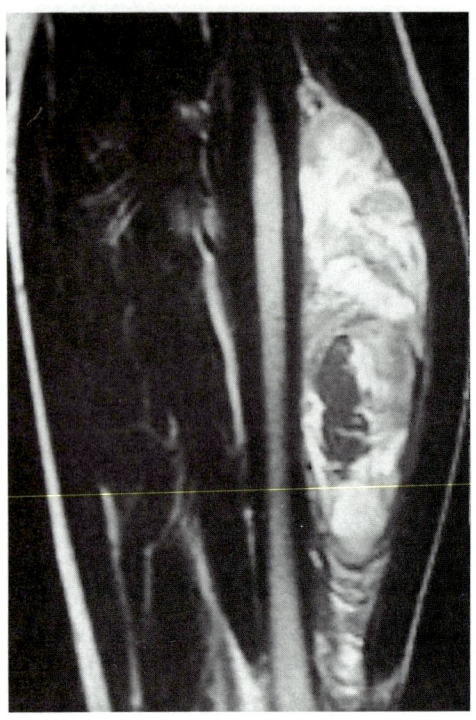

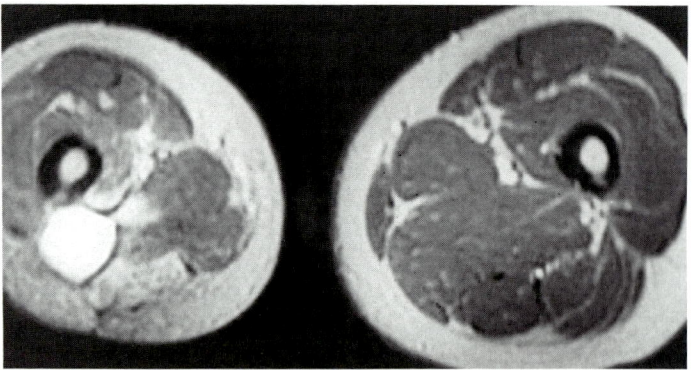

Figure 11-9
IMAGING OF MPNST
Although, irregularity, a reflection of invasion, and inhomogeneity (left) are suggestive of malignancy, some MPNSTs (right) lack these features and resemble benign nerve sheath tumors.

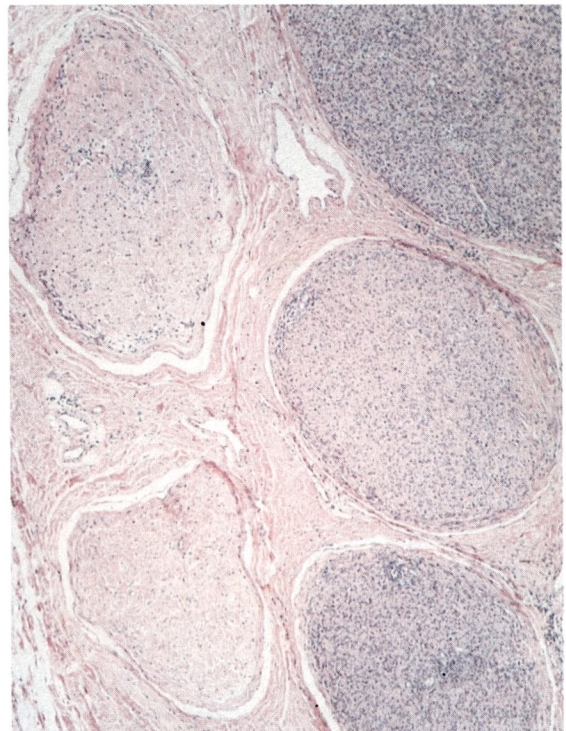

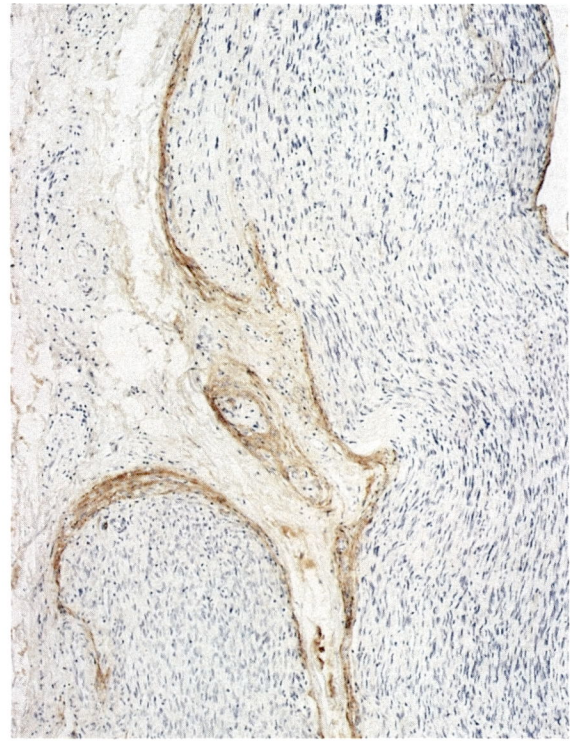

Figure 11-10
MPNST
Left: Examination of nerve margins is imperative since fascicles may be variably involved by permeating tumor cells. (Fig. 3.448 from Okazaki H, Scheithauer BW. Atlas of neuropathology, 1988. With permission from the Mayo Foundation.)
Right: In such cases, the intact perineurium, here seen on EMA stain, seems to retard extrafascicular spread.

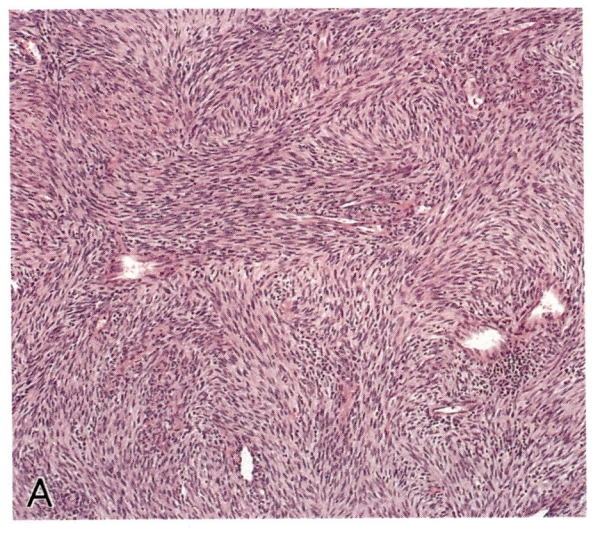

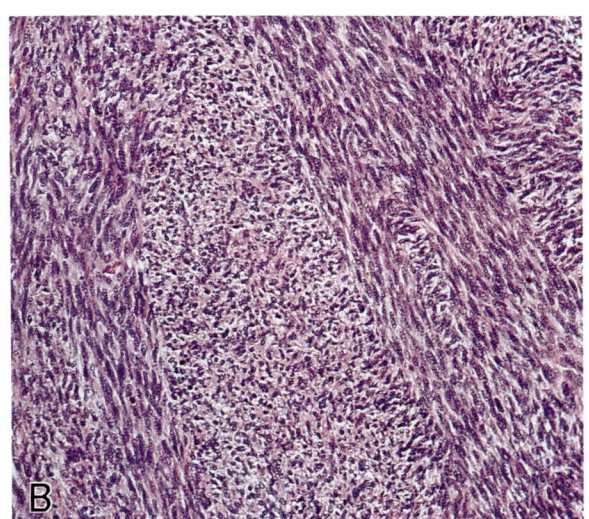

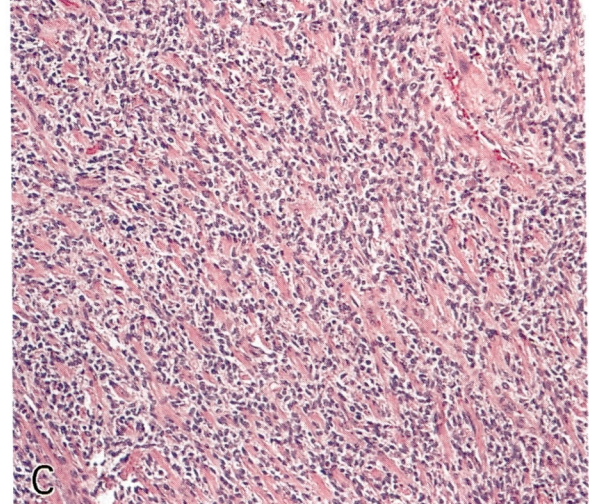

Figure 11-11

MPNST: BASIC CYTOLOGIC FEATURES

The majority of MPNSTs are composed of spindle cells disposed in sweeping fascicles (A). MPNST cells are also disposed as stiff, straight cells arrayed in herringbone pattern (B). A minority are patternless and consist of crowded, monomorphous cells without discernible processes (C), exhibit marked pleomorphism, as in this postradiation example (D), or show a storiform pattern (E).

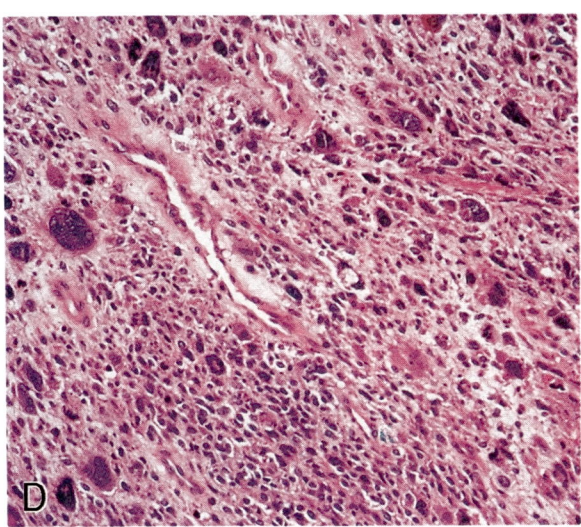

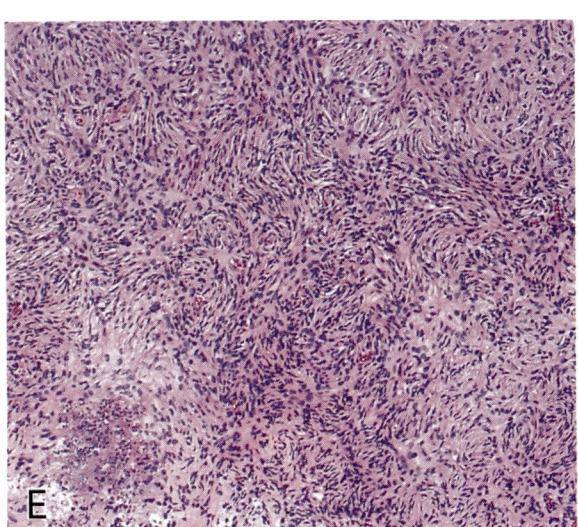

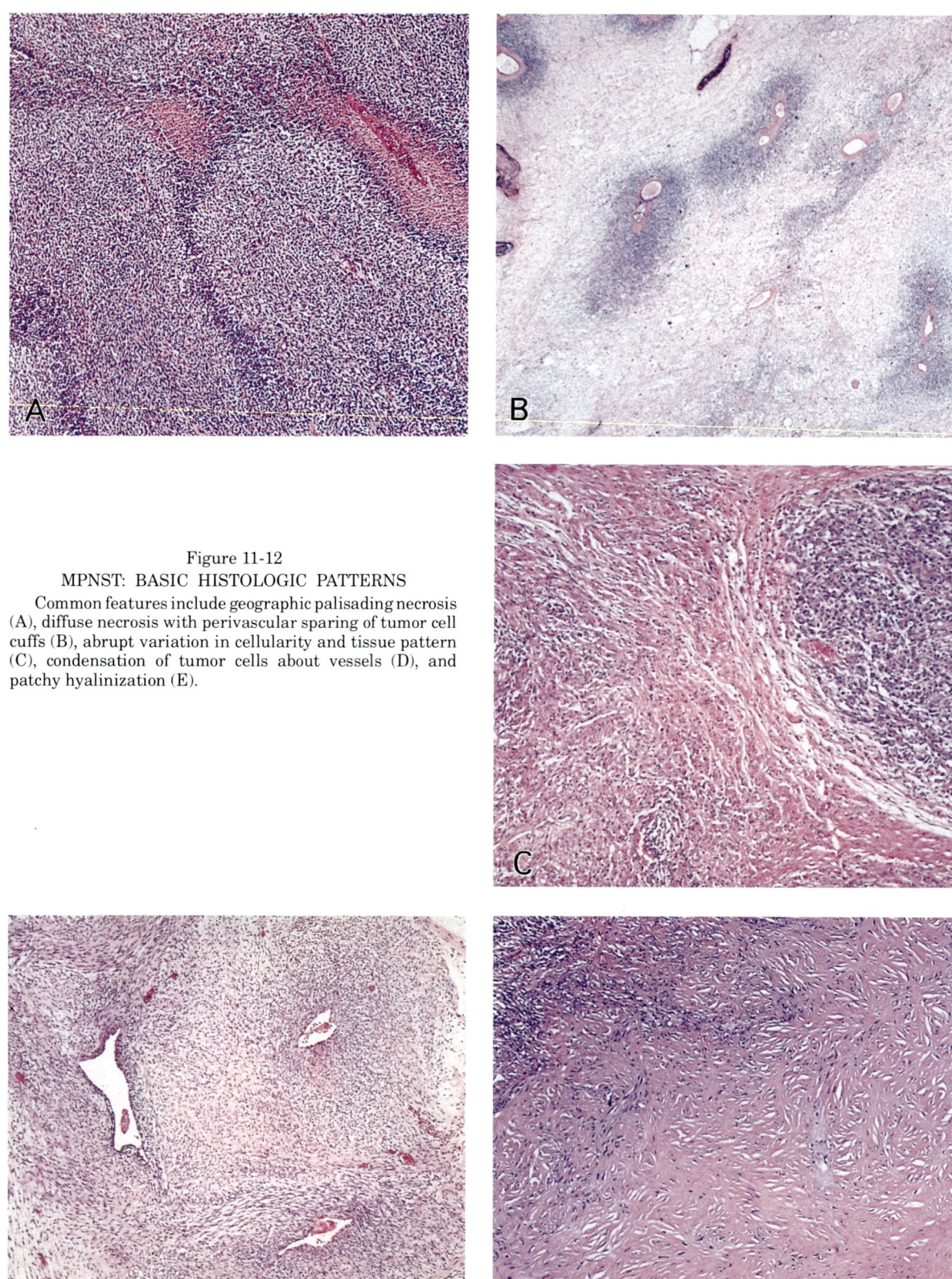

Figure 11-12
MPNST: BASIC HISTOLOGIC PATTERNS

Common features include geographic palisading necrosis (A), diffuse necrosis with perivascular sparing of tumor cell cuffs (B), abrupt variation in cellularity and tissue pattern (C), condensation of tumor cells about vessels (D), and patchy hyalinization (E).

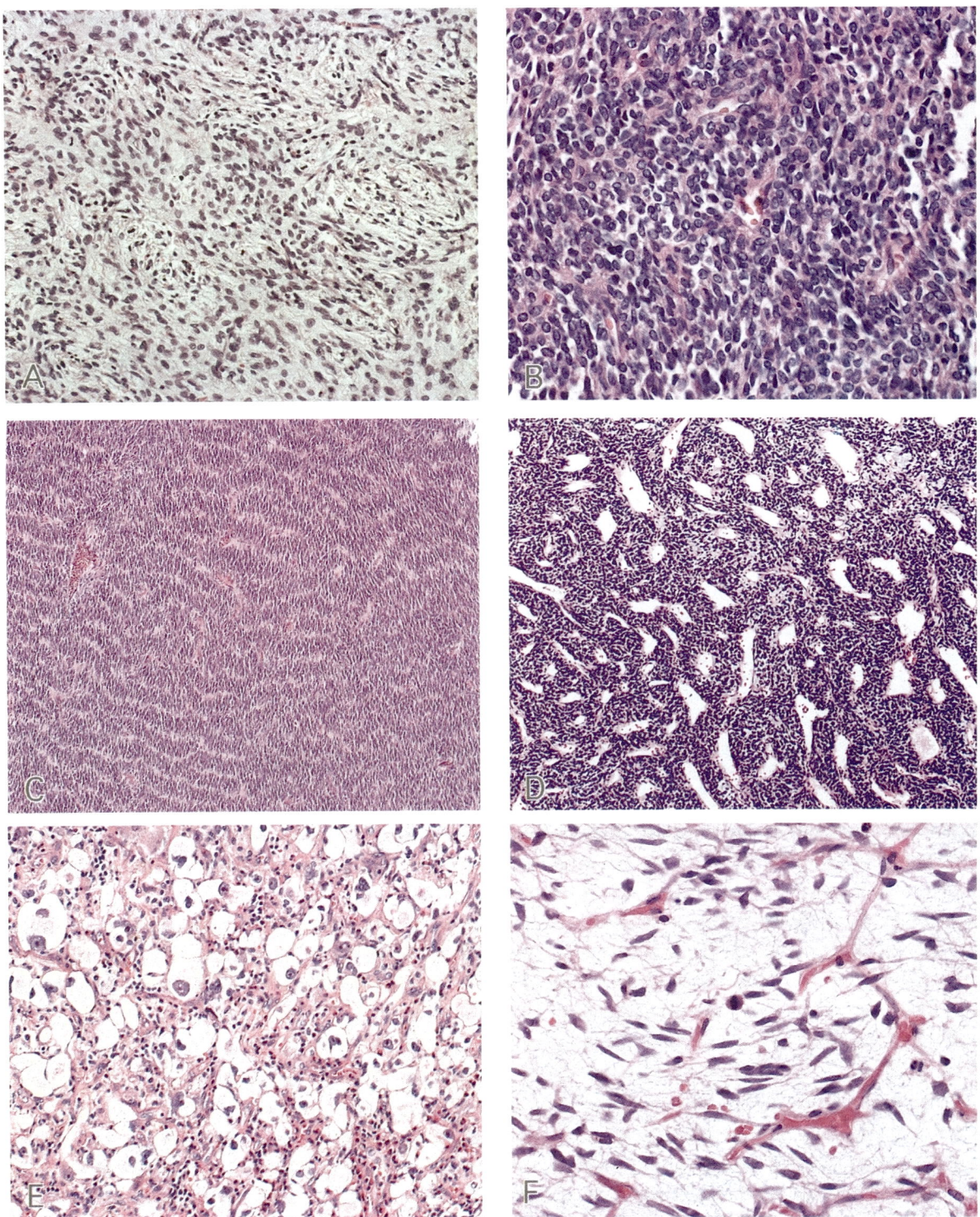

Figure 11-13
MPNST: UNUSUAL CYTOLOGIC AND HISTOLOGIC FEATURES

These include relative lack of significant cytologic atypia in an obvious high grade lesion (A), round nuclei and scant cytoplasm mimicking primitive neuroectodermal tumor (B), and a distinctly rare nuclear palisading (C). Unusual MPNST cytologic and histologic features also include hemangiopericytoma-like vasculature (D), the occurrence of giant cell patterns (E), and an appearance reminiscent of a tissue culture preparation (F).

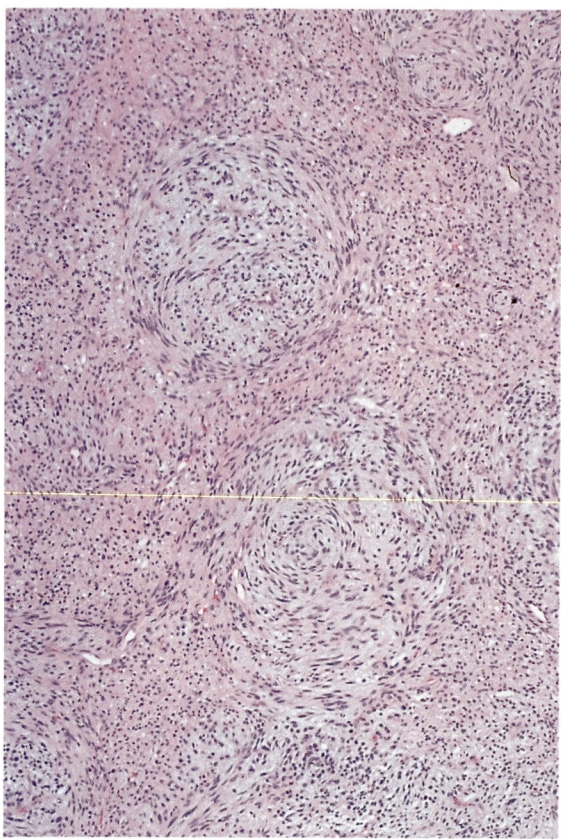

Figure 11-14
MPNST

The formation of whorls, a very unusual finding, should not be misinterpreted as tactile differentiation in MPNST. Unlike pacinian corpuscles, such whorls are generally S-100 protein immunoreactive and lack staining for epithelial membrane antigen (see also fig. 11-20).

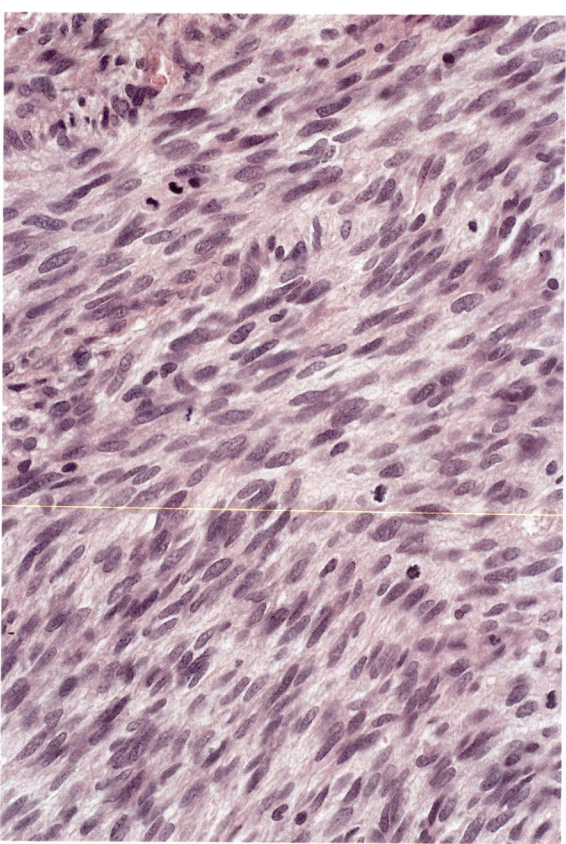

Figure 11-15
MPNST

The majority of spindle cell MPNSTs show nuclei that are tapered and exhibit a high mitotic index.

and sarcomatous foci may be either focal and limited or multifocal. We do not agree with those who simply state that the presence of mitotic figures in plexiform tumors is indicative of malignant change (19). *We distinguish low-grade MPNST from "cellular neurofibroma" by a triad of findings: 1) definite cell crowding, 2) general nuclear enlargement (at least three times the size of ordinary neurofibroma nuclei), and 3) hyperchromasia.* In the absence of these features, we accept low level mitotic activity in cellular neurofibroma, a lesion discussed in chapter 8 (fig. 11-17C) (see fig. 8-33) (56a), hence the finding of rare mitoses must not be overinterpreted as evidence of malignancy, particularly in young patients.

Unlike cellular neurofibroma and low-grade MPNST, atypical neurofibromas often lack sig-

nificant cellularity but contain scattered pleomorphic neurofibroma cells with bizarre, often hyperchromatic nuclei (see fig. 8-32) (96). Such pleomorphic cells have a degenerative appearance and may feature nuclear-cytoplasmic pseudo-inclusions. There is at present no evidence that such cytologic atypia is, in and of itself, an indication of malignant change. We have seen similar cytologic features not only in radiated neurofibromas (28) but in normal nerve subject to incidental radiotherapy (fig. 11-18). Atypical neurofibromas were previously discussed in chapter 8.

Immunohistochemical Findings. Staining for S-100 protein is a sensitive but nonspecific marker of nerve sheath tumors. Currently, there are no specific markers of benign Schwann cell neoplasms or of MPNSTs, either with or without heterologous elements. It has been reported that between 30 to 67 percent of MPNSTs contain

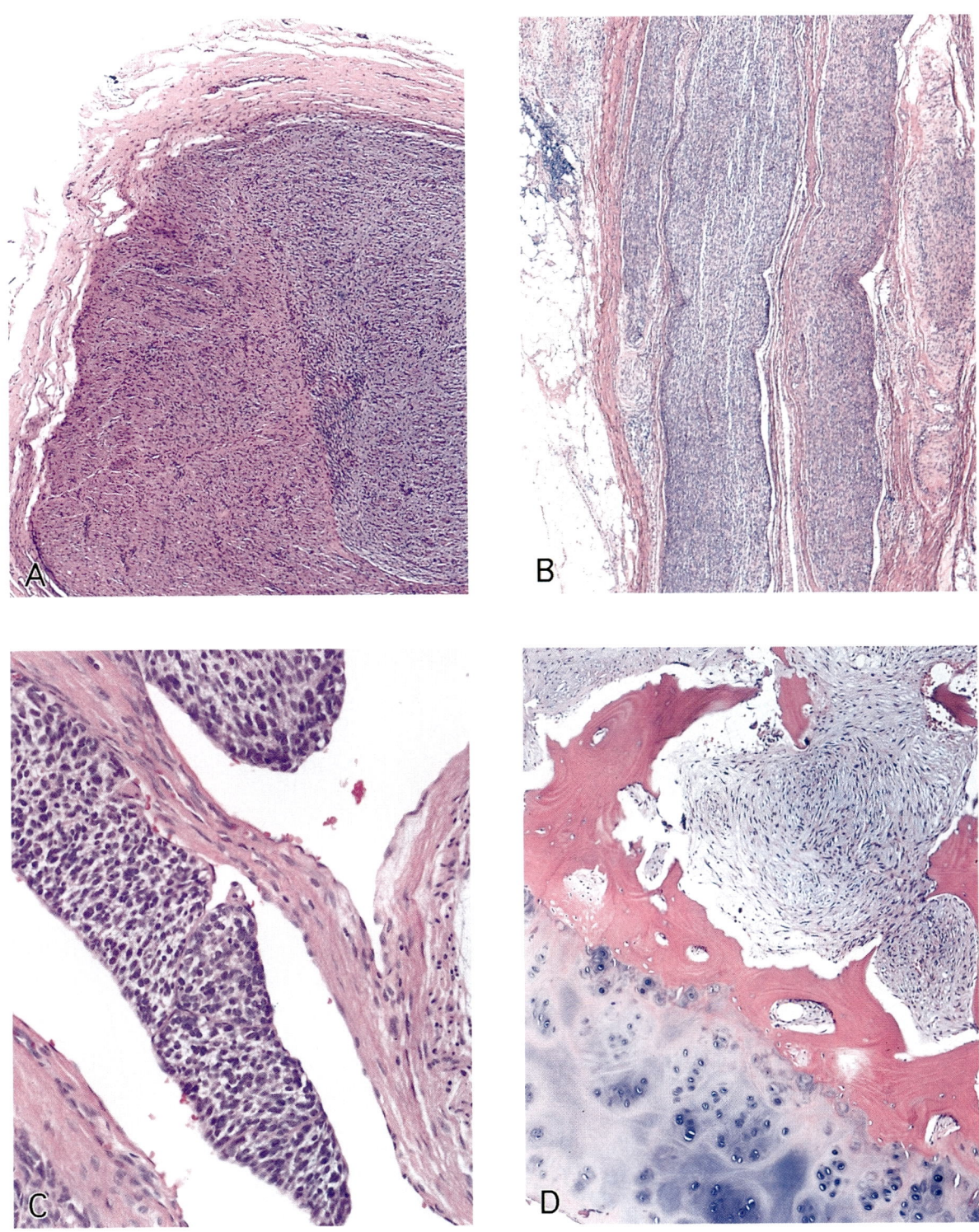

Figure 11-16
MPNST

Tumor spread by direct soft tissue extension (see fig. 11-4) is more commonly encountered than either distant intraneural extension (A - cross section, B - longitudinal section; see also figs.11-1 and 11-10) or vascular invasion (C), despite the fact that vessel invasion is considered prerequisite to metastasis. Bone invasion, here seen as permeation of trabeculae (D), may also be seen.

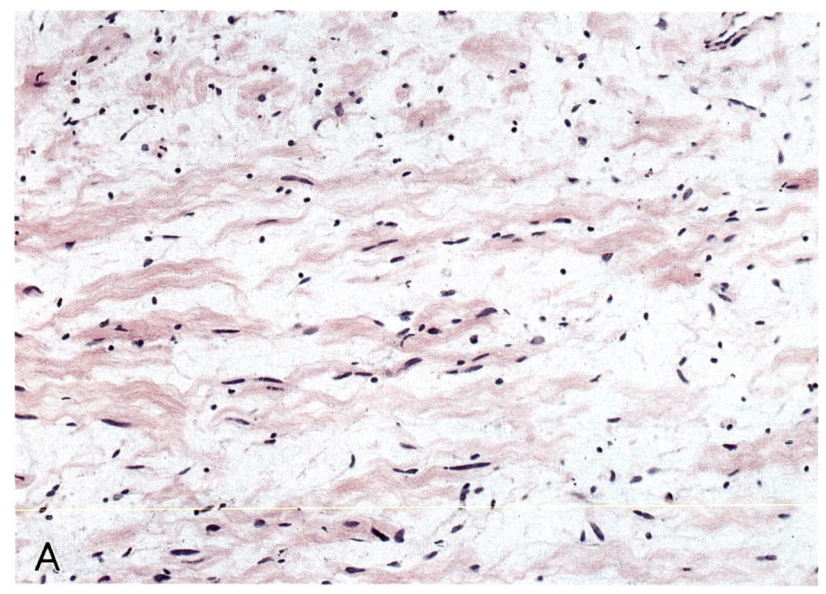

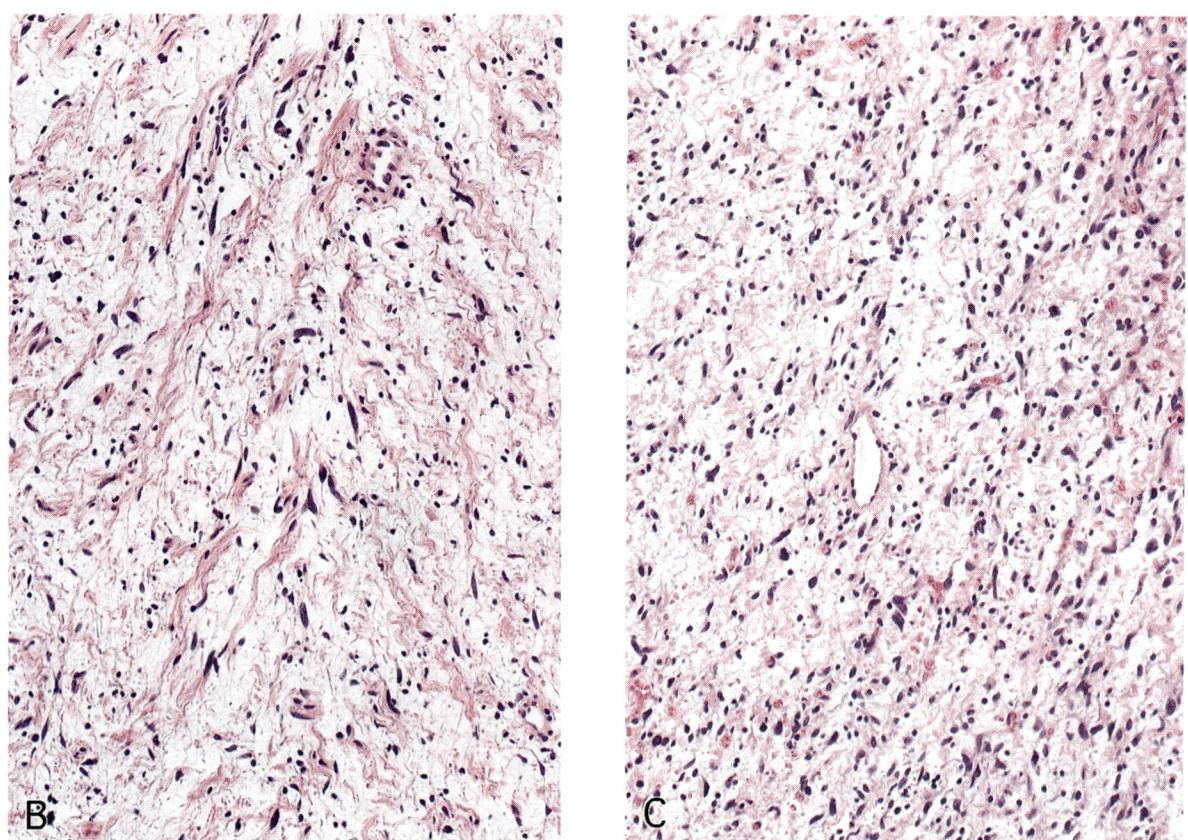

Figure 11-17
MPNST: TRANSITION FROM NEUROFIBROMA

The images are arranged to demonstrate what we consider to be transitions from neurofibroma (A) through increasingly cellular neurofibroma (B,C) to MPNST of low (D,E) to intermediate grade (F).

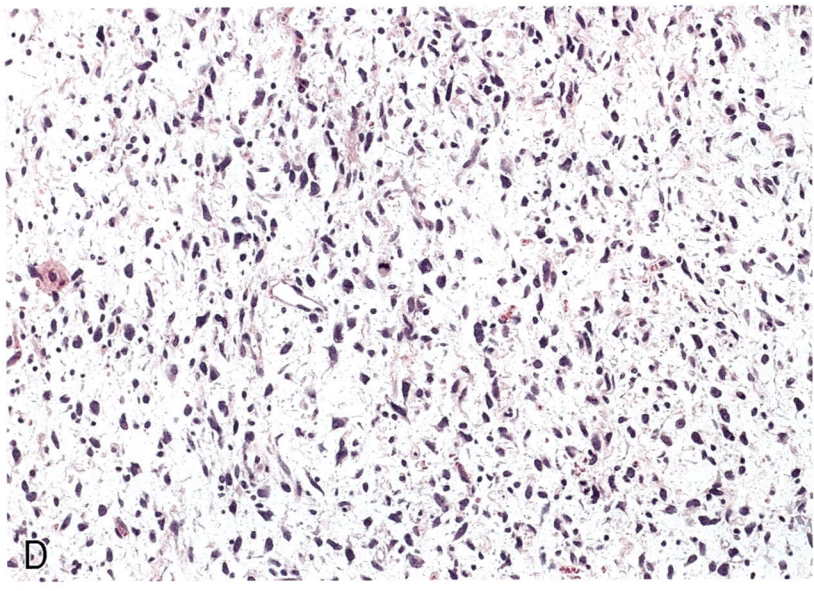

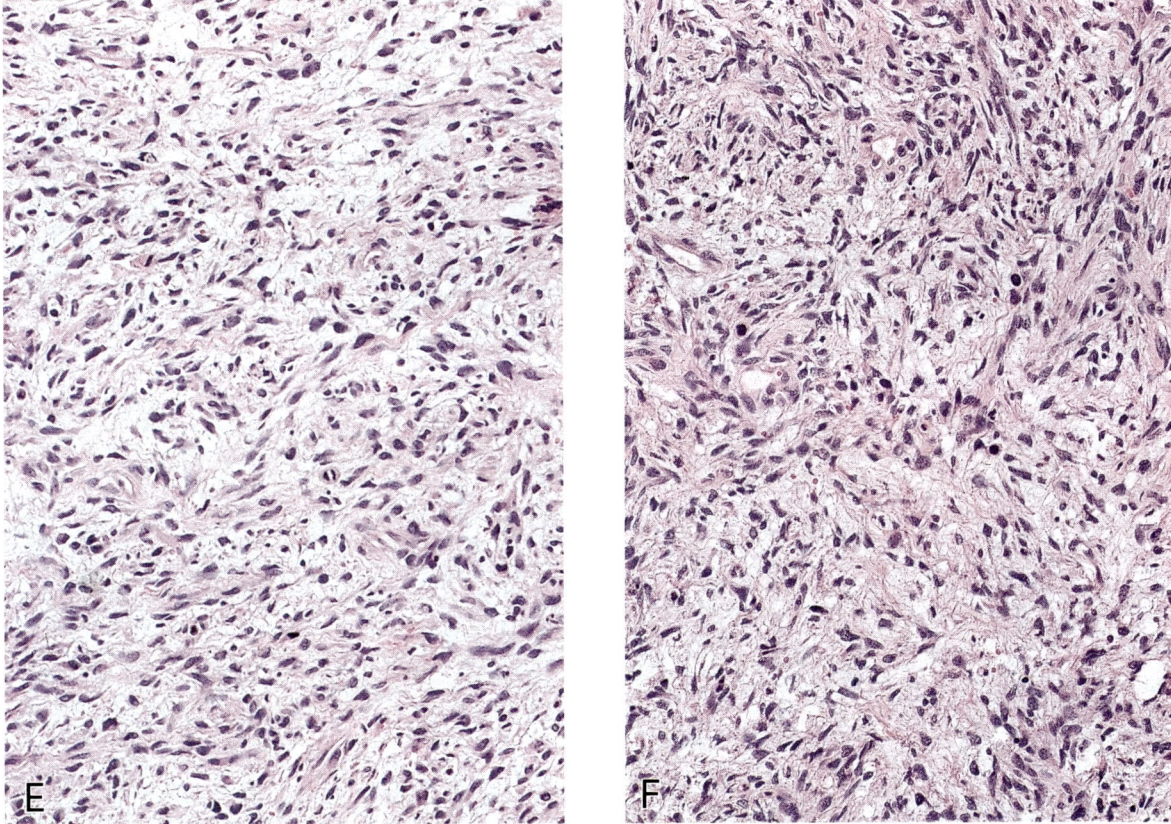

Figure 11-17 (Continued)

Criteria for transformation of neurofibroma to MPNST. We do not consider the finding of a rare mitotic figure in a normocellular neurofibroma with cytologic atypia to represent MPNST. Instead, we require the finding of hypercellularity, uniform nuclear enlargement, and hyperchromasia. Mitotic figures may or may not be present.

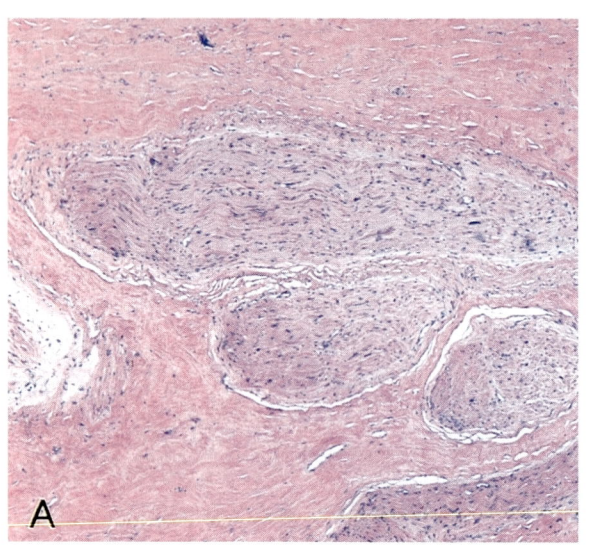

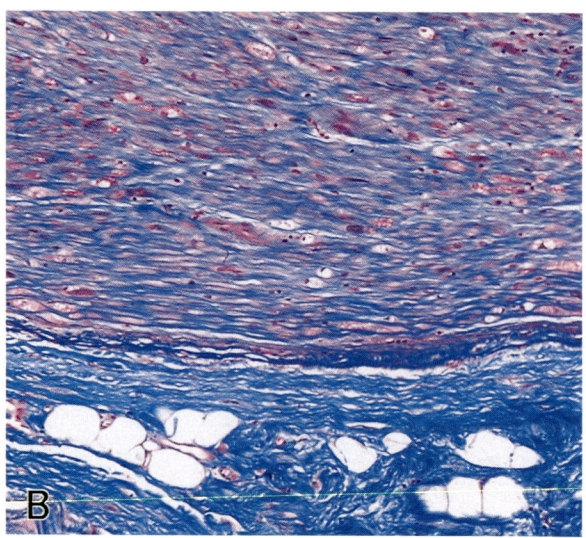

Figure 11-18

RADIATION-INDUCED EFFECT
UPON PERIPHERAL NERVE

This axillary nerve, a part of the brachial plexus subject
to radiotherapy for breast carcinoma, shows not only extensive perineural and endoneurial fibrosis (A,B, trichrome) but
loss of myelin (C, Luxol-fast blue) and axons (D, neurofilament protein) as well as nuclear atypia of Schwann cells.
When seen in the setting of a previously radiation-treated
MPNST (E), such atypical cells might be confused with
permeative sarcoma. We find such irradiation-affected non-
neoplastic cells to lack proliferative activity in terms of
mitoses and proliferation marker labeling.

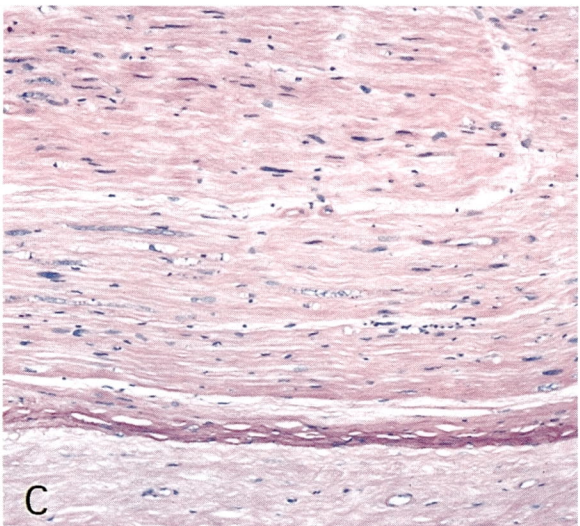

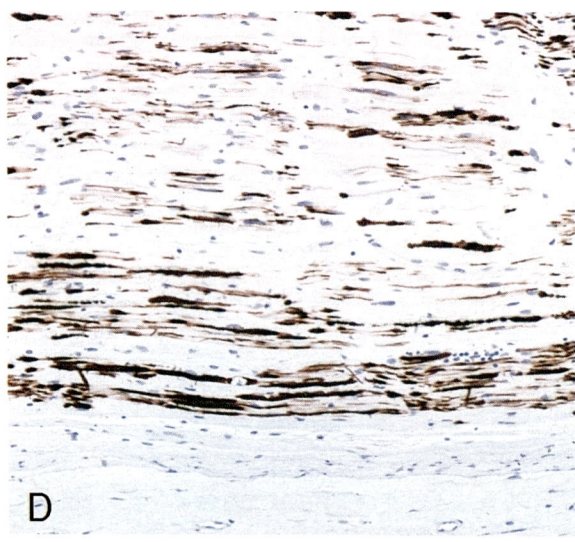

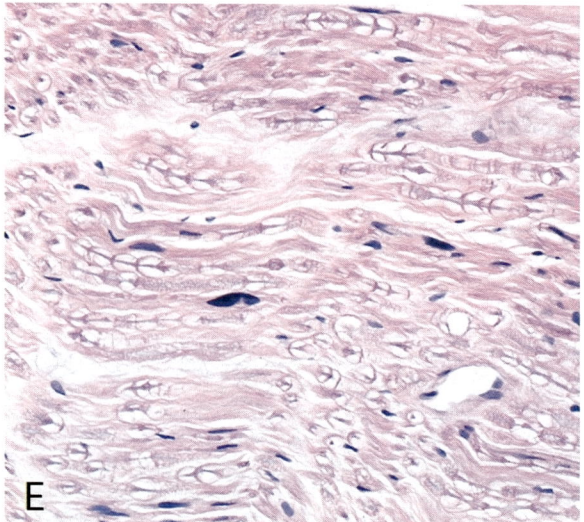

variable numbers of S-100 protein–immunoreactive cells (13,20,32,37,46,92). When present their staining is usually scattered or patchy (figs. 11-19B,C). Whereas one study of four MPNSTs (35) found S-100 protein alpha subunits to be preferentially expressed, another (47) reported an example expressing both alpha and beta forms. Thus, we consider polyclonal antisera which detect both forms of S-100 protein to be of greatest diagnostic utility. Although the frequency and intensity of S-100 protein staining does not correlate well with the histologic pattern of an MPNST of conventional type, we generally find staining to be most widespread in the uncommon low-grade examples (fig. 11-19A). MPNSTs may also show variable immunoreactivity for Leu-7 (fig. 11-19D) (46,94). Depending upon their degree of differentiation, MPNSTs may also stain for the basement membrane components such as collagen type 4 and laminin (fig. 11-19E)(7a,68). As a rule, staining is minor when compared to neurofibroma (7a) and particularly schwannoma. Although most MPNSTs are glial fibrillary acidic protein (GFAP) negative, limited staining may be seen in occasional cells of low-grade, better differentiated tumors (fig. 11-19F) (31,32,46). Epithelial membrane antigen (EMA) reactivity in MPNST, other than in MPNST with glandular differentiation (see below), is rare and suggests perineurial differentiation (fig. 11-20) (37,39–41). Virtually all soft tissue tumors, including MPNSTs, are vimentin positive (31,32). As a result, reactivity for this substance serves as little more than evidence of tissue immunoviability. Although it might be argued that MPNSTs showing only vimentin reactivity are simply fibrosarcomas, their frequent intrafascicular growth and spread, vague schwannian cytology, and occasional ultrastructural demonstration of at least some Schwann cell features, places them squarely in the MPNST spectrum.

In addition to the above-noted, commonly encountered antigens, MPNSTs may also stain for myelin basic protein (94) and nerve growth factor receptor (99).

When MPNSTs show no association with a nerve or a neurofibroma, immunohistochemistry plays an important role in diagnosis. In keeping with the observations of Wick et al. (94) and Swanson et al. (83), both of whom advocate a battery approach, employing antisera to S-100 protein and Leu-7 maximizes the identification of MPNST. Given the low frequency with which myelin basic protein, GFAP, and EMA staining are observed in MPNST, we do not recommend their routine application.

Ultrastructural Findings. The fine structural features of MPNST reflect the type and degree of differentiation of the constituent cells (figs. 11-21–11-24) (8,15,22,24,37–40,85,89). Unlike benign PNSTs in which the cells are consistently well differentiated, those in the majority of MPNSTs are undifferentiated, and electron microscopy is of no diagnostic value. In the next largest group of MPNSTs, the tumor cells are largely undifferentiated but feature inconspicuous cytoplasmic processes, rudimentary cell junctions, and wisps of basement membrane substance within the intercellular space, the only features suggesting Schwann cell differentiation (figs. 11-22, 11-23). A small proportion of MPNSTs exhibit convincing ultrastructural features of Schwann cell differentiation (fig. 11-21): arrays of relatively thick, occasionally intersecting cytoplasmic processes joined by varying numbers of rudimentary cell junctions and coated on their free surfaces by a discontinuous basement membrane. In addition to the usual cytoplasmic organelles, intermediate filaments and microtubules may be seen.

Other than tumors showing Schwann cell differentiation, a small number of MPNSTs are composed of cells with fine structural features of other nerve sheath constituents, specifically perineurial cells (fig. 11-24) and fibroblasts. Hirose et al. (41,42) have reported a small number of malignant soft tissue tumors exhibiting perineurial cell differentiation. The tumor cells expressed EMA, lacked staining for S-100 protein and Leu-7, and in most instances ultrastructurally demonstrated interdigitating cytoplasmic processes with surface pinocytotic vesicles, discontinuous basement membrane, and "primitive" cell junctions (fig. 11-24). Lastly, rare malignant spindle cell tumors originating in a major nerve are composed of cells with well-developed rough endoplasmic reticulum, a feature of fibroblastic differentiation.

Cytogenetics. MPNSTs are characterized by complex numerical and structural karyotypic changes, such as loss of chromosomal material and recombinations that lack consistency from case to case (45,61,72). At present there are about 37 cytogenetically studied cases (2,3,14,27,

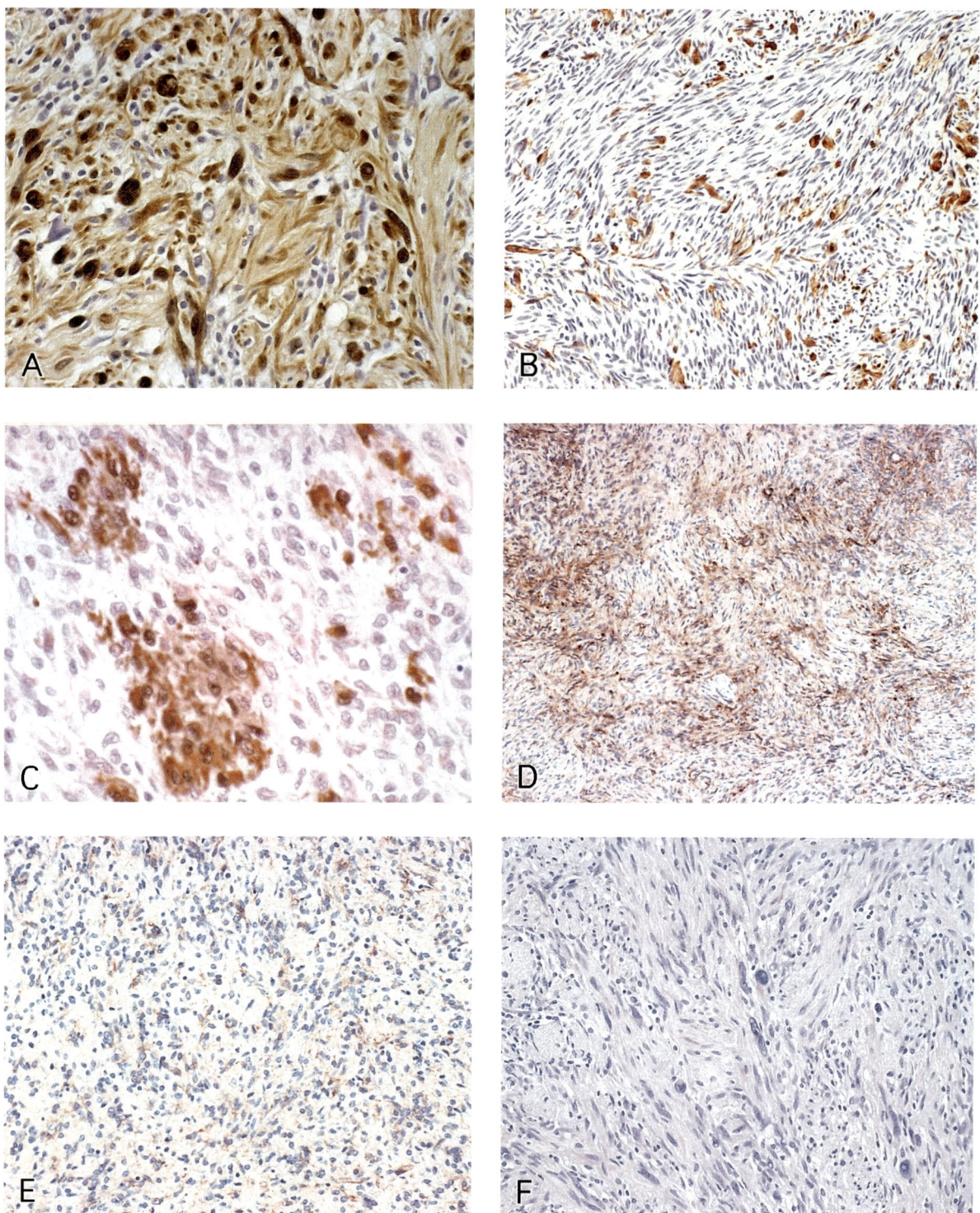

Figure 11-19
MPNST: IMMUNOPROFILE

Although staining for S-100 protein is present in only half of conventional MPNSTs, it represents the most useful marker of nerve sheath differentiation. Well-differentiated lesions may show extensive staining (A), but most tumors are high grade and show reactivity in only scattered cells (B,C). Some high-grade tumors also show reactivity in a patchy distribution (D). Staining for Leu-7 (CD57) is also of diagnostic value (E). GFAP reactivity is rarely seen, even in low-grade tumors (F).

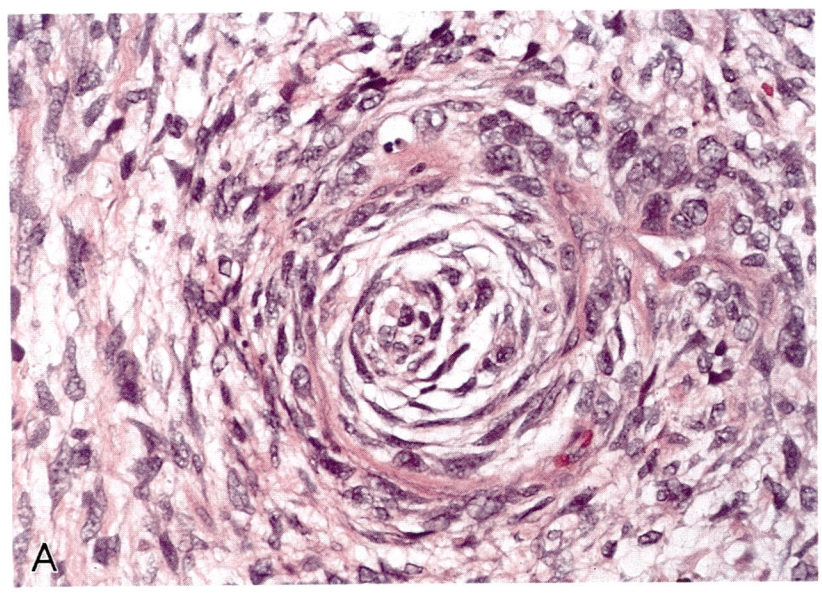

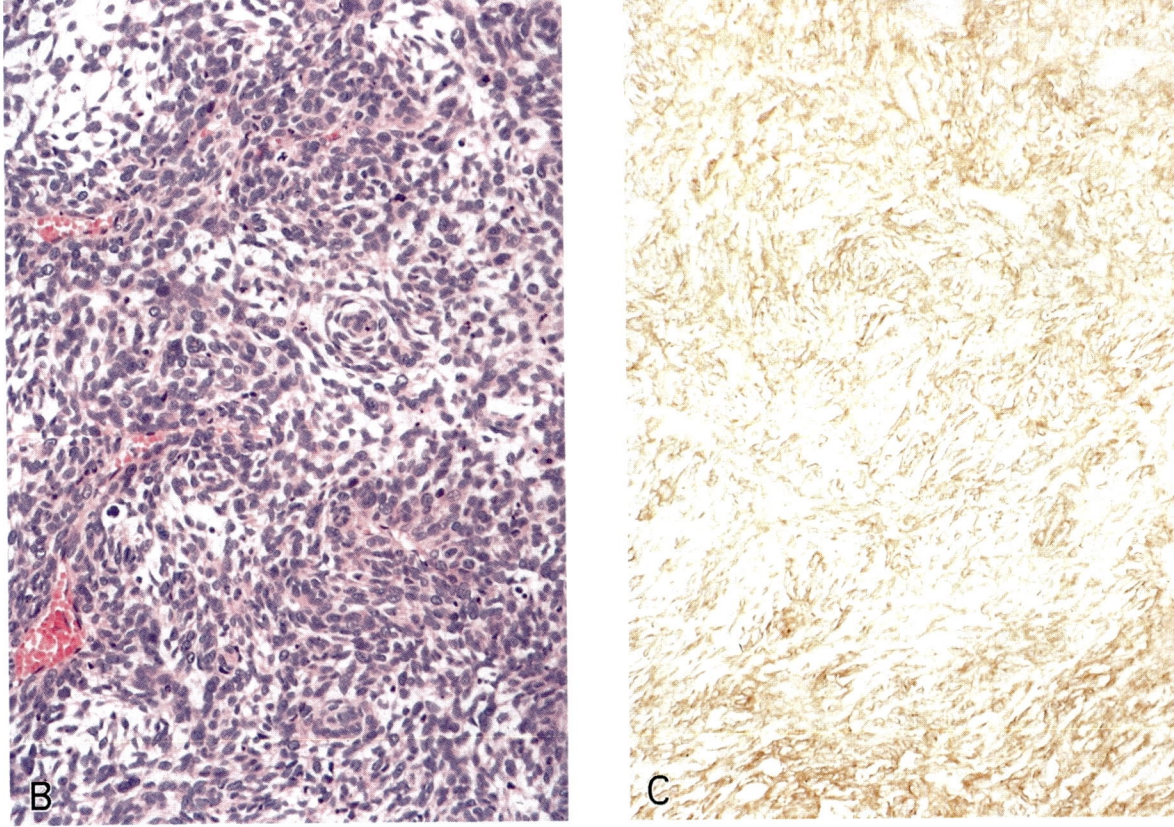

Figure 11-20

MPNST WITH PERINEURIAL CELL FEATURES

Occasional MPNSTs exhibit perineurial differentiation, such as this example with focal whorl formation (A). Yet another example (B,C) illustrates their typical EMA immunoreactivity. Their perineurial nature is also apparent on ultrastructure (see fig. 11-18). (Courtesy of Dr. T. Hirose, Tokushima, Japan.)

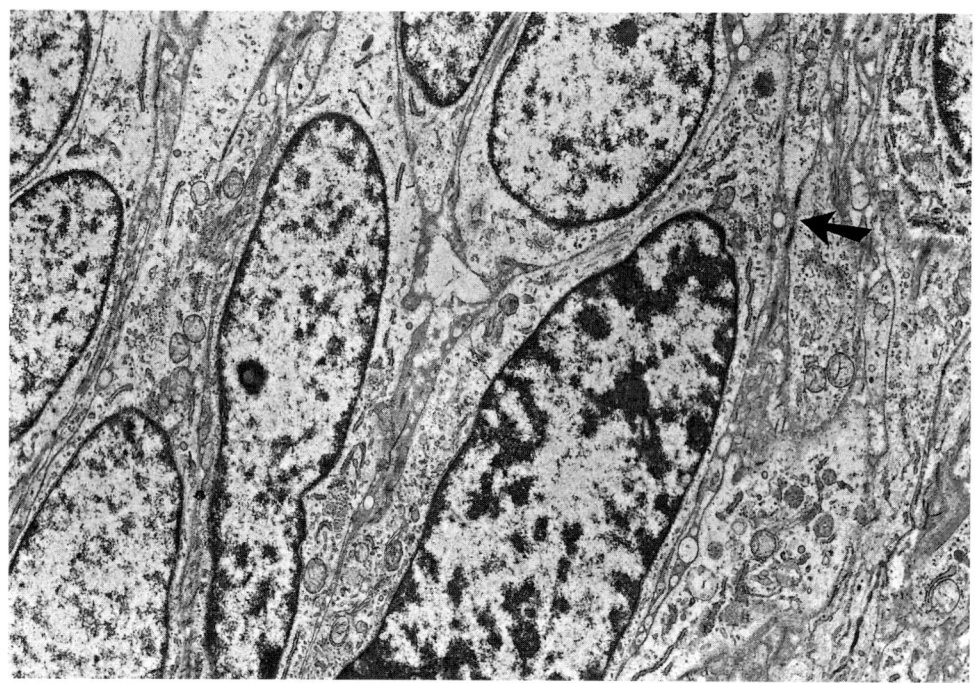

Figure 11-21
CONVENTIONAL MPNST

Spindle-shaped tumor cells with nuclei of varying size are joined by scattered rudimentary cell junctions (arrow). Note the intercellular basement membrane substance. These are characteristic diagnostic ultrastructural features of MPNST (X7,500).

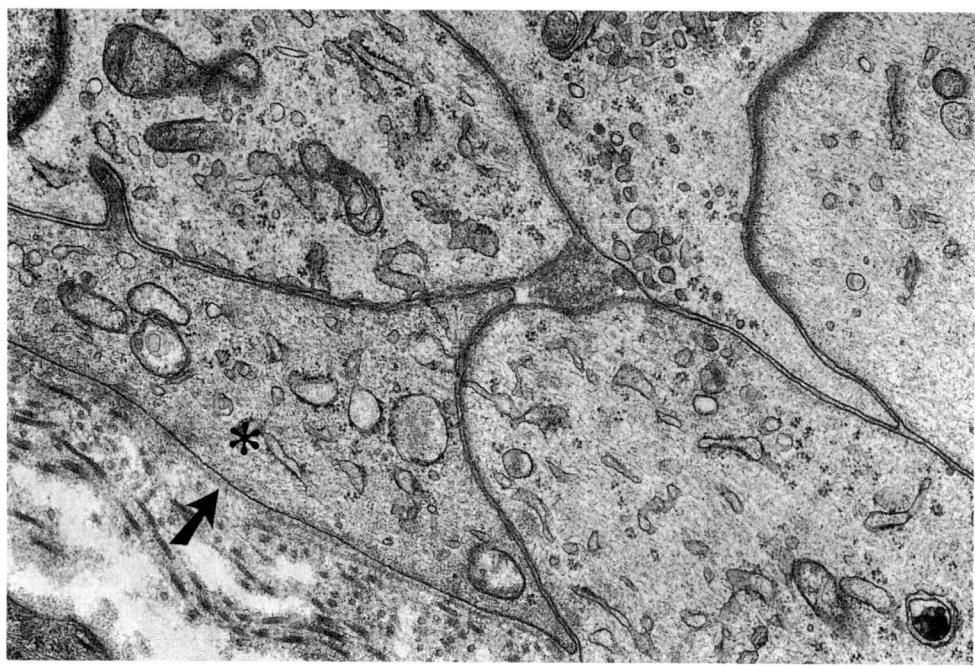

Figure 11-22
CONVENTIONAL MPNST

A cluster of obliquely sectioned cytoplasmic processes are coated by a thin basement membrane (arrow). Diffuse arrays of fine filaments as well as occasional microtubules (asterisk) are evident in the cytoplasm (X23,900).

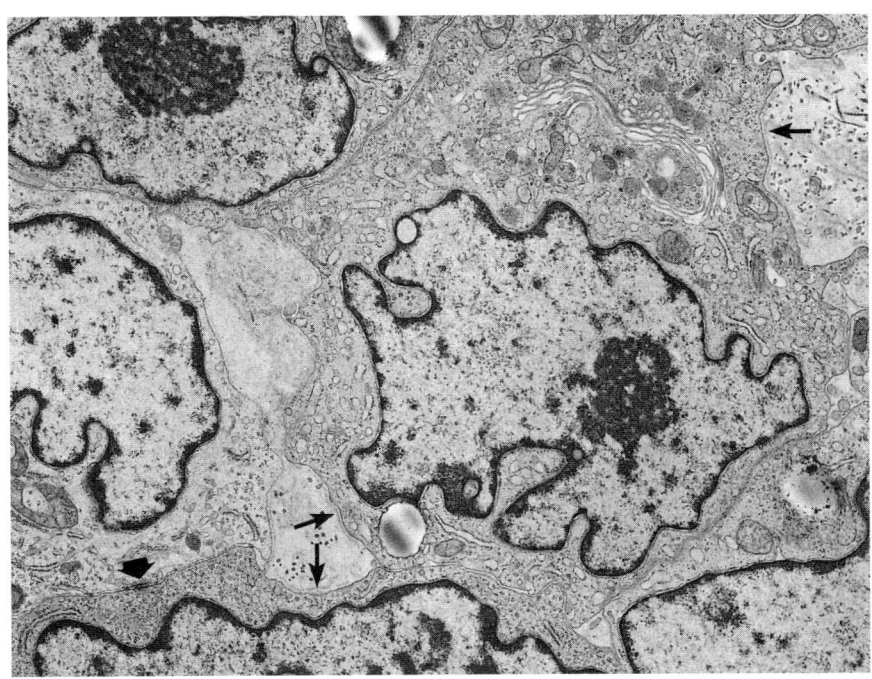

Figure 11-23
CONVENTIONAL MPNST
Cells of this poorly differentiated example with pleomorphic nuclei and large nucleoli have foci of basement membrane (arrows). The cells are joined by scattered rudimentary cell junctions (arrowhead). The presence of basement membrane and cell junctions supports a diagnosis of MPNST in the absence of structures indicating another type of sarcoma (X10,600).

Figure 11-24
MPNST WITH PERINEURIAL CELL DIFFERENTIATION
This cellular, spindle cell tumor (see fig. 11-20A) which showed EMA immunoreactivity (fig. 11-20B), has the ultrastructural features of perineurial cell differentiation as evidenced by thin cytoplasmic processes with variable numbers of pinocytotic vesicles, discontinuous basement membrane, and occasional primitive junctions. For case details see reference 42. (Courtesy of Dr T. Hirose, Saitama, Japan.)

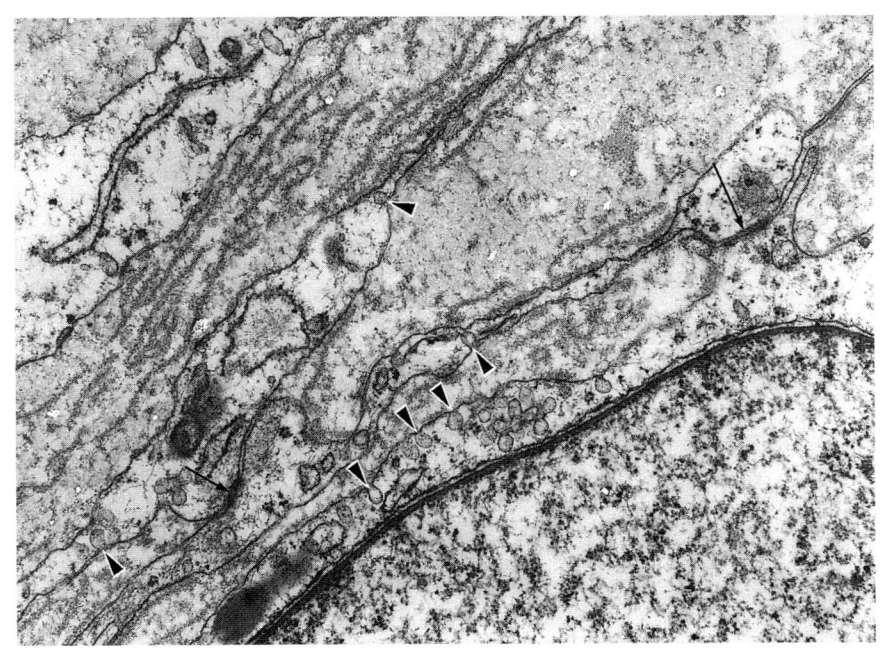

30,45,61,71,72,87) and many chromosomes have been found to be affected. Having reviewed the histologic sections of one reported case in which an identical chromosome 22 rearrangement was observed in four tumors located on the leg of one patient (27), we discount this case. Each of the four tumors was a benign schwannoma. Thus the diagnosis was schwannomatosis, not MPNST. MPNSTs often have chromosomal numbers in the triploid range (45,61). In a study of 8 tumors and a review of 20 others, Mertens et al. (61) found the most frequently affected chromosomes to be X, 1,

3, 6, 9, 11, 12, 13, 16, and 17, while Jhanwar et al. (45), in a study of 10 tumors, found preferential involvement of chromosomes X, 1, 11, 12, 14, 17, and 22. In the latter report, chromosome 17 was said to be affected in every case. Both studies found a frequent loss of both the NF1 locus (band 17q11) and the band containing the tumor suppressor gene TP53 (17p13). Based on such findings, it has been suggested that functional inactivation on the second allele of both the NF1 and p53 genes plays a role in MPNST tumorigenesis and progression (45,60).

Molecular Genetics. Evidence is accumulating that a multi-step mechanism of tumorigenesis is required for MPNST formation (60). The first of the genetic "hits" appears to involve a mutation in one or both copies of the NF1 gene, thus permitting neurofibroma formation. The second event may be a loss of one or both copies of a tumor suppressor gene on chromosome 17p. That the latter may be the p53 locus is suggested by the finding of 17p loss or deletion in nearly all malignant and in no benign PNSTs and the occurrence of point mutations in exon 4 of the p53 gene in a significant proportion of MPNSTs (60).

Immunohistochemical studies support the concept that p53 abnormalities play a role in the progression of neurofibroma to MPNST. One study (48) found that 65 percent of 26 cases of MPNST stained variably (5 to 100 percent) for p53, while none of 24 benign PNST had greater than 1 percent reactivity of tumor cells. A recent study of 28 MPNSTs and 27 neurofibromas reported similar results: 57 percent of the former and only 4 percent of the latter showed significant immunoreactivity for p53 protein (33). A slight majority of patients in both the neurofibroma and MPNST groups had NF1, but the presence of NF1 had no effect upon p53 immunoreactivity. Two of 3 radiation-induced MPNSTs were reactive for p53. It was of note that in 3 of 7 cases of MPNST in which an accompanying neurofibroma was demonstrated, no significant p53 staining was evident in the benign component. A more recent study of plexiform neurofibromas found a 13 percent frequency of p53 staining in the neurofibromatous component of MPNST-associated tumors (57).

Differential Diagnosis. Immunohistochemistry (Table 11-1) plays a pivotal role in the differential diagnosis of MPNST.

The distinction between MPNST and *cellular neurofibroma* was discussed and illustrated above (figs. 11-5, 11-6, 11-17). Similarly, their separation from *cellular schwannoma*, another benign nerve sheath tumor entering into the differential diagnosis, is discussed in chapter 7.

In the absence of an NF1 association, gross or microscopic evidence of an origin in neurofibroma, or spread within nerve fascicles, a number of soft tissue tumors are readily confused with conventional MPNST. These include monophasic (spindle cell) synovial sarcoma, leiomyosarcoma, conventional fibrosarcoma, myxofibrosarcoma (myxoid malignant fibrous histiocytoma [MFH]), storiform-pleomorphic fibrosarcoma (storiform-pleomorphic MFH), and spindle cell melanoma.

The *monophasic synovial sarcoma* of spindle cell type contains more closely packed cells with plumper nuclei than those of conventional MPNST. Furthermore, the stroma of synovial sarcoma typically features irregularly distributed, dense collagen bands of varying thickness and occasional calcifications. About 50 percent of monophasic synovial sarcomas contain cells expressing cytokeratin or EMA; such cells are usually lacking in conventional MPNSTs (69). Since S-100 protein staining is seen in about one fourth of monophasic synovial sarcomas (69), it is not a reliable marker for distinguishing this tumor from MPNST. Ultrastructurally, the cells of most monophasic synovial sarcomas differ from those of MPNST in having short bipolar processes, greater numbers of intercellular junctions, occasional small lumens with microvilli, and only inconspicuous intercellular spaces.

In contrast to the cells of conventional MPNST, those of *leiomyosarcoma* have blunt-ended nuclei and more abundant eosinophilic cytoplasm. The latter often contains longitudinal fibrils which are red in trichrome and blue in phosphotungstic acid–hematoxylin (PTAH) preparations. Since occasional leiomyosarcomas express S-100 protein (84), this antibody cannot be entirely relied upon to make the distinction from MPNST. Instead, appropriate muscle markers should be applied.

The light microscopic herringbone pattern of some MPNSTs is indistinguishable on hematoxylin and eosin (H&E) stain from that of *conventional fibrosarcoma*. Fibrosarcomas, however, lack immunoreactivity for S-100 protein and

Table 11-1

IMMUNOHISTOCHEMISTRY IN THE DIFFERENTIAL DIAGNOSIS OF MPNST

	Schwan-noma	Peri-neurioma	MPNST	Fibrosar-coma/MFH*	Leiomyo-sarcoma	Synovial Sarcoma	Epithelioid Sarcoma
Vimentin	+	+	+	+ /+	+	+	+
Cytokeratin	–	–	– (glandular +)	–	occ**	bi- and monophasic +)	+
Desmin	–	–	– (Triton +)	+ /–	+	–	
GFAP	20%	–	Rare	–	–	–	–
Muscle specific actin HHF 35	–	–	– (Triton +)	+ /–	+	–	–
HMB-45	(melanotic +)	–	–	–	–	–	–
S-100 Protein	>95%	–	50%	–	occ	occ	–
Leu-7	50–60%	–	30–40%	–	10–20%	25–40%	–
Myelin basic protein	50%	–	10%	–	–	–	–
EMA	–	+	(glandular differentiation)	–	–	bi- and monophasic +)	+
CEA	–	–	"	–	–	Glands +/–	–
Chromogranin	–	–	"	–	–	–	–
Factor VIII	–	–	(angiosarcoma differentiation)	–	–	–	–
CD34	–	+/–	"	–	occ	–	+
CD68 (KP-1)	+	+/–	+/–	–/+	–	–	–
Laminin and Collagen 4	+	+	25–30%	–	+	10%	10%

*MFH, malignant fibrous histiocytoma.
**Occ, occasional.

Leu-7. Ultrastructurally, they are devoid of surface basement membrane and show far greater development of rough endoplasmic reticulum. Rare MPNSTs may contain some myxoid stroma. These same features distinguish MPNSTs, which rarely show myxoid areas but more often contain pleomorphic cells or some cells in a storiform arrangement, from *myxofibrosarcoma* and *storiform-pleomorphic fibrosarcoma*. In both these forms of fibrosarcoma, the cells are plumper than those of MPNSTs, which only rarely show the alternating nodules of myxoid and cellular tumor so characteristic of myxofibrosarcoma.

Because both tumors are commonly S-100 protein positive, distinction from melanoma can be especially difficult. Generally, melanoma cells are more pleomorphic and often have amphophilic cytoplasm, prominent nuclear membranes and nucleoli, and intranuclear invaginations of cytoplasm. In contrast to MPNSTs, the reaction for S-100 protein is strong and diffuse; reaction for HMB-45 and A103 may also be positive.

MPNSTs that affect the gut must be distinguished from *gastrointestinal stromal tumors,* particularly the more often NF1-associated subset termed gastrointestinal autonomic nerve tumor (GANT) (21,23,36,53,63,64,74,75,90,91), a tumor discussed in more detail in chapter 13 (page 394).

Infrequently, MPNSTs exhibit areas resembling *hemangiopericytoma* (fig. 11-13) (88). In our experience this is usually a focal feature, and a more conventional spindle cell pattern is evident in other sections. The only example of MPNST we have seen displaying an exclusively hemangiopericytoma pattern (see fig. 11-13D) also expressed S-100 protein and showed an intrafascicular pattern of spread. Since basement membrane substance is commonly found in both, electron microscopy plays no significant role in the distinction of hemangiopericytoma from MPNST.

Irradiation-induced atypia also deserves mention. Therapeutic irradiation is known to affect nerve: the classic experimental study of Bergstrom (4) documented edema, myelin disintegration, axonal loss, fibrosis, and proliferation of Schwann cells and fibroblasts. Nuclear and chromosomal abnormalities have also been reported, even in association with doses as low as 200 rads (7). The finding of scattered cells exhibiting cytologic atypia, including nuclear enlargement and hyperchromasia, in an irradiated nerve should not be overinterpreted as evidence of malignant change. This differential is less problematic in nerves irradiated for non-neurogenic neoplasms (see fig. 11-18A–D) than in the assessment of a possible MPNST recurrence (see fig. 11-18E). Although no firm criteria permit the distinction of irradiation-induced atypia in Schwann cells or fibroblasts from isolated residual tumor cells or recurrent sarcoma, we have found no proliferative activity (mitoses, Ki-67 labeling) in cells exhibiting radiation-induced atypia. Interestingly, experimental evidence suggests that radiation doses of 1,000 to 2,000 rads may in fact impair the proliferative capacity of Schwann cells (7).

Recurrence and Metastasis. Rates of local tumor recurrence after surgical resection have ranged from a low of 40 percent for MPNSTs of the lower extremity and buttock (44), to 68 percent for paraspinal tumors (50). For tumors at all sites, the figure ranges from 42 (18) to 54 percent (78). There is conflicting data regarding the frequency of local recurrence in patients with and without NF1 (18,50,78).

Although the overall rate of metastasis for MPNSTs ranges from 28 (18) to 43 percent (78), a rate as high as 65 percent has been reported for lesions of the lower extremity and buttock (44) as well as for paraspinal sites (50). Two independent studies found a higher rate of metastasis in patients with NF1 (35 percent) as opposed to those without this disorder (16 percent) (18,78). This contrasts with two other studies of tumors of the buttock and lower extremities (44) and paraspinal areas (50) which found no significant difference in the metastatic rates (65 and 68 percent) for the two groups. In fact, in both studies the metastatic rate in patients without NF1 was slightly higher than that for those with NF1. The most common sites of metastasis are lung followed by bone, pleura, soft tissue, liver, and brain.

Treatment. Surgical resection is the mainstay of therapy for MPNST. Although the type of resection will vary with a lesion's anatomic location (86), wide en bloc resection is the procedure of choice for tumors involving soft tissues (44). Postoperative radiation therapy of soft tissue sarcomas including MPNST has led to a significant reduction in the incidence of local recurrence (6,77,94a). For this reason it is recommended that resection be followed by radiation therapy to the tumor bed (94a,95). The effect of such treatment varies in different series. In one recent study, adjuvant irradiation (greater than or equal to 60 Gy), as well as brachytherapy and intraoperative electron irradiation, both decreased the frequency of recurrence and significantly improved survival (94a). Similar results were obtained in a prior, smaller series (89a). To date, no chemotherapeutic regimen has proven effective in the treatment of MPNST.

Frozen Section Diagnosis. A note of caution has recently been published regarding the role of frozen section in the diagnosis of PNSTs (95). Prior to definitive therapy, it is desirable to determine whether a peripheral nerve tumor is benign or malignant. To achieve this, a biopsy is often performed prior to surgical removal. Unless the pathologist has extensive experience with soft tissue tumors, we do not think frozen sections should be relied upon to diagnose any but obvious high-grade MPNSTs. Resection of an MPNST often requires a wide en bloc procedure that may necessitate sacrifice of an involved nerve. To do this based solely upon a frozen section interpretation is problematic at best. In the mediastinum this approach is acceptable, since sacrifice of one or more thoracic spinal nerves does not result in major neurologic disability. On the other hand, a tumor in the lumbosacral region poses much more of a challenge since resection of large spinal nerves may result in significant functional deficits. If the diagnosis of cellular schwannoma is a possibility, we recommend resection of the tumor with preservation of functionally important nerves. This constitutes adequate treatment if on permanent sections the well-sampled tumor is found to be a cellular schwannoma. Alternatively, if permanent sections show the tumor to be a MPNST, either a wide local excision with or without sacrifice of nerve, or radiation therapy of the tumor bed may be undertaken.

Prognosis. The prognosis of patients with MPNST is poor, being the same as for other high-grade sarcomas. In two major studies with long-term follow-up, 63 and 68 percent of the patients died of tumor (18,44). Reported overall 5- and 10-year survival rates range from 34 to 52 percent and 23 to 34 percent, respectively (18,44, 94a). The series with more favorable overall survival rates (94a) included 10 percent low-grade tumors as well as a small number of perineurial MPNSTs. What follows is a discussion of a number of factors that appear to affect the prognosis of patients with MPNST.

Tumor Location. Location has been cited as a factor contributing to differences in prognosis of patients with and without NF1. In the series of Ducatman et al. (18), patients with this condition had a greater proportion of centrally situated tumors and a shorter survival. The effect of central location upon prognosis was recently confirmed in a study of paraspinous MPNSTs by Kourea et al. (50). The study found the 5- and 10-year survival rates (16 percent) and the rates of recurrence (65 percent) and metastasis (68 percent) differed from those of tumors occurring at all body sites (34, 23, 42, and 28 percent, respectively) (18).

Tumor Size. The series of Hruban et al. (44) reported a poorer prognosis, albeit one not sta-

tistically significant, in patients with tumors greater than 10 cm in size. In contrast, the series of Ducatman et al. (18) found a significant difference in survival at the 5 cm level.

Resection. In large series, a positive surgical margin was the principle factor determining local recurrence and a major factor determining survival (50,94a).

Histologic Subtype. The finding that perineurial MPNST is less aggressive (41,94a), specifically less likely to metastasize, remains to be confirmed. Such tumors tend to be of lower histologic grade that conventional MPNST.

Tumor Grade. The two published studies that attempted to correlate prognosis with histologic grade reported disparate results (18,67). Unfortunately, these series differ significantly, not only in the number of patients studied, but also in terms of grading methodology. The 30-patient series of Nambisan et al. (67) used a 3-grade scale: 60 percent of the tumors were grade I or II lesions; the criteria distinguishing low (grade I) and intermediate (grade II) lesions were not stated. The authors reported a statistically significant difference in recurrence-free survival between patients with tumors of grades I and II (61 percent) as compared to those with high-grade (grade III) lesions (20 percent). In contrast, in the 120-patient series of Ducatman et al. (18), tumors were graded on a 4-tier scale and consisted in large part (88 percent) of high-grade (grades III and IV) lesions. In this study, there were no statistically significant differences in patient survival by tumor grade. Although one recent study indicates that necrosis is particularly associated with recurrence and metastasis (65a), we believe that such prognostically negative factors as large tumor size and central location (often NF1 associated) may override the effects of histologic grade.

DNA Ploidy. In our experience, the majority of MPNSTs are aneuploid. A recent study of 28 MPNSTs, nearly all high grade, and 26 neurofibromas found 64 percent of MPNSTs and 33 percent of neurofibromas to be aneuploid (76). The difference was statistically significant (p=0.04), but the frequency of aneuploidy in sporadically occurring and NF1-associated tumors was not. The prognostic significance of these findings is unsettled.

Proliferation Markers. Limited data is available regarding proliferative activity in MPNST. A

327

recent series of 28 cases (76), all but two of which were high-grade tumors, found the mean and range of labeling indices to be as follows: proliferating cell nuclear antigen (PCNA) 35.7; 9–67, MIB-1 (18.5; 5–38), and percent S-phase as determined by DNA flow cytometry (12.4; 2–46). These values were of course significantly different from those of neurofibromas (p=0.001), but no differences were noted between MPNSTs occurring sporadically or in association with NF1. The prognostic utility of proliferation indices and DNA content measurement remains to be determined.

Molecular Genetics. That p53 immunoreactivity is a negative prognostic indicator is suggested by one study of 28 MPNSTs (33) in which 68 percent of tumors showed staining. Patients with p53-positive tumors had a median survival time of 18 months as compared to 82 months for those whose tumors were nonreactive (p=0.02).

Recurrence. In a study of MPNSTs of the buttock and lower extremity, 78 percent of the patients with local recurrence eventually died of tumor (44). In contrast the figure was only 31 percent in those without a local recurrence. It is not clear whether this association can be explained by the existence of occult distant metastases at the time of local recurrence, or to secondary spread from the recurrence itself.

Metastasis. The occurrence of metastases, most often to lung and at a median time of approximately 2 years, has a very negative effect on prognosis (94a). The vast majority of patients die of disease. Factors associated with metastases include tumor size, as well as histologic grade and subtype (94a) (see above).

Presence of NF1. Data from three series (18, 67,78) suggest that among patients with MPNSTs, those with NF1 have a worse prognosis than do patients with sporadically occurring tumors. The largest series, that of Ducatman et al. (18), showed significant differences in 5-year (16 versus 53 percent) and 10-year (9 versus 38 percent) survival. The poorer prognosis of NF1 patients in this series was thought to be a reflection of tumor characteristics, in that NF1-associated lesions were more often central in location (57 versus 36 percent), larger, and of higher histologic grade. Three other series found no significant difference in outcome between patients with and without NF1 (44,50,81).

MPNST VARIANTS

Epithelioid MPNST

In addition to their usual spindle cell component, otherwise conventional MPNSTs may be composed in part of polygonal and elongate cells with abundant cytoplasm, ones superficially resembling epithelial cells (102–104). We reserve the term epithelioid MPNST for tumors composed predominately or exclusively of such epithelioid cells. Less than 5 percent of MPNSTs are of this type (103). Even fewer are those purely epithelioid in composition (101,102,104).

Clinical Features. Combining data from the two largest series of epithelioid MPNSTs provides an overview of the clinicopathologic features of 40 cases (103,104). Among these, the sexes were equally represented, and mean and patient age was 38 years (range, 6 to 81 years). Most frequently affected sites were the legs, arms, and inguinal region. Laskin et al. (103) recognized two clinical presentations: in one, tumors arose in deep soft tissue; in the other, they were superficially situated in subcutaneous tissue. A nerve of origin was identified in approximately half of the cases. There was no association with NF1.

Gross and Microscopic Findings. As expected, superficially situated tumors are often smaller than 5 cm, whereas deep-seated tumors usually are larger (102–104). In addition, superficial lesions generally show greater circumscription (103). In either situation, the tumors commonly appear multinodular with a fleshy, carcinoma-like consistency (fig. 11-25). This nodular pattern persists, even at the microscopic level, wherein the epithelioid cells are variously arranged in compact sheets, loose clusters, strings, or cords separated by fibrous septa (figs. 11-26, 11-27A, 11-28A,B). On occasion, they produce mucin and lie embedded in a mucinous, hyaluronic acid–rich matrix (fig. 11-29). As a rule, the epithelioid cells are uniform, polygonal, round, or oblong, and have abundant, densely eosinophilic or plum colored cytoplasm and vesicular nuclei with prominent nucleoli (figs. 11-26, top, 11-27A, 11-28C) (102–104). Cytologic variations include pleomorphic cells, clear cells, and ones with eccentric eosinophilic cytoplasm that lends a rhabdoid appearance (fig. 11-27C)

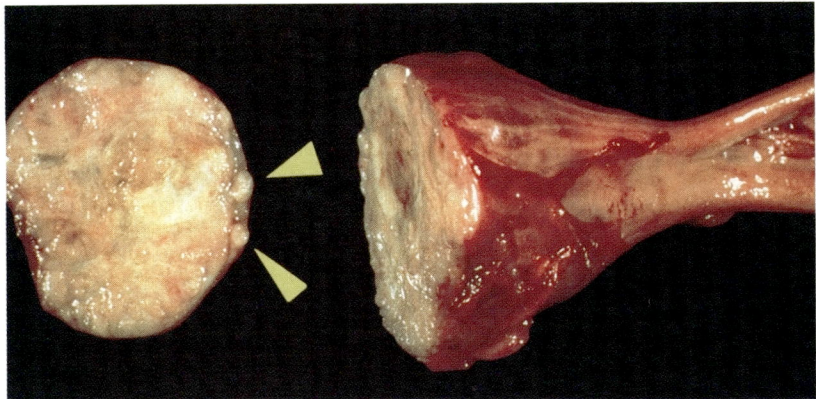

Figure 11-25
EPITHELIOID MPNST
Epithelioid MPNST involving the sciatic nerve of a 43-year-old male who noted leg pain with exercise. The lesion grew quickly over a period of 3 months and was associated with lung metastases. Note the fleshy, carcinoma-like appearance of the tumor, which unlike conventional MPNST was soft in texture. (Courtesy of Dr. W. E. Ballinger, Gainesville, FL.)

(103). In addition, a majority of the tumors contain a spindle cell element identical to that of conventional MPNST. When a lesion is purely epithelioid and devoid of a spindle cell component, the diagnosis of MPNST depends in large part upon demonstrating the origin of the tumor from nerve (102) or providing supportive immunohistochemical and ultrastructural data.

Immunohistochemical Findings. In addition to vimentin reactivity (fig. 11-30A), approximately 80 percent of epithelioid MPNSTs express S-100 protein in the form of diffuse, strong, cytoplasmic and often nuclear reactivity (fig. 11-30B,C) (103,104). We have also seen epithelioid MPNSTs reactive for Leu-7. Unlike melanomas, the tumors do not stain for the melanoma-associated antigen HMB-45 (103). In our experience, occasional epithelioid MPNSTs show cytokeratin (fig. 11-30D) or EMA reactivity (101). In addition, two examples that arose in schwannomas expressed cytokeratin (106). The frequent presence of pericellular basement membrane may be confirmed by stains for collagen 4 or laminin (fig. 11-30E). A unique epithelioid MPNST of a sciatic nerve exhibited ultrastructural as well as immunohistochemical features (co-expression of S-100 protein, EMA, and cytokeratin) of schwannian, perineurial, and squamous differentiation (101).

Ultrastructural Findings. Electron microscopy plays a role in the diagnosis of epithelioid MPNST, particularly in instances in which the results of immunostains are indeterminate. The tumors typically consist of clusters of epithelial-like cells with electron-lucent nuclei, large nucleoli, fairly numerous organelles, glycogen particles, varying numbers of cytoplasmic intermediate filaments, moderate numbers of cell junctions including small desmosomes, pericellular basement membranes which may be reduplicated, and accumulations of more diffuse basement membrane substance within narrow intercellular spaces (figs. 11-31–11-34) (100,102,104,105). In some instances, basement membrane is scant or absent. Cells containing large numbers of cytoplasmic intermediate filaments, usually vimentin, resemble rhabdoid cells at the light microscopic level (fig. 11-35). Features of true epithelial differentiation, such as tonofilaments, secretory granules, microvilli, and lumen formation, are not seen.

Differential Diagnosis. The differential diagnoses of epithelioid MPNST includes a disparate group of lesions. Distinction from *melanoma* and *clear cell sarcoma* rests upon the absence of melanin on histochemical stains, of immunoreactivity for the melanoma-associated antigen (HMB-45), and of melanosomes on electron microscopy. The exclusion of *carcinoma* is based upon finding, in epithelioid MPNSTs, strong, diffuse S-100 protein immunoreactivity and, in most instances, lack of keratin and EMA staining. *Epithelioid sarcoma* differs from superficially situated epithelioid MPNST by the greater density of the cytoplasm, cells often embedded in dense collagen, and lack of a myxoid matrix. Also, epithelioid sarcoma shows multifocal rather than discrete growth, a superficial resemblance to necrobiotic granuloma, a usual lack of S-100 protein immunoreactivity in the face of a positive keratin reaction, and the ultrastructural presence of tonofilaments. Whereas keratin may occasionally be expressed in angiosarcoma, the latter lacks S-100 protein immunoreactivity. Furthermore, *epithelioid angiosarcomas* almost always exhibit either CD34, CD31, or factor VIII

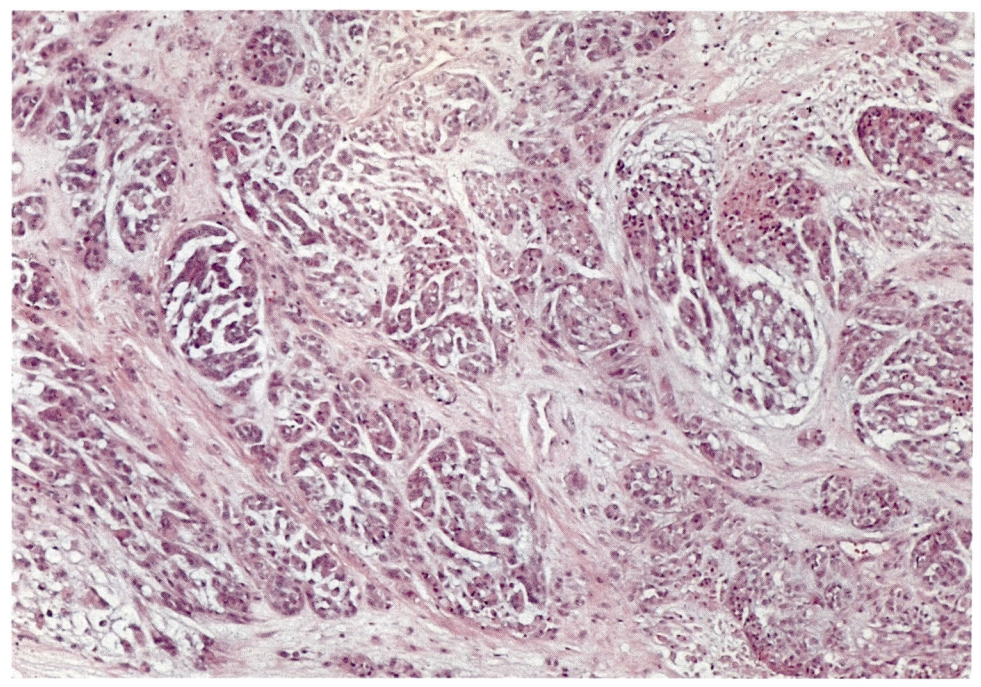

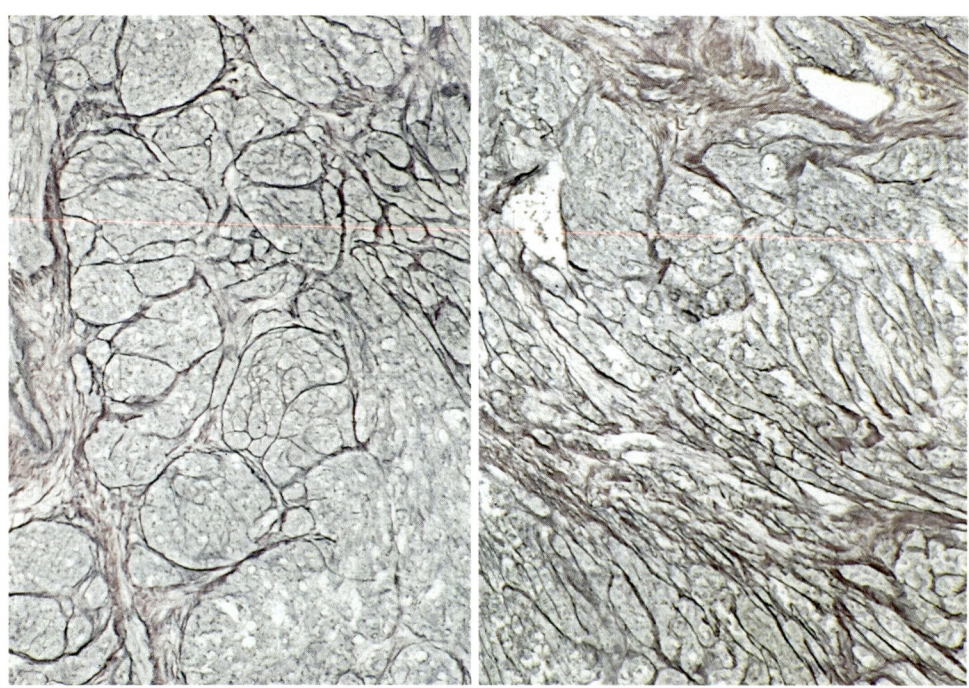

Figure 11-26
EPITHELIOID MPNST
Epithelioid MPNST showing the typical lobular growth pattern (top). A reticulin stain highlights both the lobules (bottom, left) and the intercellular pattern of a more conventional, spindle cell MPNST component of the tumor (bottom, right).

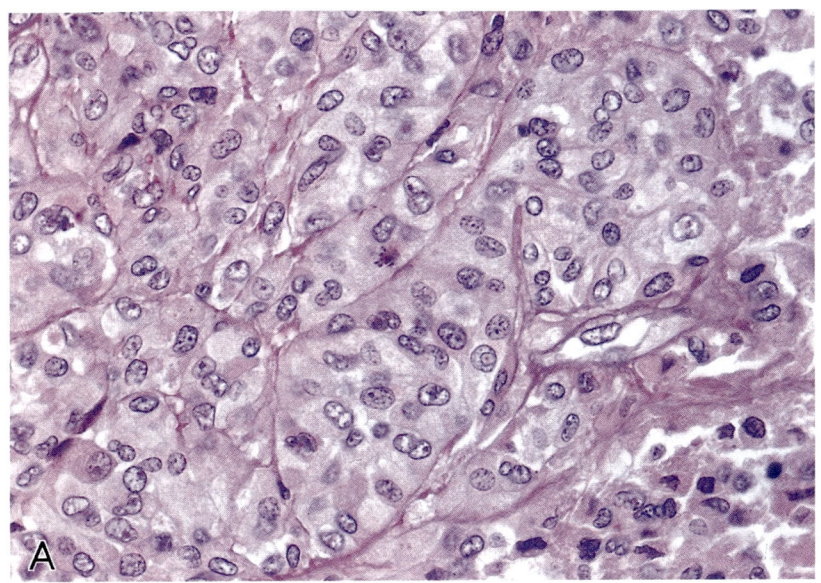

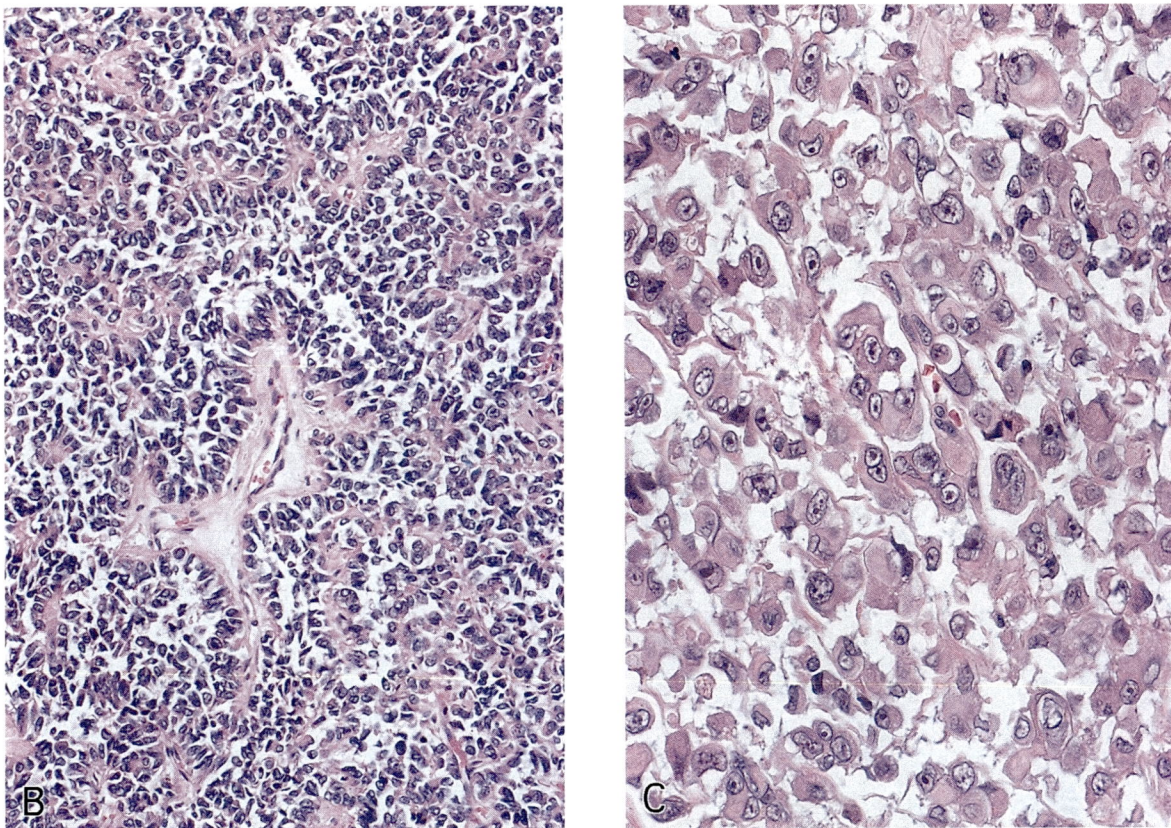

Figure 11-27
EPITHELIOID MPNST

Epithelioid MPNSTs show variation in cytology ranging from plump epithelioid cells with large round vesicular nuclei and prominent nucleoli (A), ones polarized and forming pseudopapillae (B), and cells with rhabdoid features (C).

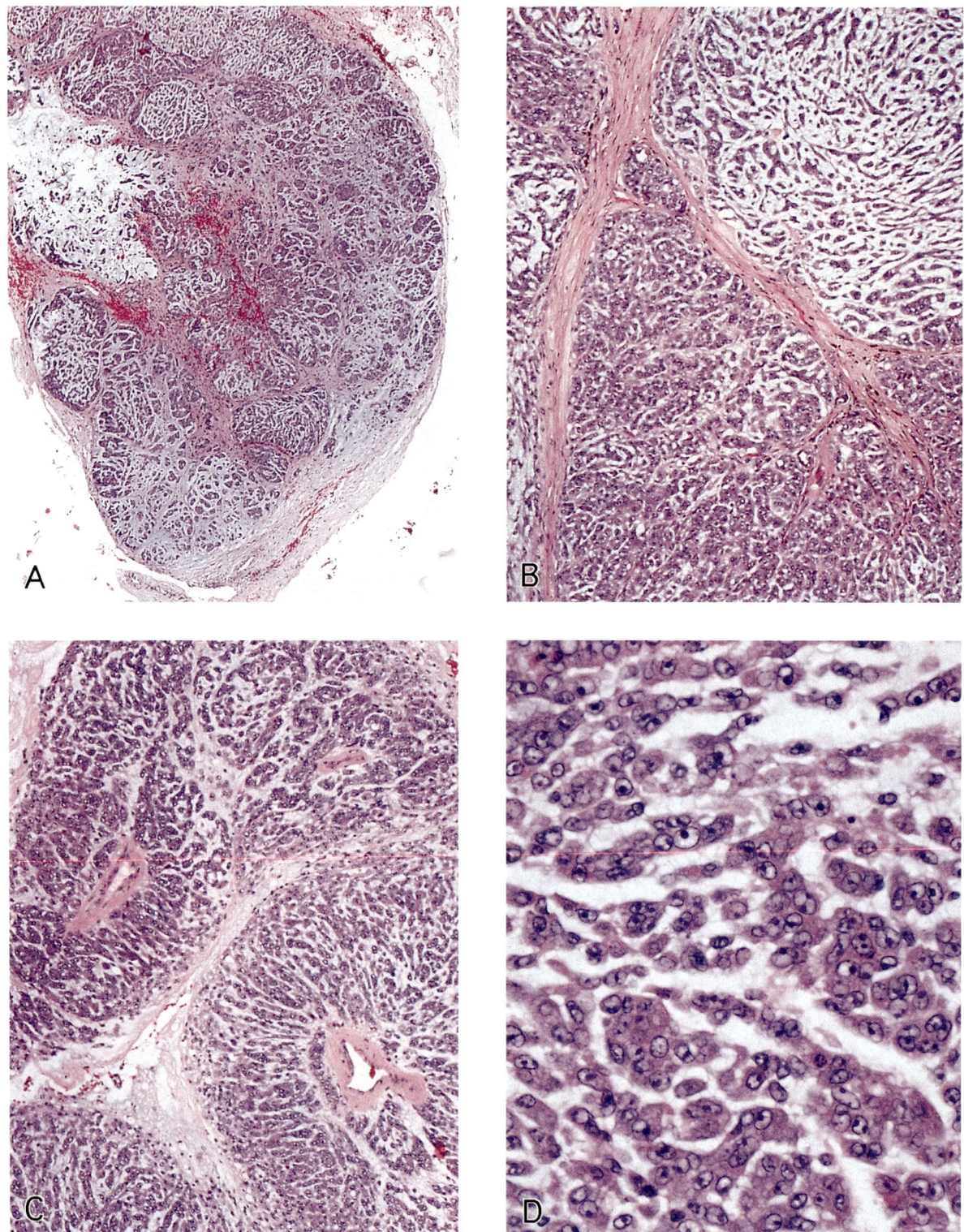

Figure 11-28
EPITHELIOID MPNST
This typically lobulated example (A) showed delicate fibrovascular septation (B) and pseudopapillae formation due to the effects of necrosis (C). Its clustered epithelioid cytology (D) was present throughout.

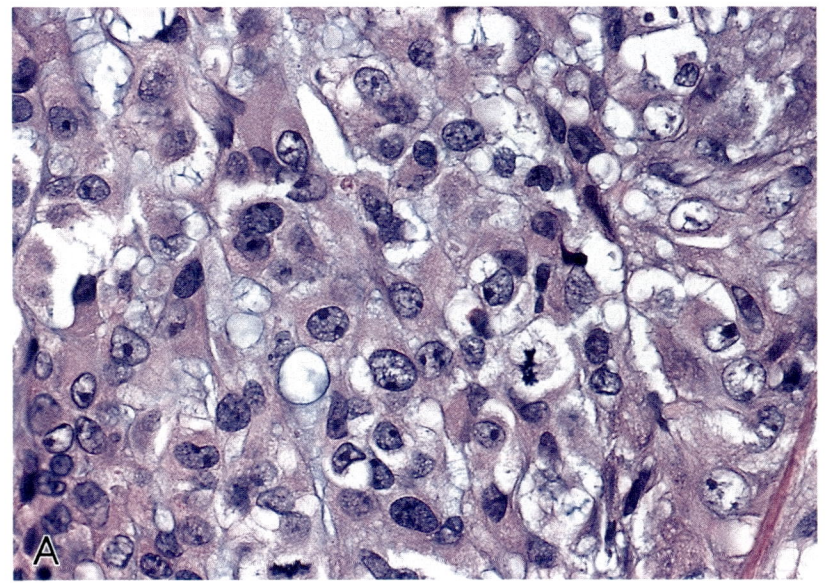

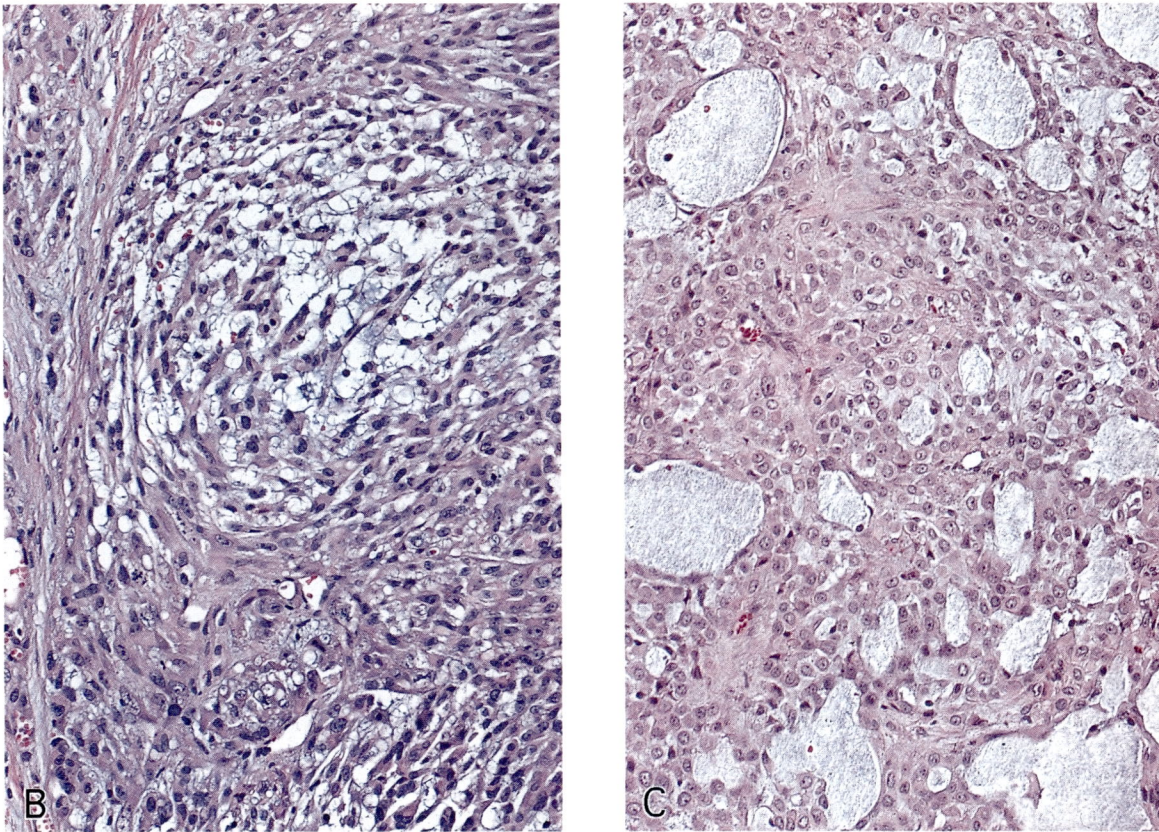

Figure 11-29
EPITHELIOID MPNST
In tumors showing mucin production (A), accumulation is largely extracellular. The mucin may form small pools within which cohesive tumor cells appear to float (B) or may accumulate in microcysts (C).

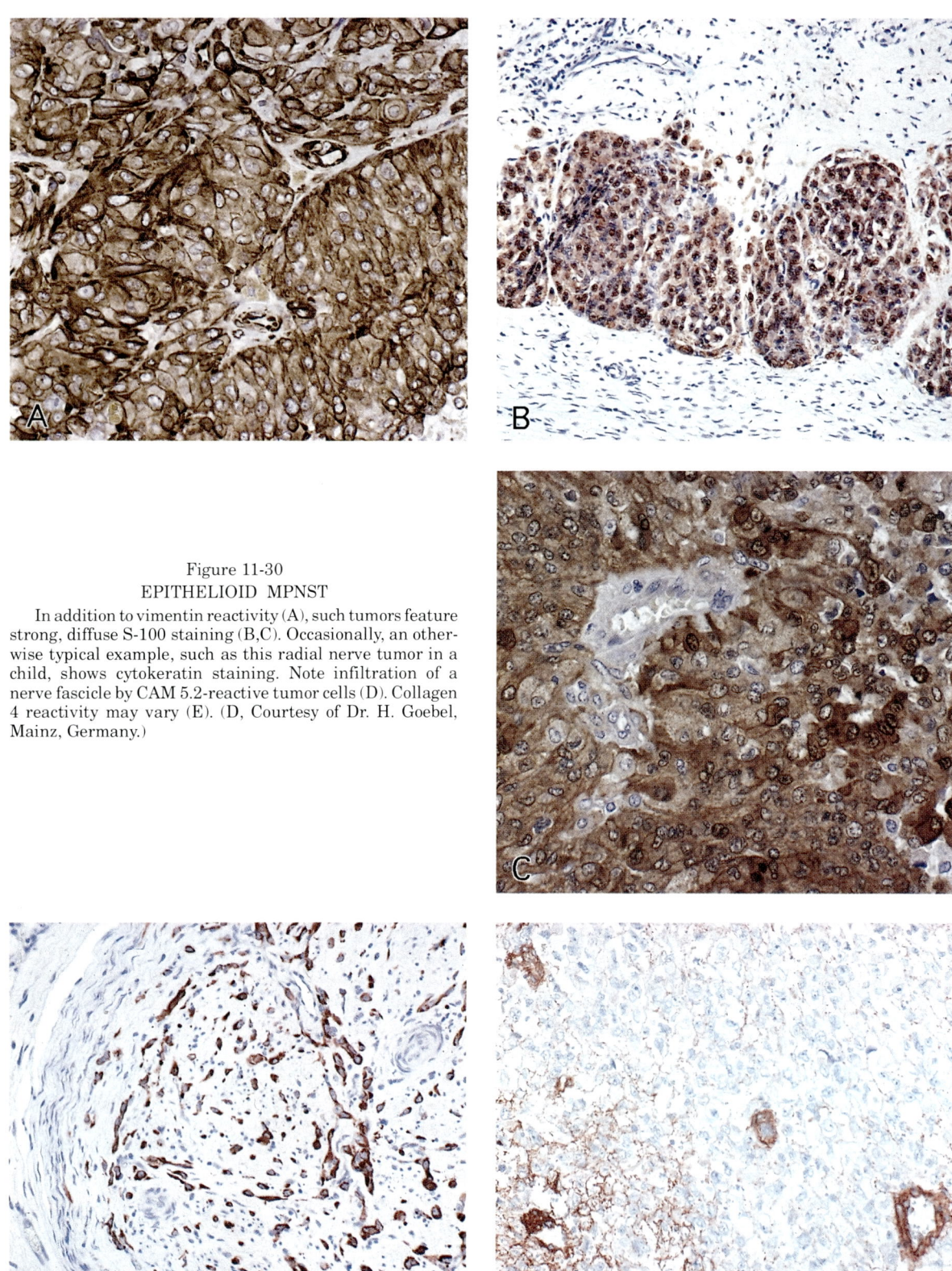

Figure 11-30
EPITHELIOID MPNST

In addition to vimentin reactivity (A), such tumors feature strong, diffuse S-100 staining (B,C). Occasionally, an otherwise typical example, such as this radial nerve tumor in a child, shows cytokeratin staining. Note infiltration of a nerve fascicle by CAM 5.2-reactive tumor cells (D). Collagen 4 reactivity may vary (E). (D, Courtesy of Dr. H. Goebel, Mainz, Germany.)

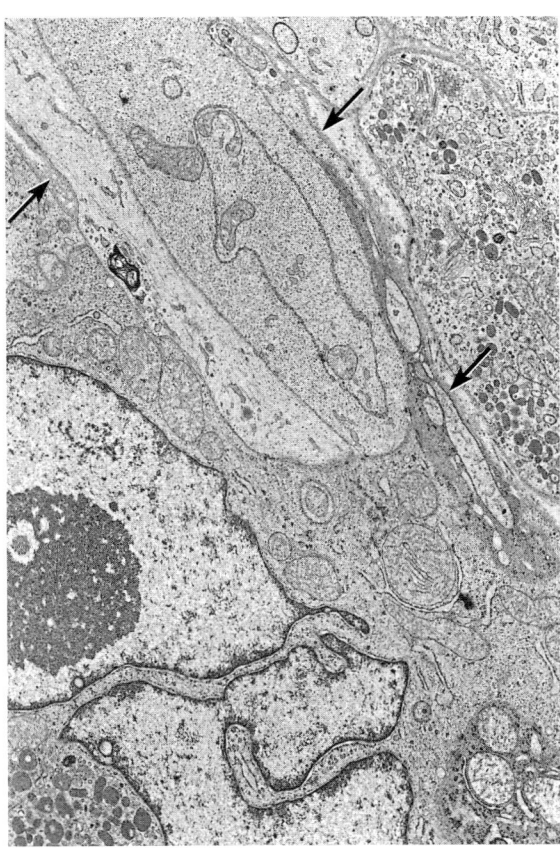

Figure 11-31
PLEXIFORM EPITHELIOID MPNST
Characteristic diagnostic ultrastructural features include large epithelioid cells with a prominent nucleolus
(lower left) and a basement membrane (arrows) (X9,700).

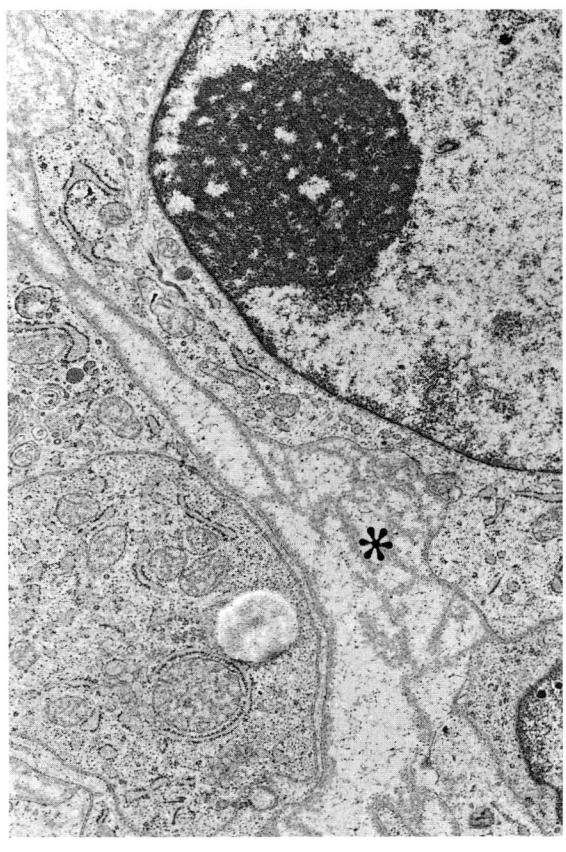

Figure 11-32
PLEXIFORM EPITHELIOID MPNST
A round nucleus containing a large nucleolus and prominent reduplicated basement membranes (asterisk) are illustrated (X14,500).

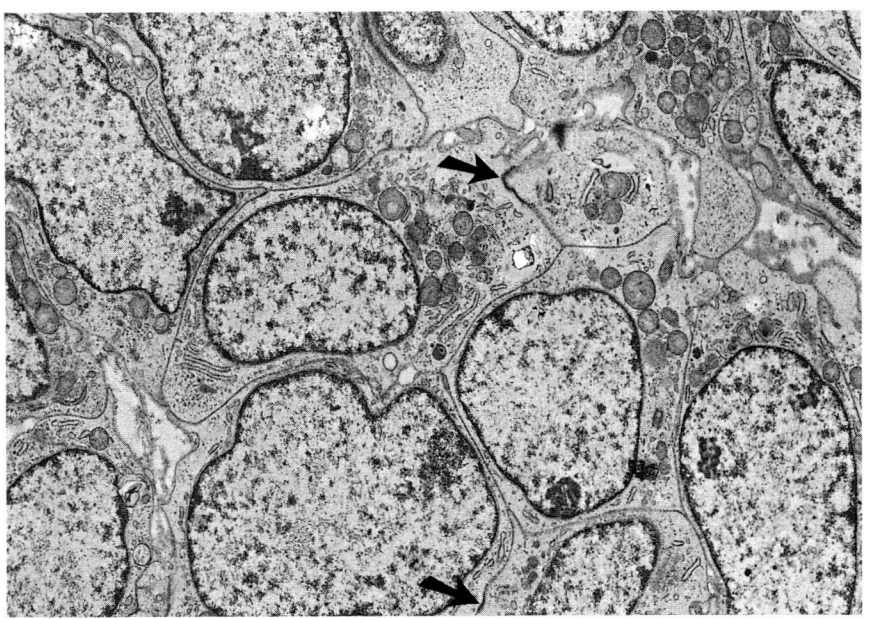

Figure 11-33
EPITHELIOID MPNST
A cluster of epithelioid
tumor cells are joined by scattered tight junction-like intercellular junctions (arrows).
Note the flocculent basement
membrane substance in the intercellular spaces (X7,200).

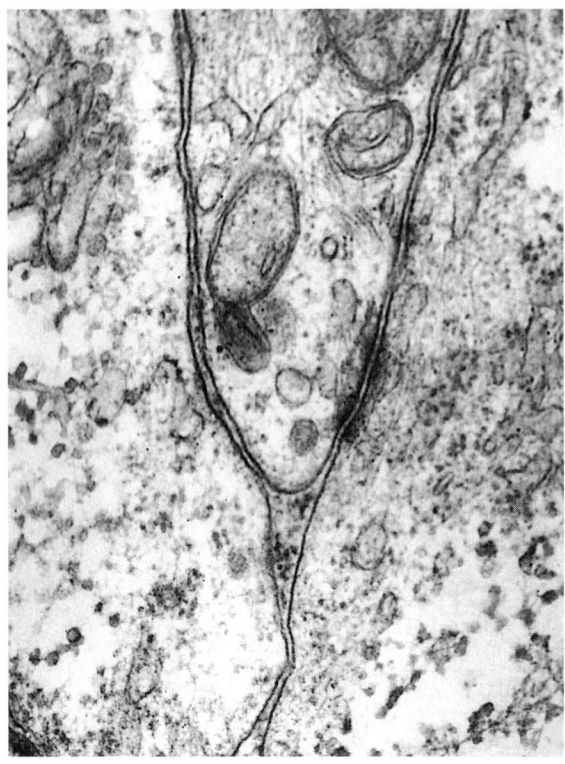

Figure 11-34
EPITHELIOID MPNST
Detail of a portion of the cytoplasm from three neoplastic epithelioid tumor cells illustrating rudimentary cell junctions, intermediate filaments, and glycogen particles (X42,000).

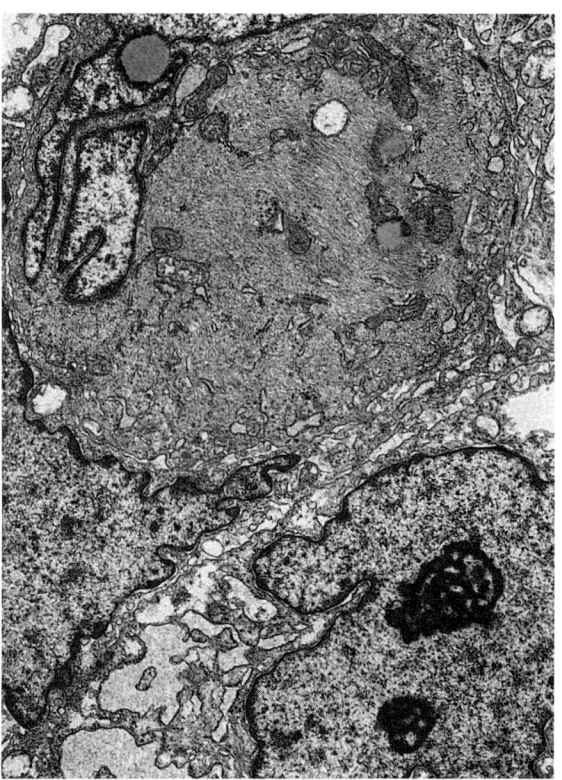

Figure 11-35
EPITHELIOID MPNST
A "rhabdoid-appearing" tumor cell with a peripherally displaced nucleus and cytoplasm distended with intermediate filaments, which were immunohistochemically shown to be vimentin (X8,700).

immunoreactivity and stain for *Ulex europaeus* lectin as well. In contrast to the *myxoid variant of malignant fibrous histiocytoma,* epithelioid MPNSTs lack the distinctive storiform pattern of spindle cells, intracellular mucin, and pleomorphic giant cells. While *extraskeletal myxoid chondrosarcoma* may also stain for S-100 protein and lacks keratin reactivity, it has not to date been reported to occur in nerve. Ultrastructurally, its cells lack a basement membrane and, in one third of cases, exhibit microtubules within cisternae of rough endoplasmic reticulum. The near total removal of mucin from epithelioid MPNST by hyaluronidase treatment also distinguishes it from the *myxoid variant of chondrosarcoma.*

Treatment and Prognosis. Most PNSTs containing epithelioid cells are regarded as clinically malignant. Their treatment is the same as for conventional MPNST. While earlier reports, based primarily upon deeply situated tumors, indicated a high mortality rate (102,104), a more

indolent behavior was noted in the series of Laskin et al. (103). Of their 16 superficial tumors, 2 recurred locally, 1 metastasized to surrounding soft tissue, and another to lung; there were no disease-related deaths in this group. Of the 10 deeply seated tumors, 1 recurred locally and 3 underwent distant metastasis; of the latter, all three patients died of tumor.

MPNST with Divergent Differentiation

Divergent differentiation in MPNST refers to the formation of neoplastic mesenchymal and epithelial elements, features unexpected in a nerve sheath tumor; this occurs in approximately 15 percent of MPNSTs (121), including ones post-irradiation (154). It is in part due to this differentiation that MPNSTs provide the most varied histology of any soft tissue neoplasm. The currently accepted explanation for divergent mesenchymal differentiation invokes the capacity of migrating neural crest cells to form not only melanocytes, ganglion cells, and Schwann cells, but to contribute to the formation of leptomeninges, bone, cartilage, and muscle of the head and face (123,128). Migrating neural crest tissue capable of such varied differentiation has been designated *"ectomesenchyme"* (123). The Schwann cell, the cell from which most MPNSTs are presumed to arise, retains this differentiating capacity, particularly in its neoplastic state. That the capacity for divergent differentiation may be a feature of neuroectoderm in general is suggested by the finding of skeletal muscle in leptomeninges (107), and by reports of myogenesis in glioma (145), medulloblastoma (142), intraocular malignant medulloepithelioma (155), and rarely in benign nerve sheath tumors (108). The occurrence of epithelial differentiation in PNSTs is less readily explainable.

MPNST with Mesenchymal Differentiation Malignant Triton Tumor

General Comments. Most of the heterologous mesenchymal elements reported to occur in MPNSTs are histologically malignant. Such sarcomatous components include rhabdomyosarcoma, chondrosarcoma, osteosarcoma, and, on rare occasion, angiosarcoma (121,134). Most frequent and extensively studied are MPNSTs showing skeletal muscle formation, a variant termed malignant "Triton" tumor. The designation was coined by Woodruff et al. (150,151) to recall the early studies of Pierre Masson, the first investigator to appreciate that rhabdomyosarcomatous elements may arise within a peripheral nerve tumor (131–133). Masson suggested that under the organizing influence of motor nerve fibers, neuroectodermal cells within neuromas may differentiate into muscle tissue. In support of this notion, he cited the experiments of Locatelli (129), who, by implantation of the sciatic nerve into soft tissue of the back, had induced the growth of supernumerary limbs in salamanders of the genus Triturus. The explanation has its problems, since it subsequently became apparent that in this model, limb regeneration is not dependent upon the presence of nervous tissue in the implant. Despite this interesting analogy, the currently accepted explanation for the occurrence of myogenic components in PNSTs is that striated muscle cells arise by metaplasia of neo-

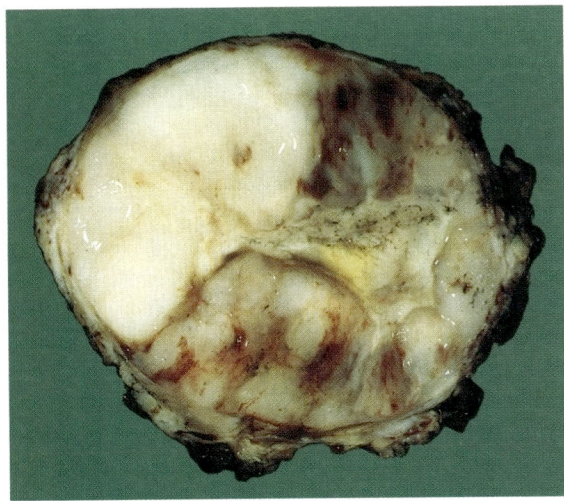

Figure 11-36
MPNST WITH DIVERGENT DIFFERENTIATION
On cut section, this malignant Triton tumor of flank is gray-tan and focally hemorrhagic. Divergent differentiation was not grossly apparent.

plastic Schwann cells. Recent confirmation of the capacity of MPNST cells to form striated muscle elements was provided by Nitikin et al. (137), who induced MPNSTs by transplacental exposure of BD1X rats to N-ethyl-N-nitrosourea. Marked by a mutant *neu* gene the cells were grown in monolayer culture and reimplanted subcutaneously into syngeneic animals. By immunohistochemical methods, myogenic differentiation was demonstrated in cells of the implant. We have not personally encountered a convincing example of "benign Triton tumor."

Clinical Features. In a review of the literature, Woodruff and Perino (153) identified 84 malignant Triton tumors. Patients ranged in age from newborn to 75 years (mean, 34 years), males and females being equally represented. Few arose in children. Most tumors arose in the head, neck, or thigh. Only 57 percent of patients had NF1 and four lesions were radiation induced. An additional postirradiation example was recently reported (154).

Gross Findings. Short of the finding of calcification (bone) or mucoid foci (glands), most MPNSTs with divergent differentiation grossly resemble conventional MPNST (fig. 11-36).

Histologic Findings. Although the rhabdomyoblasts of malignant Triton tumors vary considerably in histologic appearance (fig. 11-37),

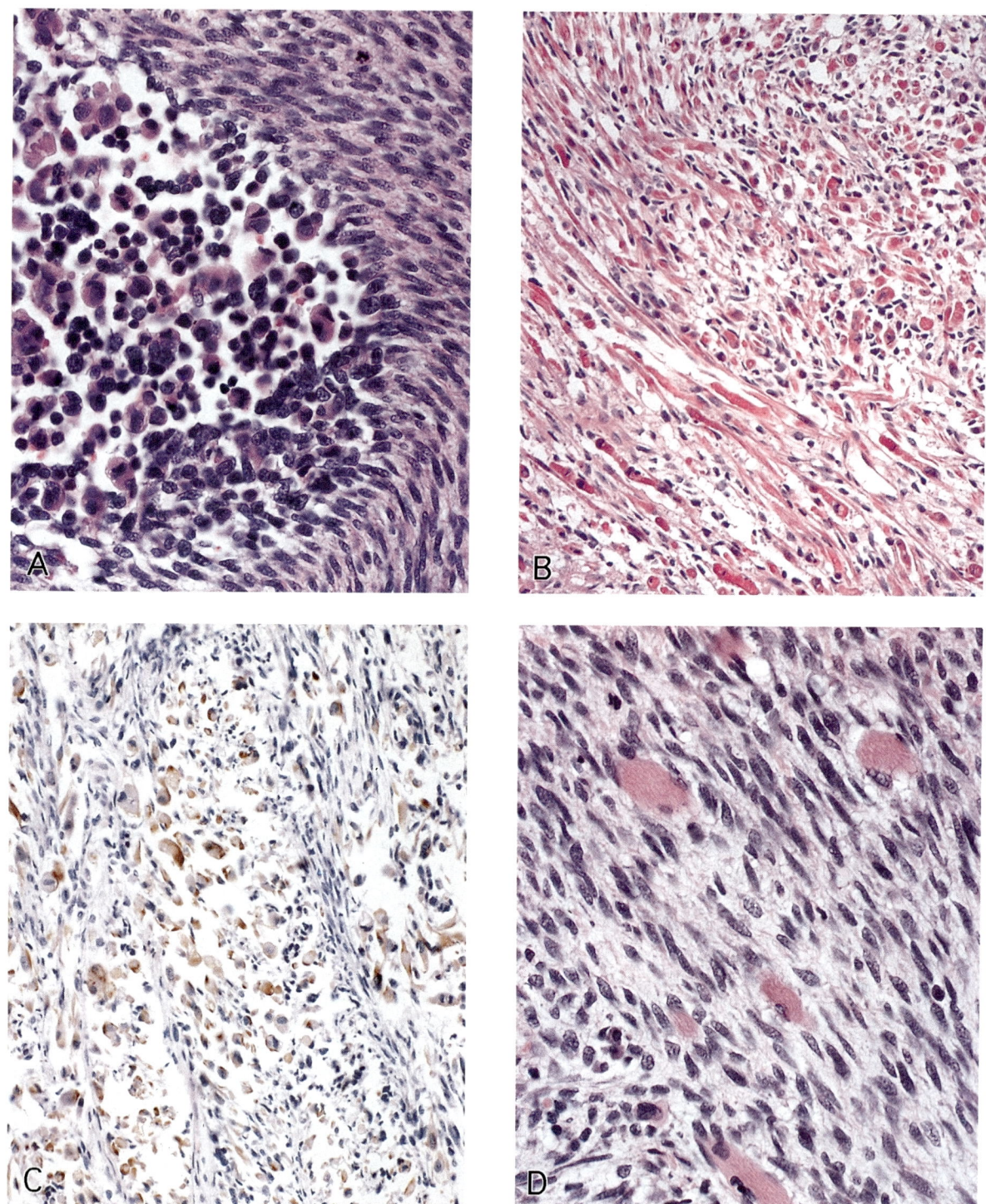

Figure 11-37
MPNST WITH RHABDOMYOBLASTIC DIFFERENTIATION

In malignant Triton tumors, the appearance of skeletal muscle elements varies. In addition to a spindle cell MPNST component, one may see clusters of rhabdomyoblasts resembling those of embryonal rhabdomyosarcoma (A). In a patient with NF1, both spindle- and strap-shaped rhabdomyoblasts are seen (B) in a tumor arising from a neurofibroma. The tumor showed pluridirectional differentiation. Muscle specific actin is a reliable marker of rhabdomyoblasts in MPNST (C). Residual normal muscle invaded by MPNST is characterized by geometric distribution of fibers and uniformity of cross striations (D).

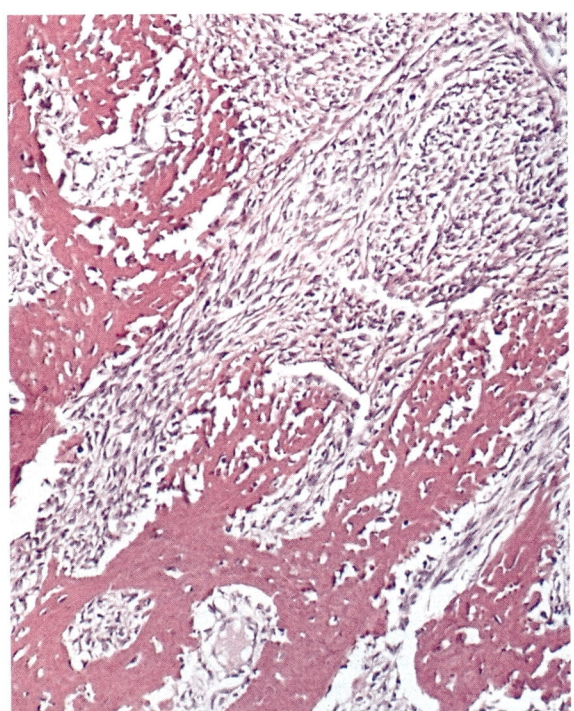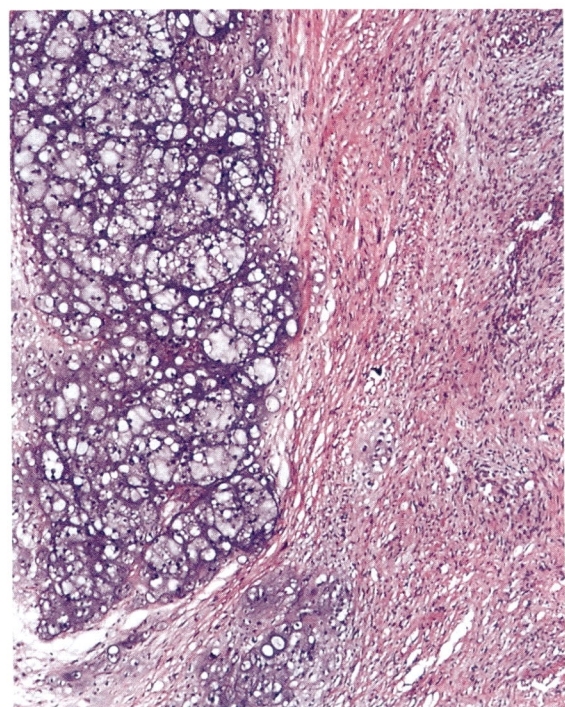

Figure 11-38
MPNST WITH SARCOMATOUS DIFFERENTIATION

An osteosarcomatous component may be seen in MPNST showing pluridirectional differentiation (left). A chondrosarcomatous component is less frequent. This femoral nerve tumor (right) invaded the underlying femoral bone and radiologically mimicked chondrosarcoma of the femur with soft tissue extension.

they resemble most closely the better differentiated cells of embryonal rhabdomyosarcoma in being round with central hyperchromatic nuclei and abundant, brightly eosinophilic cytoplasm (fig. 11-37A,B) (121,151,153). Strap-shaped myocytes are also commonly seen (fig. 11-37B). Although concentric perinuclear fibrils and cross striations are often evident on H&E stain and in phosphotungstic acid–hematoxylin (PTAH) preparations, even in their absence the myogenic nature of the cells can be confirmed by immunoreactivity for muscle markers (see below) (fig. 11-37C). The myoid cells often congregate about dilated blood vessels or lie interspersed among spindle cells which, based upon their immunoreactivity for S-100 protein, are presumed to be malignant nerve sheath cells (118). Normal muscle entrapped in MPNSTs is distinguished by its geometric fiber arrangement and by the uniform orientation of sarcomeres (fig. 11-37D). Approximately 15 percent of malignant Triton tumors contain additional mesenchymal (fig. 11-38) or even epithelial elements (fig. 11-39). Such tumors are referred to as showing "pluridirectional differentiation." As a rule, mesenchymal components are patently malignant, whereas epithelial ones are frequently benign.

Immunohistochemical and Ultrastructural Findings. The immunoprofile of the spindle cell component of MPNST with divergent differentiation is simply that of conventional MPNST. At least 50 percent of the tumors express S-100 protein. Although antibodies directed toward S-100 protein and Leu-7 are of diagnostic utility, S-100 protein staining may also be seen in embryonal rhabdomyosarcoma (114,135,143). Therefore, S-100 protein is not an absolutely reliable indicator of schwannian differentiation when faced with a myogenic tumor also exhibiting a spindle cell component. Rhabdomyoblastic differentiation in an MPNST is readily detected by the use of muscle specific antibodies such as desmin, muscle specific actin (HHF-35) (fig. 11-37C), alpha sarcomeric actin, and myogenin, as

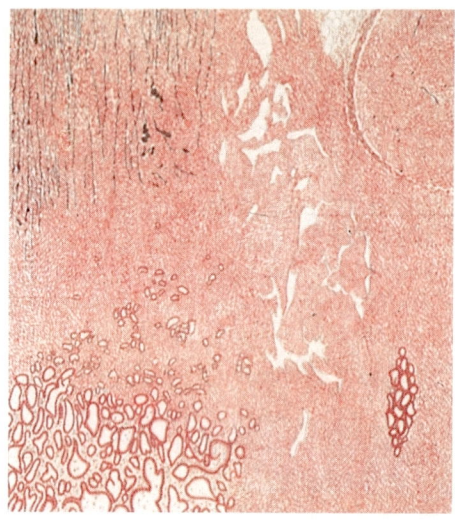

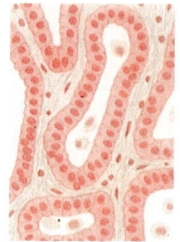 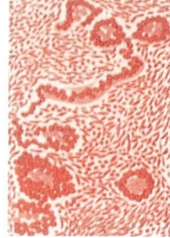

Figure 11-39
MPNST WITH EPITHELIAL DIFFERENTIATION
    Seen here is glandular differentiation as first depicted by Gàrre. With rare exception (see fig. 8-31), it occurs solely in malignant peripheral nerve sheath tumors. Reproduced from Garre C. Uber sekundar maligne Neurome. Beitr Z Klin Chir Z 1892;9:465-95.

well as by the ultrastructural finding of sarcomere formation (fig. 11-40) (111,118,121,126).

Differential Diagnosis. Rhabdomyosarcoma and leiomyosarcoma are the two tumors most likely to be misinterpreted as a malignant Triton tumor. This is especially true of *rhabdomyosarcoma of childhood* (153). As previously noted, such tumors have been reported to occasionally stain for S-100 protein (114,135,143). That a diagnosis of malignant Triton tumor cannot be reflexly made upon a positive S-100 protein reaction alone is underscored by the fact that leiomyosarcoma may also stain for this marker (112,144). It is precisely for this reason that this tumor may be mistaken for malignant Triton tumor. *Leiomyosarcoma* lacks typical rhabdomyosarcomatous features, such as round or strap cells with brightly eosinophilic cytoplasm, cytoplas-

mic cross striations, and immunoreactivity for myoglobin or alpha sarcomeric actin, and ultrastructurally has cytoplasmic arrays of actin filaments with interspersed fusiform densities.

Treatment and Prognosis. Patients with malignant Triton tumor have a poor prognosis. The treatment does not differ from that of conventional MPNST. In a survey of 67 cases, Brooks (110) noted local recurrence in 60 percent and metastases in 48 percent. Of the 84 cases reviewed by Woodruff and Perino (153), 63 percent of patients with available follow-up either died or were dying of tumor. Death usually occurred within 2 years of diagnosis. Patients with malignant Triton tumors may have a worse prognosis than those with conventional MPNSTs: the respective crude 2- and 5-year survival rates are 33 and 12 percent (111) compared to 57 and 39 percent (124).

PNST with Angiosarcoma

General Comments. Less common than malignant Triton tumors are PNSTs with angiosarcomatous elements. The neural component may be either histologically benign or malignant, and in most cases is thought to show angiosarcomatous differentation. A summary of the literature is presented in Table 11-2. There are also two reports of angiosarcoma arising within non-neoplastic peripheral nerve in patients without NF1 (109,117). Bricklin and Rushton (109) described an angiosarcoma originating from a sizable vein within the radial nerve of a 51-year-old man. We have reviewed microsections from this case. Since the vein was large and unassociated with nerve fibers, we consider the tumor to have its origin in epineurium. By definition we do not classify malignant tumors of epineurium as primary MPNSTs since they cannot be distinguished from tumors arising in connective tissue external to, but contiguous with, epineurium. The angiosarcoma reported by Conway and Smith (117) as involving the sciatic nerve of a 47-year-old man poses a greater nosologic challenge, since it is unclear whether the tumor arose from a benign schwannoma, de novo from normal nerve, or extrinsic to nerve (117). Although a focal proliferation of "schwannian cells" was noted, the authors concluded that this represented a reaction to the sarcoma. Individuals with NF1 occasionally develop angiosarcomas unrelated to nerve (136).

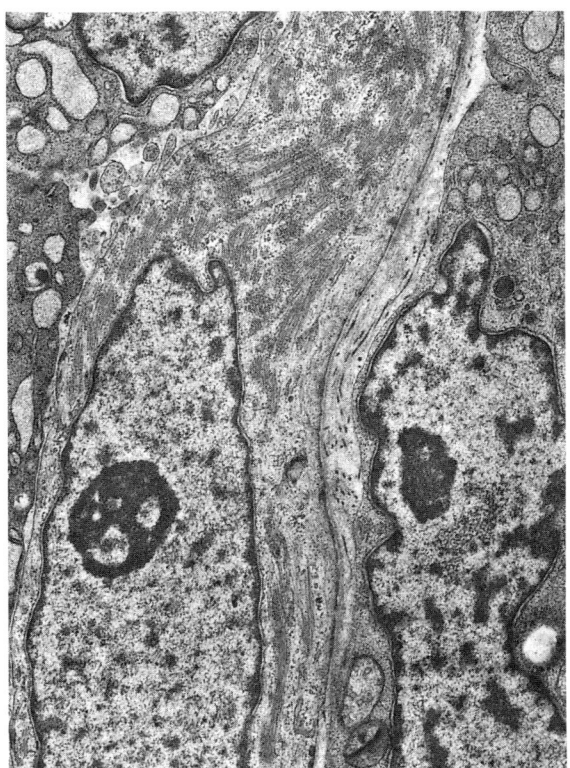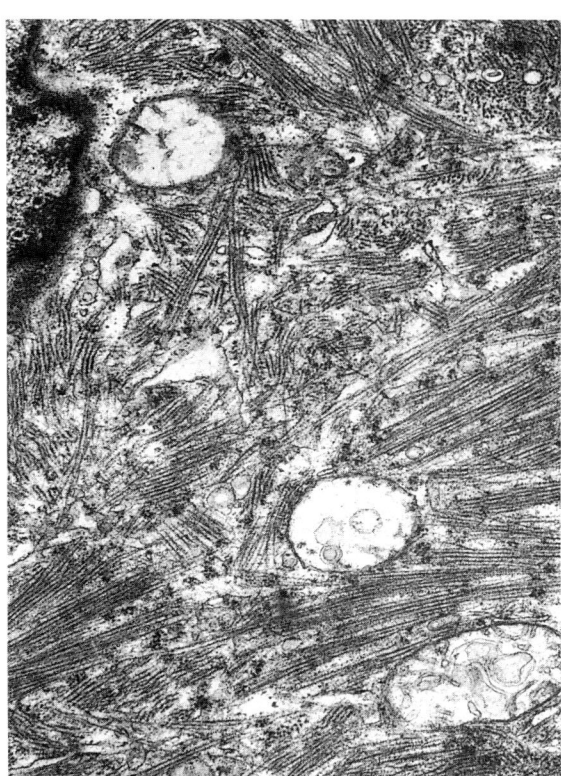

Figure 11-40
MPNST WITH RHABDOMYOBLASTIC
DIFFERENTIATION (MALIGNANT TRITON TUMOR)
Top: Portion of a neoplastic rhabdomyoblast illustrating numerous arrays of rudimentary sarcomeres (X12,300).
Bottom: Higher magnification. Stacks of 15-nm myosin filaments are evident (X28,100).

The first well-documented MPNST with angiosarcoma was that of Russell and Rubinstein (141) who described a 35-year-old man with NF1 and a femoral nerve MPNST, the peritoneal and omental metastases of which contained angiosarcoma. There are now 14 reported cases of angiosarcoma arising in PNSTs (Table 11-2) (113,115,121,127,130,134,139,141,146).

Clinical Features. Of the 14 cases of angiosarcoma arising in PNST, 13 occurred in patients with NF1. Males were primarily affected (10 to 3) (Table 11-2). Patient ages ranged from 14 to 65 years (mean, 23 years), the low mean age a reflection of the NF1 association. While most (approximately 70 percent) angiosarcomas occurring in the setting of NF1 arose in MPNSTs (113,121, 127,130,142), nearly 30 percent originated in neurofibromas (115,134,139). A neurofibromatous component was also identified in 5 of 9 MPNSTs; 6 of the 9 associated neurofibromas were of plexi-

form type (115,127,134,139). In addition to the 13 above-noted NF1-associated cases, one angiosarcoma reportedly arose in a schwannoma (146). The 14 tumors were from disparate sites, including the neck, back, upper and lower extremities, buttock, retroperitoneum, and liver. Nerves of origin were identified in 7 (50 percent). The tumors ranged from microscopic to 30 cm (mean, 10 cm).

Histologic Findings. In only 6 of the 14 reported cases was the extent of the angiosarcomatous involvement known. In one instance (121) it comprised several low-power microscopic fields within an MPNST, whereas in another (113) it represented approximately 5 percent of a 6-cm MPNST. In the remaining 4 cases it was referred to as extensive or large (115,127,134,146). Histologically, in all but the case of Trassard et al. (146) which consisted of epithelioid cells disposed in sheets and alveoli (fig. 11-41), the angiosarcoma element consisted of irregular anastomosing

Table 11-2

PERIPHERAL NERVE SHEATH TUMORS WITH ANGIOSARCOMA COMPONENT*: LITERATURE SUMMARY

Author (Ref.)	Age/ Sex	NF1	Site/Size	Assoc. NF	Assoc. MPNST	Treatment	Local Recurrence or Metastasis	Follow-up
Rubinstein (141)	35 M	+	Retroperitoneal metastasis from MPNST** of the femoral nerve	+	+	Unknown	Angiosarcoma in omental and pertioneal metastases, not in the primary tumor	DOD[†], 2 mos.
Macaulay (130)	18 M	+	Rt. axilla (radial nerve;); 15 x 15 x 5 cm	−	+	Radiation	Lung and brain metastases of angiosarcoma; metastatic adrenal MPNST and angiosarcoma	DOD, 2 mos
Chaudhuri et al. (115)	14 M	+	Lt. neck (brachial and cervical plexuses); 8 x 4.5 x 2 cm	+ (plexiform)	−	Surgical resection	Unknown	None
Prasad (139)	6 M	+	—	+	−	Unknown	Unknown	Unknown
Ducatman, et al. (121)	12 F	+	Retroperitoneum	Unknown	+	Radical excision	Recurred at 2 mos. No angiosarcoma in recurrence	DOD, 15 mos.
Lederman et al. (127)	21 M	+	Liver; Large portion of 30 cm tumor	+ (plexiform)	+	Hepatic artery embolization	Lung metastases of angiosarcoma	DOD
Brown, et al. (113)	20 M	+	Rt. neck; 6 cm (angiosarcoma was <5% of tumor)	Unknown	+	En bloc surgical resection	Unknown	None
Meis-Kindblom et al. (134)	14 M	+	Brachial plexus; 8 cm	+ (plexiform)	−	Surgery, CTX[†], XRT	Lung and bone metastases	DOD, 6 mos.
"	55 M	+	Rt. lateral neck; 5 cm	+ (previously excised)	+	Surgery, CTX, XRT	Local recurrence 7 mos. Bone metastases	DOD, 2 yrs.
"	33 F	+	Back; "Large"	+	+	Surgery	Local recurrence at 3 mos. Widespread metastases	DOD, 1 yr.
"	18 M	+	Lt. thigh - popliteal region; 10 cm	+ (plexiform)	+	Surgery (AKA), CTX, XRT	Brain metastases 1 yr.	DOD, 2 yrs.
"	22 F	+	Lt. forearm (ulnar n.); 3.5 cm	+ (plexiform)	−	Surgery, radical resection	Brain metastases 4 mos.	DOD, 4 mos.
"	21 M	+	Rt. buttock (sciatic and femoral nerve); 16 cm	+ (plexiform)	+	Surgery (hemipelvectomy)	Lung metastases 4 mos.	DOD, 15 mos.
Trassard et al. (146)	65 M	−	Lt. thigh (tibial division of sciatic nerve); 6 x 3.5 cm	− (schwannoma)	−	Surgery (total resection with partial n. sacrifice)	None	NED, 36 mos.

*Modified from table by Meis-Kindblom et al. (personal communication).

**Primary tumor with chondrosarcomatous differentiation but no angiosarcoma.

[†]CTX, chemotherapy; XRT, radiation therapy; DOD, dead of disease; NED, no evidence of disease: AKA, above knee amputation.

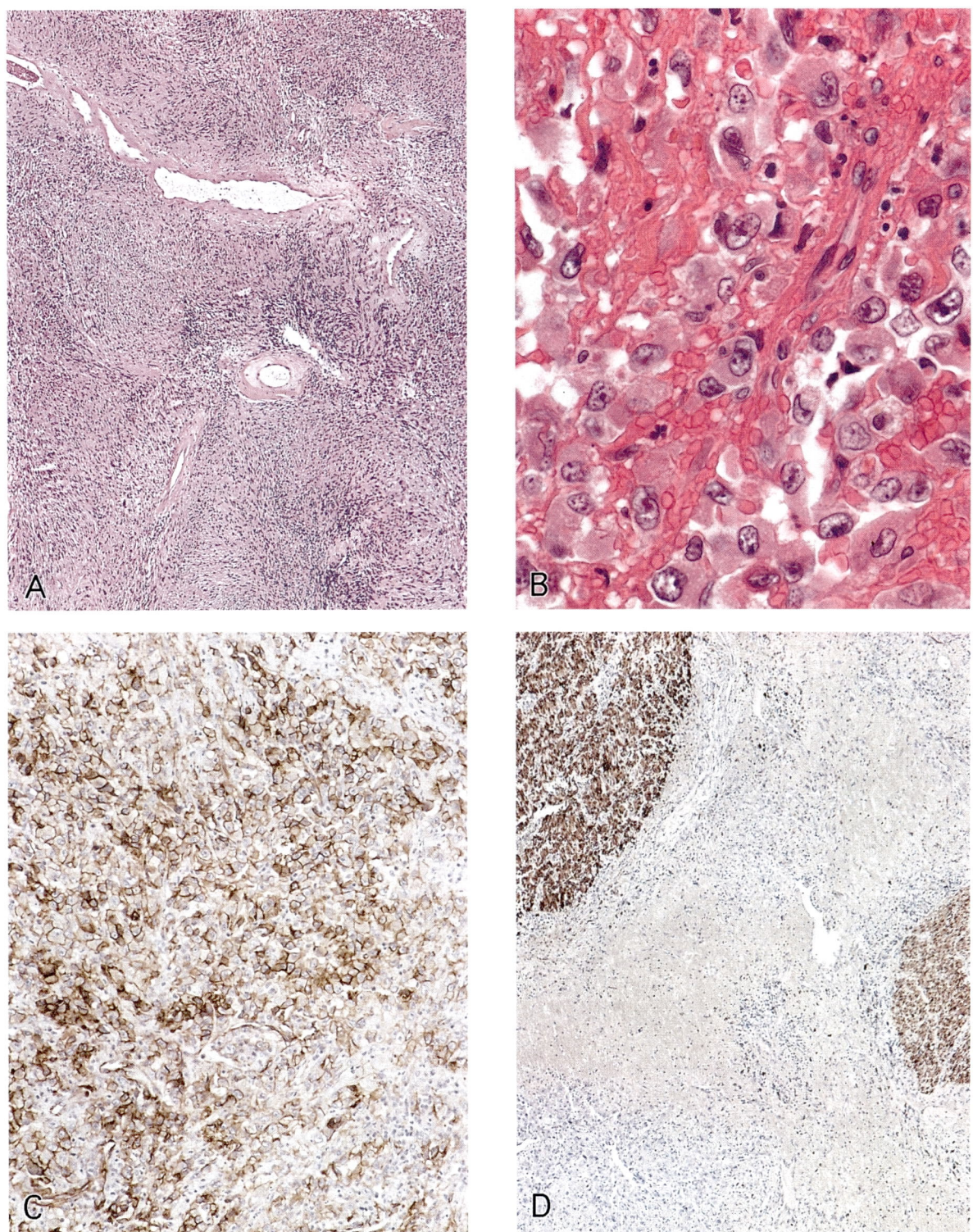

Figure 11-41
ANGIOSARCOMA ARISING IN SCHWANNOMA
Angiosarcomatous differentiation occurs in both benign and malignant PNSTs. This example arose in a benign schwannoma (A). The angiosarcoma was epithelioid (B), showed immunoreactivity for CD31 (C), and was distinct from the S-100 protein-positive schwannoma element (D). (Courtesy of Dr. J. M. Coindre, Bordeaux, France.)

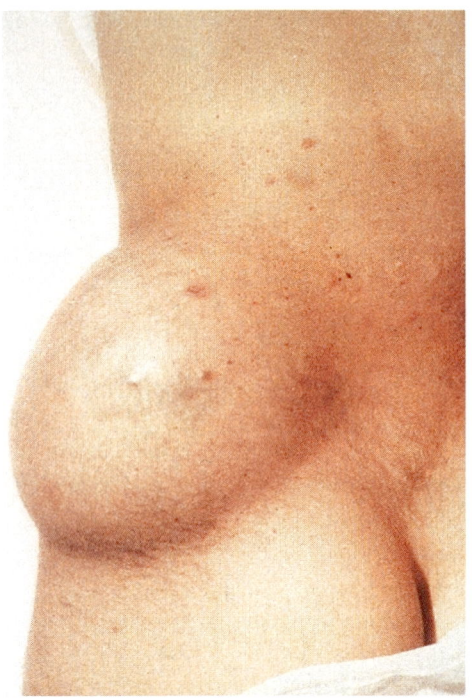

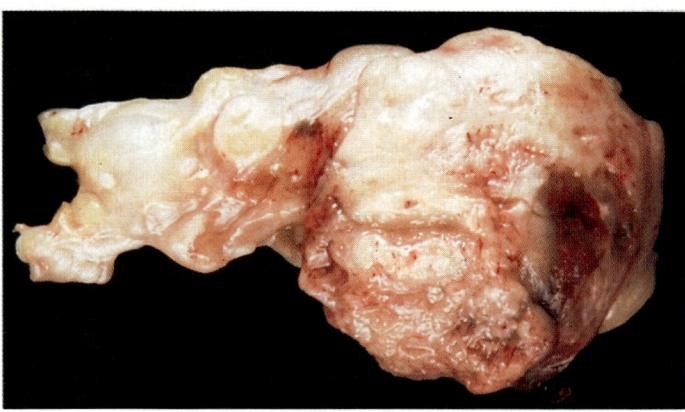

Figure 11-42
MPNST WITH EPITHELIAL DIFFERENTIATION
This MPNST of the flank occurred in an adult female with NF1. Note the large café au lait spot superior to the tumor (left). The lesion arose within the substance of a plexiform neurofibroma (above).

vascular spaces lined by flattened or plump cells with hyperchromatic nuclei. Except in one case (127), immunohistochemistry demonstrated reactivity for one or more endothelial cell markers including factor VIII-related antigen, CD31, CD34, BNH 9, or *Ulex europaeus* lectin (fig. 11-41C) (113,134). In no case did angiosarcomatous elements express S-100 protein (fig. 11-41B) (127,134,146).

Treatment and Prognosis. Although the clinical course of MPNST with angiosarcomatous differentiation is even more aggressive than that of malignant Triton tumor, the treatment is that of conventional MPNST. All but 1 (146) of 11 patients with available follow-up died of tumor; 3 developed local recurrences and 9 had distant metastases. In decreasing order of frequency, metastatic sites included lung and brain, bone, peritoneum, omentum, and adrenal gland. Survival after diagnosis ranged from 2 months to 2 years.

MPNST with Glandular Differentiation

It was Garre (122) who over a century ago first described glandular differentiation in MPNST (fig. 11-39). In an analysis of the literature, Woodruff (150a) as well as Woodruff and Christensen (152) found that 96 percent of the 25 reported glandular PNSTs had histologically malignant spindle cell components. The authors concluded that the several reports of benign glandular schwannoma previously published described conventional schwannomas with entrapped sweat glands. One case of multifocal glandular MPNST has been reported (125). The present overview is based upon these reports.

Clinical Features. Among patients with glandular MPNSTs, males and females are affected with equal frequency. They range in age from 19 months to 68 years (mean, 29 years), with a peak incidence in the fourth decade. Seventy-five percent of patients have NF1. The thigh and retroperitoneum are the most frequently involved sites, with a mean tumor size of 10 cm (fig. 11-42, left).

Gross and Microscopic Findings. In all respects, glandular MPNSTs grossly resemble their conventional counterpart (fig. 11-42, above). With the exception of one tumor in which cysts were apparent on sonogram and gross inspection, the glandular component is evident only at the microscopic level. Distributed singly or in small groups, glands often appear as islands within a background of spindle cells (fig. 11-43A). In all but a few cases, the glandular epithelium appears cytologically benign. Most glands consist

Table 11-3

GLANDULAR MPNST VERSUS BIPHASIC SYNOVIAL SARCOMA: DIFFERENTIAL DIAGNOSIS

	Glandular MPNST	Biphasic Synovial Sarcoma
Evidence of neurofibroma or origin from a nerve	Often	No
Cytologic resemblance between glandular and nonglandular cells	No	Yes
Goblet cells in glands	50%	No
Neuroendocrine cell differentiation (chromogranin staining)	91%	No
Cytokeratin	Usually present and only in glands; CK20 positive, CK7 negative	Present in glandular and often nonglandular cells; CK7 positive, CK20 negative
EMA*	In glandular cells in 67%; not present in nonglandular cells	Often present in both glandular and nonglandular cells
CEA*	Often present in glands	Infrequently present in glands

*EMA, epithelial membrane antigen; CEA, carcinoembryonic antigen.

of columnar, goblet, clear, or flattened cells. Frequently, mucin distends glandular lumens and is present within the cytoplasm of surrounding goblet cells (fig. 11-43B). In addition, extravasated mucin pools are occasionally seen within the neoplastic spindle cell stroma. Both intracellular and luminal mucin stains strongly with the PAS, Mayer's mucicarmine, and Alcian blue methods. Whereas frank squamous differentiation is uncommon (fig. 11-43C), neuroendocrine cells are frequently seen (116,148), either as single, basally situated cells in mucous glands or as the sole constituent of epithelial nests (fig. 11-43D). One fourth of malignant glandular schwannomas exhibit not only a conventional MPNST component but a rhabdomyosarcomatous component as well; such tumors are termed "pluridirectional MPNST" (fig. 11-43F) (118,120,140,148,149,152).

Immunohistochemical Findings. The glandular epithelium of these unusual tumors routinely stains for cytokeratin, EMA, and carcinoembryonic antigen (116,152). A recent study found CK20 reactivity but lack of CK7 staining (70a). In 90 percent of cases appropriately stained, the glands contain basally situated, chromogranin-positive neuroendocrine cells (fig. 11-43E). Solid clusters of neuroendocrine cells may also be seen. Such cells are frequently somatostatin- or serotonin-immunoreactive (116,148,152). The neoplastic spindle cell component shows the same immunoprofile as does conventional MPNST.

Ultrastructural Findings. Ultrastructural studies (116,119,147,148) have generally shown the glands of glandular MPNST to be of the intestinal type, featuring microvilli with a glycocalyx and core microfilaments forming rootlets. Goblet cells contain mucin droplets that vary in morphology. Neuroendocrine cells with dense core granules are also a common feature.

Differential Diagnosis. The only soft tissue tumor with which glandular MPNST is likely to be confused is *biphasic synovial sarcoma*. As indicated in Table 11-3, the distinction rests in large part upon noting the presence or absence of goblet and neuroendocrine cells as well as the differing patterns of cytokeratin and carcinoembryonic antigen expression. In approximately 20 percent of cases the spindle cell component of synovial sarcoma is immunoreactive for S-100 protein (138). As a result, this marker cannot be considered a reliable determinant for differentiating these two tumors. Their distinction is important because of the more favorable prognosis of patients with synovial sarcoma. To date, immature teratoma has not been reported to arise in nerve; in any case, the epithelial elements of glandular MPNST do not resemble immature endoderm.

Treatment and Prognosis. The treatment of patients with MPNSTs showing divergent differentiation is that of conventional MPNST. Most cases are associated with a fatal outcome. Woodruff and Christensen (152) found that 79

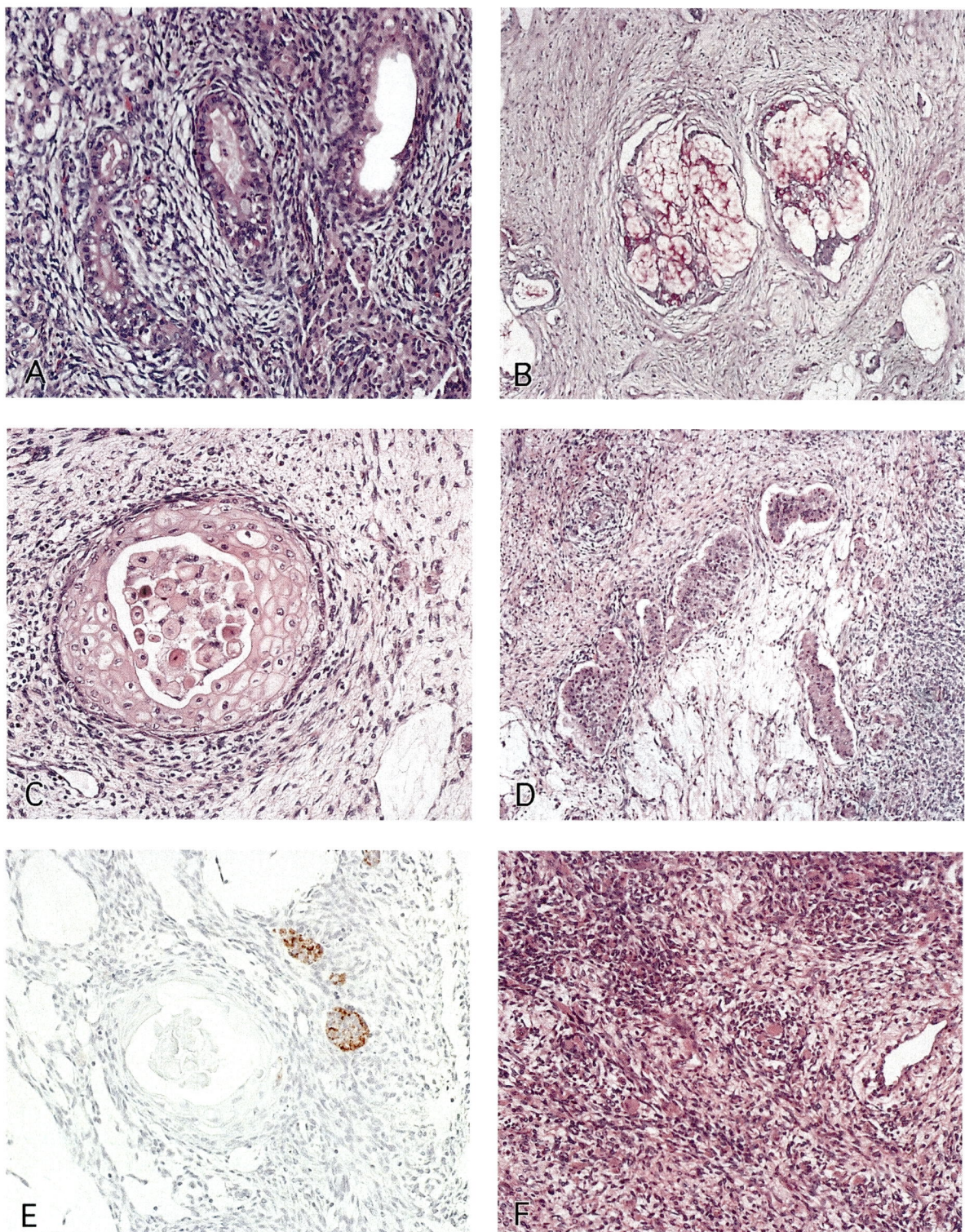

Figure 11-43
MPNST WITH EPITHELIAL DIFFERENTIATION
This remarkably diverse tumor featured glands (A) with mucin production (B), and a squamous epithelium (C), neuroendocrine cells (D) exhibiting chromogranin positivity (E), and a minor skeletal muscle component (F).

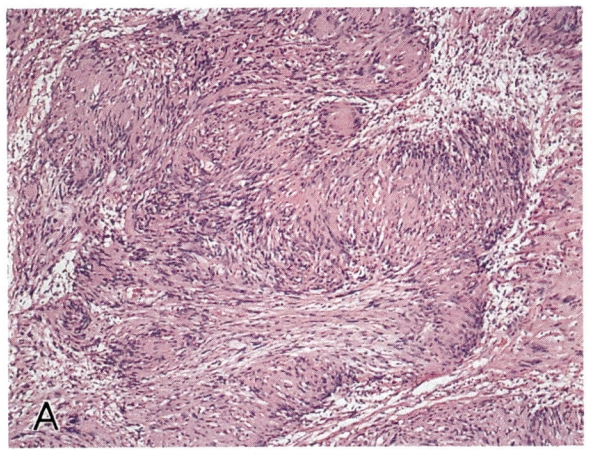

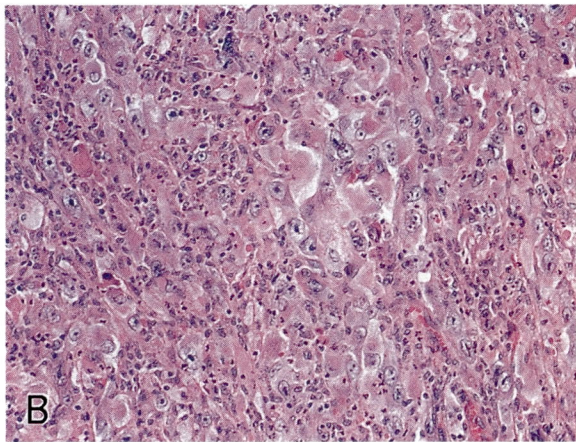

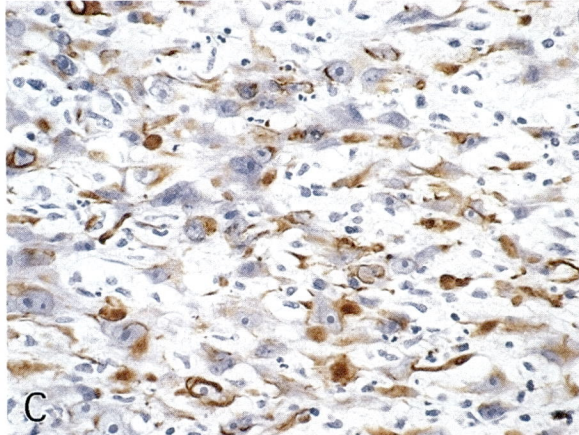

Figure 11-44
MPNST EX SCHWANNOMA
This example represented a dumbbell tumor with pelvic and intrasacral components occurring in a 31-year-old male with an 8-month history of pain. The underlying typical schwannoma showed Verocay body formation (A). Most of the lesion was composed of epithelioid MPNST (B). In addition to S-100 protein staining, the tumor also showed cytokeratin (CAM 5.2) reactivity (C). For further details, see case 2 in Woodruff et al. (163).

percent of patients with glandular MPNST died of tumor; mean survival was only 2 years.

Schwannoma with Transformation to MPNST (MPNST ex Schwannoma)

General Comments. An exceedingly rare form of MPNST is that arising in transition from schwannoma (neurilemoma). In a 1994 review of purported examples, Woodruff and co-workers found only nine acceptable cases (156–160,162–164). Substantial clinical and morphologic differences exist between these rare lesions and conventional MPNST. These include lack of an association with NF1, occurrence in an older age group, a long history of an antecedent mass (often of many years), and a predominance of malignant epithelioid or small cells within the transformed component.

Clinical Features. The nine patients ranged in age from 31 to 75 years; their mean age of 56

years exceeded by 20 years that of patients with conventional MPNST. Five patients were male and three were female; the gender of one patient was unstated. No patient had NF1. In one instance, the tumor may have been radiation induced. The lesions showed no preferential site of involvement. In four cases, the tumor was stated to have arisen in a mass that had been present for several years.

Gross and Microscopic Findings. Data regarding tumor size was available in eight cases; six lesions exceeded 5 cm in greatest dimension. One tumor was dumbbell shaped, one was multinodular, and two were bilobed. Encapsulation was mentioned in four cases; one tumor was largely cystic. When carefully examined, tan-brown, sometimes myxoid tissue alternated with or abutted cheesy or solid, gray-white tissue.

Histologically, the underlying tumors in the nine above-noted cases were classic schwannomas (figs. 11-44A, 11-45A). Antoni A and B

Table 11-4

MPNST EX SCHWANNOMA: HISTOLOGIC AND IMMUNOCYTOCHEMICAL FEATURES

Author, Year (Reference)	Histology		Immunohistochemical Findings	
	Schwannoma Type	Malignant Component	Benign Component	Malignant Component
Fowler, 1955 (157)	Conventional	Epithelioid	ND*	ND
Carstens and Schrodt, 1969 (156)	Conventional**	Round neuroepithelial cells	S-100 protein + [‡]	S-100 protein − [‡]
Hanada et al., 1982 (159)	Conventional**	Round and elongated neuroepithelial cells	S-100 protein + [‡]	S-100 protein + [‡]
Yousem et al., 1985 (164)	Conventional**	Epithelioid	S-100 protein +, keratin −, CEA −, Leu-7 − [‡]	S-100 protein +, keratin −, CEA −, Leu-7 − [‡]
Franks, 1985 (158)	Conventional	Epithelioid	S-100 protein +	S-100 protein −
Rasbridge et al., 1989 (162)	Conventional**	Epithelioid	S-100 protein +, keratin −, CEA −, MCA − [§]	S-100 protein +, keratin +, CEA- MCA − [§]
Laskin et al., 1991 (160)	Conventional	Epithelioid cells (with some stromal mucin [†,§])	S-100 protein +	S-100 protein, UK
Woodruff et al., 1994 (163)	Plexiform**	Epithelioid	ND	ND
Woodruff et al., 1994 (163)	Conventional**	Epithelioid	S-100 protein +, keratin −, CEA −, Leu-7−, desmin−, MCA−, SMA −	S-100 protein +, keratin+, CEA−, Leu-7−, desmin−, MCA−, SMA−
Nayler et al., 1996 (161)	Conventional	Epithelioid cells	S-100 protein +, cytokeratin −, EMA −	S-100 protein +, cytokeratin −, EMA −

*MCA, muscle common actin; SMA, smooth muscle actin; CEA, carcinoembryonic antigen; EMA, epithelial membrane antigen; ND, not done; UK, unknown.
**Verocay bodies present.
[†] Not indicated whether intracellular mucin present or absent.
[‡] Additional immunostaining performed in authors' laboratories.
[§] Additional information obtained subsequent to original report.

areas were present in all instances and Verocay bodies in six. In seven tumors, the malignant component was purely epithelioid, consisting of round, polygonal, or oblong cells the nuclei of which often featured prominent nucleoli (Table 11-4; fig. 11-44B). Cytoplasm was uniformly eosinophilic and dense. In two of the cases, the MPNST appeared to arise in transition from Antoni A tissue. Recently, Nayler (161) reported the same finding in a 2-cm schwannoma showing a microscopic focus of malignant transformation. Small cells resembling those of primitive neuroectodermal tumor (PNET) comprised the malignant element in the remaining two tumors (fig. 11-45B). Necrosis was evident in five cases.

Immunohistochemical Findings. Immunostains, performed in six instances (Table 11-4), showed reactivity for S-100 protein in the benign component of all lesions, as well as in the malignant element in four of six tumors. The epithelioid component of two tumors expressed keratin immunoreactivity (fig. 11-44C), a finding suggesting epithelial differentiation.

Ultrastructural Findings. We have had the opportunity to retrospectively examine one reported case (156). The benign component exhibited the classic features of schwannoma, whereas the malignant small cell element lacked specific differentiation (fig. 11-46).

Treatment and Prognosis. Based upon the behavior of this rare variant, treatment would appear to be that of conventional MPNST. The clinical outcome is poor. Of the eight patients for whom follow-up was available, four died with metastases and one due to aggressive local tumor growth. The preferred site for metastasis was the lung.

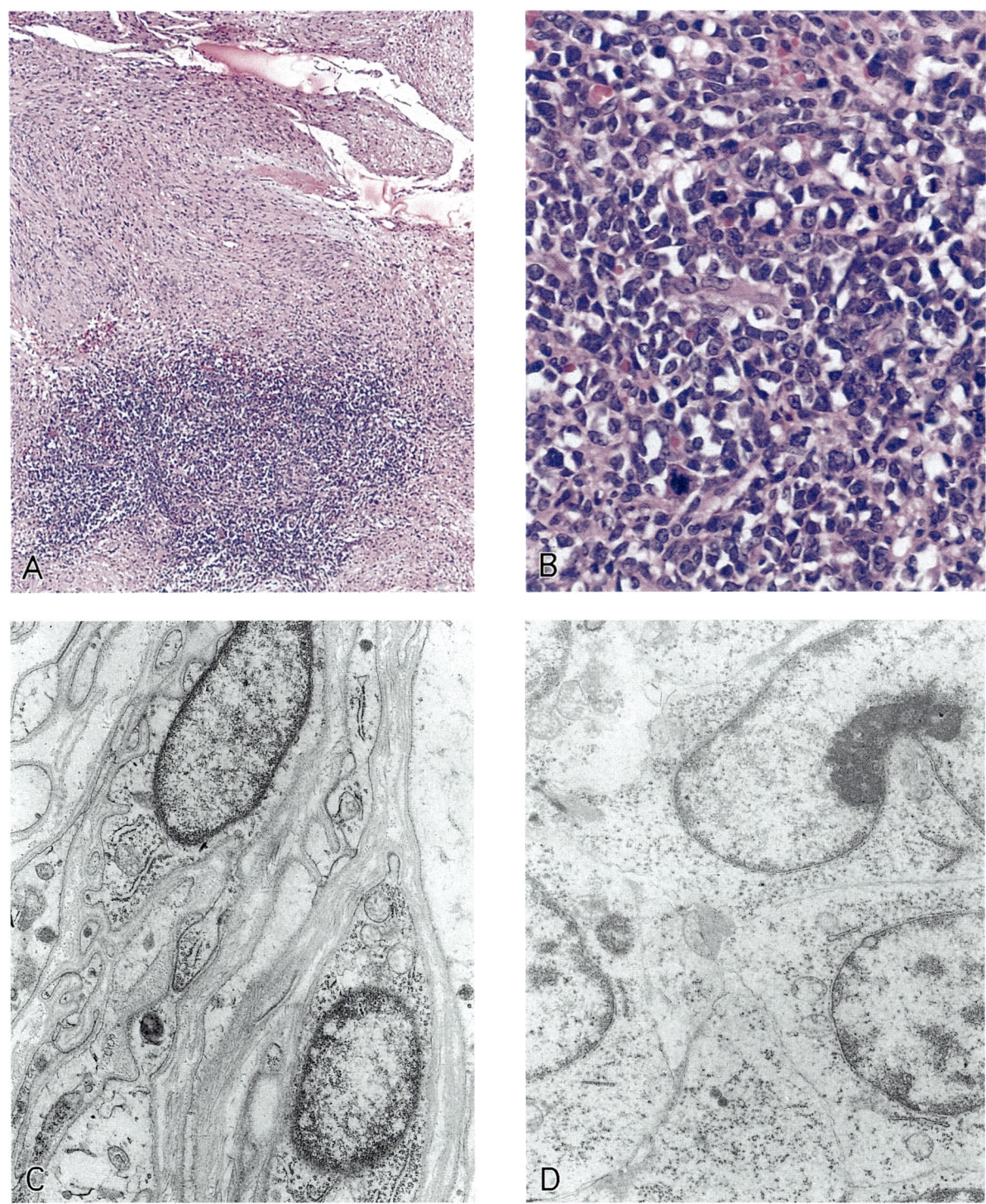

Figure 11-45
MPNST EX SCHWANNOMA

This 2.5-cm example arose at the base of the thumb in a 93-year-old female and had been present for many years. The underlying tumor was otherwise a typical schwannoma. The MPNST was a focal microscopic finding (A) and was a small cell neoplasm (B) lacking S-100 protein immunoreactivity. Although the underlying schwannoma was fully differentiated (C), electron microscopy showed the small cell component to lack specific differentiation (D) (X15,750). For clinical details see reference 163. (Courtesy of Dr. P. Carstens, Louisville, Kentucky.)

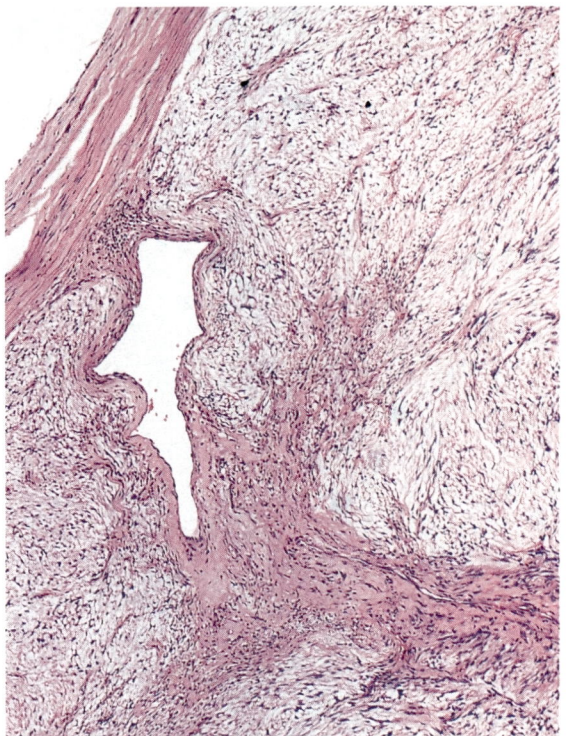 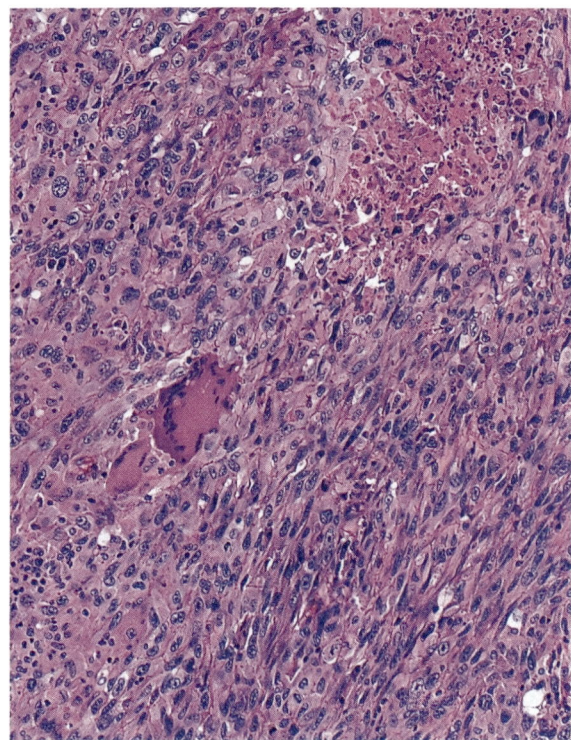

Figure 11-46
MPNST EX SCHWANNOMA
This tumor of the left leg in a 30-year-old male showed both schwannoma (left) and MPNST (right) components. The latter metastasized to inguinal lymph nodes. (Courtesy of Dr. A. Tsutsumi, Osaka, Japan.)

MPNST Arising in Association with Ganglioneuroma, Ganglioneuroblastoma, or Pheochromocytoma

MPNST ex Ganglioneuroma or Ganglioneuroblastoma

General Comments. Both ganglioneuromas and ganglioneuroblastomas contain Schwann cells which ensheath the numerous axonal processes of their ganglionic cells (176). Schwann cells contribute significantly to the bulk of both tumors and rarely serve as the source of an MPNST.

There are two situations in which MPNSTs have been reported to occur in association with ganglioneuromatous or ganglioneuroblastomatous tissue. One is when, in pure form, such tumors undergo transformation to MPNST, the other when a ganglioneuromatous portion of an ectomesenchymoma (see below) does the same.

Evidence for the development of MPNST in the latter setting is less than convincing.

MPNST developing in ganglioneuroma or ganglioneuroblastoma was first described in detail in 1984 (172,176). There are now eight known cases (Table 11-5) which fall into two clinicopathologic groups. The first consists of three infants with presumed radiation-induced MPNST (figs. 11-47, 11-48)(172,176). At initial presentation, they were 21 months of age or younger. Each had an intra-abdominal neuroblastoma or ganglioneuroblastoma which was then treated with radiation. One patient was subsequently found to have a skull metastasis histologically resembling ganglioneuroma; this also was irradiated (fig. 11-47)(176). In all three cases, after a postirradiation interval of years (7, 17, and 19 years), a high-grade malignant spindle cell tumor consistent with MPNST was found in a ganglioneuroma within the treatment

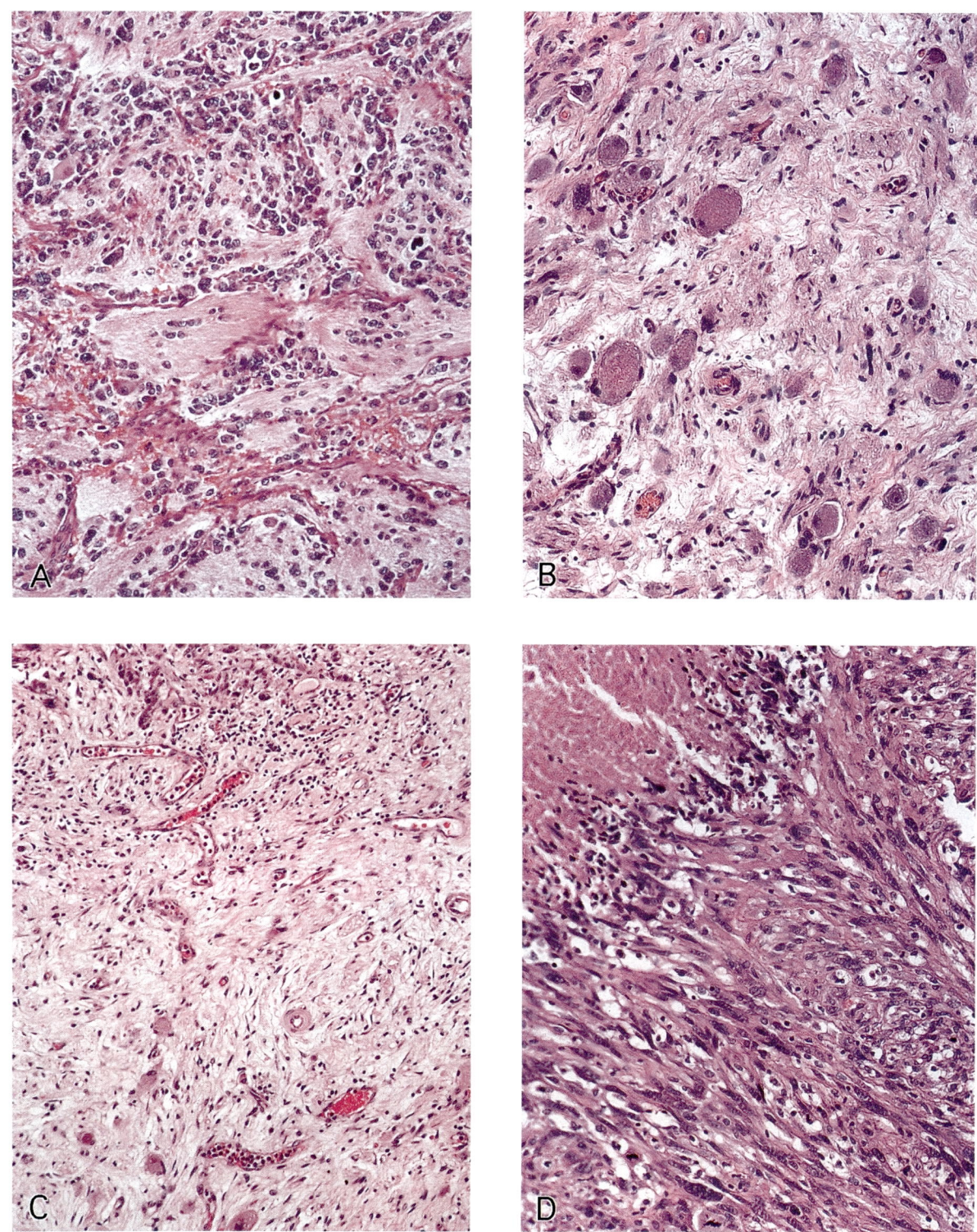

Figure 11-47
MPNST EX GANGLIONEUROMA

The primary tumor, an adrenal ganglioneuroblastoma (A) metastasized to the skull and, upon skull biopsy, was found to have matured to ganglioneuroma (B,C). After local radiotherapy, the skull lesion underwent transformation to MPNST (D). For clinical details see Table 11-5, Ricci et al. (12), case 2.

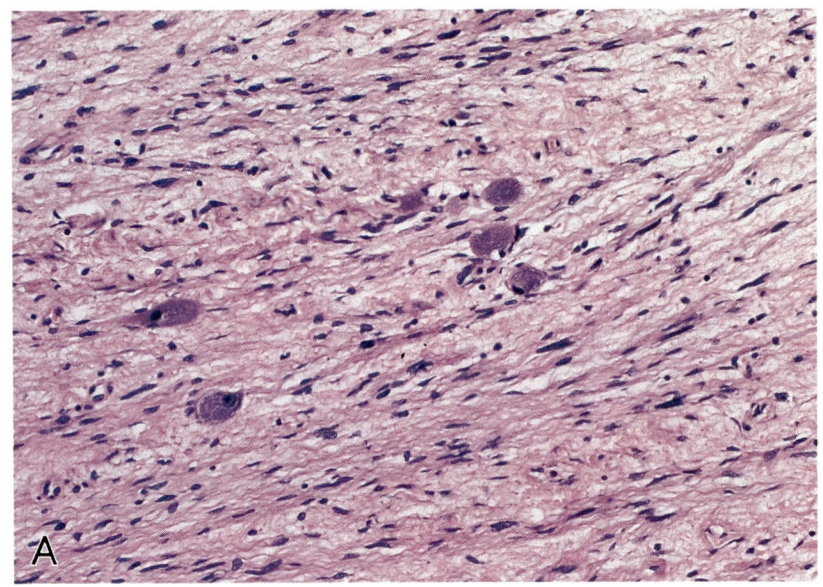

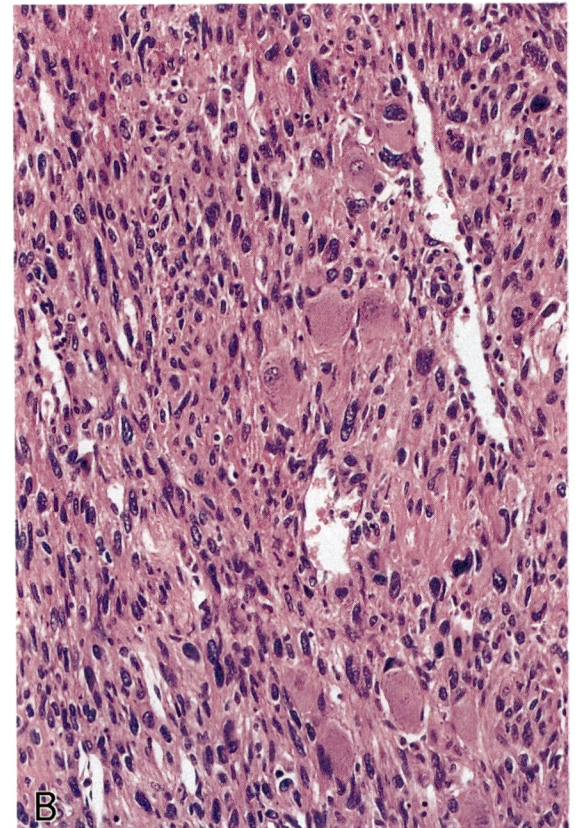
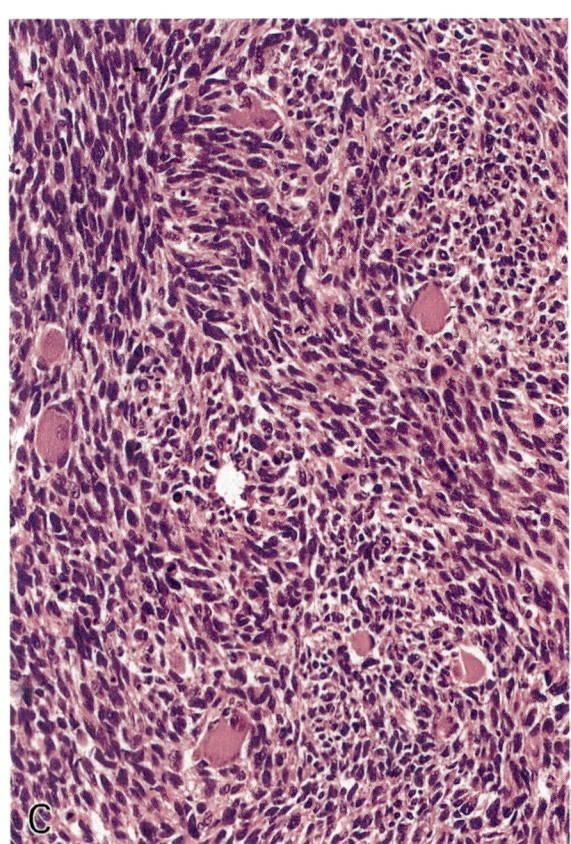

Figure 11-48
MPNST EX GANGLIONEUROMA

The primary tumor, an adrenal ganglioneuroma, underwent focal transformation to MPNST (A). Note the abrupt interface of the ganglioneuroma with the MPNST (B). The latter was a high-grade lesion (C). For clinical details see Table 11-5, Chandrasoma (2). (Courtesy of Dr. P. Chandrasoma, Los Angeles, CA.)

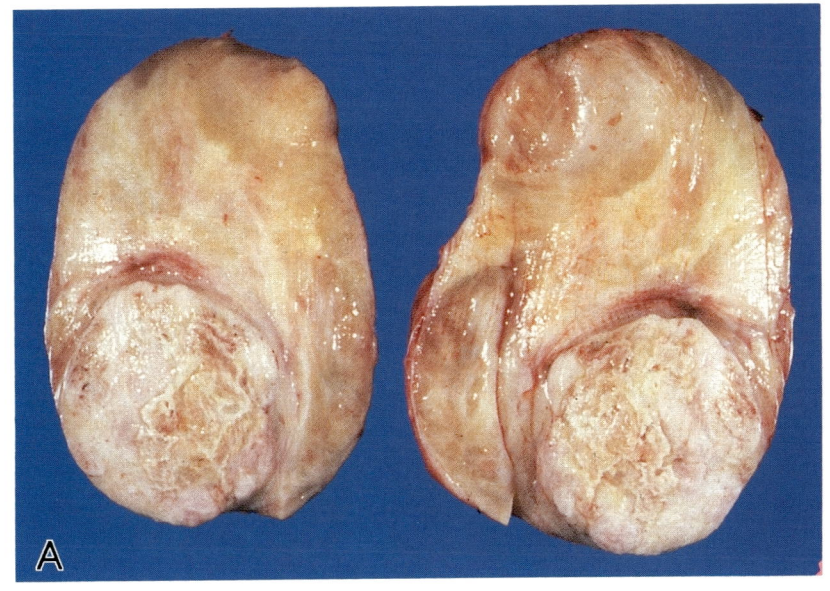

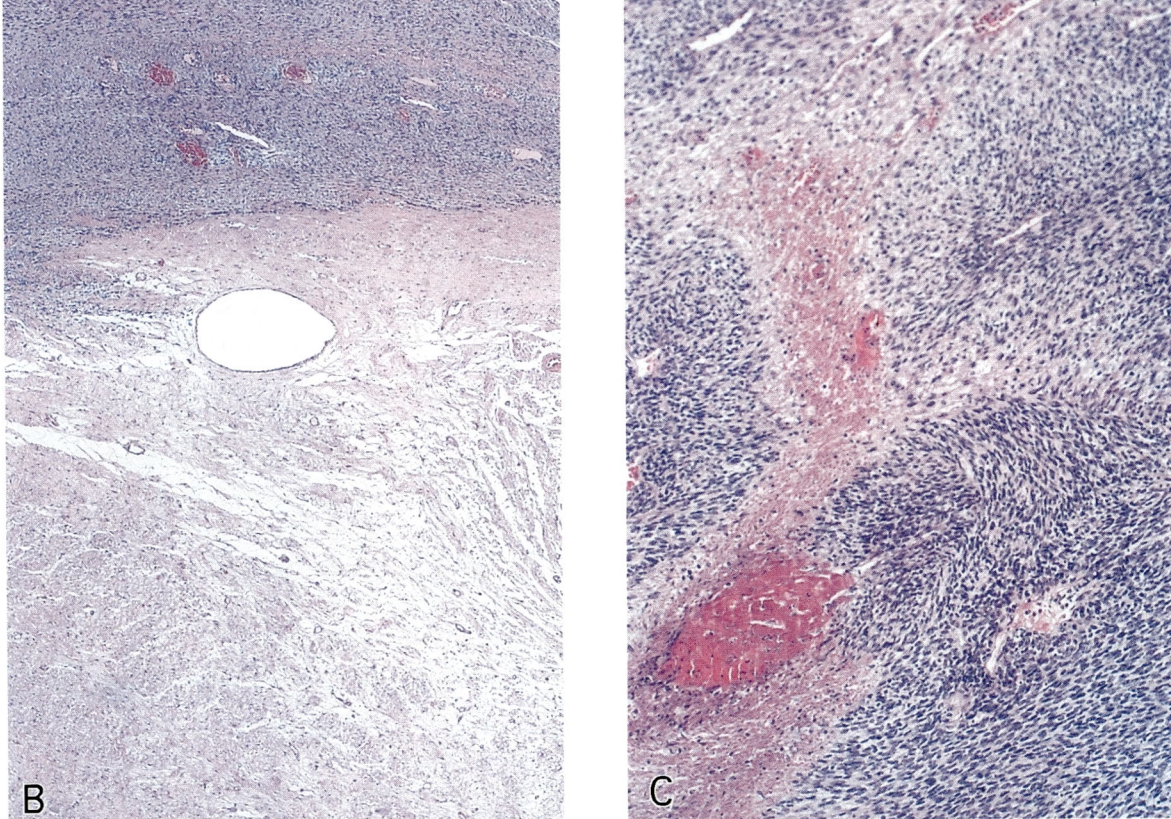

Figure 11-49

MPNST EX GANGLIONEUROMA

In this adrenal example (A), the ganglioneuroma (B) was seen to merge with the MPNST (C). Even in cellular portions of the latter, occasional ganglion cells were identified. For clinical details see Table 11-5, Ricci et al. (176), case 1.

Table 11-5

MPNST EX GANGLIONEUROMA OR GANGLIONEUROBLASTOMA: LITERATURE SUMMARY

Author (Ref.)	Age/Sex	Primary Tumor Site	Histology	Treatment	Postradiation Interval to MPNST	Secondary Tumor Site	Histology	Size	Treatment	Outcome
Ricci et al. (176)	1 yr/F	Adrenal, left	NB	Radiation therapy (2500 cGy)	17 yrs, 9 mos	Same	GN* with MPNST	13 cm	Surgical resection	Pulmonary metastases at 18 yrs, 11 mos. (treated with chemotherapy) DOD at 19 yrs, 9 mos with wide-spread metastases
	21 mos/M	Adrenal, left	GNB	Chemo- and radiation therapy	1 yr, 1 mo	Skull	GN	2.5 cm	Radiation (2000 cGy with a 970 cGy boost to the tumor bed)	8 yrs, 11 mos after the GNB and 7 yrs, 10 mos after radiation therapy to the skull GN, a para-nasal GN with MPNST was found. DOD at 9 years, 10 mos
Keller et al. (172)	14 mos/F	Retrogastric	NB	Radiation therapy (1500 cGy)	19 yrs, 4 mos	Retro-peritoneal	GN with MPNST	10 x 8 cm	Surgical resection and radiation (4500 cGY)	No follow-up
Chandrasoma et al. (166)	30/M**	Adrenal, left	GN with MPNST	Resection	N/A	Same	MPNST	11x9x8 cm	Radiation (4920 rads) and chemo-therapy	Alive with spinal metastasis at 9 mos
Fletcher et al. (168)	23/F	Thorax, paraspinal	GN with MPNST	Resection and radiation therapy (4000 cGy)	N/A					NED at 14 mos
Banks et al. (165)	15/M	Paratesticular	GN with MPNST	Resection, retroperitoneal lymph node dissection and chemotherapy	N/A					NED at 3 yrs
Damiani et al. (167)	18/F	Area of adrenal, left	GN with MPNST	Note: small area of MPNST	N/A					NED 4 yrs
Ghali et al. (169)	25/M	Retroperi-toneum	GN with MPNST	Resection	N/A	Same with left kidney, pancreas, spleen, and colon involvement	MPNST	7 cm	Resection	AWD 1 yr, 4 mos

*NB, neuroblastoma; GN, ganglioneuroma; GNB, ganglioneuroblastoma; DOD, dead of disease; AWD, alive with disease; NED, no evidence of disease; N/A, not applicable.
**HTLV III positive.

Table 11-6

MPNST EX PHEOCHROMOCYTOMA: LITERATURE SUMMARY

Author, Year (Ref.)	Age/ Sex	NF1	Gross Features	Microscopic Features (Sarcoma)	Immunohistochem-istry/Ultrastructure of Sarcoma	Treatment Follow-up
Min et al. 1988 (175)	39 F	No	Left adrenal; 35-cm encapsulated, partly hemorrhagic and necrotic tumor	Components intermingled; anaplastic spindle cell tumor with minor low-grade component	Occasional S-100 protein positivity in low-grade element; immunonegative in predominant anaplastic element; EM*: some schwannian features but mainly undifferentiated	Combination chemotherapy; DOD at 8 mos Autopsy: regional "sarcomatosis" but no metastases
Miettien and Saari 1988 (174)	38 F	No	Left adrenal; 18-cm encapsulated tumor	Spindle to round cells with some hemangiopericytoma-like pattern	Primary: many S-100 protein-positive cells. EM: schwannoma-like features; metastases: only vimentin reactive; EM: undifferentiated	Widespread metastases (liver, retroperitoneum); alive with metastases at at 18 mos
Sakaguchi et al. 1996 (177)	48 M	Yes	Left adrenal; 2-cm tumor. Right adrenal region; 8-cm tumor densely adherent to adrenal gland. Mediastinal metastasis	Left: MPNST in center of pheo; Right: both tumor components; intermingled MPNST mainly anaplastic, with chrondro-osseous differentiation	Primary: some S-100 protein-positive cells in associated "neurofibromatous nodules"; tumor negative; EM: osteosarcomatous differentiation	Mediastinal and lung metastases; radio- and chemotherapy; DOD at 3 mos; Autopsy: widespread sarcoma metastases (lungs, lymph nodes, pleura, diaphragm, spleen), cardiac tamponade; Associated gastrointestinal stromal tumors

*EM, electron microscopy; DOD, dead of disease.

field. The second clinicopathologic group consisted of five young adult patients (ages 18 to 30) without a history of prior irradiation, all of whom spontaneously developed MPNSTs within ganglioneuromas (fig. 11-49) (165–169).

Gross and Microscopic Findings. The two components of these complex lesions may be grossly distinct (fig. 11-49A). In cases in which the precursor lesion is still evident (fig. 11-49B), microscopic fields of typical ganglioneuroma may either abut or merge with sheets of crowded, hyperchromatic and mitotically active spindle cells (figs. 11-47–11-49). Occasional ganglion cells may be encountered within the malignant component of well-sampled tumors. In all three cases in which immunohistochemistry was performed, some malignant spindle cells exhibited

reactivity for S-100 protein. Four of the eight tumors had pursued a malignant course at the time of publication. Data is limited regarding clinical outcome. Two patients followed in excess of 5 years have died of tumor (Table 11-5).

Far from convincing are two reports of MPNST developing in ganglioneuromatous portions of an ectomesenchymoma (166a,169a–171,173,175a, 175b,178). The latter affect primarily infants and are complex tumors containing neuroblasts or ganglion cells as well as mesenchymal elements, often rhabdomyosarcoma (166a). Ectomesenchymomas are widely distributed in the body (169a). Their identification is of importance since typical examples are histologically malignant and associated with a poor outcome (169a). The term ectomesenchymoma is based on their assumed origin from ectomesenchyme (169b), pluripotential tissue derived from the neural crest (170). Ganglioneuroma was noted as a component in 7 of the 13 cases listed in one literature review (171). Although 2 of the 7 were said to contain an MPNST component, neither report clearly illustrates features of MPNST, and one fails to prove the presence of ganglioneuroma. Cozzutto et al. (166a) are of the opinion that to qualify as an ectomesenchymoma, the tumor should not possess histologic features of MPNST.

MPNST ex Pheochromocytoma

Least common of the MPNSTs arising in transition from tumors of neuronal type are those occurring in pheochromocytoma (174,175,177). The essential clinicopathologic features of the three cases reported to date are summarized in Table 11-6. All occurred in adults and only one was associated with NF1 (177). In two instances, presenting symptoms were entirely or partly referable to the endocrine effects of the pheochromocytoma. All three tumors involved the left adrenal gland, but in one case the lesion may have been bilateral (fig. 11-50) (177). Tumors ranged from small (2 cm) to massive, the largest (38 cm) example (175) having undergone extensive hemorrhage and necrosis. Remnants of the adrenal gland and the pheochromocytoma were identified in each case (figs. 11-50, 11-51). The location of one small MPNST within the substance of the pheochromocytoma confirmed its derivation from that tumor. To some extent, the two tumor elements were described as intermixed in all cases. Where mentioned, the lesions were encapsulated. The MPNSTs varied in their differentiation. All had a small cell or anaplastic element, but varying numbers of S-100–positive spindle cells were noted. Divergent chondroosseous differentiation was evident in one instance (fig. 11-50) (177). Yet another large, predominantly anaplastic MPNST exhibited a low-grade element (175), a finding suggesting incremental evolution of the tumor. Ultrastructural studies showed some degree of schwannian differentiation in all cases. Widespread metastases were noted in two cases. Two patients died of disease from 3 to 8 months after presentation; the other is alive with metastases at 18 months (Table 11-6). As suggested by one author (174),

MPNSTs arising in pheochromocytoma likely originate from sustentacular cells, modified Schwann cells encircling ganglionic cells.

PRIMITIVE NEUROECTODERMAL TUMOR OF PERIPHERAL NERVE

General Comments. Beginning with Stout's 1918 description of a primitive neuroectodermal tumor (PNET) of the ulnar nerve, the peripheral neuroepithelioma, a tumor now equated with PNET, was regarded as a tumor of peripheral nerve. Sixteen years elapsed before the term "peripheral neuroepithelioma" was applied to such tumors by Penfield (203). As compared to soft tissue examples unassociated with peripheral nerve, examples originating in nerve are rare. Only six cases have been reported to date (181,191, 199,208,210), while mention has been made of at least 13 additional examples (179,207,209). Affected nerves have included the sciatic, ulnar, median, radial, intercostal, lateral popliteal, and S-1 root. The six reported cases occurred in the third through the fifth decades of life, four in males and two in females. In most instances no long-term follow-up was reported, but some tumors were fatal, having metastasized distantly (195).

In the 1970s it first became evident that peripheral neuroepitheliomas also arose in soft tissues, without a nerve association. Lattes (195) reported an example occurring in the chest wall. Thereafter, Seemayer et al. (205) described two additional malignant peripheral neuroepithelial tumors, one exhibiting rosette formation; neither patient had a primary neuroblastoma at another site. Two synchronous reports emerged in 1979, one a 15-case series by Lieberman (196) who used the term "primitive neuroectodermal tumor," and another the 20-case series of Askin et al. (180) who reported 20 "malignant small cell tumor of the thoracopulmonary region of children." Both confirmed the existence of a strictly soft tissue form of peripheral neuroepithelioma. While the cell type of the tumors reported by Askin et al. was unclear to the authors, subsequent evidence of their neuroectodermal or neural nature was provided (192,197). As an aside, the term neural has been loosely used to denote both nerve sheath and neuroblastic/neuronal differentiation. With respect to PNET, it implies the latter. In addition to the above-noted forms of

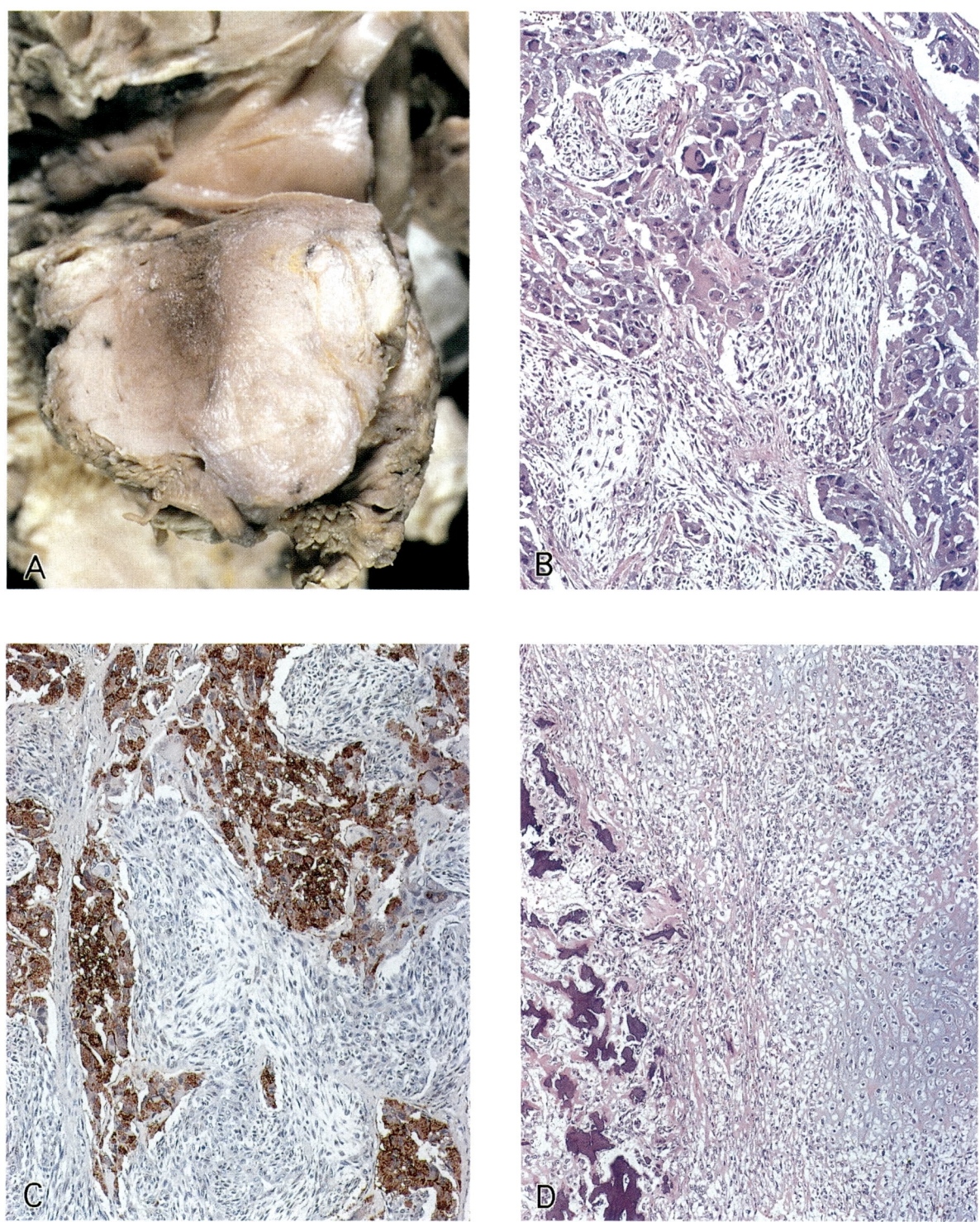

Figure 11-50
MPNST EX PHEOCHROMOCYTOMA
This mass in the right adrenal region consisted of firm tan MPNST and residual red-brown pheochromocytoma (A). Microscopically, the two components were in part admixed (B), a feature best seen on chromogranin immunostain (C). The MPNST demonstrated chondro-osseous differentiation (D). For clinical details, see Table 11-6, Sakaguchi et al. (13). (Courtesy of Dr. K. Sano, Matsumoto, Japan.)

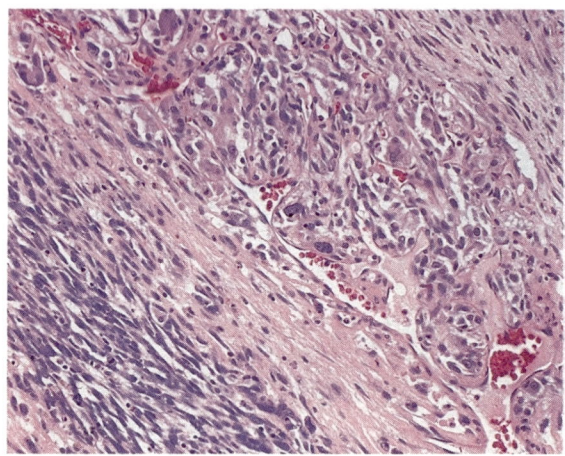

Figure 11-51
MPNST EX PHEOCHROMOCYTOMA
This massive tumor of the left adrenal gland consisted in large part of high-grade MPNST. For clinical details, see Table 11-6, Min et al. (11). (Courtesy of Dr. K.W. Min, Oklahoma City, OK.)

nerve-based and soft tissue PNET, conventional MPNST may also rarely demonstrate primitive neuroepithelial differentiation (183,184).

Histologic Findings. The PNET is a highly malignant tumor of apparent neural crest origin. It exhibits neural differentiation only in the sense that it closely resembles but is less well differentiated than neuroblastoma (fig. 11-52). Histologically, PNETs consist of poorly differentiated, small, round cells disposed in a lobular pattern and often showing a somewhat fibrillar background. Although some degree of Homer-Wright rosette formation may be seen (fig. 11-52B,D), ganglionic differentiation is rarely observed (182, 184,190,192,204,212). Nucleoli are typically small or inconspicuous (fig. 11-52B,D) (185,200). Cytoplasmic glycogen may be present in optimally fixed tissue.

Immunohistochemical Findings. Most PNETs express neuron-specific enolase (NSE) and the glycoprotein CD99 (p30/32MIC2) as identified by the monoclonal antibodies HBA71 and 013 (187,189,202). In the appropriate setting, CD99 reactivity (fig. 11-52, right) is a more specific marker of PNET than is NSE. Its expression is also seen in Ewing's sarcoma, the osseous counterpart of PNET (186,188), and in a variety of other neoplasms (193,206). Lastly, occasional synaptophysin and rare neurofilament protein reactivity may be expressed by PNET.

Ultrastructural Findings. Electron microscopy (fig. 11-53) reveals rounded cells with variable numbers of short microtubule-containing neuritic processes. Cytoplasm is scant and contains few, occasionally pleomorphic dense-core granules (fig. 11-53, right). Glycogen is also present in some cases (201).

Cytogenetics. On genetic analysis, most soft tissue PNETs demonstrate a reciprocal translocation of chromosomes 11 and 22 (q21:q12) (213), an alteration also seen in Ewing's sarcoma (211). To date, no cytogenetic evaluation of a nerve-based PNET has been reported.

Differential Diagnosis. The principal differential diagnosis of nerve-based PNET is *neuroblastoma*. Clinicopathologic distinctions are summarized in Table 11-7.

Treatment and Prognosis. PNETs are both locally aggressive (180) and capable of widespread metastases. Common sites of metastatic spread include the lungs, bone, and lymph nodes (198). The reported 3-year disease-free survival rate of patients with initially localized tumors is 56 percent (194).

MALIGNANT GRANULAR CELL TUMOR

Definition. This is a histologically or clinically malignant counterpart of the benign granular cell tumor, a lesion of probable peripheral nerve sheath origin composed of granular cells which are immunoreactive for S-100 protein and contain large numbers of secondary lysosomes. The tumor is also known as *malignant granular cell schwannoma*.

General Comments. Since Ravich and Stout's (246) original description of a malignant granular cell tumor (GCT) in the urinary bladder, there have been over 30 bona fide examples reported (214–217,219,221–223,225–230,230a,232–235,238–240, 242–249,251,253,255,256,258–261). Critical reviews of the literature (225,238) have rejected many of the earlier reported cases since their morphologic features were more suggestive of alveolar soft part sarcoma or rhabdomyosarcoma.

By convention, GCTs are classified as malignant when their constituent cells are cytologically malignant or when a morphologically benign GCT metastasizes to regional lymph nodes, distant sites, or otherwise causes a patient's death. By this definition, morphologically benign examples

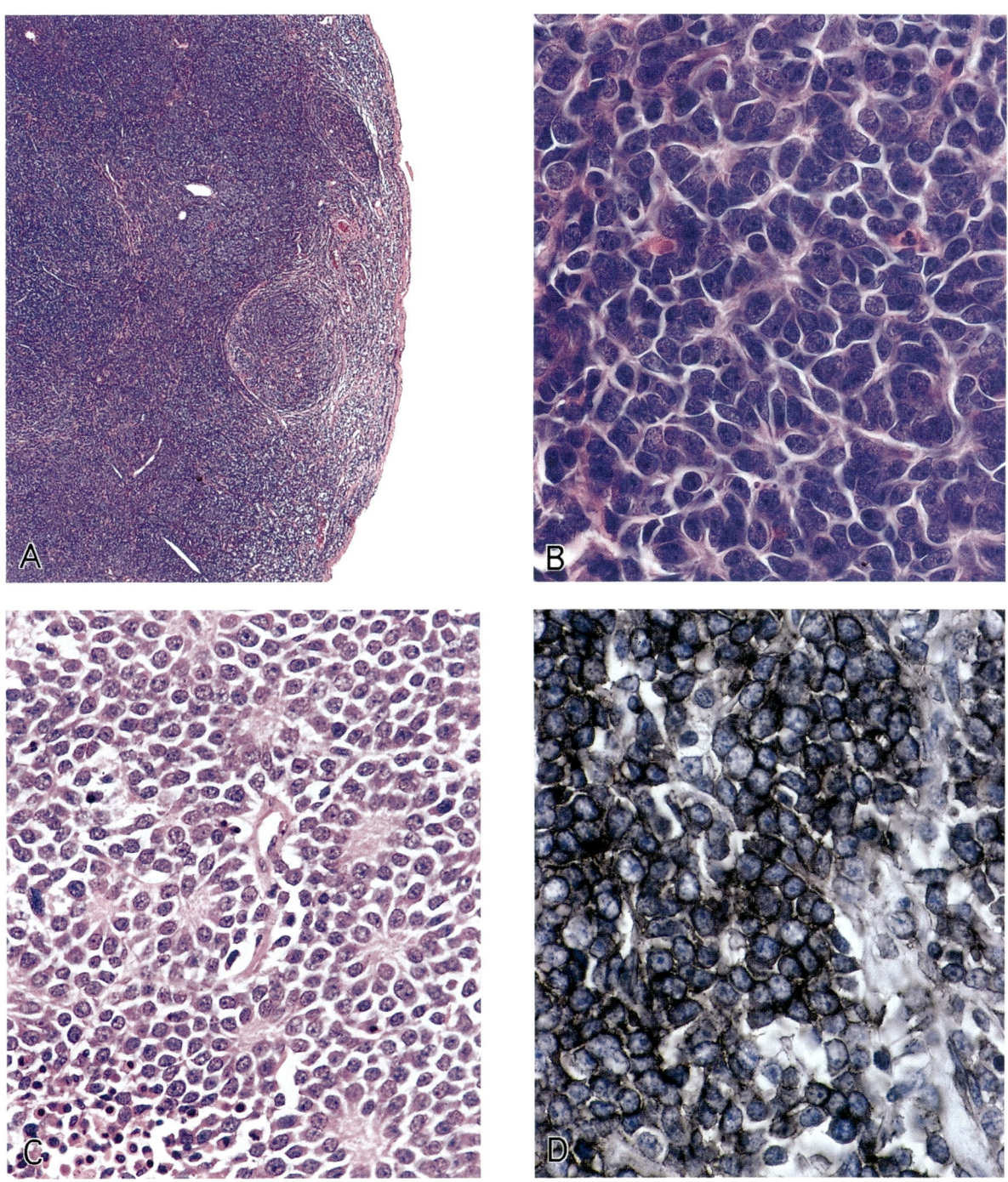

Figure 11-52
PNET

A,B: This cervical nerve root lesion occurred in a 20-year-old female. Dumbell-shaped with both an intradural and extradural foraminal component, it involves both epineurium and nerve fascicles (A). Its cytologic features are typical and include vague rosette formation (B).

C,D: This typical highly cellular example which arose in the left S-1 nerve root of a 40-year-old male (C) shows chromatin to be more coarse and nucleoli to be more prominent than in neuroblastomas of comparable cellularity. Well-formed Homer-Wright rosettes are a conspicuous feature. Strong membrane immunoreactivity for CD99 (D), the MIC2 gene product, is helpful in the differential diagnosis of PNET in that such immunoreactivity is lacking in neuroblastoma. (Courtesy of Dr. P. C. Burger, Baltimore, MD.)

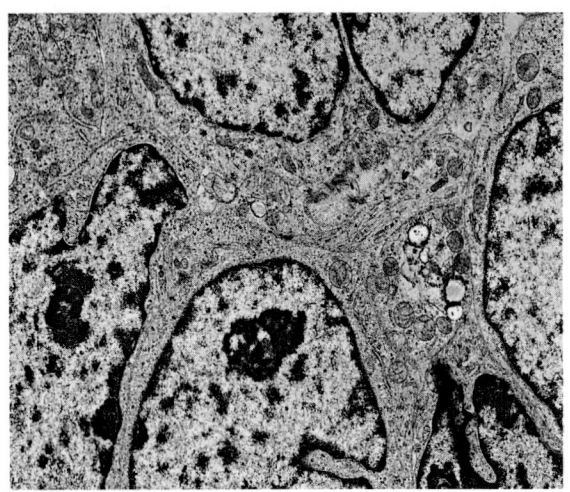
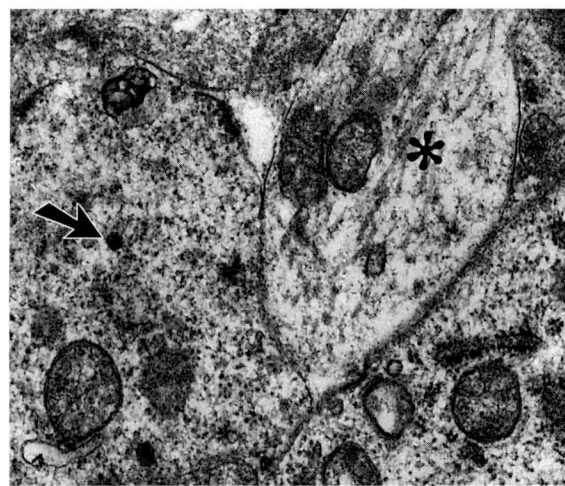

Figure 11-53
PNET
The ultrastructural features of this poorly differentiated tumor (left) include the formation of occasional microtubule-containing processes and the presence (*) of rare dense-core granules (right, arrow). (Left, X10,000; right, X32,100)

Table 11-7

NEUROBLASTOMA AND PERIPHERAL PNET: DIFFERENTIAL DIAGNOSIS

	Neuroblastoma	Peripheral PNET
Age	<5 years	>10 years
Location	Adrenal, sympathetic ganglia	Soft tissue, thoracopulmonary region, bone
Neurotransmitters	Adrenergic	Cholinergic
Metabolite excretion	Present	Absent
Immunohistochemistry		
Vimentin	<5%	+
013	−	+
Chromogranin A	~10%	−
Synaptophysin	+	occasional
Nerve growth receptor	+	+
Neuron specific enolase	+	+
Neurofilament protein	+	rare
Keratin	−	<5%
S-100 protein	−	Occasional
Leu-7	+ 40%	+ 40%
MHC*(beta$_2$ microglobulin)	−	Frequent
Ultrastructure	Frequent, long neurites, few to numerous neruosecretory granules	Abortive neurites, few pleomorphic granules
Chromosomal abnormalities	del 1 (q-), HSRs, DMs	Reciprocal translocation 11:22
Oncogenes	N-*myc*	c-*myc*
Survival		
Local disease	80%	50%
Disseminated disease	20%	10%

*MHC, major histocompatibility complex; DMs = double minutes; HSRs = homogeneously stained regions.

represent nearly 90 percent of malignant GCTs. Since cytologically bland GCTs may behave in an aggressive manner, many investigators have focused upon even minor cytologic features that might provide a clue to the biologic potential of otherwise benign-appearing examples. One recent large series successfully applied histologic criteria to the determination of malignancy (230a). As a result, we require the presence of histologic malignancy rather than atypia before designating a GCT morphologically malignant.

Clinical Features. The age and sex distributions of benign and malignant GCTs coincide. The peak incidence for malignant GCT is in the fourth through the sixth decades, with a mean patient age of 50 years and a female sex predilection (1.4 to 1). Malignant GCTs have not been reported to occur in children, the youngest patient being 23 years of age (243). In our review of the literature, malignant GCTs occur at almost all sites. Head and neck tumors are less frequent than among benign GCTs. Instead, the trunk and extremities are most often affected; the thigh is the single most common site of malignant GCT. Several lesions involved deep soft tissues: one was intrapelvic (244) and two were vulvar (240,248). Oral mucosa examples are also uncommon. It is of note that at least two malignant GCTs reportedly involved identifiable large nerves, specifically the sciatic and radial nerves (253,260). Little data is available regarding the imaging characteristics of malignant GCT (230).

Gross Findings. Grossly, malignant GCTs present either as relatively circumscribed or clearly infiltrative masses (fig. 11-54A,B), usually measuring 4 to 15 cm in greatest dimension (214). Malignant GCTs as small as 1 cm have been reported (230a). Gross association with a nerve is rare. Firm to hard on palpation, their cut surface is variously gray, white, or yellow. On occasion, areas of necrosis are grossly apparent.

Histologic Findings. As a whole, malignant GCTs consist of sheets or irregular packets of polygonal to somewhat spindle-shaped cells with abundant eosinophilic cytoplasm containing PAS-positive, diastase-resistant granules (figs. 11-54C, 11-55A). Like benign GCT, malignant examples often contain spherical, PAS-positive cytoplasmic globules (figs. 11-54C, 11-55A). Similarly staining angulate bodies may be seen within accompanying histiocytes. Although some ma-

lignant GCTs are virtually indistinguishable from their benign counterpart (see below) (260), histologically malignant examples generally show at least three of the following: marked cellularity, pleomorphism, a high nuclear: cytoplasmic ratio, nucleolar prominence, readily identifiable mitoses, prominent spindling of tumor cells, and frequent foci of necrosis (230a). Mitotic figures are generally absent in benign GCTs (fig. 11-54C). The same is true of areas of necrosis (fig. 11-55D).

Clinically malignant but histologically benign GCTs cannot be diagnosed on the basis of their microscopic features alone. Although benign GCTs generally consist of a uniform population of cytologically bland granular cells, it has been suggested that even mild to moderate pleomorphism in a largely benign-appearing tumor should prompt consideration of malignancy (248). This may be true. Nonetheless, given the implications for treatment, we are reluctant to make a diagnosis of malignant GCT in such instances unless there are two or more low-power fields wherein most cells have enlarged, pleomorphic, vesicular or hyperchromatic nuclei with prominent nucleoli. Mitotic figures may or may not be present but alone do not indicate malignant change. Fortunately, in our experience the histologic changes upon which a diagnosis of malignant GCT can be made in this setting are often obvious and widespread. Attention to the growth characteristics is also of diagnostic utility. Although limited invasion of surrounding soft tissue cannot be interpreted as malignant behavior, destructive growth and lymphatic or vascular invasion are features of malignant GCT.

In those instances in which malignant GCTs were subject to aspiration or exfoliative cytologic study, it was not possible to distinguish a benign from a malignant process (224,226).

Immunohistochemical Findings. Like those of their benign counterparts, the cells of malignant GCTs consistently express S-100 protein (fig. 11-55B) (227,230a,233,259,261), vimentin, and neuron-specific enolase (NSE) (230a). Reactivity for carcinoembryonic antigen has also been reported (226), although the frequency and significance of this unexpected finding has not been determined. By definition, stains for muscle markers are negative. Despite uniform immunoreactivity of benign GCTs for KP-1 (CD 68), a macrophage marker (236), only a minority of

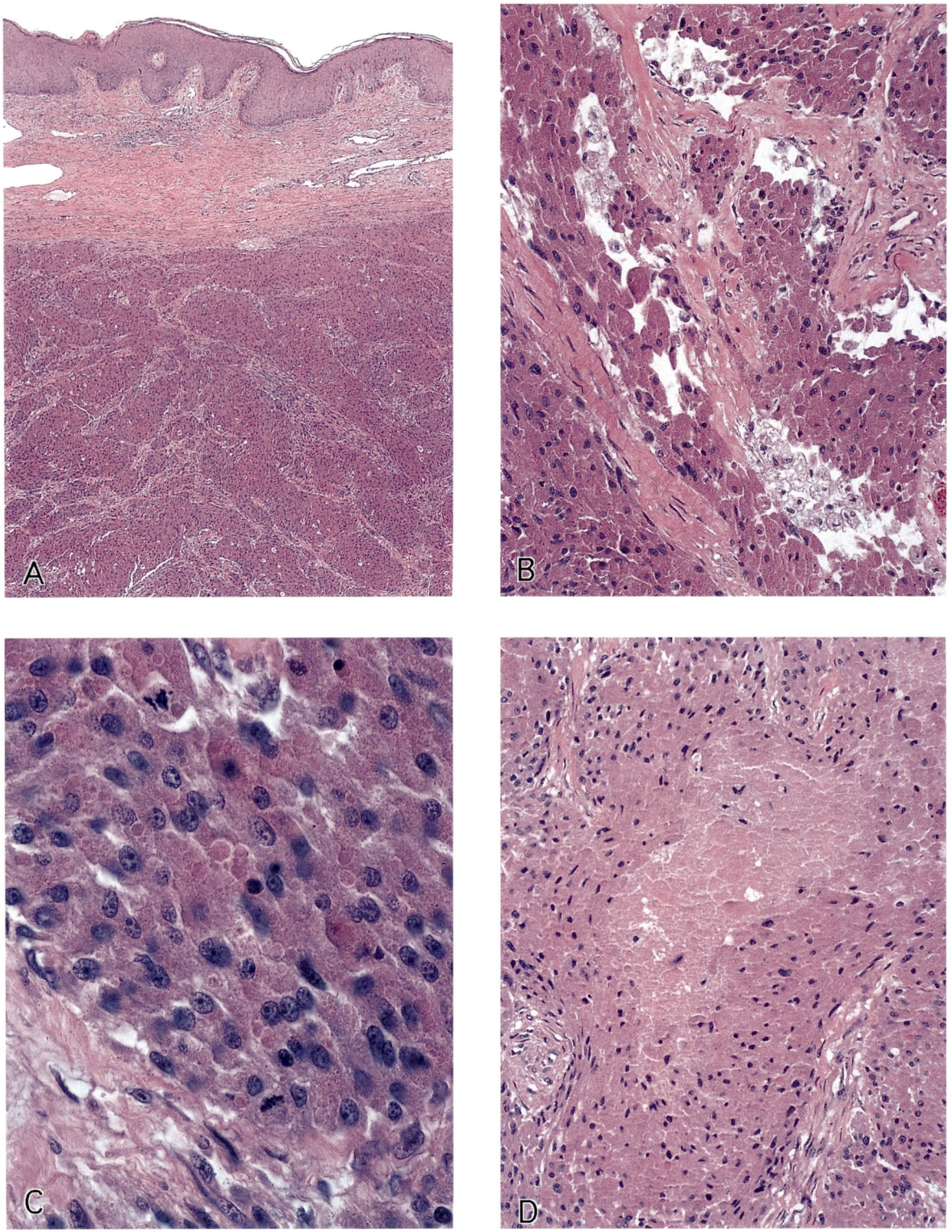

Figure 11-54

MALIGNANT GRANULAR CELL TUMOR

This cellular, infiltrative example (A,B) arose in the thigh of a 31-year-old female. Note conspicuous mitotic activity (C) and focal necrosis (D). (Figures 11-54 and 11-55 are from the same patient.)

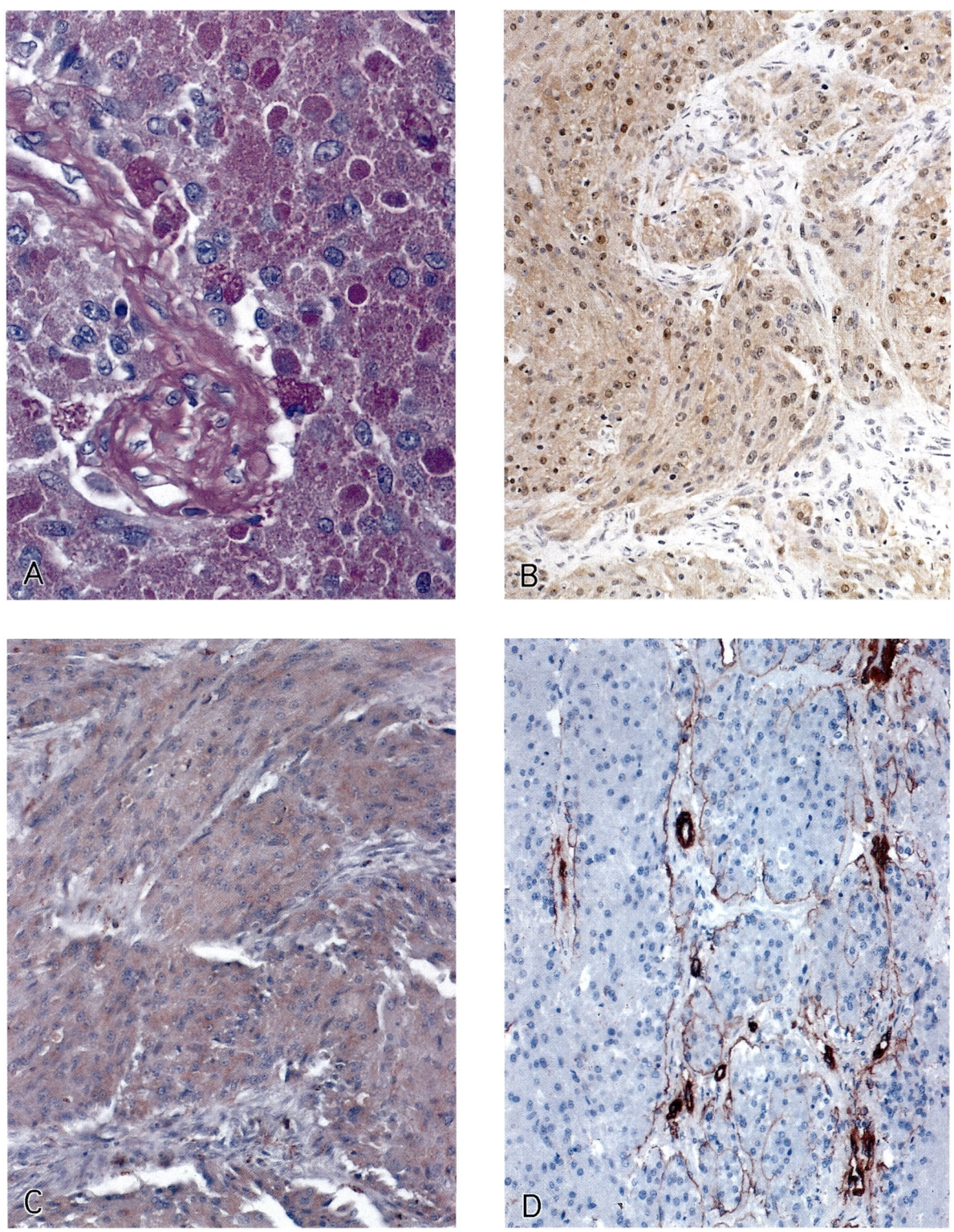

Figure 11-55
MALIGNANT GRANULAR CELL TUMOR

This lesion showed not only prominence of globules (see fig. 11-54C) which are PAS positive (A), but also immunoreactivity for S-100 protein (B) and CD68 (C). Collagen 4 reactivity outlines cell lobules (D).

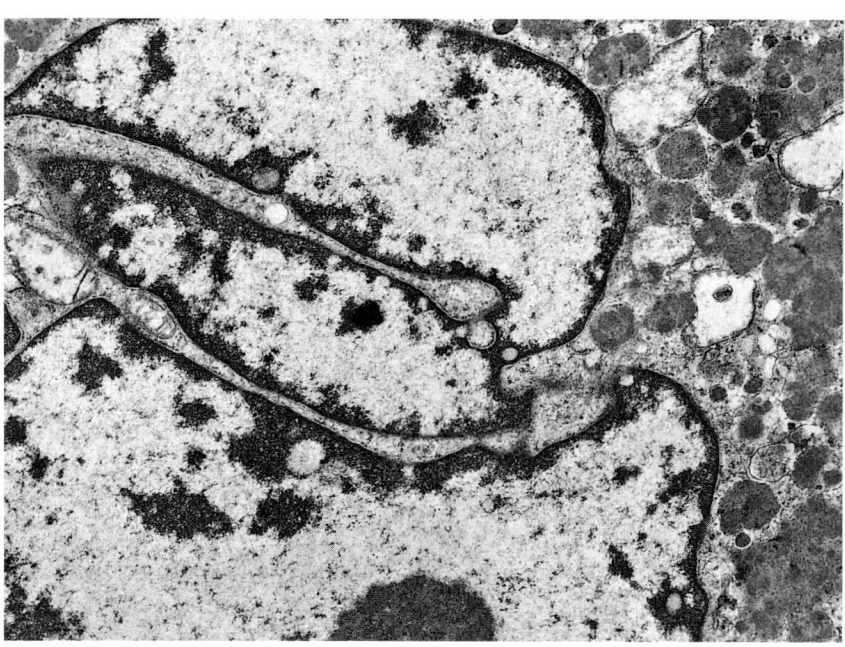

Figure 11-56
MALIGNANT GRANULAR
CELL TUMOR
Portion of a neoplastic tumor cell with a pleomorphic nucleus and numerous cytoplasmic secondary lysosomes, features diagnostic for GCT (X10,100).

malignant GCTs are reactive (fig. 11-55C) (230a). Similarly, collagen 4 reactivity is occasionally seen outlining cell lobules (fig. 11-54D).

Immunoreactivity for proliferation markers may aid in the identification of GCTs likely to exhibit malignant behavior. In one large series, fully half of histologically malignant tumors exhibited labeling indices of 10 to 50 percent (230a); in addition, nearly 70 percent showed extensive p53 protein staining.

Electron Microscopic Findings. Aside from the presence of large pleomorphic nuclei, clumped and marginated chromatin, and often multiple, large nucleoli (fig. 11-56) (223,231,233,259–261), the ultrastructural features of morphologically malignant GCT are identical to those described in the benign GCT section. Lysosomes fill the cells. Specialized junctions are lacking and individual cells or grouped cells are often surrounded by basement membrane.

Differential Diagnosis. The two major considerations in the differential diagnosis of morphologically malignant GCTs are leiomyosarcoma and alveolar soft part sarcoma. In the past there was concern about the distinction of malignant GCT and *pleomorphic rhabdomyosarcoma*, but this has been largely negated by the definition of GCT as being immunonegative for muscle markers. Conversely, rhabdomyosarcomas are, with but few exceptions (218,241,252), S-100 protein

negative. *Granular cell leiomyosarcoma* (257) may be indistinguishable from malignant GCT on routine immunohistochemical stains. Whenever muscle differentiation is suspected we recommend the use of a panel of antibodies designed to identify smooth or striated muscle cells: desmin, muscle common actin (HHF 35), smooth muscle actin, myogenin, and sarcomeric actin. The distinction of malignant GCT from *alveolar soft part sarcoma* poses little difficulty, since the organoid or alveolar growth pattern that characterizes the latter is absent in GCT (220). Lack of S-100 protein expression in alveolar soft part sarcoma also distinguishes the lesions. An additional helpful clue is the finding of PAS-positive, diastase-resistant crystalline structures in the cytoplasm of about one fourth of alveolar soft part sarcomas (254). Such crystalloids have a distinctive rhomboid appearance on electron microscopy (237). Obviously the differential diagnosis of clinically malignant but histologically benign GCT is the same as that of benign GCT (see chapter 9).

Treatment and Prognosis. Wide en bloc excision is the treatment of choice in the management of malignant GCT. There is no evidence indicating that radiotherapy or chemotherapy are effective treatment modalities. Indeed, one malignant GCT reportedly increased in size during a 5500 cGy course of radiation; the patient subsequently died with generalized metastases (216).

Malignant GCTs are aggressive lesions that often recur locally before spreading to regional lymph nodes or other sites. The lung is the most common site of distant spread, being involved in nearly half of all reported clinically malignant GCTs. In the majority of instances, metastases developed within 2 years of initial tumor resection; in one case, however, it was 5 years after (35). Generalized metastases have been described as occurring in five cases (216,219,222, 246,258). The prognosis of patients with malignant GCTs is poor. In a literature review of 31 clinically malignant examples with available follow-up (214–216,219,221–223,225–228,233–235,238,240,242–249,253,256,258–261) we found that 58 percent of patients had died of tumor. Most of these patients died within 3 years, although one survived for 6 years, and two died only after 8 years. Of five patients with histologically malignant but nonmetastatic tumors (229,232,239,249,250), none died of tumor.

A recent large AFIP series (230a) found a number of clinical, gross, and histologic features to be associated with survival, including old patient age, larger tumor size, malignant histology (three or more of the criteria noted above), vesicular nuclei with large nucleoli, increased mitotic activity, and necrosis. When subject to multivariate analysis, only increasing age and Ki67 values of greater than or equal to 10 percent were adverse factors with respect to survival; older age was the only parameter significantly related to metastases, and none were significant with respect to local tumor recurrence.

REFERENCES

Primary Malignant Peripheral Nerve Sheath Tumor

1. Albert A, Albisu J, Gutierrez-Hoyos A, Tovar JA. Malignant abdominal schwannoma associated with von Recklinghausen's neurofibromatosis. Z Kinderchir 1981;33:93–6.

2. Becher R, Wake N, Gibas Z, Ochi H, Sandberg AA. Chromosome changes in soft tissue sarcomas. JNCI 1984;72:823–31.

3. Bello MJ, de Campos JM, Kusak ME, et al. Clonal chromosome aberrations in neuromas. Genes Chromosomes Cancer 1993;6:206–11.

4. Bergstrom R. Changes in peripheral nerve tissue after irradiation with high energy protons. Acta Radiol 1962;58:301–12.

5. Best PV. Malignant triton tumor in the cerebellopontine angle. Report of a case. Acta Neuropathol 1987;74:92–6.

5a. Bhargava R, Parham DM, Lasater OE, Chari RS, Chen G, Fletcher BD. MR imaging differentiation of benign and malignant peripheral nerve sheath tumors: use of the target sign. Pediatr Radiol 1997;27:124–9.

6. Brennan MF, Hilaris B, Shiu MH, et al. Local recurrence in adult soft tissue sarcoma. A randomized trial of brachytherapy. Arch Surg 1987;122:1289–93.

7. Cavanagh JB. Effects of x-irradiation on the proliferation of cells in peripheral nerve during Wallerian degeneration in a rat. Br J Radiol 1968;41:275–81.

7a. Chanoki M, Ishii M, Fukai K, et al. Immunohistochemical localization of type I, III, IV, V, and VI collagens and laminin in neurofibroma and neurofibrosarcoma. Am J Dermatol 1991;13:365–73.

8. Chen KT, Latorraca R, Fabich D, Padgug A, Hafez GR, Gilbert EF. Malignant schwannoma. A light microscopic and ultrastructural study. Cancer 1980;45:1585–93.

9. Conley FK, Rubinstein LJ, Spence AM. Studies on experimental malignant nerve sheath tumors maintained in tissue and organ culture systems. II. Electron microscopy observations. Acta Neuropath (Berl) 1976;34: 293–310.

10. Crowe FW, Schull WJ, Van Neel J. A clinical, pathological, and genetic study of multiple neurofibromatosis. Springfield, Illinois: Charles C. Thomas, 1956.

11. D'Agostino AN, Soule EH, Miller RH. Primary malignant neoplasms of nerves (malignant neurilemomas) in patients without manifestations of multiple neurofibromatosis (von Recklinghausen's disease). Cancer 1963;16:1003–14.

12. D'Agostino AN, Soule EH, Miller RH. Sarcomas of the peripheral nerves and somatic soft tissues associated with multiple neurofibromatosis (von Recklinghausen's disease). Cancer 1963;16:1015–27.

13. Daimaru Y, Hashimoto H, Enjoji M. Malignant peripheral nerve sheath tumors (malignant schwannomas). An immunohistochemical study of 29 cases. Am J Surg Pathol 1985;9:434–44.

14. Decker HJ, Cannizzaro LA, Mendez MJ, et al. Chromosomes 17 and 22 involved in marker formation in neurofibrosarcomas. Hum Genet 1990;85:337–42.

15. Dickersin GR. The electron microscopic spectrum of nerve sheath tumors. Ultrastruct Pathol 1987;11:103–46.

16. Ducatman BS, Scheithauer BW. Post-irradiation neurofibrosarcoma. Cancer 1983;51:1028–33.

17. Ducatman BS, Scheithauer BW, Piepgras DG, Reiman HM. Malignant peripheral nerve sheath tumors in childhood. J Neuro-Oncology 1984;2:241–8.

18. Ducatman BS, Scheithauer BW. Piepgras DG, Reiman HM, Ilstrup DM. Malignant peripheral nerve sheath tumor. A clinicopathologic study of 120 cases. Cancer 1986;57:2006–21.

19. Enzinger FM, Weiss SW. Benign tumors of peripheral nerves. In: Enzinger FM, Weiss SW, eds. Soft tissue tumors. 3rd ed. St. Louis: C.V. Mosby, 1995:821–88.

20. Enzinger FM, Weiss SW. Malignant tumors of peripheral nerves. In: Enzinger FM, Weiss SW, eds. Soft tissue tumors. 2nd ed. St. Louis: C.V. Mosby, 1988:781–815.

21. Erlandson RA. Gastrointestinal autonomic nerve (GAN) tumor: plexosarcoma. In: Diagnostic transmission electron microscopy of tumors. New York: Raven Press, 1994:381–4.

22. Erlandson RA. Synovial sarcoma. In: Diagnostic transmission electron microscopy of tumors. New York: Raven Press, 1994:775.

23. Erlandson RA, Klimstra DS, Woodruff JM. Subclassification of gastrointestinal stromal tumors based on evaluation by electron microscopy and immunohistochemistry. Ultrastruct Pathol 1996;20:373–93.

24. Erlandson RA, Woodruff JM. Peripheral nerve sheath tumors: an electron microscopic study of 43 cases. Cancer 1982;49:273–87.

25. Ernst H, Rittinghausen S, Wahnschaffe U, Mohr U. Induction of malignant peripheral nerve sheath tumors in European hamsters with 1, 1-dimethylhydrazine (UDMH). Cancer Lett 1987;35:303–11.

26. Fletcher CD. Peripheral neuroectodermal tumors. In: Fletcher CD, ed. Diagnostic histopathology of tumors. Edinburgh: Churchill Livingstone, 1995:1221–50.

27. Fletcher JA, Kozakewich HP, Hoffer FA, et al. Diagnostic relevance of clonal cytogenetic aberrations in malignant soft-tissue tumors. N Engl J Med 1991;324:436–42.

28. Foley KM, Woodruff JM, Ellis FT, Posner J. Radiation induced malignant and atypical PNST. Ann Neurol 1980;7:311–8.

29. Franks AJ. Epithelioid neurilemoma of the trigeminal nerve: an immunohistochemical and ultrastructural study. Histopathology 1985;9:1339–50.

30. Glover TW, Stein CK, Legius E, Andersen LB, Brereton A, Johnson S. Molecular and cytogenetic analysis of tumors in von Recklinghausen neurofibromatosis. Genes Chromosomes Cancer 1991;3:62–70.

31. Gould VE, Moll R, Moll I, Lee I, Schwechheimer K, Franke WW. The intermediate filament complement of the spectrum of nerve sheath neoplasms. Lab Invest 1986;55:463–74.

32. Gray MH, Rosenberg AE, Dickersin GR, Bhan AK. Glial fibrillary acidic protein and keratin expression by benign and malignant nerve sheath tumors. Hum Pathol 1989;20:1089–96.

33. Halling KC, Scheithauer BW, Halling AC, et al. p53 expression in neurofibroma and malignant peripheral nerve sheath tumor. An immunohistochemical study of sporadic and NF1-associated tumors. Am J Clin Pathol 1996;106:282–8.

34. Han DH, Kim DG, Chi JG, Park SH, Jung HW, Kim YG. Malignant triton tumor of the acoustic nerve. Case report. J Neurosurg 1992;76:874–7.

35. Hayashi K, Takahashi K, Sonobe H, Ohtsuki Y, Taguchi K. The distribution of alpha and beta subunits of S-100 protein in malignant schwannoma arising in neurofibromatosis of von Recklinghausen's disease. Virchows Arch [A] 1987;411:515–21.

36. Herrera GA, DeMoraes HP, Grizzle WE, Han SG. Malignant small bowel neoplasm of enteric plexus derivation (plexosarcoma). Dig Dis Sci 1984;29:275–84.

37. Herrera GA, Pinto de Moraes H. Neurogenic sarcoma in patients with neurofibromatosis (von Recklinghausen's disease). Light, electron microscopy, and immunohistochemistry study. Virchows Arch [A] 1984;403:361–76.

38. Herrera GA, Reimann BE, Salinas JA, Turbat EA. Malignant schwannoma presenting as malignant fibrous histiocytomas. Ultrastruct Pathol 1982;3:253–61.

39. Hirose T, Hasegawa T, Kudo E. Malignant peripheral nerve sheath tumors: an immunohistochemical study in relation to ultrastructural features. Hum Pathol 1992;23:865–70.

40. Hirose T, Sano T, Hizawa K. Heterogeneity of malignant schwannomas. Ultrastruct Pathol 1988;12:107–16.

41. Hirose T, Scheithauer BW, Sano T. Malignant perineurioma. A study of 8 cases [Abstract]. Mod Pathol 1997.

42. Hirose T, Sumitomo M, Kudo E, et al. Malignant peripheral nerve sheath tumor (MPNST) showing perineurial cell differentiation. Am J Surg Pathol 1989;13:613–20.

43. Hope DG, Mulvihill JJ. Malignancy in neurofibromatosis. Adv Neurol 1981;39:33–56.

44. Hruban RH, Shiu MH, Senie RT, Woodruff JM. Malignant peripheral nerve sheath tumors of the buttock and lower extremity. A study of 43 cases. Cancer 1990;66:1253–65.

45. Jhanwar SC, Chen Q, Li FP, Brennan MF, Woodruff JM. Cytogenetic analysis of soft tissue sarcomas. Recurrent chromosome abnormalities in malignant peripheral nerve sheath tumors (MPNST). Cancer Genet Cytogenet 1994;78:138–44.

46. Johnson TL, Lee MW, Meis JM, Zarbo RJ, Crissman JD. Immunohistochemical characterization of malignant peripheral nerve sheath tumors. Surg Pathol 1991;4:121–35.

47. Kikuchi A, Akiyama M, Han-Yaku H. Solitary cutaneous malignant schwannoma. Immunohistochemical and ultrastructural studies. Am J Dermatopathol 1991;15:15–9.

48. Kindblom LG, Ahlden M, Meis-Kindblom JM, Stenman G. Immunohistochemical and molecular analysis of p53, MDM2, proliferating cell nuclear antigen and Ki67 in benign and malignant peripheral nerve sheath tumours. Virchows Arch 1995;427:19–26.

49. Koestner A, Swenberg JA, Wechsler W. Transplacental production of ethylnitrosourea of neoplasm of the nervous system in Sprague-Dawley rats. Am J Pathol 1971;63:37–56.

50. Kourea HP, Bilsky MH, Leung DH, Lewis JJ, Woodruff JM. Subdiaphragmatic and intrathoracic paraspinal malignant peripheral nerve sheath tumor. A clinicopathologic study of 25 patients and 26 tumors. Am J Cancer 1998;82:2191–203.

51. Krumerman MS, Stingle W. Synchronous malignant glandular schwannomas in congenital neurofibromatosis. Cancer 1978;41:2444–51.

52. Kudo M, Matsumoto M, Terao H. Malignant nerve sheath tumor of acoustic nerve. Arch Pathol Lab Med 1983;107:293–7.

53. Lauwers GY, Erlandson RA, Casper ES, Brennan MF, Woodruff JM. Gastrointestinal autonomic nerve tumors. A clinicopathological, immunohistochemical, and ultrastructural study of 12 cases. Am J Surg Pathol 1993;17:887–97.

54. Leslie MD, Cheung KY. Malignant transformation of neurofibromas at multiple sites in a case of neurofibromatosis. Postgrad Med J 1987;63:131–3.

55. Levy D, Khatib R. Intestinal neurofibromatosis with malignant degeneration: report of a case. Dis Colon Rectum 1960;3:140–4.

56. Lewis JJ, Brennan MR. Soft tissue sarcomas. Curr Probl Surg 1996;33:817–72.

56a. Lin BT, Weiss LM, Medeiros LJ. Neurofibroma and cellular neurofibroma with atypia. Am J Surg Pathol 1997;21:1443–9.

57. McCarron KF, Goldblum JR. Plexiform neurofibroma with and without associated malignant peripheral nerve sheath tumor: a clinicopathologic and immunohistochemical analysis of 54 cases [Abstract]. Mod Pathol 1997;10:11A.

58. McLean CA, Laidlaw JD, Brownbill DS, Gonzales MF. Recurrence of acoustic neurilemoma as a malignant spindle-cell neoplasm. Case report. J Neurosurg 1990;73:946–50.

59. Meis JM, Enzinger FM, Martz KL, Neal JA. Malignant peripheral nerve sheath tumors (malignant schwannomas) in children. Am J Surg Pathol 1992;16:694–707.

60. Menon AG, Anderson KM, Riccardi VM, et al. Chromosome 17p depletions and p53 gene mutations associated with the formation of malignant neurofibrosarcoma in von Recklinghausen neurofibromatosis. Proc Natl Acad Sci 1990;87:5435–9.

61. Mertens F, Rydholm A, Bauer HF, et al. Cytogenetic findings in malignant peripheral nerve sheath tumors. Intl J Cancer 1995;61:793–8.

62. Miettinen M, Saari A. Pheochromocytoma combined with malignant schwannoma: unusual neoplasm of the adrenal medulla. Ultrastruct Pathol 1988;12:513–27.

63. Min KW. Myenteric plexomas and pheochromocytomas in neurofibromatosis type-1 [Abstract]. Mod Pathol 1997;10:60A.

64. Min KW, Balaton AJ. Small intestinal stromal tumors with skeinoid fibers in neurofibromatosis: report of 4 cases with ultrastructural study of tissue retrieved from paraffin blocks. Ultrastruct Pathol 1993;17:307–14.

65. Min KW, Clemens A, Bell J, Dick H. Malignant peripheral nerve sheath tumor and pheochromocytoma. A composite tumor of the adrenal. Arch Pathol Lab Med 1988;112:266–70.

65a. Miracco C, Montesco MC, Santopietro R, et al. Proliferative activity, angiogenesis, and necrosis in peripheral nerve sheath tumors: a quantitative evaluation for prognosis. Mod Pathol 1996;9:1108–17.

66. Mrak RE, Flanigan S, Collins CL. Malignant acoustic schwannoma. Arch Pathol Lab Med 1994;118:557–61.

67. Nambisan RN, Rao U, Moore R, Karakousis CP. Malignant soft tissue tumors of nerve sheath origin. J Surg Oncol 1984;25:268–72.

68. Ogawa K, Oguchi M, Yamabe H, Nakashima Y, Hamashima Y. Distribution of collagen type IV in soft tissue tumors. An immunohistochemical study. Cancer 1986;58:269–77.

69. Ordonez NG, Mahfouz SM, Mackay B. Synovial sarcoma: an immunohistochemical and ultrastructural study. Hum Pathol 1990;21:733–49.

70. Preston FW, Walsh WS, Clarke TH. Cutaneous neurofibromatosis (von Recklinghausen's disease): clinical manifestations and incidence of sarcoma in 61 male patients. Arch Surg 1952;64:813–27.

70a. Rao SK, Scheithauer BW, Nascimento AG. Cytokeratin expression in the glandular elements of synovial sarcomas and malignant peripheral nerve sheath tumors. Mod Pathol 1999 (in press).

71. Rey JA, Bello MJ, Kusak ME, de Campos JM, Pestana A. Involvement of 22q12 in a neurofibrosarcoma in

neurofibromatosis type 1. Cancer Genet Cytogenet 1993;66:28–32.

72. Riccardi VM, Elder DW. Multiple cytogenetic aberrations in neurofibrosarcomas complicating neurofibromatosis. Cancer Genet Cytogenet 1986;23:199–209.

73. Ricci A Jr, Parham DW, Woodruff JM, Callihan T, Green A, Erlandson RA. Malignant peripheral nerve sheath tumors arising from ganglioneuromas. Am J Surg Pathol 1984;8:19–29.

74. Sakaguchi N, Sano K, Makoto I, Baba T, Fukuzawa M, Hotchi M. A case of von Recklinghausen's disease with bilateral pheochromocytoma—malignant peripheral nerve sheath tumors of the adrenal and gastrointestinal autonomic nerve tumors. Am J Surg Pathol 1996;20:889–97.

75. Schaldenbrand JD, Appelman HD. Solitary solid stromal gastrointestinal tumors in von Recklinghausen's disease with minimal smooth muscle differentiation. Hum Pathol 1994;15:229–32.

76. Scheithauer BW, Halling KC, Nascimento AG, Hill EM, Sim FH, Katzmann JA. Neurofibroma and malignant peripheral nerve sheath tumor: a proliferation index and DNA ploidy study [Abstract]. Pathol Res Pract 1995;191:771.

76a. Seppala MT, Haltia MJ. Spinal malignant nerve sheath tumor or cellular schwannoma? A striking difference in prognosis. J Neurosurg 1993;79:528–32.

77. Shiu MH, Turnbull AD, Nori D, Hajdu S, Hilaris B. Control of locally advanced extremity soft tissue sarcomas by function-saving resection and brachytherapy. Cancer 1984;53:1385–92.

78. Sordillo PP, Helson L, Hajdu SI, et al. Malignant schwannoma—clinical characteristics, survival, and response to therapy. Cancer 1981;47:2503–9.

79. Sorensen SA, Mulvihill JJ, Nielsen A. Long-term follow-up of von Recklinghausen neurofibromatosis. Survival and malignant neoplasms. N Engl J Med 1986;314:1010–5.

80. Stefanko SZ, Vuzevski VD, Maas AI, Van Vroonhoven CC. Intracerebral malignant schwannoma. Acta Neuropathol 1986;71:321–5.

81. Storm FK, Eilber FR, Mirra J, Morton DL. Neurofibrosarcoma. Cancer 1980;45:126–9.

82. Stout AP. Tumors of the peripheral nervous system. Atlas of Tumor Pathology, Section II, Fascicle 6. Washington D.C.: Armed Forces Institute of Pathology, 1949.

83. Swanson PE, Scheithauer BW, Wick MR. Peripheral nerve sheath neoplasms: clinicopathologic and immunochemical observations. In: Rosen PP, Fechner RE, eds. Pathology annual. Stamford, CT: Appleton and Lange, 1995:1–82.

84. Swanson PE, Stanley MW, Scheithauer BW, Wick MR. Primary cutaneous leiomyosarcoma. A histologic and immunohistochemical study of 9 cases, with ultrastructural correlation. J Cutan Pathol 1988;15:129–41.

85. Taxy JB, Battifora H, Trujillo Y, Dorfman HD. Electron microscopy in the diagnosis of malignant schwannoma. Cancer 1981;48:1381–91.

86. Thomas JE, Piepgras DG, Scheithauer BW, Onofrio BM, Shives TC. Neurogenic tumors of the sciatic nerve. A clinicopathologic study of 35 cases. Mayo Clin Proc 1983;58:640–7.

87. Travis JA, Sandberg AA, Neff JR, Bridge JA. Cytogenetic findings in malignant Triton tumor. Genes Chromosomes Cancer 1994;9:1–7.
88. Tsuneyoshi M, Daimaru Y, Enjoji M. Malignant hemangiopericytoma and other sarcomas with hemangiopericytoma-like pattern. Pathol Res Pract 1984;178:446–53.
89. Tsuneyoshi M, Enjoji M. Primary malignant peripheral nerve tumor (malignant schwannomas). Acta Pathol Jpn 1979;29:363–75.
89a.Vauthey JN, Woodruff JM, Brennan MF. Extremity malignant peripheral nerve sheath tumors (neurogenic sarcomas): a 10-year experience. Ann Surg Oncol 1995;2:126–31.
90. Walker P, Dvorak AM. Gastrointestinal autonomic nerve (GAN) tumor: ultrastructural evidence for a newly recognized entity. Arch Pathol Lab Med 1986;110:309–16.
91. Walsh NM, Bodurtha A. Auerbach's myenteric plexus. A possible site or origin for gastrointestinal stromal tumors in von Recklinghausen's neurofibromatosis. Arch Pathol Lab Med 1990;114:522–5.
92. Weiss SW, Langloss JM, Enzinger FM. Value of S-100 protein in the diagnosis of soft tissue tumors with particular reference to benign and malignant Schwann cell tumors. Lab Invest 1983;49:299–308.
93. White HR Jr. Survival in malignant schwannoma. An 18-year study. Cancer 1971;27:720–9.
94. Wick MR, Swanson PE, Scheithauer BW, Manivel JC. Malignant peripheral nerve sheath tumor. An immunohistochemical study of 62 cases. Am J Clin Pathol 1987;87:425–33.
94a.Wong WM, Hirose T, Scheithauer BW, Schild SE, Gunderson LL. Malignant peripheral nerve sheath tumor: analysis of treatment outcome. Int J Radiat Oncology Biol Phys 1998;42:351–60.
95. Woodruff JM. The pathology and treatment of peripheral nerve sheath tumors and tumor-like conditions. CA Cancer J Clin 1993;43:290–308.
96. Woodruff JM, Horten BC, Erlandson RA. Pathology of peripheral nerves and paragangliomas. In: Silverberg SG, ed. Principles and practice of surgical pathology. New York: John Wiley and Sons, 1983:1503–20.
97. Woodruff JM, Selig AM, Crowley K, Allen PW. Schwannoma with malignant transformation. A rare, distinctive peripheral nerve tumor. Am J Surg Pathol 1994;18:882–95.
98. Yamashiro S, Nagashiro S, Mimata C, Kuratsu J, Ushio Y. Malignant trigeminal schwannoma associated with xeroderma pigmentosum—case report. Neurol Med Chir (Tokyo) 1994;34:817–20.
99. Yasuda T, Sobue G, Ito T, et al. Human peripheral nerve sheath neoplasm: expression of Schwann cell-related markers and their relation to malignant transformation. Muscle Nerve 1991;14:812–9.

Epithelioid MPNST

100. Alvira MM, Mandybur TK, Menefee MG. Light microscopic and ultrastructural observations of a metastasizing malignant epithelioid schwannoma. Cancer 1976;38:1977–82.
101. Axiotis CA, Merino MJ, Tsokos M, Yang JJ. Epithelioid malignant peripheral nerve sheath tumor with squamous differentiation: a light microscopic, ultrastructural, and immunohistochemical study. Surg Pathol 1990;3:301–8.
102. DiCarlo EF, Woodruff JM, Bansal M, Erlandson RA. The purely epithelioid peripheral nerve sheath tumor. Am J Surg Pathol 1986;10:478–90.
103. Laskin WB, Weiss SW, Brathauer GL. Epithelioid variant of malignant peripheral nerve sheath tumor (malignant epithelioid schwannoma). Am J Surg Pathol 1991;15:1136–45.
104. Lodding P, Kindblom LG, Angervall LG. Epithelioid malignant schwannoma. A study of 14 cases. Virchows Arch [A] 1986;409:433–51.
105. Taxy JB, Battifora H. Epithelioid schwannoma: diagnosis by electron microscopy. Ultrastruct Pathol 1981;2:19–24.
106. Woodruff JM, Selig AM, Crowley K, Allen PW. Schwannoma (neurilemoma) with malignant transformation. A rare, distinctive peripheral nerve tumor. Am J Surg Pathol 1994;18:882–95.

MPNST with Divergent Differentiation

107. Ambler MW. Striated muscle cells in the leptomeninges in cerebral dysplasia. Acta Neuropathol 1977;40:269–71.
108. Azzopardi JG, Eusebi V, Tison V, Betts BM. Neurofibroma with rhabdomyomatous differentiation: benign "Triton" tumour of the vagina. Histopathology 1983;7:561–72.
109. Bricklin AS, Rushton HW. Angiosarcoma of venous origin arising in the radial nerve. Cancer 1977;39:1556–8.
110. Brooks JJ. Malignant schwannomas with divergent differentiation including "Triton" tumor. In: William CJ, Krikouan JG, Green MR, Raghavan D, eds. Textbook of uncommon cancer. New York: John Wiley and Sons, 1988:653–68.
111. Brooks JJ, Freeman M, Enterline HT. Malignant Triton tumors. Natural history and immunohistochemistry of nine new cases with literature review. Cancer 1985;55:2543–9.
112. Brown DC, Theaker JM, Banks PM, Gatter KC, Mason DY. Cytokeratin expression in smooth muscle and smooth muscle tumors. Histopathology 1987;11:477–86.
113. Brown RW, Tornos C, Evans HL. Angiosarcoma arising from malignant schwannoma in a patient with neurofibromatosis. Cancer 1992;70:1141–4.
114. Chang Y, Dehner LP, Egbert B. Primary cutaneous rhabdomyosarcoma. Am J Surg Pathol 1990;14:977–82.
115. Chaudhuri B, Ronan SG, Manaligod JR. Angiosarcoma arising in a plexiform neurofibroma: a case report. Cancer 1980;46:605–10.
116. Christensen WN, Strong EW, Bains MS, Woodruff JW. Neuroendocrine differentiation in the glandular peripheral nerve sheath tumor. Pathologic distinction from the biphasic synovial sarcoma with glands. Am J Surg Pathol 1988;12:417–26.
117. Conway JD, Smith MB. Hemangio-endothelioma originating in a peripheral nerve. Report of a case. Ann Surg 1951;134:138–41.
118. Daimaru Y, Hashimoto H, Enjoji M. Malignant Triton tumors: a clinicopathologic and immunohistochemical study of nine cases. Hum Pathol 1984;15:768–77.

119. DeSchryver K, Santa Cruz DJ. So-called glandular schwannoma: ependymal differentiation in a case. Ultrastruct Pathol 1984;6:167–75.

120. Despres S, Doliveux P, Laurent M, Nezelof C. Neurofibrosarcome a differentiation glandulaire: a propus d'une observation. Arch Anat Pathol 1973;21:59–62.

121. Ducatman BS, Scheithauer BW. Malignant peripheral nerve sheath tumor with divergent differentiation. Cancer 1984;54:1049–57.

122. Garre C. Uber sekundar maligne Neurome. Beitr Z Klin Chir Z 1892;9:465–95.

123. Horstadius SD. The neural crest. Its properties and derivations in the light of experimental research. New York: Hafner Publishing Co., 1969.

124. Hruban RH, Shiu MH, Senie RT, Woodruff JM. Malignant peripheral nerve sheath tumors of the buttock and lower extremity. A study of 43 cases. Cancer 1990;66:1253–69.

125. Krumerman MS, Stingle W. Synchronous malignant glandular schwannomas in congenital neurofibromatosis. Cancer 1978;41:2444–51.

126. Lagace R. Triton tumor (malignant schwannoma with rhabdomyoblastic differentiation). Ultrastruct Pathol 1987;11:777–80.

127. Lederman SM, Martin EC, Laffey KT, Lefkowitch JH. Hepatic neurofibromatosis, malignant schwannoma, and angiosarcoma in von Recklinghausen's disease. Gastroenterology 1987;92:234–9.

128. Le Douarin NM, Smith J. Development of the peripheral nervous system from the neural crest. Ann Rev Cell Biol 1988;4:375–404.

129. Locatelli P. Formation de Membres Surnumeraires. CR Assoc des Anotomistes, 20 e reunion Turin, 1925:279–82.

130. Macaulay RA. Neurofibrosarcoma of the radial nerve in von Recklinghausen's disease with metastatic angiosarcoma. J Neurol Neurosurg Psychiatry 1978;41:474–8.

131. Masson P. Human tumors. Detroit: Wayne State University Press, 1970:1107–9.

132. Masson P. Recklinghausen's neurofibromatosis. Sensory neuromas and motor neuromas. Libman Anniversary Volumes 2. New York: International Press, 1932:793–802.

133. Masson P, Martin J. Rhabdomyomes des nerfs. Bull Assoc Fr Cancer 1938;27:751–67.

134. Meis-Kindblom JM, Kindblom LG, Enzinger FM. Angiosarcoma arising in von Recklinghausen's disease (NF1): report of additional cases.

135. Mierau GW, Berry PJ, Orsini EN. Small round cell neoplasms: can electron microscopy and immunohistochemical studies accurately subclassify them? Ultrastruct Pathol 1985;9:99–111.

136. Millstein DI, Tang CK, Campbell EW Jr. Angiosarcoma developing in a patient with neurofibromatosis (von Recklinghausen's disease). Cancer 1981;47:950–4.

137. Nikitin AY, Lennartz K, Pozharisski KM, Rajewsky MF. Rat model of the human "Triton" tumor: direct genetic evidence for the myogenic differentiation capacity of schwannoma cells using the mutant neu gene as a cell lineage marker. Differentiation 1991;48:33–42.

138. Ordonez NG, Mahfouz SM, Mackay B. Synovial sarcoma: an immunohistochemical and ultrastructural study. Hum Pathol 1990;21:733–49.

139. Prasad SB. von Recklinghausen's disease with angiosarcoma in a child. J Indian Med Assoc 1983;81:138–42.

140. Rose SC, Wilkins MJ, Birch R, Evans DJ. Malignant peripheral nerve sheath tumor with rhabdomyoblastic and glandular differentiation: immunohistochemical features. Histopathology 1992;21:287–90.

141. Rubinstein LJ. Tumeurs et hamartomes dans la neurofibromatose centrale. In: Michaux L, Feld M, eds. Les Phakomatoses cérébrales. Paris: SPEI Editeurs, 1963:427–51.

142. Russell DS, Rubinstein LJ. Pathology of tumours of the nervous system. 5th ed. Baltimore: Williams & Wilkins, 1989:769–84.

143. Schmidt D, Steen A, Voss C. Immunohistochemical study of rhabdomyosarcoma: unexpected staining with S-100 protein and cytokeratin [Letter]. J Pathol 1989;157:83.

144. Swanson P, Stanley ME, Scheithauer BW, Wick MR. Primary cutaneous leiomyosarcoma. A histologic and immunohistochemical study of 9 cases with ultrastructural correlation. J Cutan Pathol 1988;15:129–41.

145. Tomlinson FH, Scheithauer BW, Kelly PJ, Forbes GS. Subependymoma with rhabdomyosarcomatous differentiation: report of a case and literature review. Neurosurgery 1991;28:761–8.

146. Trassard M, LeDoussal V, Bui BN, Coindre JM. Angiosarcoma arising in a solitary schwannoma (neurilemoma) of sciatic nerve. Am J Surg Pathol 1996;20:1412–7.

147. Uri AK, Witzleben CL, Raney RB. Electron microscopy of glandular schwannoma. Cancer 1984;53:493–7.

148. Warner TF, Louie R. Malignant nerve sheath tumor containing endocrine cells. Am J Surg Pathol 1983;7:583–90.

149. Wong SY, Teh M, Tan YD, Best PV. Malignant glandular Triton tumor. Cancer 1991;67:1076–83.

150. Woodruff JM. Origin of Triton tumor [Letter]. Am J Dermatopathol 1993;15:411–2.

150a. Woodruff JM. Peripheral nerve tumors showing glandular differentiation (glandular schwannomas). Cancer 1976;37:2399–413.

151. Woodruff JM, Chernik N, Smith M, Millett W, Foote F. Peripheral nerve tumors with rhabdomyosarcomatous differentiation (malignant "Triton" tumors). Cancer 1973;32:426–39.

152. Woodruff JM, Christensen WN. Glandular peripheral nerve sheath tumors. Cancer 1993;72:3618–28.

153. Woodruff JM, Perino G. Non-germ cell or teratomatous malignant tumors showing additional rhabdomyoblastic differentiation, with emphasis on the malignant Triton tumor. Semin Diagn Surg Pathol 1994;11:69–81.

154. Yakulis R, Manack L, Murphy AI Jr. Postradiation malignant Triton tumor. A case report and review of the literature. Arch Pathol Lab Med 1996;120:541–8.

155. Zimmerman LE, Font RL, Anderson SR. Rhabdomyosarcomatous differentiation in malignant intraocular medulloepitheliomas. Cancer 1972;30:817–35.

Schwannoma with Malignant Transformation

156. Carstens PH, Schrodt GR. Malignant transformation of a benign encapsulated neurilemoma. Am J Clin Pathol 1969;51:144–9.

157. Fowler M. A malignant neurilemoma. Med J Aust 1955;1:236–7.

158. Franks AJ. Epithelioid neurilemoma of the trigeminal nerve: an immunohistochemical and ultrastructural study. Histopathology 1985;9:1339–50.
159. Hanada M, Tanaka T, Kanayama S, Takami M, Kimura M. Malignant transformation of intrathoracic ancient neurilemoma in a patient without von Recklinghausen's disease. Acta Pathol Jpn 1982;32:527–36.
160. Laskin WB, Weiss SW, Brathauer GL. Epithelioid variant of malignant peripheral nerve sheath tumor (malignant epithelioid schwannoma). Am J Surg Pathol 1991;15:1136–45.

161. Nayler SJ, Leiman G, Omar T, Cooper K. Malignant transformation in a schwannoma. Histopathology 1996;29:189–92.
162. Rasbridge SA, Browse NL, Tighe JR, Fletcher CD. Malignant nerve sheath tumor arising in a benign ancient schwannoma. Histopathology 1989;14:525–8.
163. Woodruff JM, Selig AM, Crowley K, Allen PW. Schwannoma with malignant transformation. A rare, distinctive peripheral nerve tumor. Am J Surg Pathol 1994;18:882–95.
164. Yousem SA, Colby TV, Urich H. Malignant epithelioid schwannoma arising in a benign schwannoma. A case report. Cancer 1985;55:2799–803.

MPNST Arising in Association with Ganglioneuroma or Ganglioneuroblastoma

165. Banks E, Yum M, Brodhecker C, Goheen M. A malignant peripheral nerve sheath tumor in association with a paratesticular ganglioneuroma. Cancer 1989;64:1738–42.
166. Chandrasoma P, Shibata D, Radin R, Brown LP, Koss M. Malignant peripheral nerve sheath tumor arising in an adrenal ganglioneuroma in an adult male homosexual. Cancer 1986;57:2022–5.
166a. Cozzutto C, Comelli A, Bandelloni R. Ectomesenchymoma. Virchows Arch [A] 1982;398:185–95.
167. Damiani S, Manetto V, Carrillo G, DiBlasi A, Nappi O, Eusebi V. Malignant peripheral nerve sheath tumor arising in a de novo ganglioneuroma. A case report. Tumori 1991;77:90–3.
168. Fletcher CD, Fernando IN, Braimbridge MV, McKee PH, Lyall JR. Malignant nerve sheath tumor arising in a ganglioneuroma. Histopathology 1988;12:445–8.
169. Ghali VS, Gold JE, Vincent RA, Cosgrove JM. Malignant peripheral nerve sheath tumor arising spontaneously from retroperitoneal ganglioneuroma: a case report, review of the literature, and immunohistochemical study. Hum Pathol 1992;23:72–5.
169a. Hajlvassiliou CA, Carachi E, Simpson WJ, Young DG. Ectomesenchymoma: one or two tumors? Case report and review of literature. J Ped Surg 1997;32:1351–5.
169b. Holimon JL, Rosenblum WI. "Gangliorhabdomyosarcoma": a tumor of ectomesenchyme. J Neurosurg 1971;34:417–22.
170. Karcioglu Z, Someren A, Mathes SJ. Ectomesenchymoma: a malignant tumor of migrating neural crest (ectomesenchyme) remnants showing ganglionic, schwannian, melanocytic, and rhabdomyoblastic differentiation. Cancer 1977;39:2486–96.
171. Kawamoto EH, Weidner N, Agostini RM, Jaffe R. Malignant ectomesenchymoma of soft tissue. Report of two cases and review of the literature. Cancer 1987;59:1791–802.

172. Keller SM, Papazoglou S, McKeever P, Baker A, Roth JA. Late occurrence of malignancy in a ganglioneuroma 19 years following radiation therapy to a neuroblastoma. J Surg Oncol 1984;25:227–31.
173. Kodet R, Kasthuri N, Marsden HB, Coad NA, Raafat F. Gangliorhabdomyosarcoma: a histopathological and immunohistochemical study of three cases. Histopathology 1986;10:181–93.
174. Miettinen M, Saari A. Pheochromocytoma combined with malignant schwannoma: unusual neoplasm of the adrenal medulla. Ultrastruct Pathol 1988;12:513–27.
175. Min KW, Clemens A, Bell J, Dick H. Malignant peripheral nerve sheath tumor and pheochromocytoma. A composite tumor of the adrenal. Arch Pathol Lab Med 1988;112:266–70.
175a. Mouton SC, Rosenberg HS, Cohen MC, Emms M. Malignant ectomesenchymoma in childhood. Ped Pathol Lab Med 1996;16:607–24.
175b. Naka A, Matsumoto S, Shirae T, Itoh T. Ganglioneuroblastoma associated with malignant mesenchymoma. Cancer 1975;36:1050–6.
176. Ricci A Jr, Parham DM, Woodruff JM, Callihan T, Green A, Erlandson RA. Malignant peripheral nerve sheath tumors arising from ganglioneuromas. Am J Surg Pathol 1984;8:19–29.
177. Sakaguchi N, Sano K, Ito M, Baba T, Fukuzawa M, Hotchi M. A case of von Recklinghausen's disease with bilateral pheochromocytoma—malignant peripheral nerve sheath tumors of the adrenal and gastrointestinal autonomic nerve tumors. Am J Surg Pathol 1996;20:889–97.
178. Shuangshoti S, Chutchavaree A. Parapharyngeal neoplasm of mixed mesenchymal and neuroepithelial origin. Arch Otolaryngol 1980;106:361–4.

Peripheral Neuroepithelioma

179. Abell MR, Hart WR, Olson JR. Tumors of the peripheral nervous system. Hum Pathol 1970;1:503–51.
180. Askin FB, Rosai J, Sibley RK, Dehner LP, McAlister WH. Malignant small cell tumor of the thoracopulmonary region in childhood. Cancer 1979;43:2438–51.
181. Bolen JW, Thorning D. Peripheral neuroepithelioma: a light and electron microscopic study. Cancer 1980;46:2456–62.
182. Cavazzana AO, Fassina AS, Ninfo V. Peripheral primitive neuroectodermal tumors. In: Ninfo V, Chung EB, Cavazzana AO, eds. Tumors and tumor-like lesions of soft tissues. New York: Churchill Livingston, 1991:229–58.
183. DiCarlo EF, Woodruff JM, Bansal M, Erlandson RA. The purely epithelioid malignant peripheral nerve sheath tumor. Am J Surg Pathol 1986;10:478–90.
184. Enzinger FM. Case twelve. In: Proceedings of Forty-Ninth Annual Anatomic Pathology Slide Seminar of the American Society of Clinical Pathologists. Chicago: ASCP, 1983:90–6.
185. Erlandson RA. Diagnostic transmission electron microscopy of tumors. New York: Raven Press, 1994:665–71.

186. Fellinger EJ, Garin-Chesa P, Glasser DB, Huvos AG, Rettig WJ. Comparison of cell surface antigen HBA71 (p30/32MIC2), neuron-specific enolase, and vimentin in the immunohistochemical analysis of Ewing's sarcoma of bone. Am J Surg Pathol 1992;16:746–55.

187. Fellinger EJ, Garin-Chesa P, Su SL, DeAngelis P, Lane JM, Rettig WJ. Biochemical and genetic characterization of HBA71 Ewing's sarcoma cell surface antigen. Cancer Res 1991;51:336–40.

188. Fellinger EJ, Garin-Chesa P, Triche TJ, Huvos AG, Rettig WJ. Immunohistochemical analysis of Ewing's sarcoma cell surface antigen p30/32MIC2. Am J Pathol 1991;139:317–35.

189. Garin-Chesa P, Fellinger EJ, Huvos AG, Rettig WJ, Beresford HR, Molamed MR. Immunohistochemical analysis of neural adhesion molecules (NCAM): differential expression in small round cell tumors of childhood and adolescence. Am J Pathol 1991;139:275–86.

190. Gonzalez-Crussi F, Wolfson SL, Misugi K, Nakajima T. Peripheral neuroectodermal tumors of the chest wall in childhood. Cancer 1984;54:2519–27.

191. Harper PG, Pringle J, Souhami RL. Neuroepithelioma—a rare malignant peripheral nerve tumor of primitive origin: report of two new cases and a review of the literature. Cancer 1981;48:2282–7.

192. Hashimoto H, Enjoji M, Nakajima T, Kiryu H, Daimaru Y. Malignant neuroepithelioma (peripheral neuroblastoma). A clinicopathologic study of 15 cases. Am J Surg Pathol 1983;7:309–18.

193. Hess E, Cohen C, DeRose PB, Yost BA, Costa MJ. Nonspecificity of p30/32MIC2 immunolocalization with the 013 monoclonal antibody in the diagnosis of Ewing's sarcoma: application of an algorithmic immunohistochemical analysis. Appl Immunohistochem 1997;5(2):94–103.

194. Jurgens H, Bier V, Harms D, et al. Malignant peripheral neuroectodermal tumors. A retrospective analysis of 42 patients. Cancer 1988;61:349–57.

195. Lattes R. Case 9. In: Soft tissue tumors. American Society of Clinical Pathologists. Chicago: ASCP, 1973:49–52.

196. Lieberman PH. Case twenty-one. In: Proceedings of the Forty-Fifth Annual Anatomic Pathology Slide Seminar of the American Society of Clinical Pathologists. Chicago: ASCP, 1979:100–5.

197. Linnoila RI, Tsokos M, Triche TJ, Marangos PJ, Chandra RS. Evidence for neural origin and PAS-positive variants of the malignant small cell tumor of thoracopulmonary region ("Askin tumor"). Am J Surg Pathol 1986;10:124–33.

198. Marina NM, Etcubanas E, Parham DM, Bowman LC, Green A. Peripheral primitive neuroectodermal tumor (peripheral neuroepithelioma) in children. A review of the St. Jude experience and controversies in diagnosis and management. Cancer 1989;64:1952–60.

199. Nesbitt KA, Vidone RA. Primitive neuroectodermal tumor (neuroblastoma) arising in sciatic nerve of a child. Cancer 1976;37:1562–70.

200. Nesland JM, Sobrinho-Simões MA, Holm R, Johannessen JV. Primitive neuroectodermal tumor (peripheral neuroblastoma). Ultrastruct Pathol 1985;9:59–64.

201. Papierz W, Alwasiak J, Kolasa P, et al. Primitive neuroectodermal tumors: ultrastructural and immunohistochemical studies. Ultrastruct Pathol 1995;19:147–66.

202. Pappo AS, Douglass EC, Meyer WH, Marina N, Parham DM. Use of HBA71 and anti-b2-microglobulin to distinguish neuroepithelioma from neuroblastoma. Hum Pathol 1993;24:880–5.

203. Penfield W. Tumors of the sheaths of the nervous system. In: Penfield W, ed. Cytology and cellular pathology of the nervous system. New York, 1932:953–90.

204. Schmidt D, Harms D, Burdach S. Malignant peripheral neuroectodermal tumours of childhood and adolescence. Virchows Arch [Pathol Anat] 1985;406:351–65.

205. Seemayar TA, Thelmo WL, Bolande RP, Wiglesworth FW. Peripheral neuroectodermal tumors. Perspect Pediatr Pathol 1975;2:151–72.

206. Stevenson AJ, Chatten J, Bertoni F, Miettinen M. CD99 (p30/32MIC2) neuroectodermal/Ewing's sarcoma antigen as an immunohistochemical marker. Appl Immunohistochem 1994;2(4):231–40.

207. Stout AP. Case 6. In: Seminar on tumors of the soft tissues. American Society of Clinical Pathologists. Chicago: ASCP, 1953:18–9.

208. Stout AP. A tumor of the ulnar nerve. Proc NY Pathol Soc 1918;18:2–11.

209. Stout AP. Tumors of the peripheral nerve system. Atlas of Tumor Pathology, 1st Series, Fascicle 6. Washington, D.C.: Armed Forces Institute of Pathology, 1949.

210. Stout AP, Murray MR. Neuroepithelioma of the radial nerve with a study of its behaviour in vitro. Rev Canad de Biol 1942;1:651–9.

211. Turc-Carel C, Aurias A, Mugneret F, et al. Chromosomes in Ewing's sarcoma. I. An evaluation of 85 cases of remarkable consistency of t(11:22)(q24:q12). Cancer Genet Cytogenet 1988;32:229–38.

212. Voss BL, Pysher TJ, Humphrey BG. Peripheral neuroepithelioma in childhood. Cancer 1984;54:3059–64.

213. Whang-Peng J, Triche TJ, Knutset T, Miser J, Kao-Shan S, Tsai S. Cytogenetic characterization of selected small round cell tumor of childhood. Cancer Genet Cytogenet 1986;21:185–208.

Malignant Granular Cell Tumor

214. Al-Sarraf M, Loud AV, Vaitkevicius VK. Malignant granular cell tumor. Histochemical and electron microscopic study. Arch Pathol 1971;91:550–8.

215. Busanny-Caspari Von W, Hammar CH. Zur Malignitat der sogenannten Myoblastenmyome. Zentralblatt Fur Pathologie und Pathologische Anatomie 1958;98:401–6.

216. Cadotte M. Malignant granular cell myoblastoma. Cancer 1974;33:1417–22.

217. Ceelen von W. åber die Natur der sogenannten Myoblastenmyome (zugleich ein Bericht über eine maligne Myoblastengeschwulst). Zentralblatt für Pathologie und Pathologische Anatomie 1949;85:289–300.

218. Chang Y, Dehner LP, Egbert B. Primary cutaneous rhabdomyosarcoma. Am J Surg Pathol 1990;14:977–82.

219. Chetty R, Kalan MR. Malignant granular cell tumor of the breast. J Surg Oncol 1992;49:135–7.

220. Christopherson WH, Foote FW Jr, Stewart FW. Alveolar soft part sarcomas. Structurally characteristic tumors of uncertain histogenesis. Cancer 1952;5:100–11.

221. Crawford ES, DeBakcy ME. Granular cell myoblastoma: two unusual cases. Cancer 1953;6:786–9.

222. Dunnington JH. Granular cell myoblastoma of the orbit. Arch Ophthalmol 1948;40:14–22.

223. Finkel G, Lane B. Granular cell variant of neurofibromatosis: ultrastructure of benign and malignant tumors. Hum Pathol 1982;13:959–63.

224. Franzen S, Stenkvist B. Diagnosis of granular cell myoblastoma by fine-needle aspiration biopsy. Acta Pathol Microbiol Scand 1968;72:391–5.

225. Gamboa LG. Malignant granular cell myoblastoma. Arch Pathol 1955;60:663–8.

226. Geisinger KR, Kawamoto EH, Marshall RB, Ahl ET, Cooper MR. Aspiration exfoliative cytology including ultrastructure of a malignant granular-cell tumor. Acta Cytologica 1985;29:593–7.

227. Gleason-Jordan IO, Mirra JM, Mahendra T, Pathmarajah C. Case report 676: malignant granular cell tumor (schwannoma, myoblastoma), disseminated. Skeletal Radiol 1991;20:529–32.

228. Haustein von UF. Malignes metastasierendes Granularzellmyblastom Abrikosow mit symptomatische Dermatomyositis. Dermatologische Monatsschrift 1974;160:318–28.

229. Hunter DT, Dewar JP. Malignant granular-cell myoblastoma: report of a case and review of literature. Am Surg 1960;26:554–9.

230. Hurrell MA, McLean C, Desmond P, Tress BM, Kaye A. Malignant granular cell tumour of the sciatic nerve. Australas Radiol 1995;39:86–9.

230a. Fanburg-Smith JC, Meis-Kindblom JM, Fante R, Kindblom LG. Malignant granular cell tumor of soft tissue. Diagnostic criteria and clinicopathologic correlation. Am J Surg Pathol 1998;22:779–94.

231. Kindblom LG, Olsson KM. Malignant granular cell tumor. A clinicopathologic and ultrastructural study of a case. Pathol Res Pract 1981;172:384–93.

232. Kirschner H. Uber einen Fall von maligne entartetem myoblastenmyom de mamma. Bruns' Beitrage zur Klinischen Chirugie 1962;204:87–94.

233. Klima M, Peters J. Malignant granular cell tumor. Arch Pathol Lab Med 1987;111:1070–3.

234. Kubac G, Doris I, Ondro M, Davey PW. Malignant granular cell myoblastoma with metastatic cardiac involvement: case report and echocardiogram. Am Heart J 1980;100:227–9.

235. Kuchemann Von K. Malignes Granuläres Neurom (Granularzell-myoblastom). Fallbericht und Literaturfbersicht. Zentrablatt für Pathologie und Pathologische Anatomie 1971;114:426–34.

236. Kurtin PJ, Bonin DM. Immunohistochemical demonstration of the lysosome associated glycoprotein CD 68 (KP-1) in granular cell tumors and schwannomas. Hum Pathol 1994;25:1172–8.

237. Lieberman PH, Brennan MF, Kimmel M, Erlandson RA, Garin-Chesa P, Flehinger BY. Alveolar soft-part sarcoma. A clinicopathologic study of half a century. Cancer 1989;63:1–13.

238. MacKenzie DH. Malignant granular cell myoblastoma. J Clin Pathol 1967;20:739–42.

239. Madhaven M, Aurora AL, Sen SB. Malignant granular cell myoblastoma—report of a case. Indian J Cancer 1974;11:360–3.

240. Magori von A, Szegvari M. Rezidivierender und metastasierender Abrikossoff—Tumor der Vulva. Zentralbl Allg Pathol 1973;117:265–73.

241. Mierau GW, Berry PJ, Orsini EN. Small round cell neoplasms: can electron microscopy and immunohisto-chemical studies accurately subclassify them? Ultrastruct Pathol 1985;9:99–111.

242. Nitze von H. Das sogenannte Myoblastenmyom und seine Maligne Verlaufsform. Z Laryngol Rhinol Otol 1966;45:740–7.

243. Obiditsch-Mayer I, Salzer-Kuntschik M. Malignes, "gekorntzelliges Neurom" sogenanntes, Myoblastenmyom, des Oesophagus. Beit Pathol Anat 1961;125:357–73.

244. O'Donovan DG, Kell P. Malignant granular cell tumor with intraperitoneal dissemination. Histopathology 1989;14:417–9.

245. Powell EB. Granular cell myoblastoma. Arch Pathol 1946;42:517–24.

246. Ravich A, Stout AP, Ravich RA. Malignant granular cell myoblastoma involving the urinary bladder. Ann Surg 1945;121:361–72.

247. Remaggi PL, Galetti G, Balli R. Considerazioni istomorfologiche sui mioblastomiomi maligni in occasione di uni caso interessante il massiccio maxillofacciale. Minerva Otorinolaringologica 1968;18:275–86.

248. Robertson AJ, McIntosh W, Lamont P, Guthrie W. Malignant granular cell tumour (myoblastoma) of the vulva: report of a case and review of the literature. Histopathology 1981;5:69–79.

249. Ross RC, Miller TR, Foote FW Jr. Malignant granular cell myoblastoma. Cancer 1952;5:112–21.

250. Salvadori B, Talamazzi F. Sul mioblastomioma granulocellulare maligno. Tumori 1967;53:645–9.

251. Saperstein AL, Lusskin R, Doniguian AE, Thomas PA, Battista AF. Malignant granular cell tumor mimicking herniated nucleus pulposus. Clin Orthop 1996;324:244–50.

252. Schmidt D, Steen A, Voss C. Immunohistochemical study of rhabdomyosarcoma: unexpected staining with S-100 protein and cytokeratin [Letter]. J Pathol 1989;157:83.

253. Shimamura K, Osamura RY, Ueyama Y, et al. Malignant granular cell tumor of the right sciatic nerve. Cancer 1984;53:524–9.

254. Shipkey FH, Lieberman PH, Foot FW, Stewart FW. Ultrastructure of alveolar soft part sarcoma. Cancer 1964;17:821–30.

255. Simsir A, Osborne BM, Greenebaum E. Malignant granular cell tumor: a case report and review of the recent literature. Hum Pathol 1996;27:853–8.

256. Steffelaar JW, Nap M, Haelst UJ. Malignant granular cell tumor: report of a case with special reference to carcinoembryonic antigen. Am J Surg Pathol 1982;6:665–72.

257. Suster S, Rosen LB, Sanchez JL. Granular leiomyosarcoma of the skin. Am J Dermatopathol 1988;10:234–9.

258. Svejda J, Horn V. A disseminated granular cell pseudotumour: so-called metastasizing granular cell myoblastoma. J Pathol Bacteriol 1958;76:343–8.

259. Troncoso P, Ordonez N, Raymond A, Mackay B. Malignant granular cell tumor: immunocytochemical and ultrastructural observations. Ultrastruct Pathol 1988;12:137–44.

260. Usui M, Ishii S, Yamawaki S, Sasaki T, Minami A, Hizawa K. Malignant granular cell tumor of the radial nerve: an autopsy observation with electron microscopic and tissue culture studies. Cancer 1977;39:1547–55.

261. Uzoaru I, Firfer B, Ray V, Hubbard-Shepard M, Rhee H. Malignant granular cell tumor. Arch Pathol Lab Med 1992;116:206–8.

12

SECONDARY NEOPLASIA

This chapter deals primarily with involvement of peripheral nerve by other than primary neoplasms. The spectrum of involvement is broad, ranging from carcinoma, sarcoma, and melanoma to hemopoietic neoplasia. The mechanism of nerve involvement varies from direct extension of nearby neoplasms to metastasis from a remote primary. Also included is a discussion of metastasis to nerve sheath tumors.

METASTASES AND DIRECT EXTENSION OF NEOPLASMS TO NERVE

Definition. Involvement of a nerve is by direct extension from a nearby tumor or by metastasis from a distant primary. The tumor may involve one or more compartments of nerve.

General Comments. Since early descriptions of nerve involvement by infiltrating or metastatic neoplasms (19,39), its occurrence in association with carcinoma, sarcoma, neurotropic melanoma, and leukemia-lymphoma has become increasingly recognized. Depending in large part upon the nature of the neoplasm, patterns of nerve involvement vary. They include simple compression or encompassment of nerve, infiltration of epineurial tissue, perineurial extension, and involvement of the endoneurium (5). Whereas small nerve involvement is common, secondary disease affecting large nerves, such as the sciatic, is not.

The "perineurial space" serves as the primary conduit for spread of infiltrating malignant tumors within peripheral nerve. It is the anatomic region most often involved when invasion of small nerves is noted in surgical specimens. Although only a potential space, it is readily accessed by infiltrating tumor due to the loose attachment of perineurium to surrounding epineurium. Although the space was once thought to be lymphatic (25), no lining cells are demonstrable. It is, nonetheless, a potential space, one demonstrated to communicate with the subarachnoid space in experiments involving the injection of dyes (36,43) and local anesthetic (46). It is not only by way of the perineurial space that malignant cells, notably carcinoma cells, may enter a nerve. Tumor can also infiltrate the perivascular sleeve of the transperineurial arterial system whereby arterioles pass into the endoneurium to link epineurial nutrient vessels with the endoneurial capillary plexus (7). It is by this route that neoplastic cells, particularly lymphoma-leukemia cells, gain direct access to the endoneurium. Carcinoma and sarcoma far less often involve endoneurium. The patterns of peripheral nerve involvement exhibited by carcinoma, sarcoma, melanoma, and leukemia-lymphoma are sufficiently distinctive to warrant their separate discussion.

Carcinoma

General Comments. Carcinomas are by far the most common neoplasms secondarily involving nerve. In the majority of instances neural involvement is by direct extension into perineurium or the potential space surrounding it. Although most commonly observed in association with adenocarcinoma of the prostate, adenoid cystic carcinoma of salivary glands (fig. 12-1), and ductal carcinoma of the breast, perineurial invasion may be seen with virtually any type of carcinoma (23). One study of head and neck carcinomas (4) found the incidence of perineurial invasion in squamous carcinomas of the skin, lip, and oral mucosa to be as high as that of adenoid cystic carcinoma. Particularly detailed descriptions of tumor spread are found in the head and neck literature (4,13–15,23,28,38).

Having gained access to the perineurial space, tumors may track proximal or distal, i.e., toward or away from the central nervous system (CNS). A study of 83 squamous carcinomas of the head and neck associated with neural invasion (13) found the size of the primary tumor to be at least 2.5 cm, and its extent of perineurial spread to be a distance of 1 cm or less. Growth and spread of tumor within the perineurial space, whether proximal, distal, or both, is continuous and unassociated with "skip areas." Extensive proximal spread is of particular clinical importance in that it brings the tumor within reach of the CNS, thus setting the stage for leptomeningeal spread (meningeal

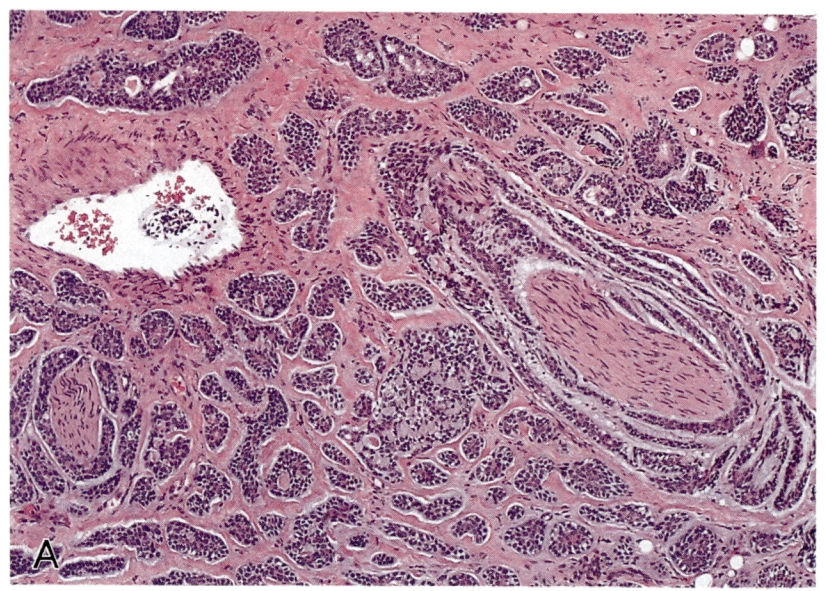

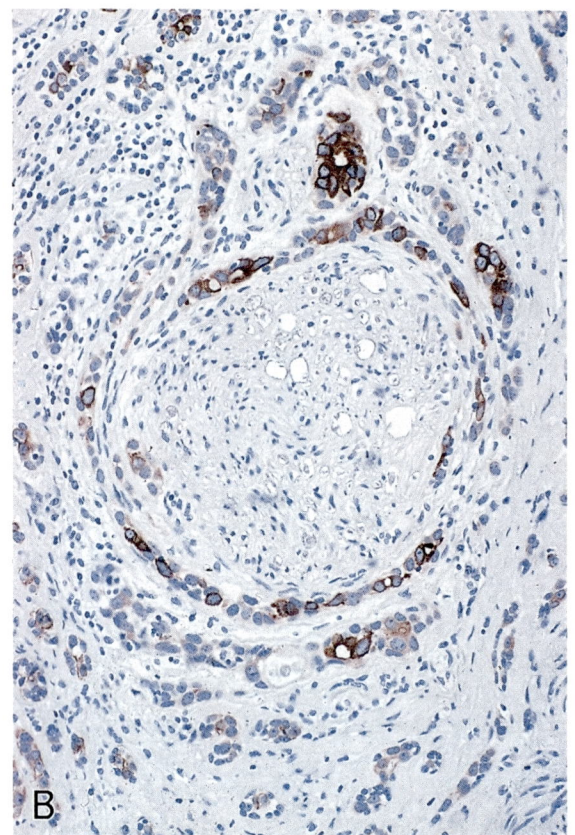
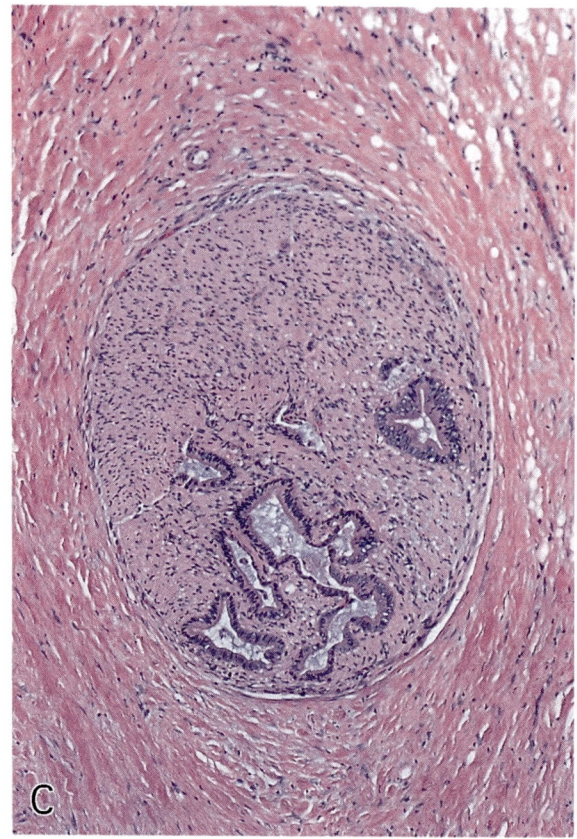

Figure 12-1
CARCINOMA INVOLVING PERIPHERAL NERVE

Adenoid cystic carcinoma (A,B). Invasion of the epineurium and perineurial space is a conspicuous feature of this tumor. Focal endoneurial spread is most apparent on a cytokeratin stain (B). Cholangiocarcinoma showing extension within the endoneurium (C).

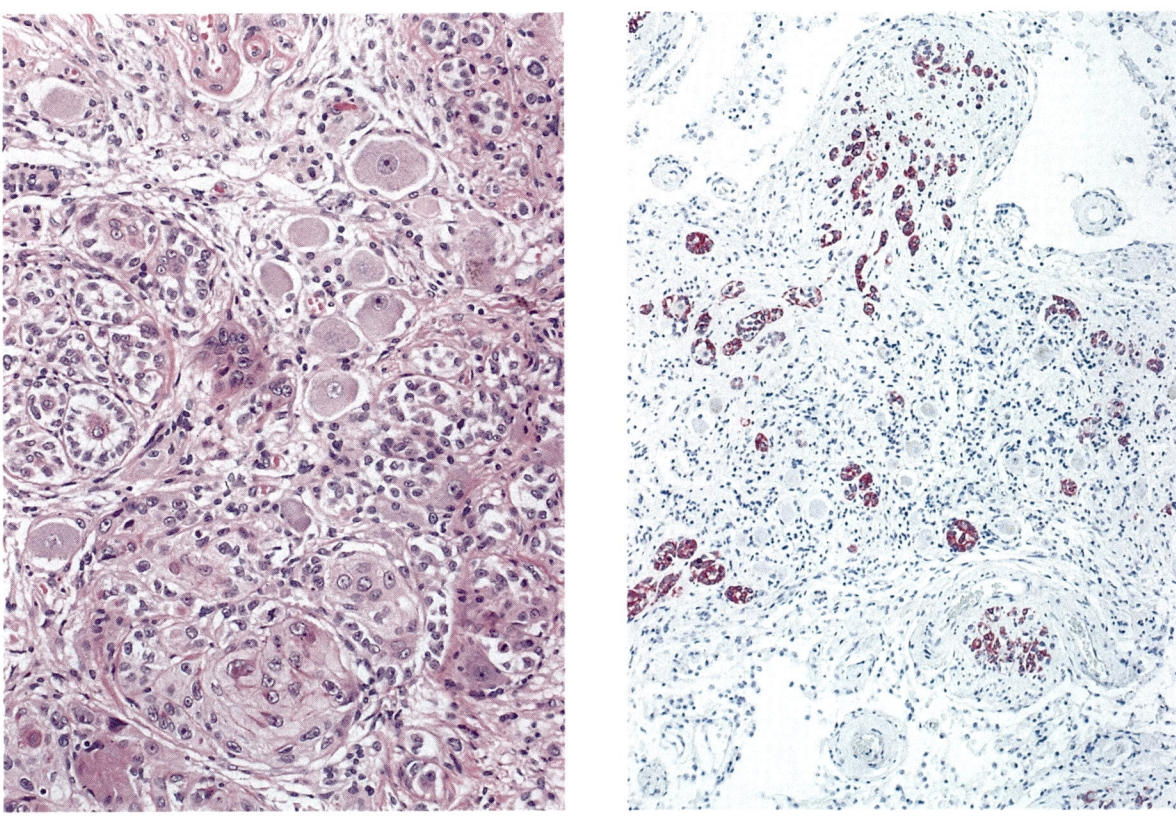

Figure 12-2
CARCINOMA INVOLVING SENSORY GANGLION
Note extension of carcinoma (left) into exiting nerve fascicle and on immunostain for keratin (right).

carcinomatosis) (4,29). Carcinomas uncommonly involve the endoneurium (3,4,23,38). Possible routes of endoneurial invasion include direct extension through perineurium, as well as growth of tumor within perivascular sleeves of the transperineurial arteriolar system (7). Tumoral compression of such vessels may underlie the occasional finding of associated nerve necrosis (15). Whereas endoneurium of peripheral nerves is infrequently involved by carcinoma (fig. 12-1), sensory ganglia are less resistant (fig. 12-2) (32). Their susceptibility to metastasis is attributed to their fenestrated vasculature, a feature which also underlies the lack of a blood-ganglion barrier in ganglia.

Clinical Features. Carcinomatous involvement of nerves may or may not be clinically apparent. Subjective complaints of burning, stinging, and shooting pain in a region known to be affected by a primary tumor (4) are highly suggestive of neoplastic extension along a nerve. Numbness in the distribution of a nerve is even more significant (4). Sensory symptoms may precede recognition of a primary tumor by months. Conversely, relatively asymptomatic persistence of carcinoma within nerves has been reported to occur years after removal of the primary tumor (4).

Differential Diagnosis. Perineurial or endoneurial nerve involvement by benign proliferative epithelial processes has been reported. Examples include florid fibrocystic disease of breast (47), benign prostatic hypertrophy (12), vasitis nodosa (55), and benign gallbladder lesions (15a). Glandular inclusions of nerve in normal tissue are also rarely seen, such as in prostate (12) or pancreas (18). The process may occur spontaneously or, as in the case of vasitis nodosa (fig. 12-3), may be a postoperative phenomenon wherein reactive epithelial cells presumably gain access to the nerve through the traumatically disrupted perineurial sheath. As a rule, affected nerves are small.

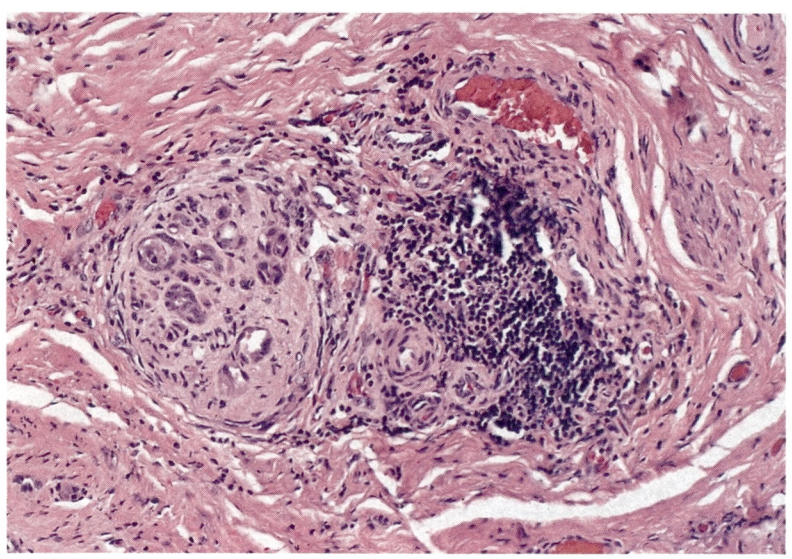

Figure 12-3
BENIGN INTRANEURAL
GLANDULAR INCLUSIONS
An example of this phenomenon is vasitis nodosa. (Courtesy of Dr. P. Johnson, Tucson, Arizona.)

Sarcoma

Not surprisingly sarcomas secondarily affecting peripheral nerve most often originate in surrounding soft tissue. The frequency and mechanism of nerve involvement were addressed by Barber et al. (5) in a study of 98 extremities amputated for soft tissue sarcoma. Thirty-nine percent were found to grossly affect peripheral nerve. The manner in which they did so ranged from simple displacement, to firm adherence, encasement without invasion and, in 10 percent of cases, to presumed nerve invasion based on the presence of localized or diffuse nerve enlargement. Histologic confirmation of neural invasion was apparent in 11 percent of cases, and invasion was limited to the epineurium in over half. No correlation could be made with symptoms, which included pain, numbness, weakness, palsy, and paresthesias. Of the 50 patients with such complaints, symptoms could be explained on the basis of gross and microscopic findings in only 46 percent; in 27 percent of cases with histologically documented neural invasion, there were no corresponding neurologic symptoms.

Invasion of the fascicles of large peripheral nerves by soft tissue sarcoma is generally associated with a high-grade tumor. In most instances the tumor destroys the epineurium and infiltrates perineurial space (fig. 12-4, left). Endoneurial involvement is far less common (fig. 12-4, right). Upon gaining access to the "perineurial space,"

sarcomas may extend great distances. For example, Barber et al. (5) described a high-grade fibrosarcoma which extended within the median nerve from the level of the wrist to within 2.5 cm of the brachial plexus. We have observed a similar case (fig. 12-3), an angiosarcoma of pelvic soft tissues which entered the perineurial space of small nerves, extended within the space into the right sciatic nerve above the level of the sciatic foramen, descended along the sciatic nerve in the buttock and thigh for a distance of 25 cm, and continued within the tibial nerve to a point 2 cm above the ankle. Both nerves were markedly enlarged due to circumferential epineurial expansion as well as to limited invasion of perineurium (fig. 12-5). Such extensive invasion typically results in cylindrical nerve enlargement. In the few examples of extensive transneural spread that we have studied, all nerve compartments, including endoneurium, were involved by sarcoma. Secondary involvement of nerve by high-grade sarcoma may lead to parenchymal hemorrhage and necrosis. On rare occasion, the result is focal, near-total destruction of a major nerve and a profound functional deficit.

Sarcomas primary in epineurium are rare. We have observed an example of clear cell sarcoma of the sciatic nerve, grossly resembling a malignant peripheral nerve sheath tumor (MPNST), but growing exclusively in an extrafascicular pattern (fig. 12-6).

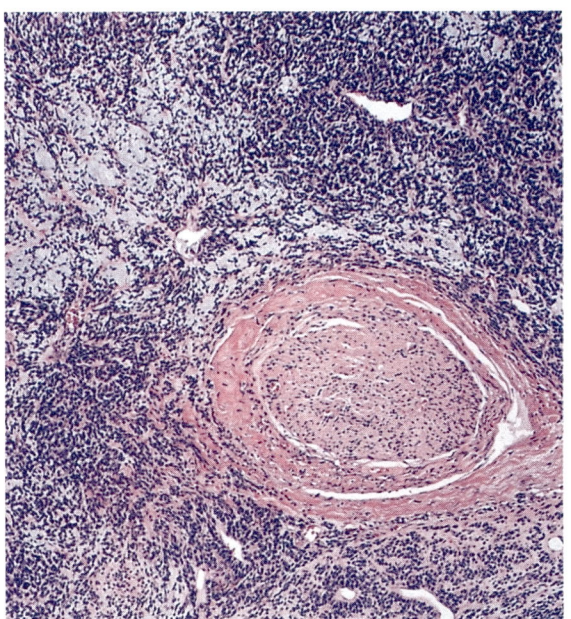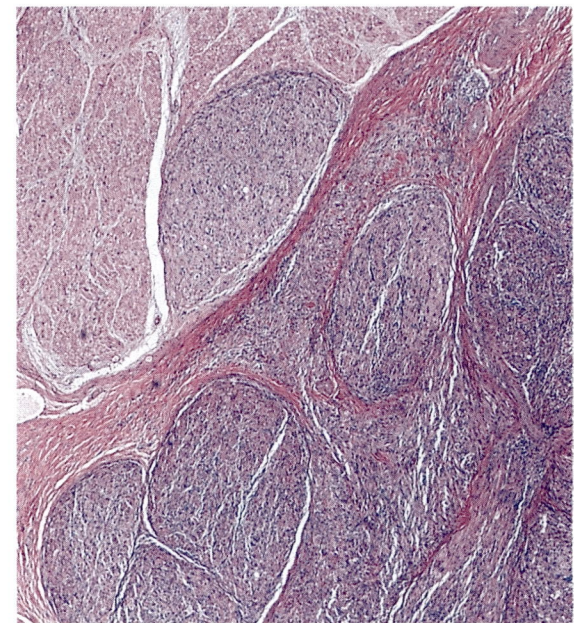

Figure 12-4
SARCOMA INVADING NERVE SHOWS PRIMARILY EPINEURIAL INVOLVEMENT
Involvement of epineurium is far more often secondary from a surrounding soft tissue tumor than a primary process. Secondary involvement is illustrated by an example of a large hemangiopericytoma of the brachial plexus region (left). Sarcomas such as this leiomyosarcoma of the pelvis in a 54-year-old female (right) only infrequently invade the endoneurium.

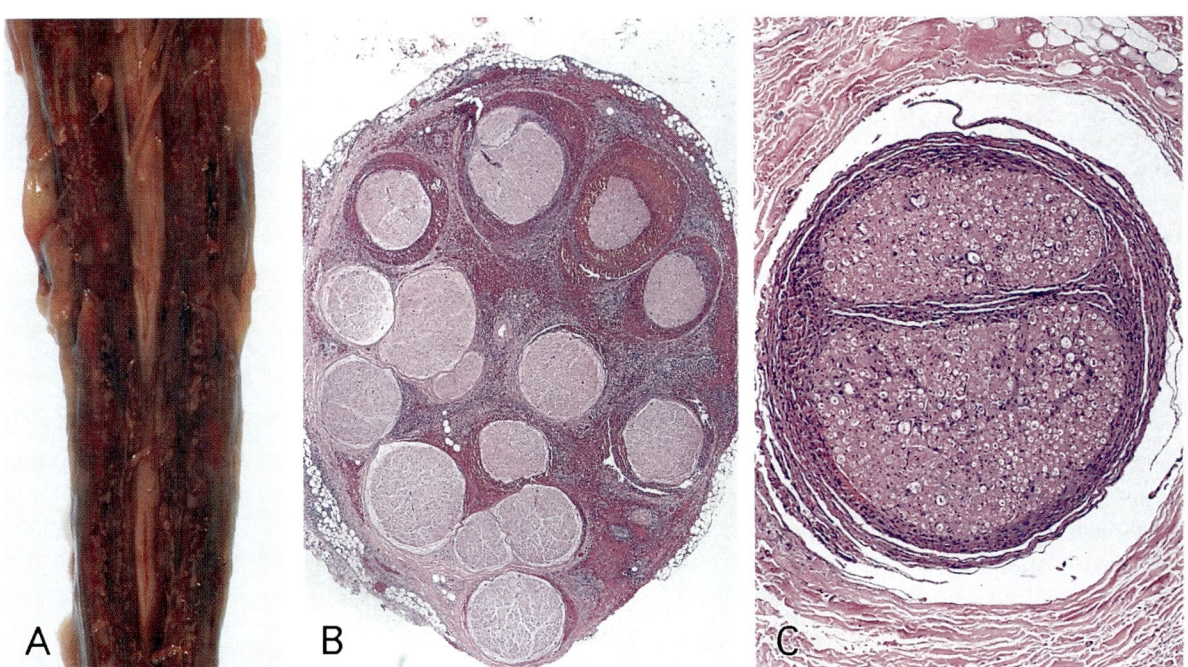

Figure 12-5
ANGIOSARCOMA INVOLVING NERVE
This example arising in the rectal wall of an adult male showed dramatic distal extension in sciatic nerve perineurium and epineurium to the level of the tibial nerve (A). Cross sections of the tibial nerve (B) show spread of tumor along perineurium (B) with general sparing of endoneurium (C).

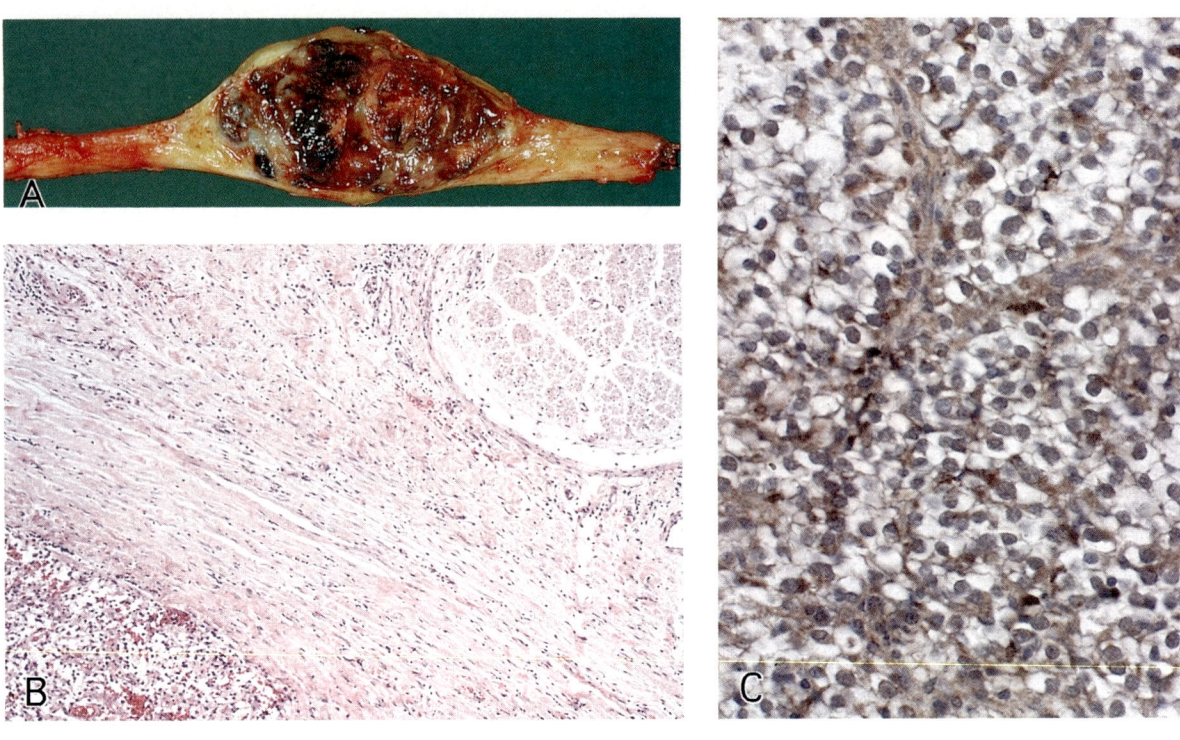

Figure 12-6
SARCOMA WITHIN EPINEURIUM

The occurrence of sarcoma within epineurium is illustrated by a clear cell sarcoma arising in the sciatic nerve of a 13-year-old female. Although the tumor grossly resembled MPNST (A), its pattern of growth was almost entirely extrafascicular (B). The histology and its HMB-45 immunoreactivity was typical of clear cell sarcoma (C). The lesion subsequently metastasized to an adrenal gland.

Neurotropic Melanoma

General Comments. First described by Conley et al. (17), desmoplastic melanoma is a spindle cell variant of cutaneous melanoma associated with inconspicuous, junctional, intraepidermal aggregates of atypical melanocytes, and an invasive, nonpigmented, and variably collagenized component. Sites primarily affected are the head and neck (8,31). Desmoplasia is thought to reflect the capacity of invasive melanoma cells to undergo "adaptive fibroplasia" (17,48,49). Ultrastructurally, such cells contain both well-developed rough endoplasmic reticulum and, in many but not all instances, rare melanosomes (26). Cytoplasmic intermediate filaments and microtubules may also be seen (51). Reed and Leonard (Reed and Leonard, oral communication, 1979) first brought attention to a subset of desmoplastic melanomas exhibiting neurotropism, i.e., invasion and extension along peripheral nerve, and coined the term neurotropic melanoma. Such tumors have since been well characterized (1,26,27,31,33–35,37,41,

51–53). They arise in sun-exposed skin of the head and neck, often lack a recognizable intraepidermal (in situ) component, and occasionally extend along peripheral nerves for significant distances. Some exhibit intracranial spread. Cells of both ordinary desmoplastic melanoma and the neurotropic type exhibit "neuroid" features, as evidenced by a tendency to form "nerve-like" cell bundles and a pericellular basement membrane (22,51).

Clinical Features. Neurotropic melanomas show a distinct tendency to affect males, in a ratio of 2 to 1. Mean patient age in a reported group of 37 patients was 56 years (31,41,51–53). Eighty-four percent of these tumors arose in the head and neck. In decreasing order of frequency affected sites were lip, temple, inferior dental nerve, forehead, cheek, neck, ear, nose, buccal mucosa, and chin. Other sites included the lower extremity and vulva. Sun exposure was a common denominator. Although occasional examples presented with peripheral nerve impairment or as a mass associated with neuropathy (31), the clinical presentation of the neurotropic tumors did not differ from that of ordinary desmoplastic melanoma. Neurotropic melanomas are highly malignant, showing a propensity to local recurrence and metastasis. Of the 37 cases referred to above, approximately two thirds of the patients developed local recurrences. In addition, roughly 50 percent died of disease, often with metastasis, or were terminally ill with tumor. Deaths occurred between 19 months and 9 years after initial diagnosis. The lung and brain were frequent sites for metastasis, whereas regional lymph nodes were only infrequently involved.

Histologic Findings. Morphologic features of neurotropic melanoma include strands, fascicles, or nodules of variably atypical, amelanotic spindle cells forming a poorly circumscribed dermal and occasionally subcutaneous infiltrate. Overlying epidermis or squamous mucosa often contains atypical basal melanocytes. The neoplastic nuclei are elongate and exhibit either uniformly dense or marginated chromatin with prominent nucleoli. Cytoplasm is moderate to abundant, faintly eosinophilic, afibrillar, and nonstriated. Cell margins are often ill-defined. Epithelioid and multinucleate tumor cells may be seen and mitoses are usually evident. The intercellular stroma is variably collagenized. Invasion of nerves by fascicles of tumor cells is best seen in deep portions of the tumor. Affected nerves, whether small or large (fig. 12-7), retain their overall shape but appear enlarged by layers of spindle tumor cells filling the perineurial space and occasionally involving endoneurium. In most instances affected nerves are surrounded by layers or nodules of neoplastic cells (fig. 12-7C). Given their hyperchromasia and larger nuclear size, tumor cells are readily distinguished from normal Schwann cells (fig. 12-7A).

Immunohistochemical Findings. Usually, but not invariably, the tumor cells of neurotropic melanoma are immunoreactive for S-100 protein (fig. 12-7B) (37a). Unlike ordinary cutaneous melanomas, desmoplastic melanomas are typically HMB-45 negative (37a).

Ultrastructural Findings. At the ultrastructural level, the amelanotic, plump spindle cells of neurotropic melanoma feature abundant rough endoplasmic reticulum, intermediate filaments, scant melanosomes, and cytoplasmic processes, often with focal basement membranes and rudimentary cell junctions (26).

Differential Diagnosis. The differential diagnosis of neurotropic melanoma includes MPNST as well as soft tissue sarcomas secondarily involving nerve. It is uncommon to find *MPNSTs* confined to the substance of a nerve and lacking significant extrafascicular extension. As a rule, the distinction between neurotropic melanoma and MPNST is difficult. Helpful clues include the presence in neurotropic melanoma cells of amphophilic cytoplasm, larger and more elongate nuclei, and a stronger and more diffuse reactivity for S-100 protein. Neurotropic melanomas occasionally involve cranial nerves. Although in the past such examples were often erroneously regarded as MPNSTs (20,42), the cytologic features of most are indistinguishable from neurotropic melanoma. Furthermore, several were associated with an overlying, longstanding, pigmented skin lesion (31). The current approach is to regard most cranial nerve tumors of this description as nerve-centered examples of neurotropic melanoma. The malignant epithelioid schwannoma of superficial soft tissues described by Enzinger and Weiss (24) is now also regarded as a neurotropic melanoma.

As previously noted, invasion of a peripheral nerve by a *soft tissue sarcoma* usually represents direct extension from a nearby, sizable, high-grade soft tissue neoplasm. It is not readily mistaken for a tumor of cutaneous origin, since primary neurotropic melanomas are rarely larger than 2 to 3 cm. Furthermore, most sarcomas invasive of nerve destroy neural tissue rather than cause nerve enlargement with preservation of its normal contour, as is the case with neurotropic melanoma. Lastly, when subject to immunohistochemical and ultrastructural study, the differentiation of most sarcomas becomes apparent.

Lymphoma-Leukemia

Mononeuropathies or polyneuropathies are commonly observed in association with hemopoietic tumors, which may be localized or widespread and involve nerve roots, ganglia, and cranial or peripheral nerves (fig. 12-8) (11,45). Microscopically, the process is often diffuse but nonuniform in distribution. Epineurial invasion may be seen but, unlike in carcinomatous involvement of peripheral nerve, infiltrates often affect the subperineurial zone, endoneurial

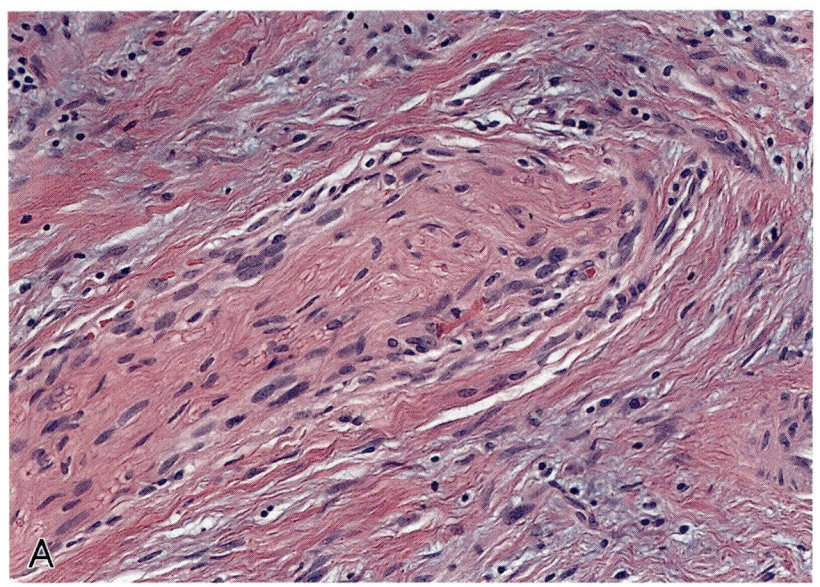

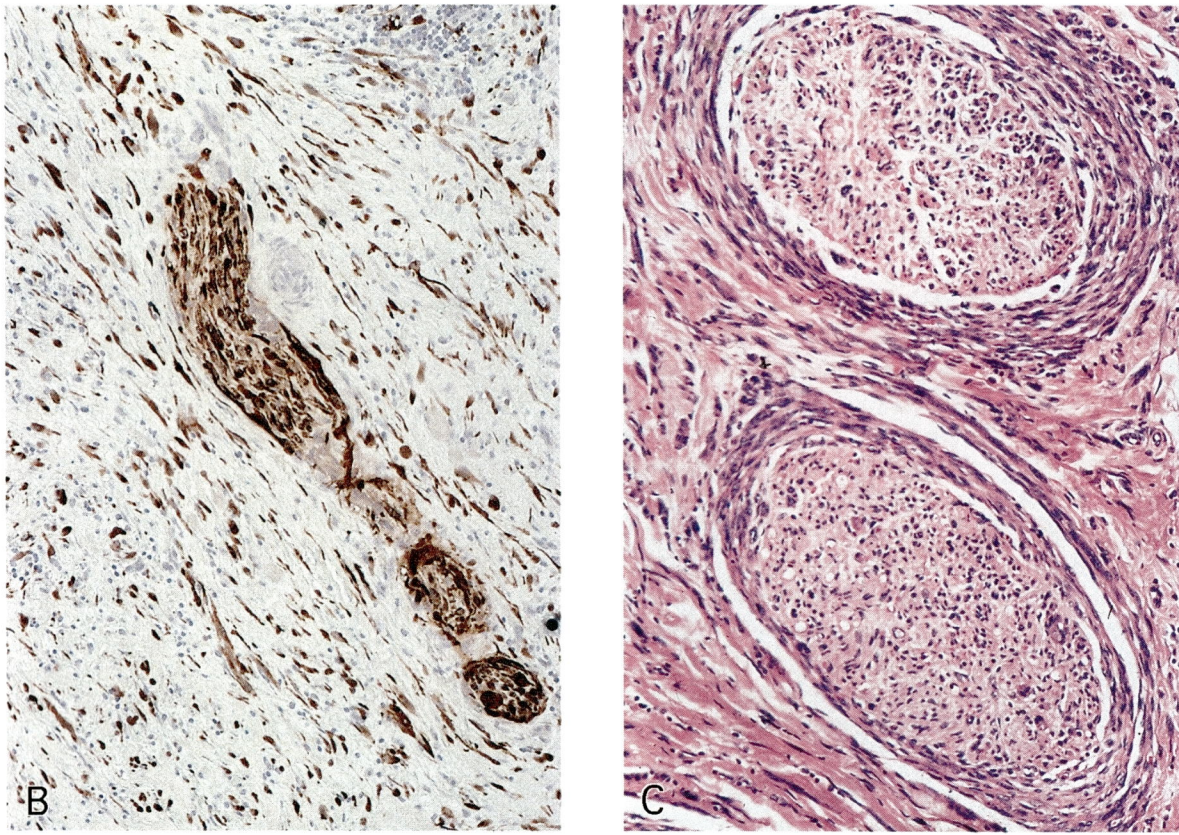

Figure 12-7
NEUROTROPIC MELANOMA

Intimate involvement of a small dermal nerve is seen (A). Permeation of dermal connective tissue and invasion of all nerve compartments is readily apparent on S-100 immunostain. Such tumors permeate epineurium, concentrate in perineurium, and may extend into endoneurium (B). In larger nerves such tumors permeate epineurium and concentrate in perineurium (C).

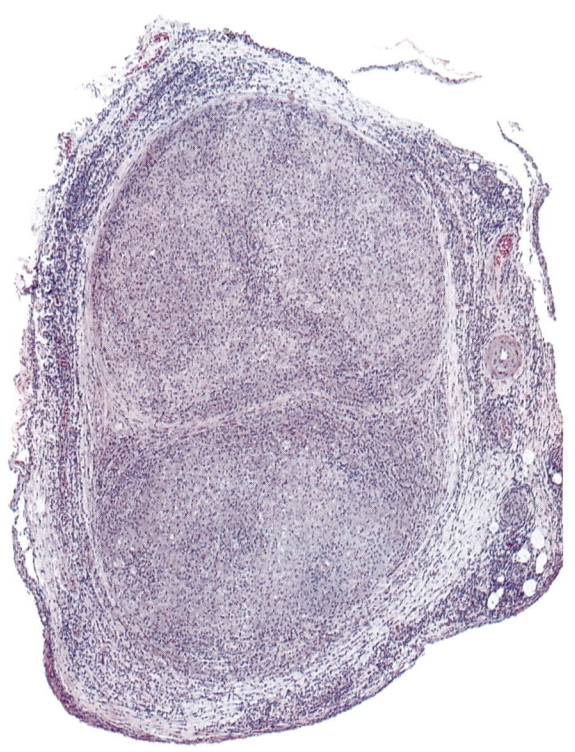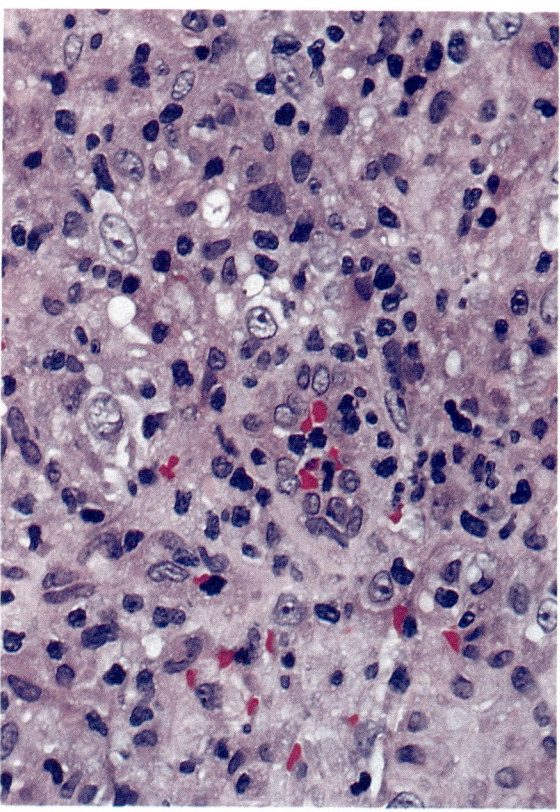

Figure 12-8
LYMPHOMA INVOLVING NERVE
Nerve roots (left) and ganglia are most often involved. Lymphoma infiltrates all compartments of these structures (right).

septa, and the endoneurium itself (fig. 12-8). Axonal degeneration and myelin loss commonly result.

In most instances, nerve involvement by lymphoma, including angiotropic lymphoma (angioendotheliomatosis) and leukemia, occur in a setting of systemic disease. Nerve involvement following CNS lymphoma has rarely been described (50). Nevertheless, non-Hodgkin's lymphomas occasionally involve nerve in the absence of disease elsewhere (see chapter 10, figs. 10-11, 10-12) as in sciatic mononeuropathy (44). So-called neurolymphomatosis (9,30), a disorder characterized by extensive, apparently selective peripheral nerve involvement, is poorly understood.

Miscellaneous

Primitive neuroectodermal tumors (PNET) of soft tissue origin may also involve all nerve compartments (fig. 12-9).

METASTASES TO NERVE SHEATH TUMOR

Metastasis of one tumor to another is rare and seen in only 0.1 percent of random autopsies (6); most reported cases were encountered at autopsy. Among tumors that metastasize to another, breast and lung carcinomas are most common and are nearly equal in frequency (2). Most recipient tumors are benign. Although the vast majority are thyroid adenomas and adrenal adenomas or meningiomas (2,10,16), schwannomas may also be affected (fig. 12-10) (16,40). Renal cell carcinomas comprise 70 percent of malignant recipient tumors. Common to most recipient tumors is slow growth, a factor causing them to be at protracted risk of metastatic involvement. A high lipid content, as is often seen in meningioma, schwannoma, and renal cell carcinoma, is also considered a predisposing factor

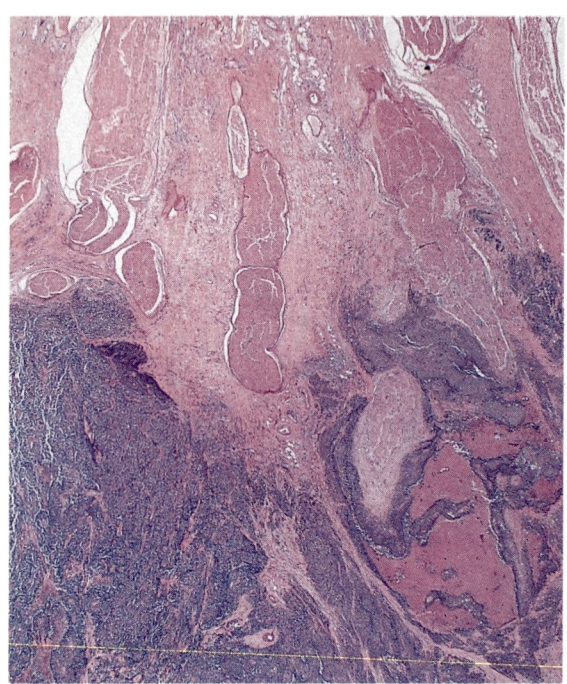
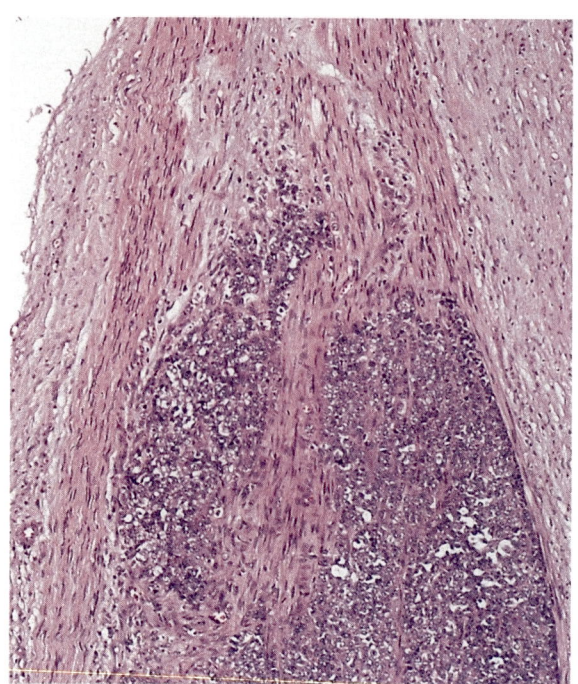

Figure 12-9
PRIMITIVE NEUROECTODERMAL TUMOR INVOLVING NERVE
Although, strictly speaking, PNET is not a soft tissue sarcoma, it may involve all nerve compartments by direct extension.

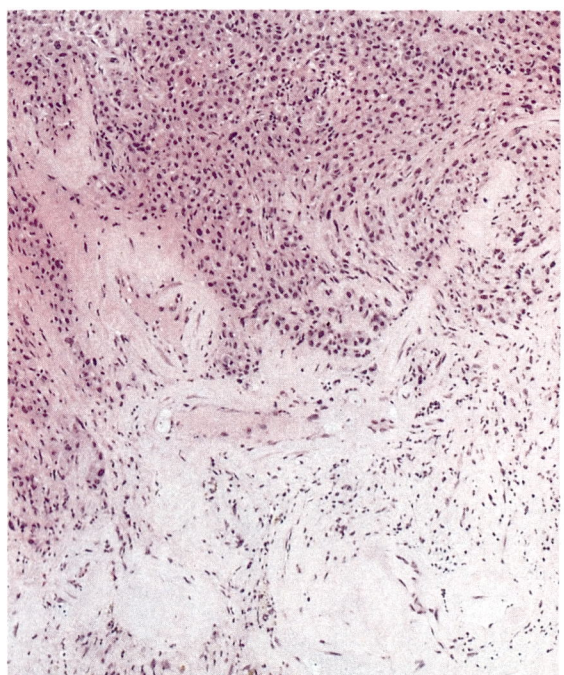
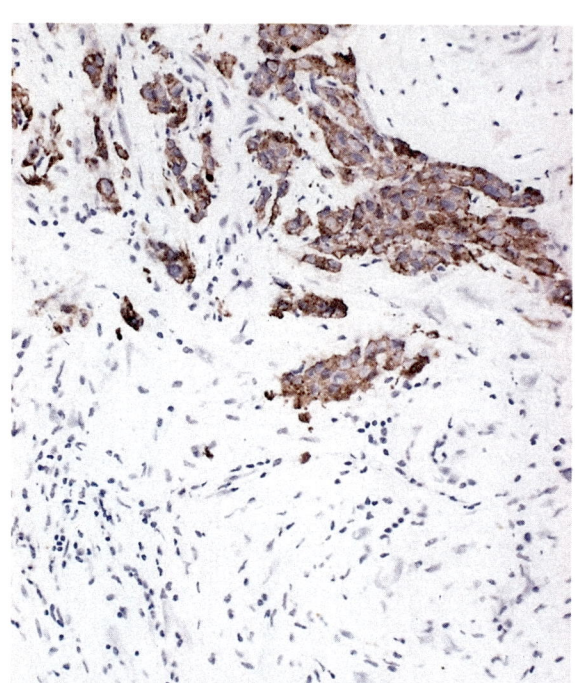

Figure 12-10
METASTASIS TO NERVE SHEATH TUMOR
Occurring in an elderly man with a lung mass, this schwannoma from the region of the elbow (left) was the recipient of a large cell undifferentiated carcinoma. Note staining for cytokeratin (right). (Courtesy of Dr. E. Venza, Bassano del Grappa, Italy.)

(54), as are common hormonal attributes, such as the presence of steroid hormone receptors in breast carcinoma and meningioma (21). Metastasis to schwannoma must be distinguished from the exceedingly rare occurrence of malignant transformation of schwannoma (MPNST ex schwannoma), which is discussed in detail in chapter 11.

REFERENCES

1. Ackerman AB, Godomski J. Neurotrophic malignant melanoma and other neurotrophic neoplasms in the skin. Am J Dermatopathol 1984;6:63–80.
2. Arnold AC, Hepler RS, Badr MA, et al. Metastases of adenocarcinoma of the lung to optic nerve sheath meningioma. Arch Ophthalmol 1995;113:346–51.
3. Asbury AK, Johnson PC. Pathology of the peripheral nerve. Philadelphia: WB Saunders Co, 1977.
4. Ballantyne AJ, McCarten AB, Ibanez ML. The extension of cancer of the head and neck through peripheral nerves. Am J Surg 1963;106:651–67.
5. Barber JR, Coventry MB, McDonald JR. Spread of soft tissue sarcomata of extremities along peripheral nerve trunks. J Bone Joint Surg 1957;39:534–40.
6. Barz H. The incidence of metastatic carcinomas in meningiomas: a report of four cases. Zentralbl Allg Pathol 1983;127:367–74.
7. Beggs J, Johnson PC, Olafsen A, Watkins CJ, Cleary C. Transperineurial arterioles in human sural nerve. J Neuropathol Exp Neurol 1991;50:704–18.
8. Beenken S, Byers R, Smith L, Goepfert H, Shallenberger R. Desmoplastic melanoma.Histologic correlation with behavior and treatment. Arch Otolaryngol Head Neck Surg 1989;115:374–9.
9. Borit A, Altrocchi PH. Recurrent polyneuropathy and neurolymphomatosis. Arch Neurol 1971;24:40–9.
10. Bucciero A, Del basso de Caro M, Vizioli L, Carraturo S, Cerillo A, Tedeschi G. Metastasis of breast carcinoma to intracranial meningioma. Case report and review of the literature. J Neurosurg Sci 1992;36:169–72.
11. Burger PC, Scheithauer BW, Vogel FS. Surgical pathology of the central nervous system and its coverings. 3rd ed. New York: Churchill Livingstone, 1991:359–65.
12. Carstens PH. Perineural glands in normal and hyperplastic prostates. J Urol 1980;123:686–8.
13. Carter RL, Foster CS, Dinsdale EA, Pittam MR. Perineural spread by squamous carcinomas of the head and neck: a morphological study using antiaxonal and antimyelin monoclonal antibiotics. J Clin Pathol 1983;36:269–75.
14. Carter RL, Pittam MR, Tanner NS. Pain and dysphagia in patients with squamous carcinomas of the head and neck: the role of perineurial spread. J Roy Soc Med 1982;75:598–606.
15. Carter RL, Tanner NS, Clifford P, Shaw HJ. Perineurial spread in squamous cell carcinomas of the head and neck: a clinicopathological study. Clin Otolaryngol 1979;4:271–81.
15a. Cavazza A, Asioli S, Martella EM, DeMarco L, Gardini G. [Neural infiltration in benign gallbladder lesions. Description of a case.] Pathologica 1998;90:42–5.
16. Chambers PW, Davis RL, Buck FS. Metastases to primary intracranial meningiomas and neurilemomas. Arch Pathol Lab Med 1980;104:350–4.
17. Conley J, Lattes R, Orr W. Desmoplastic malignant melanoma (a rare variant of spindle cell melanoma). Cancer 1971;28:914–36.
18. Costa J. Benign epithelial inclusions in pancreatic nerves [Letter]. Am J Clin Pathol 1977;67:306–7.
19. Cruveilhier J. Maladies nes nerfs. Anatomic Pathologique du Dorps Humain. 2nd ed. Pt. 35. Paris: J.B. Bailliére, 1816:1829–42.
20. David DJ, Speculand B, Vernon-Roberts B, Sach RP. Malignant schwannoma of the inferior dental nerve. Br J Plast Surg 1978;31:323–33.
21. Di Bonito L, Bianchi C. Metastase d'un cancer mammaire dans un meningiome. Arch Anat Cytol Pathol 1978;26:175–6.
22. DiMaio SM, Mackay B, Smith JL, Dickersin GR. Neurosarcomatous transformation in malignant melanoma. An ultrastructural study. Cancer 1982;50:2345–54.
23. Dodd GD, Dolan PA, Ballantyne AJ, Ibanez ML, Chau P. The dissemination of tumors of the head and neck via the cranial nerves. Radiol Clin North Am 1970;8:445–61.
24. Enzinger FM, Weiss SW. Soft tissue tumors. 1st ed. St. Louis: CV Mosby, 1983:644–8.
25. Ernst P. åber das Wachstum und die Verbeitung bösartige Geschwuhste ins besoderes des Krebses in den Nerven. Beitr Pathol Anat 1907;7(Suppl):29–51.
26. From L, Hanna W, Kahn HJ, Gruss J, Marks A, Baumal R. Origin of the desmoplasia in desmoplastic malignant melanoma. Hum Pathol 1983;14:1072–80.
27. Gentile RD, Donovan DT. Neurotrophic melanoma of the head and neck. Laryngoscope 1985;95:1161–6.
28. Goepfert H, Dichtel WJ, Medina JE, Lindberg RD, Luna MD. Perineurial invasion in squamous cell skin carcinoma of the head and neck. Am J Surg 1984;148:542–7.
29. Gonzalez-Vitale JC, Garcia-Bunuel R. Meningeal carcinomatosis. Cancer 1976;37:2906–11.
30. Guberman A, Rosenbaum H, Braciale T, Schlaepfer WW. Human neurolymphomatosis. J Neurol Sci 1978;36:1–12.
31. Jain S, Allen PW. Desmoplastic malignant melanoma and its variants. A study of 45 cases. Am J Surg Pathol 1989;13:358–73.
32. Johnson PC. Hematogenous metastases of carcinoma to dorsal root ganglia. Acta Neuropathologica 1977;38:171–2.
33. Khalil MK, Duguid WP. Neurotropic malignant melanoma of right temple with orbital metastasis: a clinicopathological case report. Br J Ophthalmol 1987;71:41–6.

34. Kossard S, Doherty E, Murray E. Neurotropic melanoma. A variant of desmoplastic melanoma. Arch Dermatol 1987;123:907–12.

35. Labrecque PG, Hu CH, Winkelmann RK. On the nature of desmoplastic melanoma. Cancer 1976;38:1205–13.

36. Larson DL, Rodin AE, Roberts DK, O'Steen WK, Rapperport AS, Lewis SR. Perineurial lymphatics: myth or fact? Am J Surg 1966;112:488–92.

37. Lee JY, Kapadia SB, Musgrave RH, Futrell WJ. Neurotropic malignant melanoma occurring in a stable burn scar. J Cutan Pathol 1992;19:145–50.

37a. Longacre TA, Egbert BM, Rouse RV. Desmoplastic and spindle cell malignant melanoma. An immunohistochemical study. Am J Surg Pathol 1996;20:1489–500.

38. Mark GJ. Basal cell carcinoma with intraneurial invasion. Cancer 1977;40:2181–7.

39. Neumann E. Secondare cancroid infiltration des nervus mentalis bei einem fall von lippincroid. Arch Pathol Anat 1862;24:24–201.

40. Ni K, Dehner LP. Schwannoma with metastatic carcinoma of the breast: an unconventional form of glandular peripheral nerve sheath tumor. Hum Pathol 1995;26:457–9.

41. Reed RJ, Leonard DD. Neurotropic melanoma. A variant of desmoplastic melanoma. Am J Surg Pathol 1979;3:301–11.

42. Robertson I, Cook MG, Wilson DF, Henderson DW. Malignant schwannoma of cranial nerves. Pathology 1983;15:421–9.

43. Rodin AE, Larson DL, Roberts DK. Nature of the perineurial space invaded by prostatic carcinoma. Cancer 1967;20:1772–9.

44. Roncaroli F, Poppi M, Riccioni L, Frank F. Primary non-Hodgkin's lymphoma of the sciatic nerve followed by localization in the central nervous system: case report and review of the literature. Neurosurgery 1997;40:618–22.

45. Russell DS, Rubinstein LJ. Nervous system involvement by lymphomas, histiocytoses and leukemias. In: Russell DS, Rubinstein LJ, eds. Pathology of the nervous system. 5th ed. Baltimore: Williams & Wilkins, 1989:608–15.

46. Selander D, Sjostrand J. Longitudinal spread of intraneurally injected local anesthetics. Acta Anaesthesiol Scand 1978;22:622–34.

47. Taylor HB, Norris JH. Epithelial invasion of nerves in benign diseases of the breast. Cancer 1967;20:2245–9.

48. Valensi QJ. Desmoplastic malignant melanoma. A light and electron microscopic study of two cases. Cancer 1979;43:1148–55.

49. Valensi QJ. Desmoplastic malignant melanoma: a report on two additional cases. Cancer 1977;39:286–92.

50. VanBolden V, Kline DG, Garcia CA, VanBolden RN. Isolated radial nerve palsy due to a metastasis from a primary malignant lymphoma of the brain. Neurosurgery 1987;21:905–9.

51. Warner TF, Ford CN, Hafez GR. Neurotropic melanoma of the face invading the maxillary nerve. J Cutan Pathol 1985;12:520–7.

52. Warner TF, Lloyd RC, Hafez GR, Angevine JM. Immunocytochemistry of neurotropic melanoma. Cancer 1984;53:254–7.

53. Warner TF, Hafez GR, Finch RE, Brandenberg JH. Schwann cell features in neurotropic melanoma. J Cutan Pathol 1981;8:177–87.

54. Wolintz AH, Mastri A. Metastasis of carcinoma of lung to sphenoid ridge meningioma. NY State J Med 1970;70:2592–8.

55. Zimmerman KG, Johnson PC, Paplanus SH. Nerve invasion by benign proliferating ductules in vasitis nodosa. Cancer 1983;51:2066–9.

◇◇◇

13

NEUROFIBROMATOSIS

Neurofibromatosis is one of a group of neuro-cutaneous disorders which includes tuberous sclerosis, neurocutaneous melanosis, hypomelanosis of Ito, incontinentia pigmenti, and Sturge-Weber syndrome. Collectively, these have also been referred to as "phakomatoses," a term derived from the Greek phakos, meaning a lentil or birthmark. All but Sturge-Weber syndrome, which is rarely familial, have an autosomal dominant pattern of inheritance, and only neurofibromatosis shows prominent involvement of the peripheral nervous system.

Neurofibromatosis is characterized by multiple lesions, often of diverse type, affecting a variety of tissues. These include hyperplasias, hypoplasias, hamartomas, and neoplasms, both benign and malignant. The majority of lesions are neuroectodermal or mesenchymal in nature. All races and both sexes are equally affected. Although the existence of as many as eight variants of neurofibromatosis has been proposed (55), the disorder occurs in two principal genetic and clinicopathologic forms. Termed neurofibromatosis types 1 and 2 (NF1 and NF2), each is characterized by distinctive abnormalities; overlap is minor. Both conditions result from genetic alterations of separate tumor suppressor genes. The risk of malignancy is ten times higher in patients with either form. The salient features of NF1 and NF2 are summarized in Table 13-1. The need to distinguish these conditions, both conceptually and in practical terms, has long been recognized (79). Since the unqualified use of the term "neurofibromatosis" no longer provides diagnostic precision, the variant under consideration should always be specified.

NEUROFIBROMATOSIS 1 (NF1)

General Manifestations. The full expression of this frequently occurring disorder, also termed *peripheral neurofibromatosis* or *von Recklinghausen's disease,* has long been recognized (fig. 13-1) (56). The mutation responsible for this most common form of neurofibromatosis is in a large gene on the long arm and near the centromere of chromosome 17 (3,37,72,76). Its precise location (17q11.2) is close to the gene for nerve growth-factor receptor (65). Spanning 350 kb of genomic DNA and consisting of 60 exons, it encodes neurofibromin, a 2818 amino acid protein. Evidence suggests that the NF1 gene functions in part as a tumor suppressor gene and that it may play a role in cell proliferation and differentiation (22,73). Its product is normally expressed in many different tissues.

Sparing no races and showing a population incidence of 1 in 3,000, NF1 is one of the most common human mendelian disorders. Approximately half of affected individuals have a family history of the disorder since inheritance is autosomal dominant. Penetrance is high but expression is variable (57). The remainder of cases appear to be sporadic in occurrence, thus attesting to the high mutation rate of the NF1 gene. Although the penetrance of NF1 is 100 percent, slightly over half of patients are only mildly affected.

According to Gutmann et al. (22a), a clinical diagnosis of NF1 can be made if a patient has two or more of the findings listed in Table 13-2. Of these, none in isolation is pathognomonic of NF1. Concordant manifestations have been reported, not only in affected monozygotic twins (2), but also in members of the same family (64). As a rule, however, the expression of NF1 is variable, even among affected members of the same family.

Among the earliest manifestations of NF1, congenital in some cases, are smooth contoured, pigmented cutaneous macules termed café-au-lait spots (fig. 13-2). These may enlarge and become more darkly pigmented over time. Occasional macules are two-toned with both dark and pale areas. Axillary freckling, a form of pigmentation affecting intertriginous skin, is of particular diagnostic significance (fig. 13-3). Pigmentation in café-au-lait spots and freckles is not due to an increase in melanocytes; rather, it is due to an excess of melanin in the form of melanosome-containing phagolysosomes. Referred to as macro-melanosomes (fig. 13-4) (31) or melanin macroglobules (48), such lysosomes are not limited to melanocytes, but may also be seen in keratinocytes, Langerhans cells, and macrophages. In

Table 13-1

COMPARATIVE FEATURES OF NEUROFIBROMATOSIS 1 AND 2

	NF1 (Peripheral Form; von Recklinghausen's Disease)	NF2 (Central Form)
Incidence	1/3,000	1/40,000
Prevalence	60/100,000	0.01/100,000
Inheritance	Autosomal dominant	Autosomal dominant
Sporadic occurrence	50%	50%
Chromosome location	17q11.2	22q12
Encoded protein	Neurofibromin	Merlin (schwannomin)
Café-au-lait spots -one or more -six or more	Often multiple and large About 90% of patients At least 70% of patients	Small, rarely more than 6 40% of patients
Cutaneous neurofibromas	Most patients	Rare
Cutaneous schwannomas	Not associated	70%
Multiple Lisch nodules	Very common	Not associated
Cataracts	Not associated	60 to 80%
Skeletal malformations	Common	Not associated
Astrocytomas (optic, cerebellar, cerebral)	Moderate incidence	Infrequent
Pheochromocytoma	Occasionally seen	Not associated
Malignant peripheral nerve sheath tumor	Approximately 2%	Not seen
Intellectual impairment	Associated	Not associated
Vestibular schwannoma	Not associated	Most cases (usually bilateral)
Meningioma	Uncommon	Common
Spinal cord ependymoma	Not associated	Common
Meningioangiomatosis	Not associated	Occasional
Schwannosis	Not associated	Common
Glial hamartomas	Occasional	Very common
Syringomyelia	Not associated	Associated
Posterior subcapsular cataracts	Not associated	Common
Ganglioneuroma	Occasional	Not associated
Gastrointestinal autonomic nerve tumor (GANT)	Occasional	Not associated
Paraganglioma, including duodenal gangliocytic variant	Occasional	Not associated
Foregut carcinoid tumor, including duodenal calcifying somatostatinoma	Occasional	Not associated
Juvenile xanthogranuloma	Occasional	Not associated
Rhabdomyosarcoma	Occasional	Not associated
Juvenile leukemia (CML)	Occasional	Not associated

fair-skinned people, café-au-lait spots and freckles are light tan, their color truly resembling that of coffee laced with milk. On the other hand, in brown or black individuals, such pigmented lesions are dark brown or black (fig. 13-3). Since café-au-lait spots are commonly found in normal persons and in unrelated diseases, such as the McCune-Albright syndrome (polyostotic fibrous dysplasia), their size, contour, and number must be taken into account when considering a clinical diagnosis of NF1 (Table 13-2). For instance, the presence of six macules, each measuring at least 1.5 cm, is required for diagnosis in an adult patient (8). An equal number of macules greater than 5 mm in diameter is required in prepubertal patients (22a). The number of café-au-lait spots

Table 13-2

DIAGNOSTIC CRITERIA FOR NEUROFIBROMATOSIS 1*

The patient should have two or more of the following:

1.   Six or more café-au-lait spots
     1.5 cm or larger in postpubertal individuals
     0.5 cm or larger in prepubertal individuals

2.   Two or more neurofibromas of any type or one or more plexiform neurofibroma

3.   Freckling in the axilla or groin

4.   Optic glioma (tumor of the optic pathway)

5.   Two or more Lisch nodules (benign iris hamartomas)

6.   A distinctive bony lesion
     Dysplasia of the sphenoid bone
     Dysplasia or thinning of the long bone cortex

7.   A first-degree relative with NF1

*Table 1 from Gutmann DH, Aylsworth A, Carey JC, et al. The diagnostic evaluation and multidisciplinary management of neurofibromatosis 1 and neurofibromatosis 2. JAMA 1997;278:51–7.

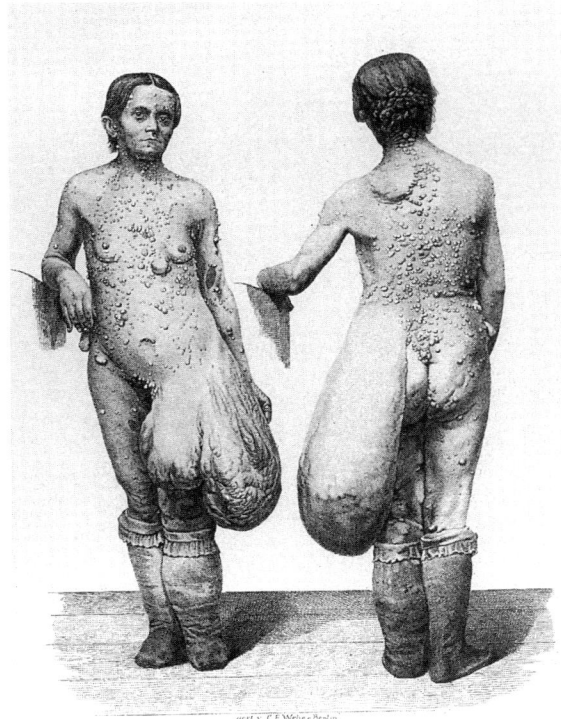

Figure 13-1
NEUROFIBROMATOSIS TYPE 1
(VON RECKLINGHAUSEN'S DISEASE)
AS DEPICTED IN VIRCHOWS'
"KRANKHAFTE GESCHWÜLSTE," 1856 (71)
   In addition to the obvious cutaneous neurofibromas, most concentrated on the trunk, occasional café-au-lait spots, and massive "elephantiasis neuromatosa," the illustration captures the typical NF1 facies.

and freckles may increase over time. At diagnosis, nearly all patients have at least one café-au-lait spot of diagnostic size, and two thirds have six or more such spots (68). Although occasional individuals with proven NF1 may appear to have few or no café-au-lait spots, their presence may be demonstrated by examination of the skin under ultraviolet light. The typical NF1 facies includes a broad forehead, triangular face, and dark infraorbital discoloration (figs. 13-1, 13-7, 13-19A).

Pigmented iris hamartomas, termed Lisch nodules, are also a common feature of NF1 (fig. 13-5) (36). Although perhaps an overestimate, they are thought to occur in 95 percent of NF1 patients over 6 years of age (34). Visualized on slit lamp examination as brown, frequently bilateral nodules, they must be distinguished from other nevi of the iris.

Like café-au-lait spots, neurofibromas are hallmark lesions of NF1 (figs. 13-6–13-18). The pathologic spectrum of neurofibromas is discussed and illustrated in detail in chapter 8. They are composed not only of Schwann cells, but of perineurial-like cells, fibroblasts, and cells with features intermediate between perineurial-like cells and fibroblasts. This cellular heterogeneity has prompted some to suggest that neuro-

fibromas are polyclonal (15) and perhaps hamartomatous in nature. Recent evidence based upon active and inactive X chromosomes in the individual tumors suggests that neurofibromas are monoclonal (66). As currently understood, all NF1 patients harbor one nonfunctional NF1 gene (germline mutation) in every cell in the body (22). Neurofibromas are assumed to arise as a result of a second, somatic mutation (22). Thereafter, malignant transformation of neurofibroma to malignant peripheral nerve sheath tumor (MPNST) (17) appears to be related to loss or mutation of one or more tumor suppressor genes. As previously discussed in the chapter on MPNST, aberrant expression of the p53 gene, a tumor suppressor gene on the short arm of chromosome 17, has been shown to occur in the transition of neurofibroma to MPNST (24,43).

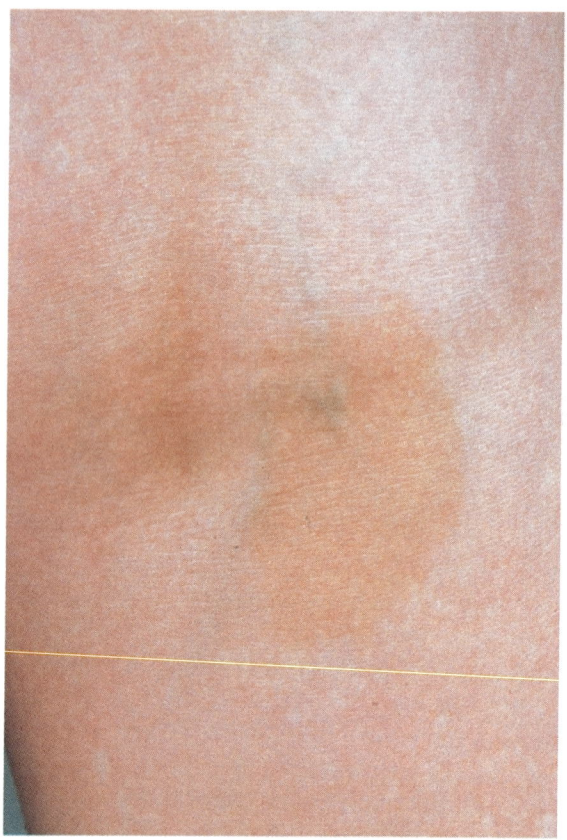
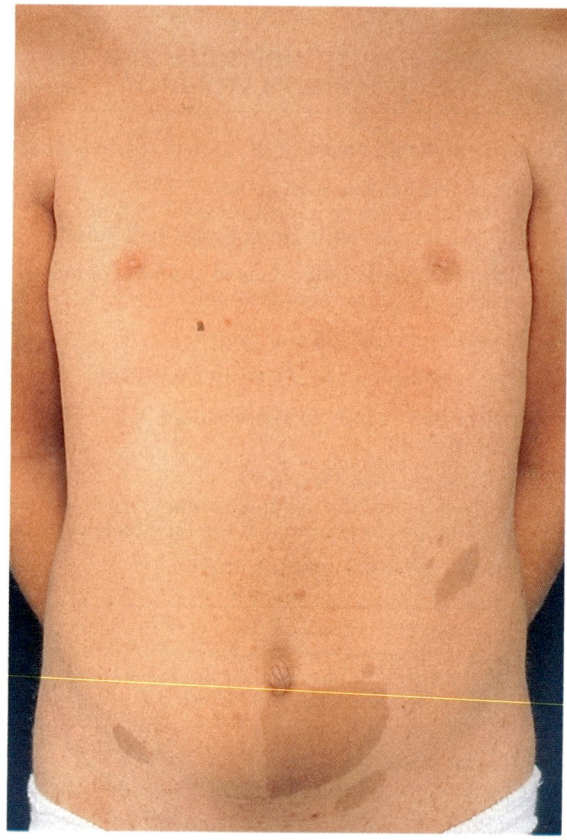

Figure 13-2
CAFÉ-AU-LAIT SPOTS IN NF1

Often oval or oblong in configuration, these hyperpigmented lesions are discrete and clearly demarcated from surrounding skin. Subtle examples could easily be missed (left) whereas others are obvious (right). Sharp demarcation of a lesion in the midline (right) suggests a dermatomal distribution. Clinical experience suggests that hyperpigmentation extending across the midline is associated with an increased risk of MPNST development.

Although neurofibromas may occasionally be present at birth, most develop in later life. In most instances they first appear around puberty, other lesions emerging thereafter. Hyperpigmentation may be seen overlying massive soft tissue neurofibromas (see fig. 8-30A), but their locations do not necessarily coincide. Both peripheral and visceral nerves may be affected by neurofibromas, small nerves of skin and subcutaneous tissue are preferentially involved. A single localized neurofibroma is of no significance in terms of establishing a diagnosis of NF1.

Four clinically and morphologically distinct variants of neurofibroma occur in NF1 (see chapter 8): 1) cutaneous lesions of localized and diffuse type; 2) localized intraneural tumors of peripheral nerves; 3) plexiform neurofibromas typically in-

volving major nerve trunks (78); and 4) massive soft tissue neurofibromas. Whereas solitary neurofibromas of localized intraneural type, even sizable tumors arising in a nerve root, are usually sporadic in occurrence, multiple examples are typically NF1-associated (figs. 13-7, 13-8D) (23). The same is true of large, diffuse cutaneous neurofibromas (see fig. 8-5). Numerous localized cutaneous neurofibromas (fig. 13-7, left), plexiform examples (figs. 13-1, 13-8–13-18), and massive soft tissue variants (fig. 13-10D; see also fig. 8-30) are generally considered diagnostic of NF1.

In those instances in which a plexiform neurofibroma occurs in a patient without other stigmata of NF1 or a family history, the tumor may be the result of a local somatic mutation (55). The latter mechanism appears to be the basis of

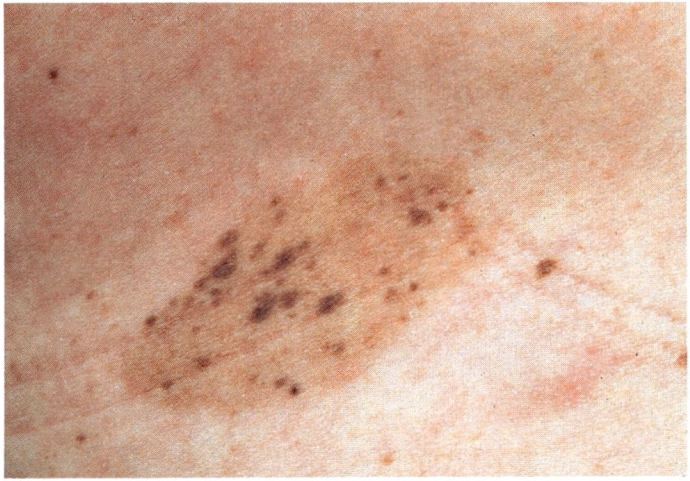

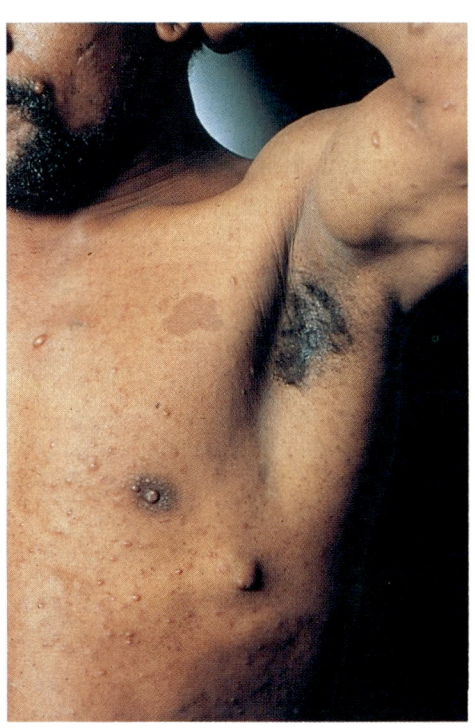

Figure 13-3
FRECKLING IN NF1

Often affecting the axilla (above), groin, or both, these lesions may be bilateral or unilateral. In individuals not generally freckled, their finding is highly suggestive of NF1. Nonintertriginous skin is unaffected. Both café-au-lait spots and axillary freckling may be more deeply pigmented in blacks (right).

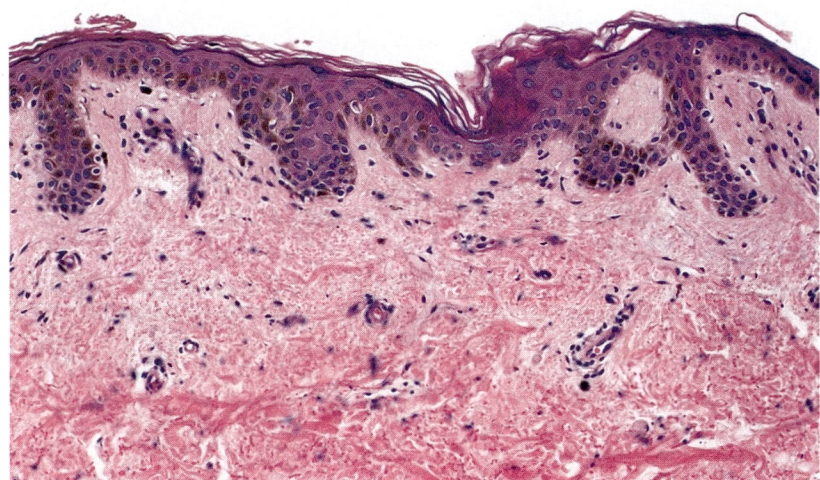

Figure 13-4
CAFÉ-AU-LAIT SPOT IN NF1

In this example, in contrast to most café-au-lait macules, there is also a slight elongation of rete ridges and a slight increase in the number of intraepidermal melanocytes.

so-called localized or *segmental neurofibromatosis,* an anatomically limited form of NF1 (53). Such cases often feature cutaneous or subcutaneous neurofibromas as well as café-au-lait spots limited to one portion of the body, typically one limb or even single dermatome (fig. 13-11). These patients do not transmit the condition to their progeny and develop disease complications only in the distribution of the affected nerve. Other localized

forms of NF1 include hemifacial hypertrophy (fig. 13-19B,C) and visceral neurofibromatosis (see below). On only slim evidence, macrodystrophia lipomatosa (see chapter 6) has been included by some in the spectrum of localized NF.

Visceral Neurofibromas. Neurofibromas may affect viscera in a variety of ways. They may be solitary or multiple, and sporadic or NF1 associated. So-called visceral neurofibromatosis is a

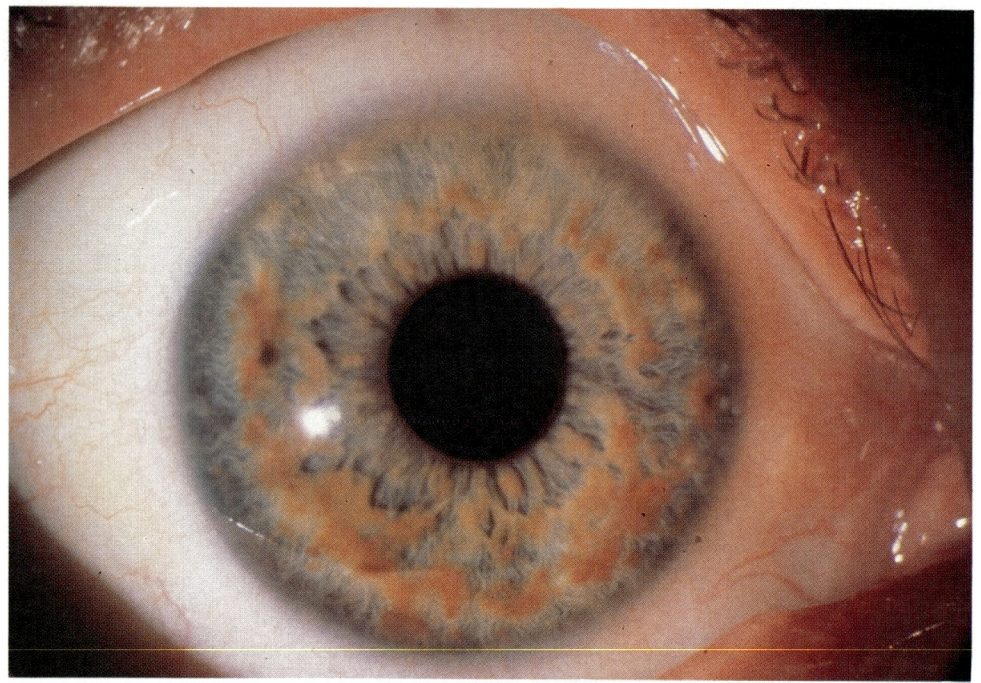

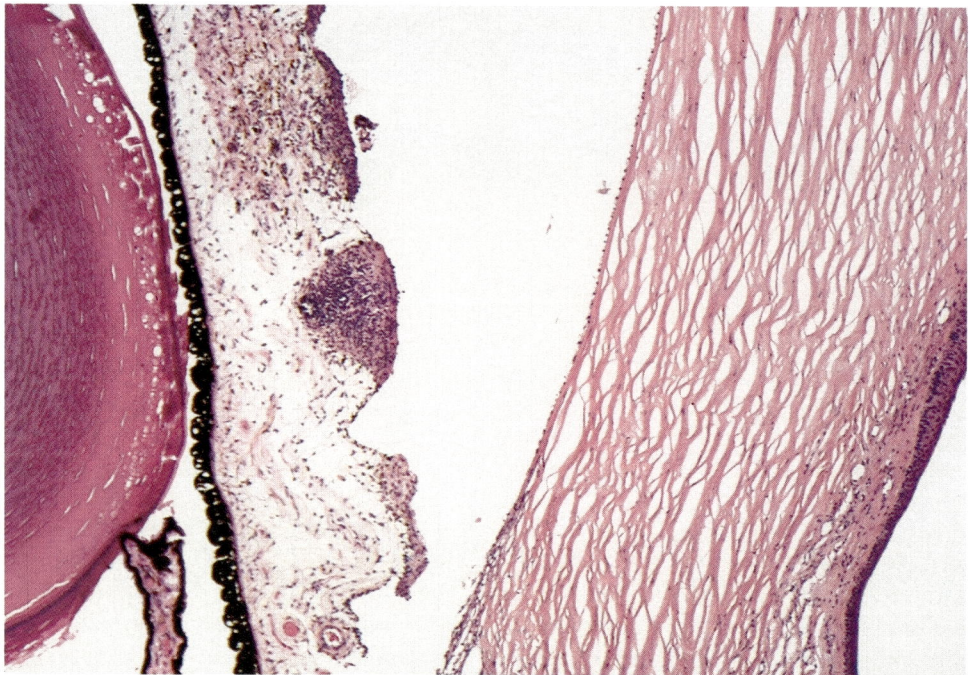

Figure 13-5
LISCH NODULES OF THE IRIS IN NF1

Top: Unlike iris freckles, these lesions are elevated above the surface of the iris. They also affect the entire area of the iris rather than the inner or outer circumference.

Bottom: A sagittal section of the eye shows the nodules to be multiple and to lie on the anterior aspect of the iris.

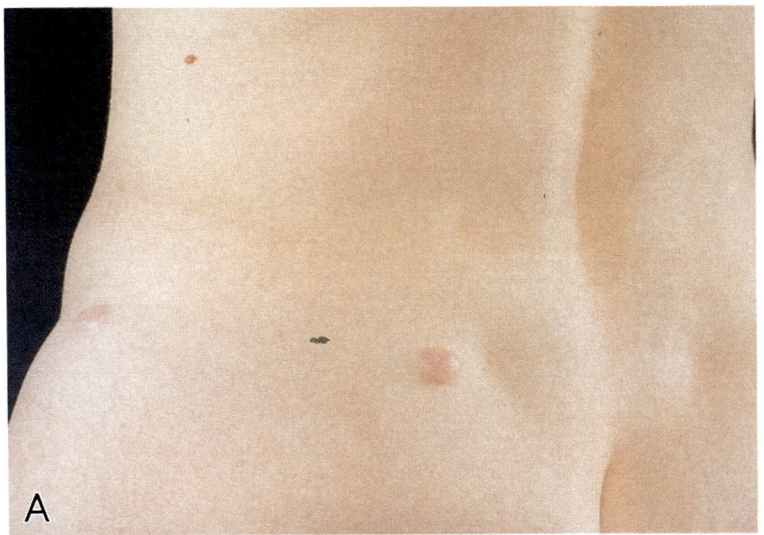

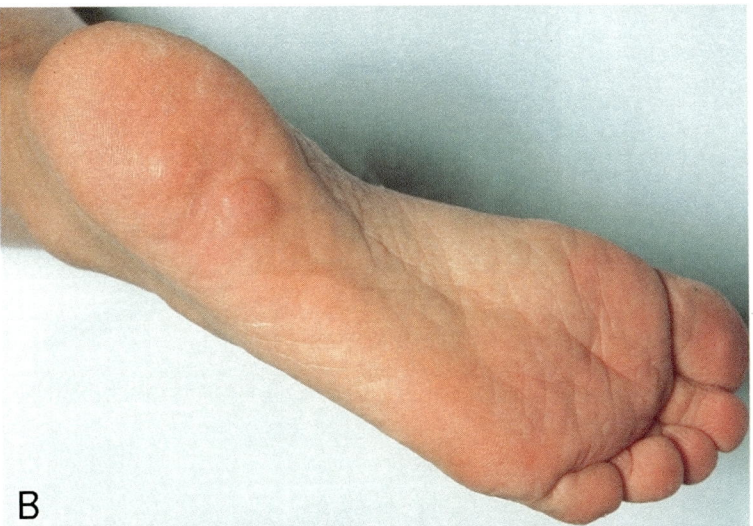

Figure 13-6
LOCALIZED CUTANEOUS
NEUROFIBROMAS IN NF1

Unlike plexiform examples, these dermal and subcutaneous neurofibromas are dome-shaped, discrete, and movable (A). Neurofibromas affecting the palm or sole (B) are rare outside the setting of NF1 and are thought to be associated with an increased risk of intracranial neoplasms. Neurofibromas of the areola (C) may become manifest or enlarge during pregnancy.

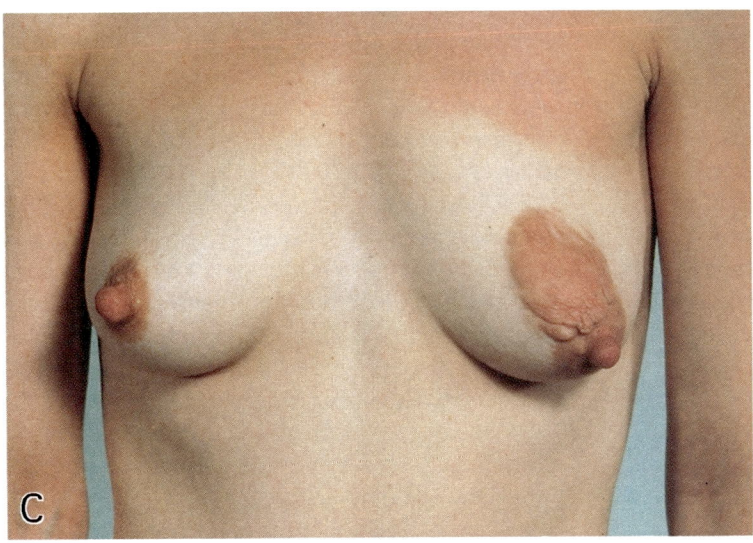

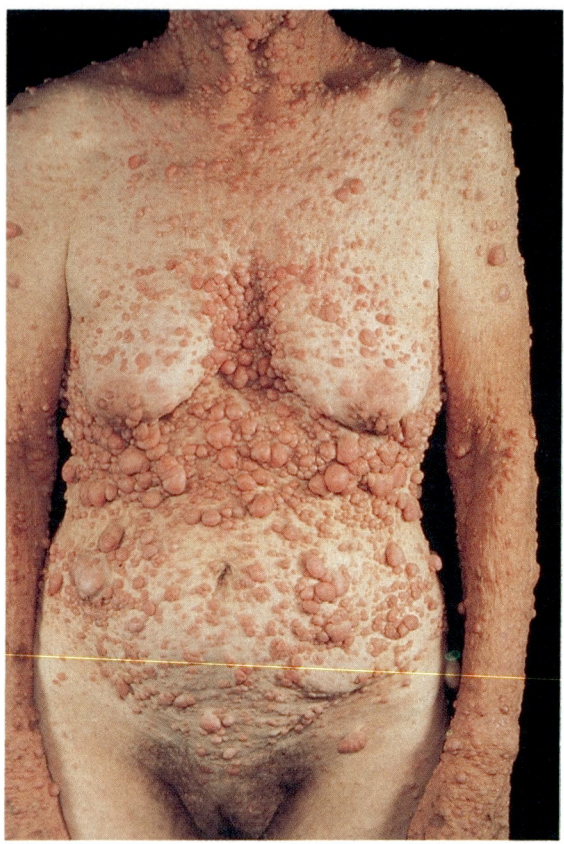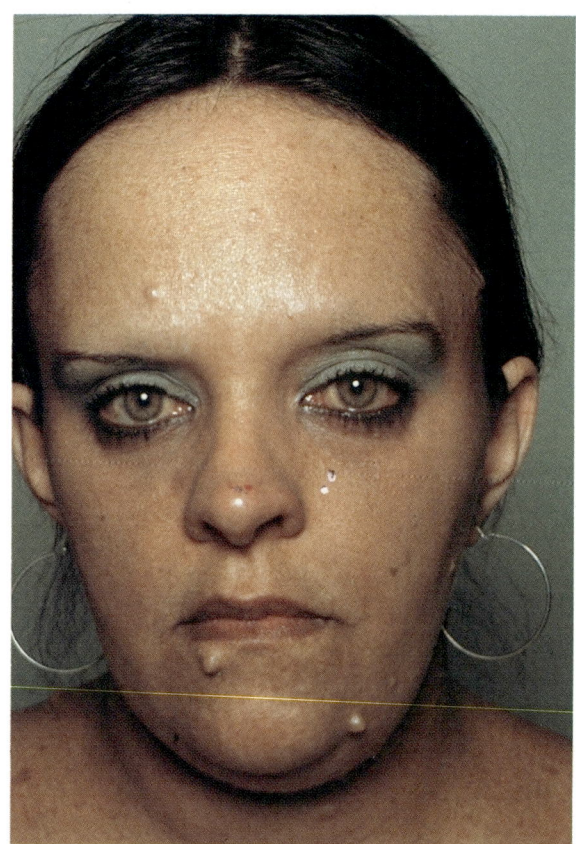

Figure 13-7
INNUMERABLE LOCALIZED CUTANEOUS NEUROFIBROMAS IN NF1
Left: Such nodular to pedunculated cutaneous examples most often affect the trunk.
Right: Neurofibromatosis 1 is occasionally associated with typical facial features, including a triangular configuration, a broad forehead, and deep-set eyes with infraorbital discoloration (see fig. 13-1).

rare condition in which patients often exhibit few external manifestations of NF1. The basis of visceral neurofibromatosis is unclear but it may be a reflection of anatomically selective NF1 gene expression or nerve growth factor effect (18). Aside from visceral neurofibromatosis as the sole manifestation of NF1, various organ systems may be affected in the generalized form of the disease (figs. 13-12–13-18). Primarily involved is the gastrointestinal tract, which shows great case-to-case variation (figs. 13-13–13-16) (18,27). The upper gastrointestinal tract (esophagus, stomach, and small bowel) is most often affected (fig. 13-14; see also fig. 8-15C), but colonic and rectal lesions may also be seen (fig. 13-16, left). Hepatic neurofibromas have also been reported (fig. 13-16, right) (38,50). Urinary bladder involvement is rare (figs. 13-17, 13-18).

The spectrum of NF1-associated gastrointestinal lesions includes ganglioneuromatosis, neurofibromas of both localized and plexiform type, gastrointestinal stromal tumors, and various neuroendocrine neoplasms. Ganglioneuromatosis, subtle or focal and localized or diffuse, results in a Hirschsprung-like picture in children and in pseudo-obstruction or megacolon in adults. It is characterized by an increase in ganglion cells and their processes which affects primarily the submucosal plexus. When impressive, "giant ganglia" may form. As in multiple endocrine neoplasia (MEN) IIb, the mucosa may also be involved, particularly the lower lamina propria (see fig. 5-15C). The degree to which the myenteric plexus is affected varies from markedly hypertrophic to diminished (18). The distinction of NF1 and MEN IIb-associated ganglioneuromatosis is discussed

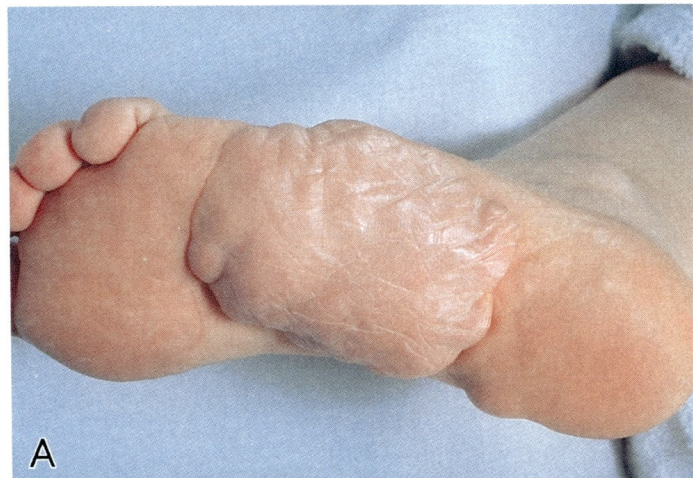
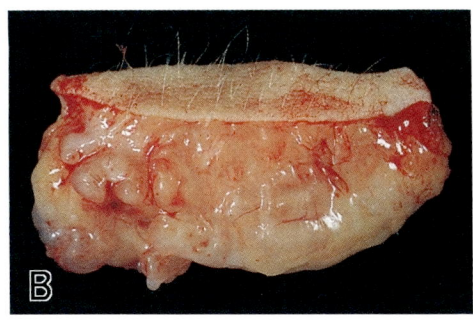
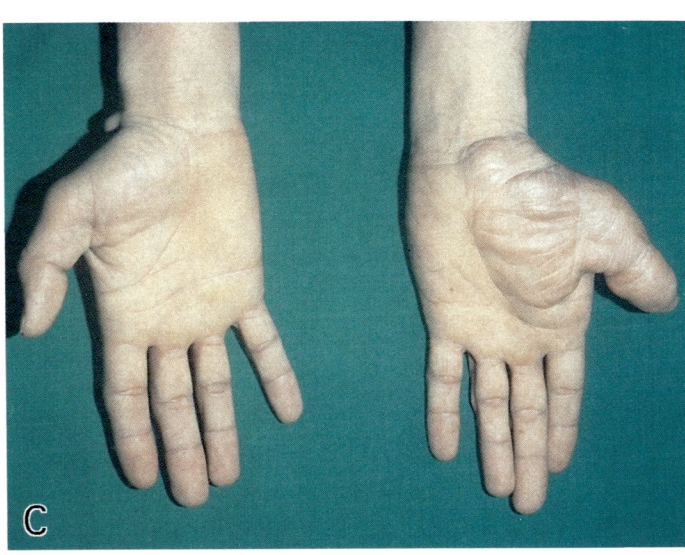
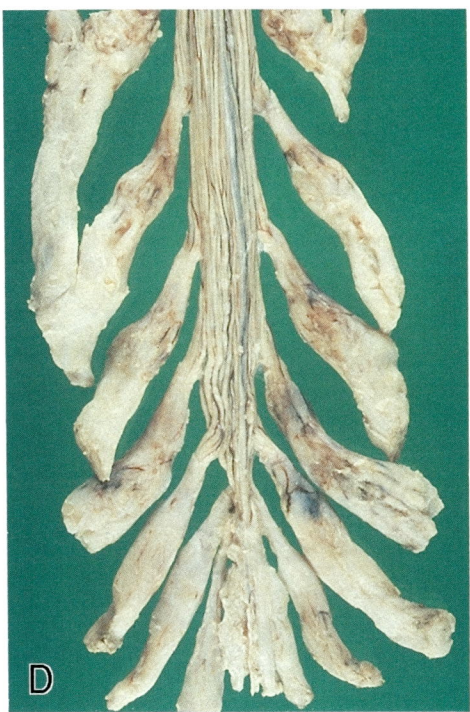

Figure 13-8
PLEXIFORM NEUROFIBROMA

Soft and compressible, these lesions are often likened to a "bag of worms" (A). Large plexiform neurofibromas massively enlarge nerves and often have intervening diffuse neurofibromatous tissue (B). Distal lesions, such as this median nerve tumor (C) may produce massive digital enlargement ("localized gigantism"). Neurofibromatous involvement of multiple spinal nerve roots is limited to NF1. Note the abrupt tapering of affected nerves as the process approaches the transition zone to spinal cord (D). (C,D: Figs. 3.437 and 3.441 from Okazaki H, Scheithauer BW. Atlas of neuropathology, 1988. With permission from the Mayo Foundation.)

in chapter 5. Neurofibromas in the gastrointestinal tract usually occur in the stomach and small bowel. Unlike solitary, often sporadic examples, those of NF1 are often multiple or grouped (fig. 13-14) or are large and diffuse with transmural involvement and a plexiform component (fig. 13-15). The latter often include the presence of mucosal ganglion cells. The plexiform component varies considerably in size and extent, but often involves both the submucosal and myenteric plexuses as well as the serosa. In a superficial biopsy, the microscopic distinction between such lesions and the ganglioneuromatosis described above may be difficult. Much less common are visceral neurofibromas affecting the heart (52), larynx (51), or genitourinary tract (figs. 13-17, 13-18). Multiple intestinal neurofibromas unassociated with NF1 have been described in association with a reciprocal translocation of chromosomes 12 and 14 (6a,70). In addition to

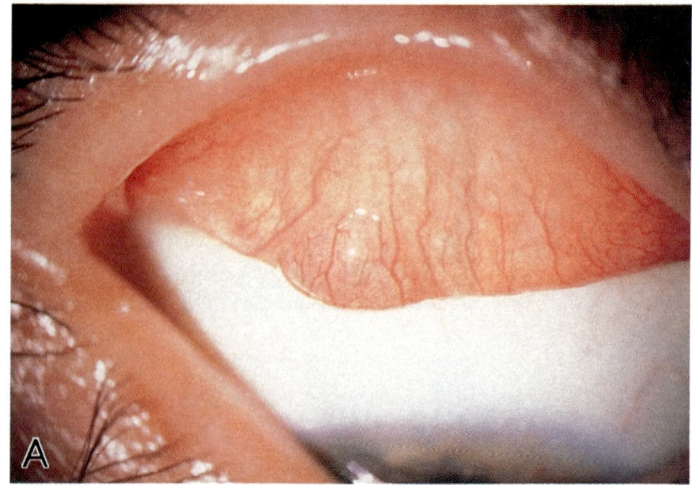

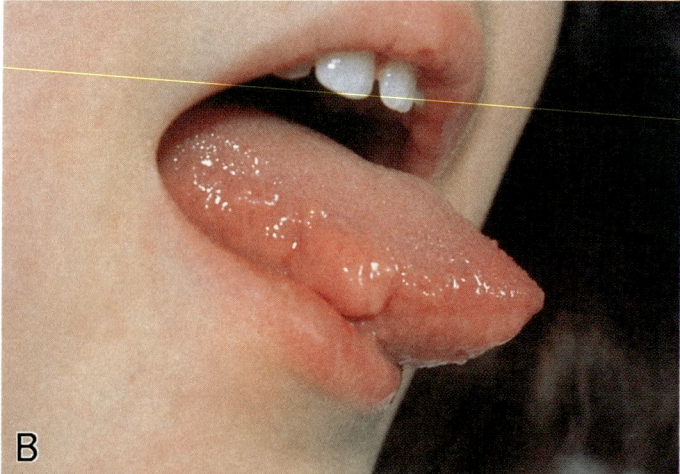

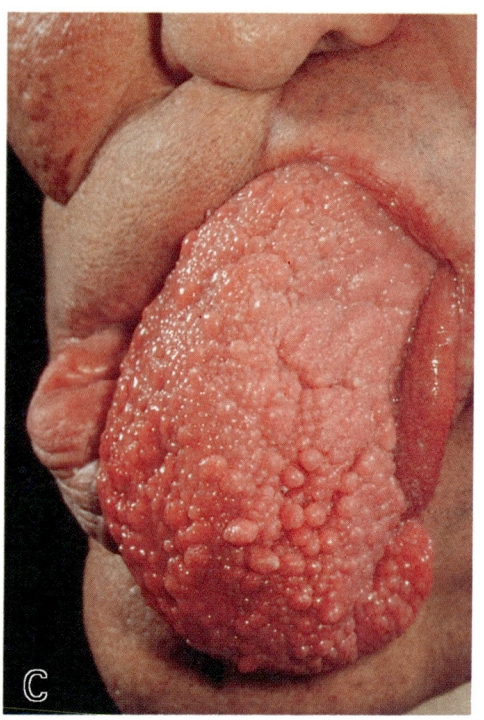

Figure 13-9
NEUROFIBROMA OF
MUCOUS MEMBRANES IN NF1

Illustrated are an unbiopsied, presumably plexiform neurofibroma that produced nodularity of the conjunctival mucosa (A) and a similar tumor of the tongue. Lesions of the tongue may be relatively localized (B) or extensive (C), extending down through the root of the tongue into the neck. Such extensive lesions may interfere with glutition and cause severe disability. The facial features of this severely affected patient are illustrated in fig. 13-18C.

neurofibroma, rare examples of visceral purported MPNST (19,20,33) and of leiomyoma (18, 27) have also been reported in NF1. Patients with neurofibromatosis are also prone to develop gastrointestinal stromal tumors (GIST). One variant, termed *gastrointestinal autonomic nerve tumor (GANT),* represents a sizable proportion of NF1-associated examples (fig. 13-20) (26,32, 44,45,60,62,75,77). Most GANTs affect the small bowel and stomach. GANTs are composed of spindle and epithelioid cells occasionally exhibiting whorling, and are commonly immunoreactive for neuron-specific enolase, occasionally for neurofilament protein, and rarely for synaptophysin or S-100 protein (12). Although GANT

and other GISTs were once thought to be derived from cells of the myenteric plexus (4,77), recent work has shown the majority of them to have immunophenotypic characteristics of the intestinal interstitial cells of Cajal (26a,31a). These characteristics include staining for CD117 (c-kit) and CD34. Ultrastructurally, GANTs feature processes with synapse-like terminations, dense- core granules, and vesicles (12,26,32,75). So-called skeinoid fibers (44,45) are seen in some of the tumors. As a whole, GISTs are clinically aggressive, with recurrence, peritoneal seeding, and distant metastases (32). A variety of gastrointestinal neuroendocrine tumors are also associated with NF1 (Table 13-1).

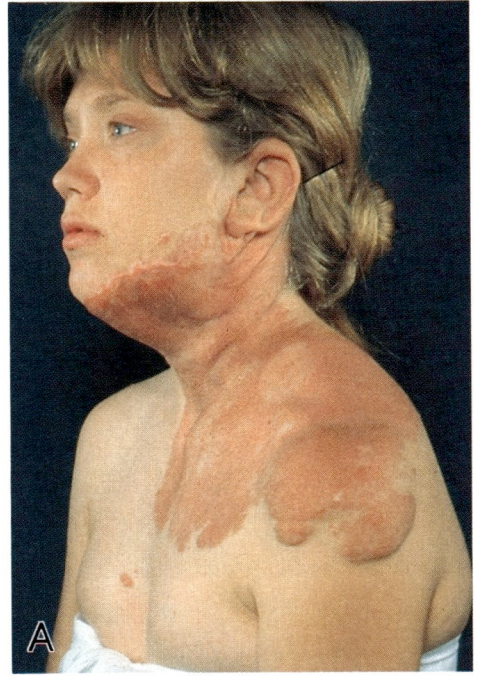

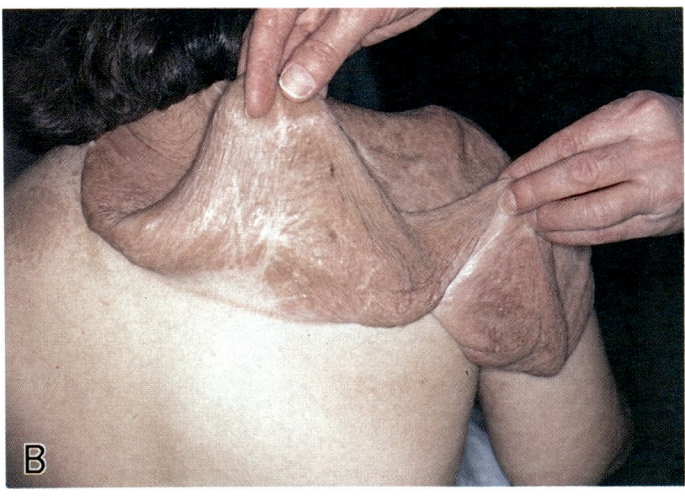

Figure 13-10
MASSIVE NEUROFIBROMAS IN NF1
These soft tissue lesions range from plaques (A) to cape-like flaps (B) and pendulous facial lesions (C). Only rarely do massive diffuse examples affect an entire limb, a lesion once referred to as "elephantiasis neuromatosa" (D) (see also fig. 13-1). Microsections of massive soft tissue neurofibromas typically consist of both diffuse and plexiform components.

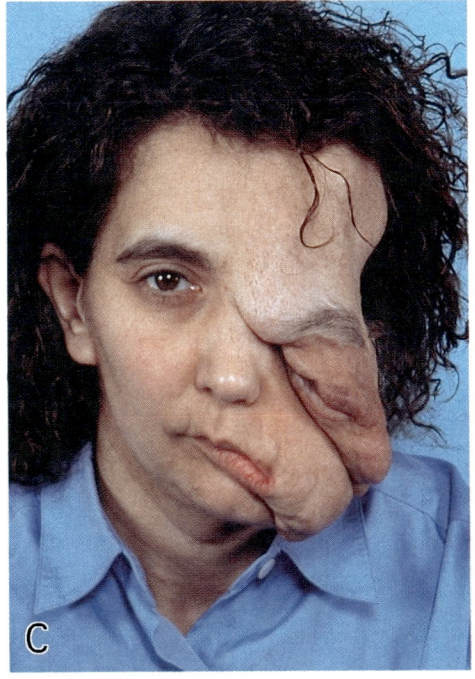

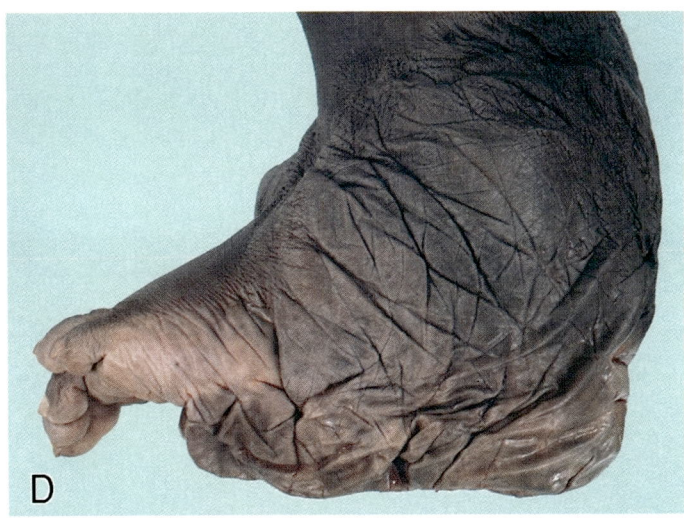

Other NF1-Associated Tumors. Miscellaneous tumors associated with NF1 include bilateral pheochromocytoma, duodenal paraganglioma and carcinoid tumor (10,63,67), rhabdomyosarcoma (29), juvenile chronic myelogenous leukemia (fig. 13-16, right) (46,80), juvenile xantho- granuloma (46,80), and nonossifying fibroma of bone (fibrous cortical defect).

NF1 and the Central Nervous System. Among central nervous system (CNS) neoplasms, nearly all are neuroectodermal in nature. Astrocytomas are by far the most common and include

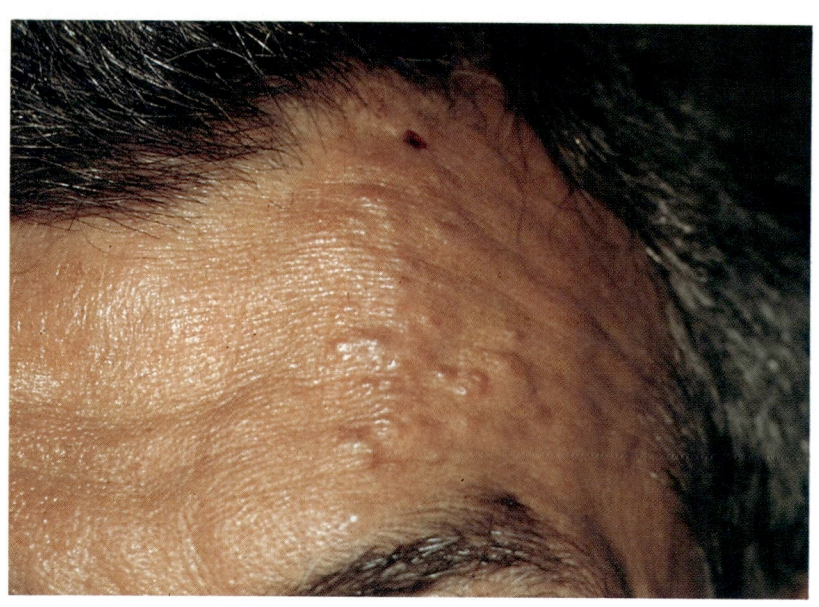

Figure 13-11
SEGMENTAL
NEUROFIBROMATOSIS
Localized to one body part or even a single dermatome, this rare variant of NF1 results from a local somatic mutation. This example affects a portion of the trigeminal nerve distribution.

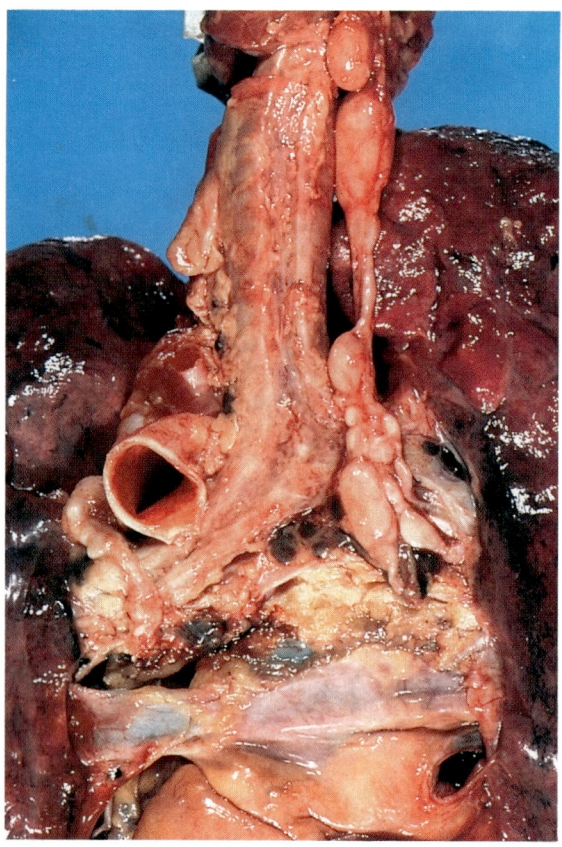

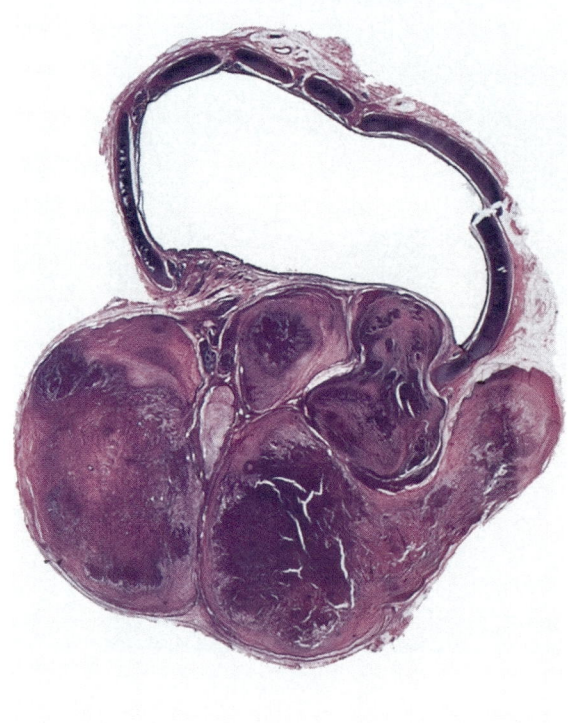

Figure 13-12
VISCERAL PLEXIFORM NEUROFIBROMAS IN NF1

Although plexiform tumors usually arise in soft tissues where they resemble a "bag of worms," nerves in body cavities and viscera may also be affected. Illustrated here are two examples, including an extensive plexiform neurofibroma involving the right vagus nerve and its branches (left), and one involving the posterior trachea (right).

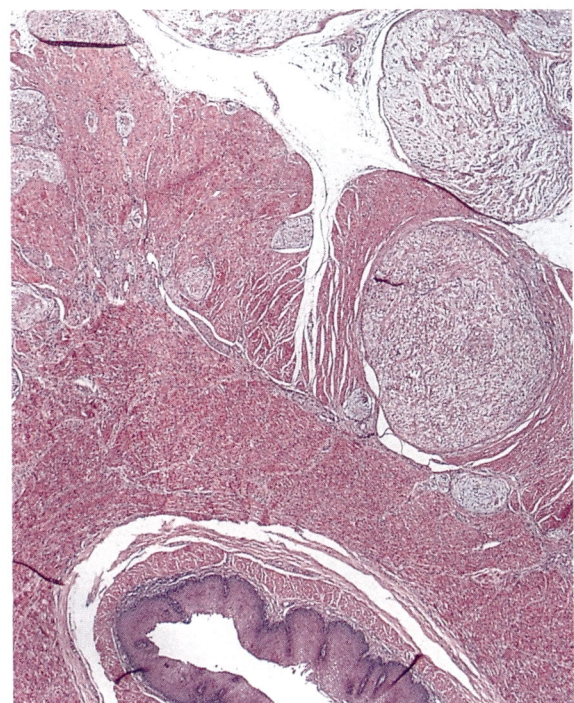

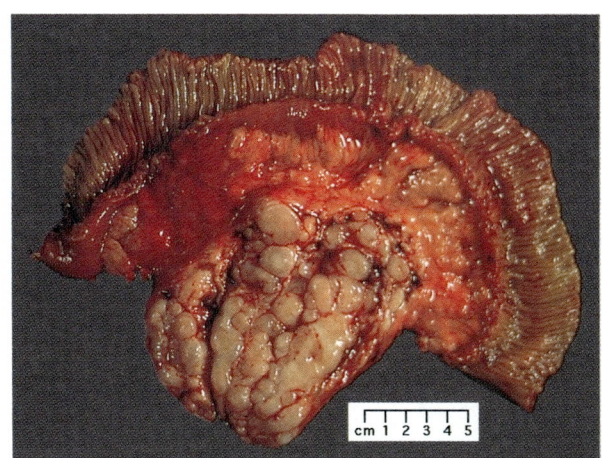

Figure 13-13
VISCERAL PLEXIFORM NEUROFIBROMAS IN NF1
A plexiform tumor affecting the muscularis of the esophagus (left). Another example fills the small bowel mesentery (below).

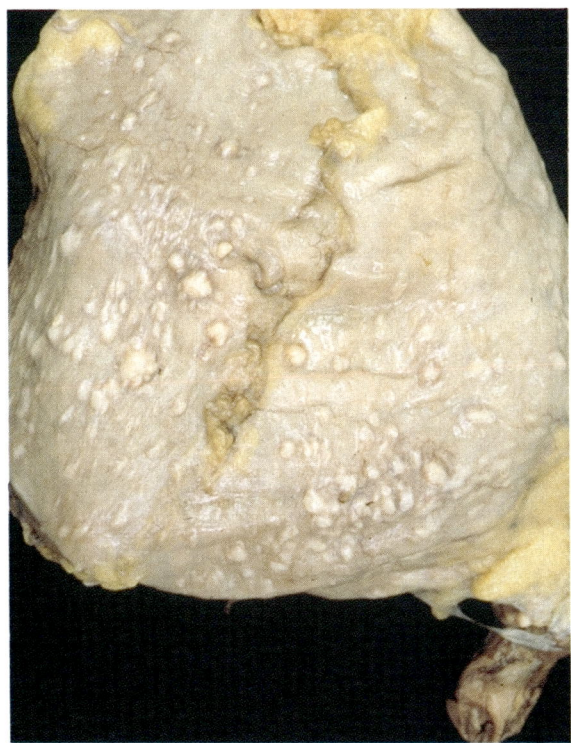

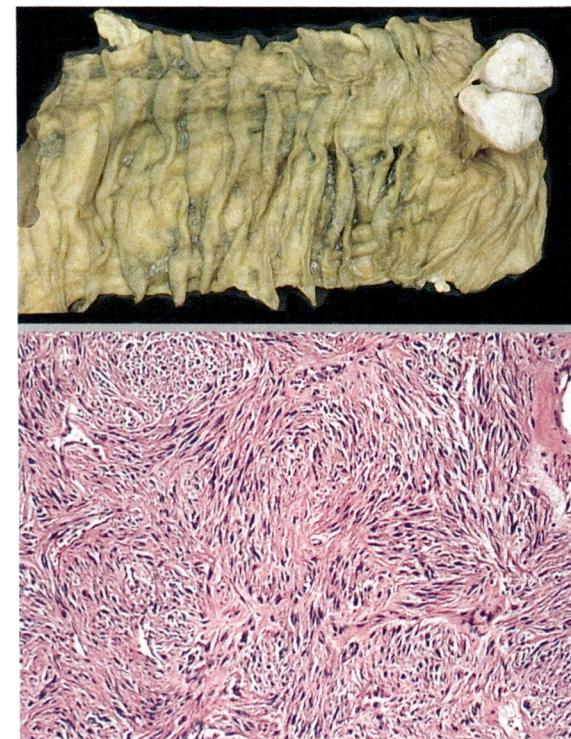

Figure 13-14
GASTROINTESTINAL NEUROFIBROMAS IN NF1
Such lesions are usually multifocal as illustrated by a patient with numerous gastric mucosal examples (left) and a jejunal submucosal example (right).

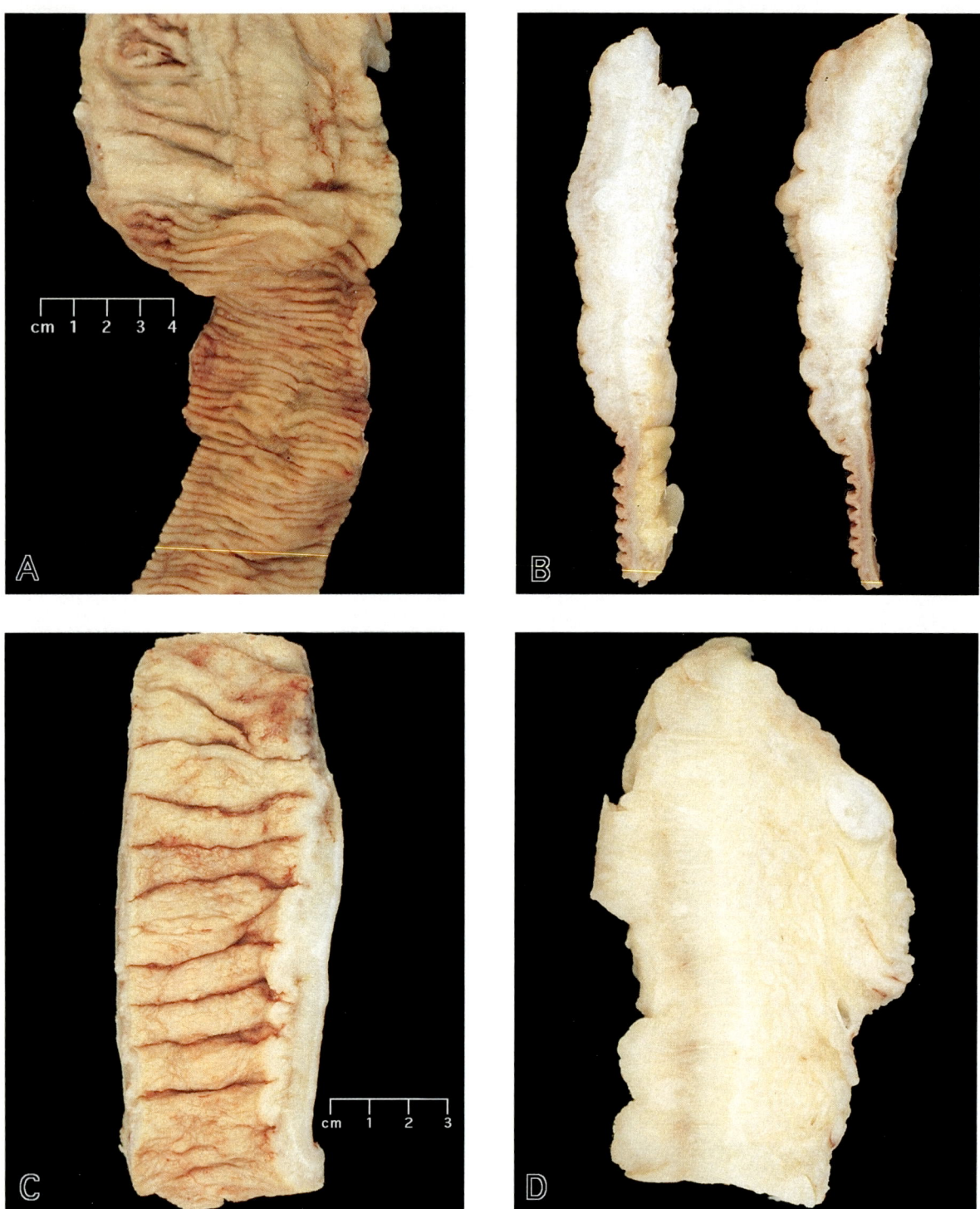

Figure 13-15
SMALL BOWEL NEUROFIBROMAS IN NF1

This 27-year-old female presented with small bowel obstruction. Note the abrupt transition of normal to markedly enlarged small bowel (A,B), coarsening of mucosal folds (C), and the presence of an obvious plexiform component in the serosa (D). Microsections show involvement of the mucosa by ganglioneuromatous tissue (E), diffuse and plexiform intraneural involvement of the submucosa (F), myenteric plexus over-run by tumor (G), and serosal and intramuscular plexiform neurofibroma (H). (Courtesy of Dr. W. Stahr, Cape Giradeau, MO.)

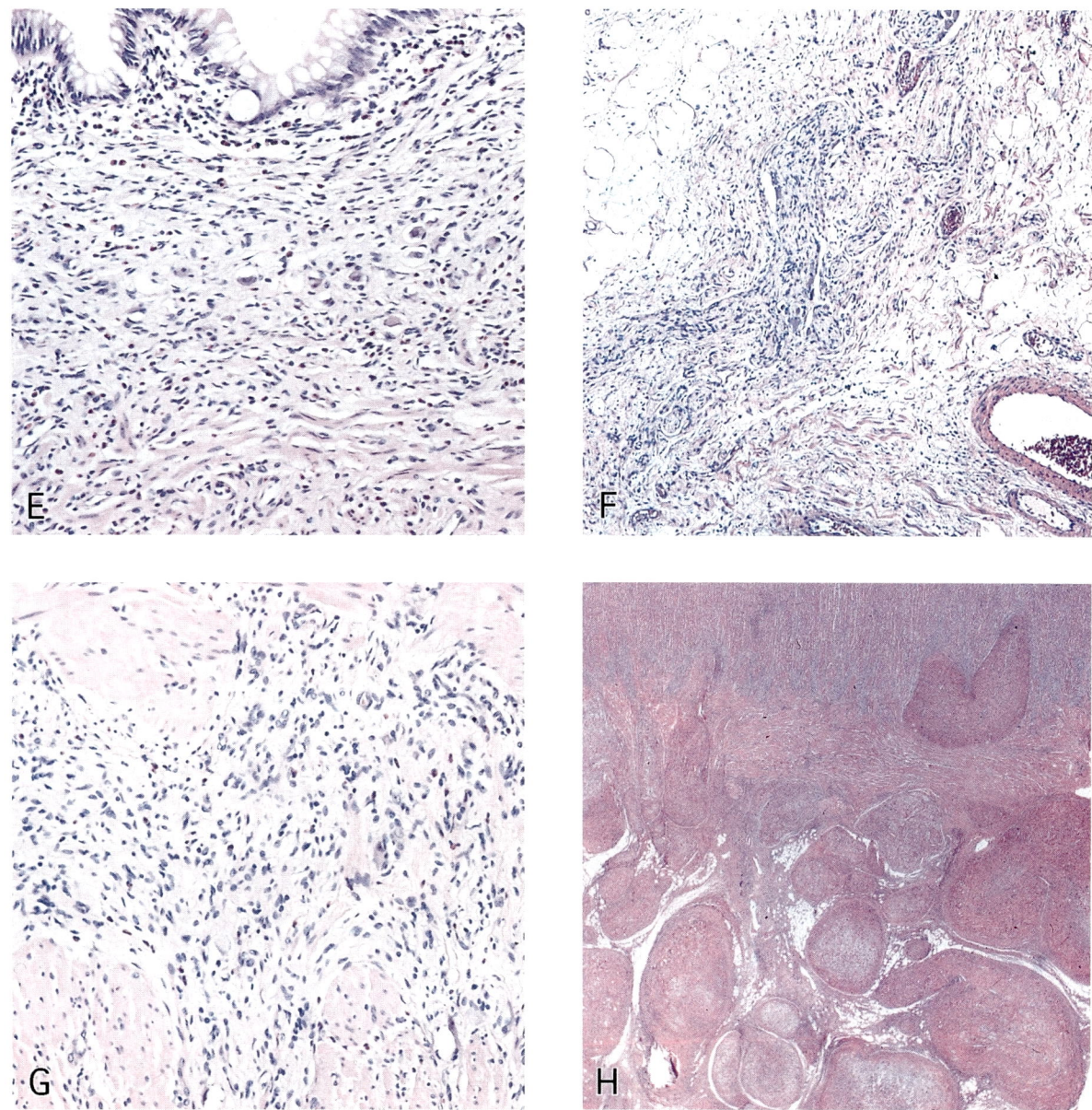

Figure 13-15 (Continued)

unilateral or bilateral optic gliomas (fig. 13-21A,B), the most frequently occurring glioma in NF1 (5,6,9,34,35,39,40), as well as cerebral (30, 58), brain stem, and cerebellar examples (1,30, 42,49,59,74). The majority are pilocytic astrocytomas. Given the presence of optic gliomas in as many as 15 percent of patients, as well as their early age at presentation (80 percent are diagnosed by age 11 when computerized tomography [CT] scans are routinely performed), such tu-

mors are an important element in the diagnosis of NF1 (35). They may involve the intraorbital optic nerve, the chiasm, or both. Bilateral optic nerve gliomas are said to occur only in NF1 (7). In addition to pilocytic astrocytomas, which are relatively benign and preferentially affect the optic apparatus (fig. 13-21A,B), thalamus (fig. 13-21C), and cerebellum, ordinary diffuse or fibrillary astrocytomas also occur in the setting of NF1. Of these, fully half exhibit malignant behavior (30).

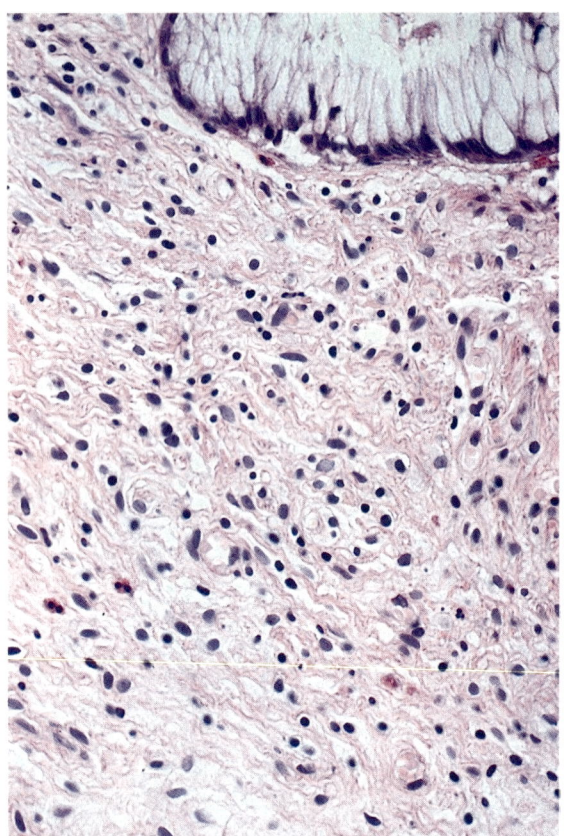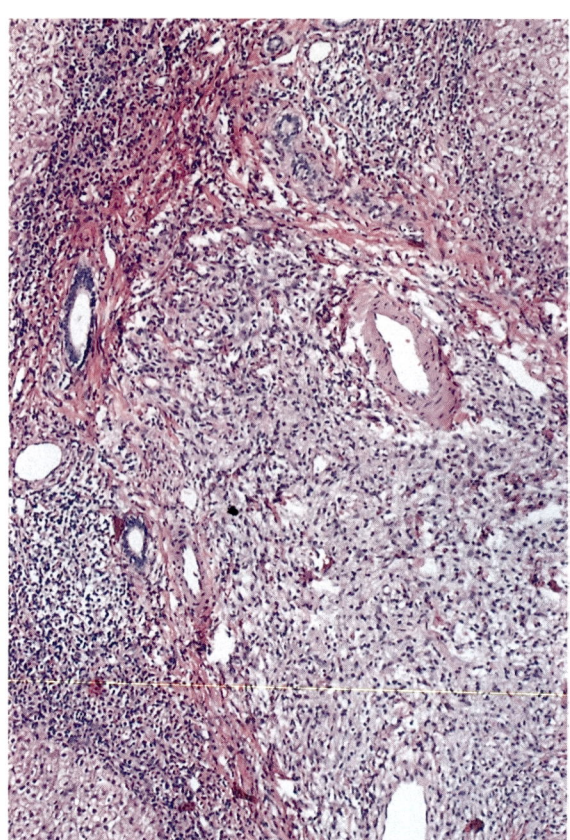

Figure 13-16
GASTROINTESTINAL TRACT NEUROFIBROMAS IN NF1
Left: Superficial biopsies, such as of the colon, may show infiltration of the lamina propria and muscularis mucosa.
Right: Hepatic involvement is rare; note the coexisting infiltrate of juvenile chronic myelogenous leukemia. (Courtesy of Dr. J. Ludwig, Rochester, MN.)

Although tumors of the CNS are relatively common in NF1, they differ both in type and distribution from those of NF2 (Table 13-1).

Patients with NF1 also develop neuroglial hamartomas or malformations such as gliofibrillary nodules (fig. 13-21D) (58), retinal glial hamartomas, and aqueductal stenosis. Other abnormalities encountered in association with NF1 include macrocephaly, short stature, learning disabilities, epilepsy, and hydrocephalus. In addition to the endocrine effects of pheochromocytoma, endocrinopathy in the setting of NF1 also includes precocious puberty. Both are perhaps due to hypothalamic dysfunction.

Miscellaneous NF1-Associated Lesions.
Less frequently occurring manifestations of NF1 are skeletal and other mesodermal dysplasias. The bony dysplasias include "scalloping" of ver-

tebral bodies (fig. 13-22A); kyphoscoliosis (fig. 13-22B,C), anteroposterior indentation or fusion of vertebrae; overgrowth of long bones; dysplastic underdevelopment of long bones with tibial bowing, bone cysts, fractures, and orbital malformation due to dysplasia or absence of portions of the sphenoid or frontal bones (fig. 13-19A,B), which result in facial asymmetry and proptosis; and pseudoarthroses (40). Massive osseous and soft tissue overgrowth may be particularly disfiguring (fig. 13-19C,D). Congenital pseudoarthroses, 50 to 90 percent of which occur in NF1, affect primarily the tibia and fibula (13). Lower thoracic acute-angular scoliosis occurs almost exclusively in NF1 (28,69). Mesodermal dysplasias also affect arteries (14,21,54,61), wherein they produce a range of intimal changes including hyperplasia and fibrosis (61), which result in

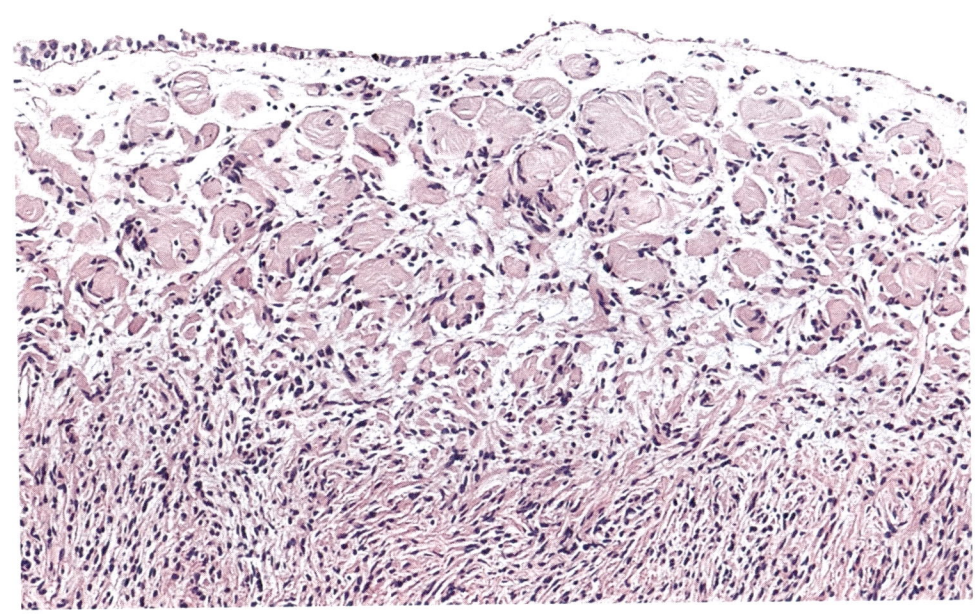

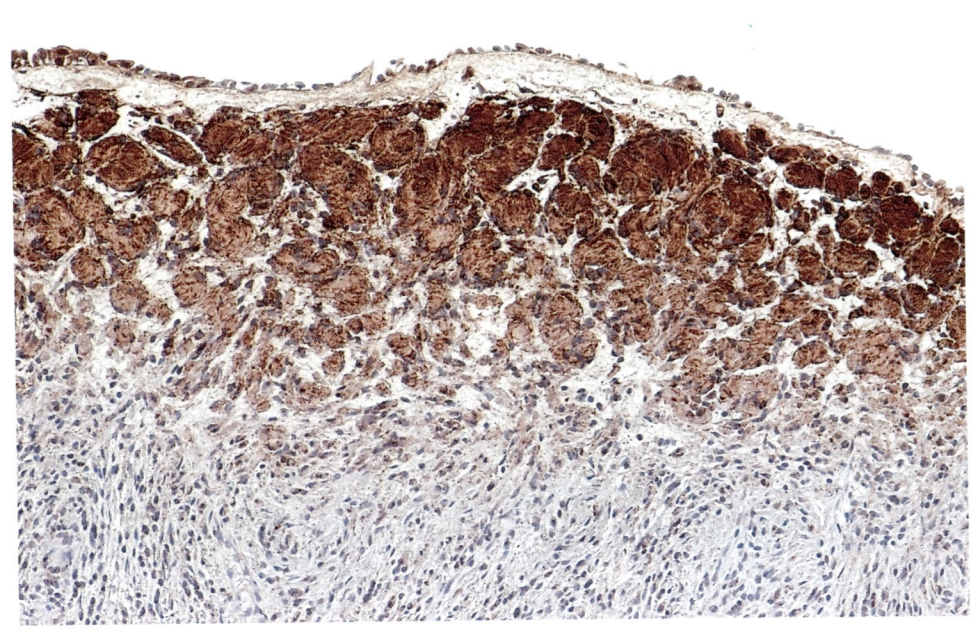

Figure 13-17

NEUROFIBROMA OF URINARY BLADDER IN NF1

Top: A conspicuous feature of this case was the diffuse presence of pseudo-meissnerian corpuscles beneath the urothelium.
Bottom: The corpuscle-like structures are strongly immunoreactive for S-100 protein.

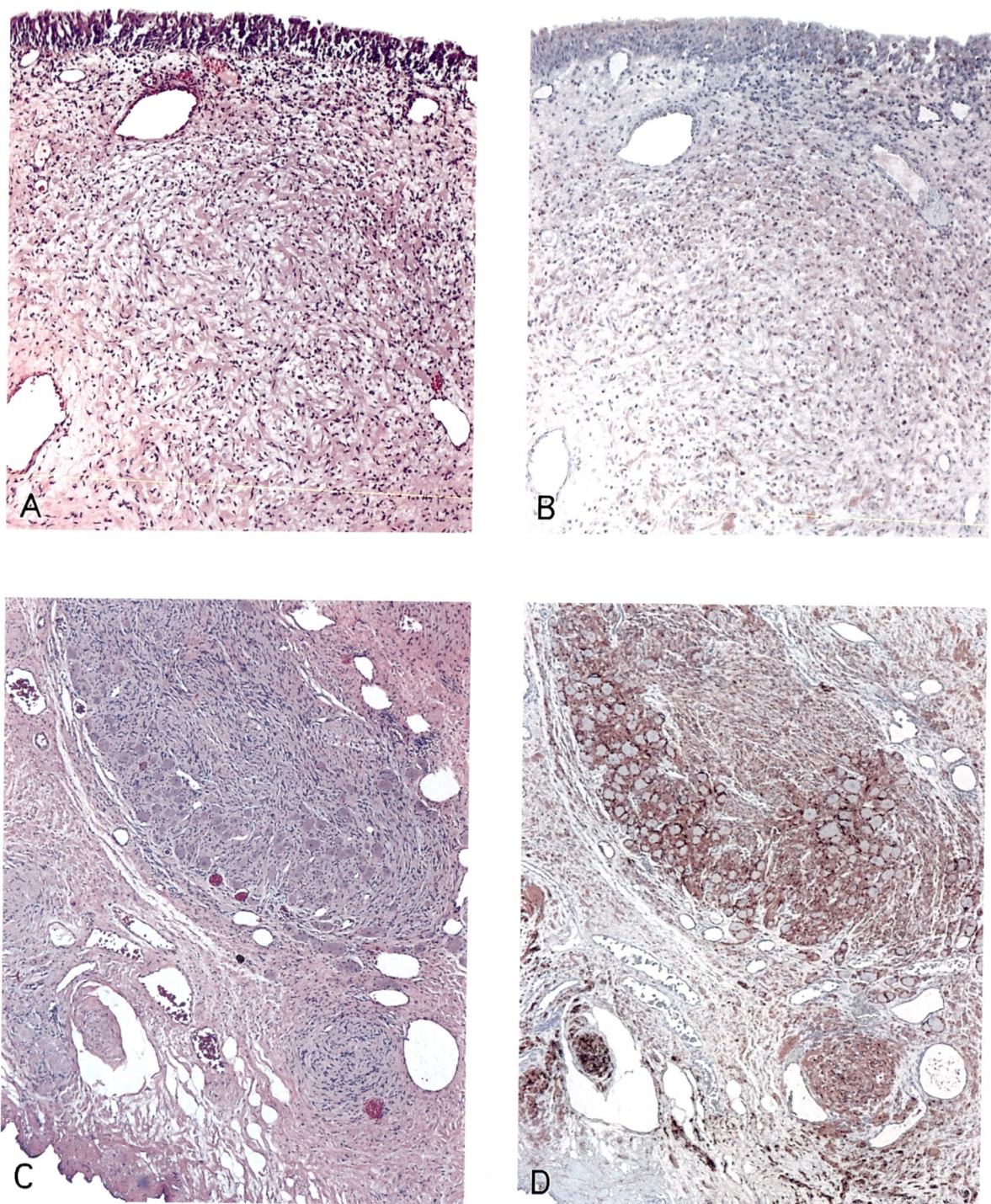

Figure 13-18

NEUROFIBROMA OF URINARY BLADDER IN NF1

Note the diffuse involvement of the mucosa (A; B, S-100 protein stain) and serosal plexiform neurofibroma involving an autonomic ganglion (C; D, S-100 protein stain).

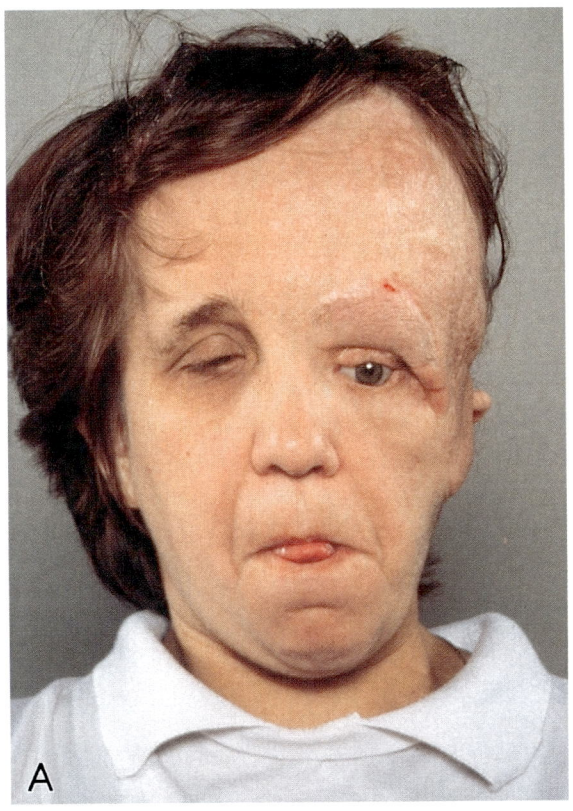

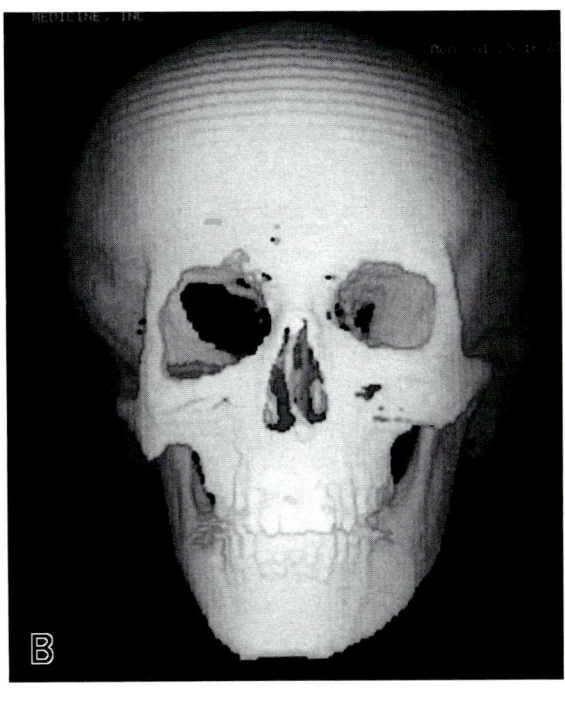

Figure 13-19
OSSEOUS DYSPLASIAS IN NF1

Dysplasia of the sphenoid with enlargement of the superior orbital fissure (B) often results in facial asymmetry and proptosis (A). Massive hemifacial skeletal and soft tissue overgrowth may also be seen in NF1 (C). Such extreme examples are rare. The osseous abnormalities are clearly evident on radiographs (D). The affected tongue of this patient is illustrated in fig. 13-9C.

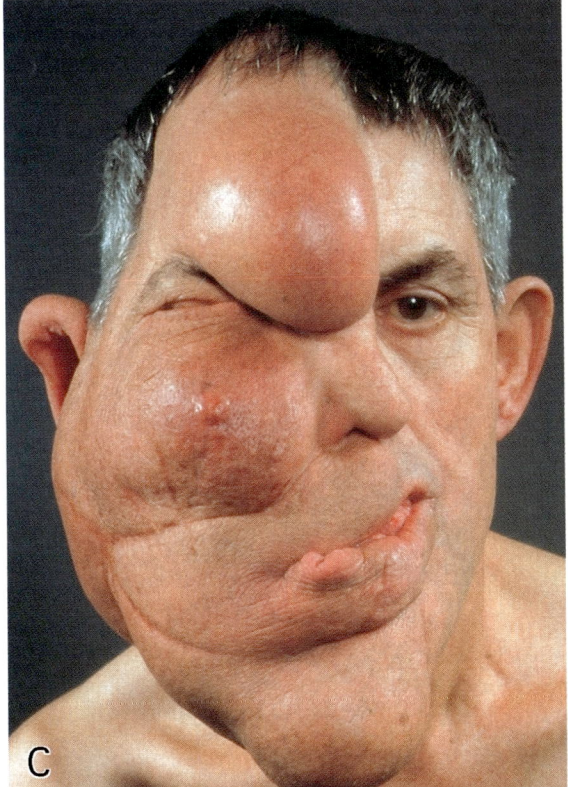

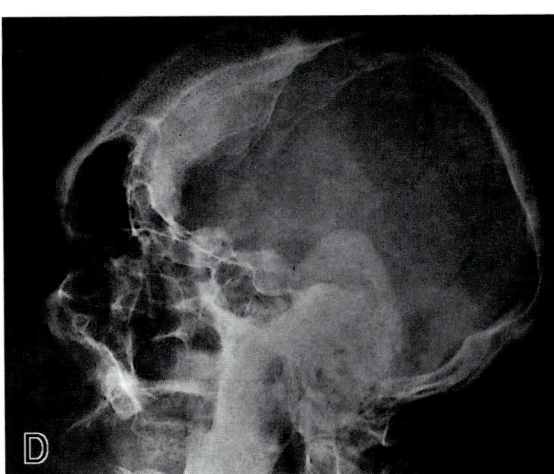

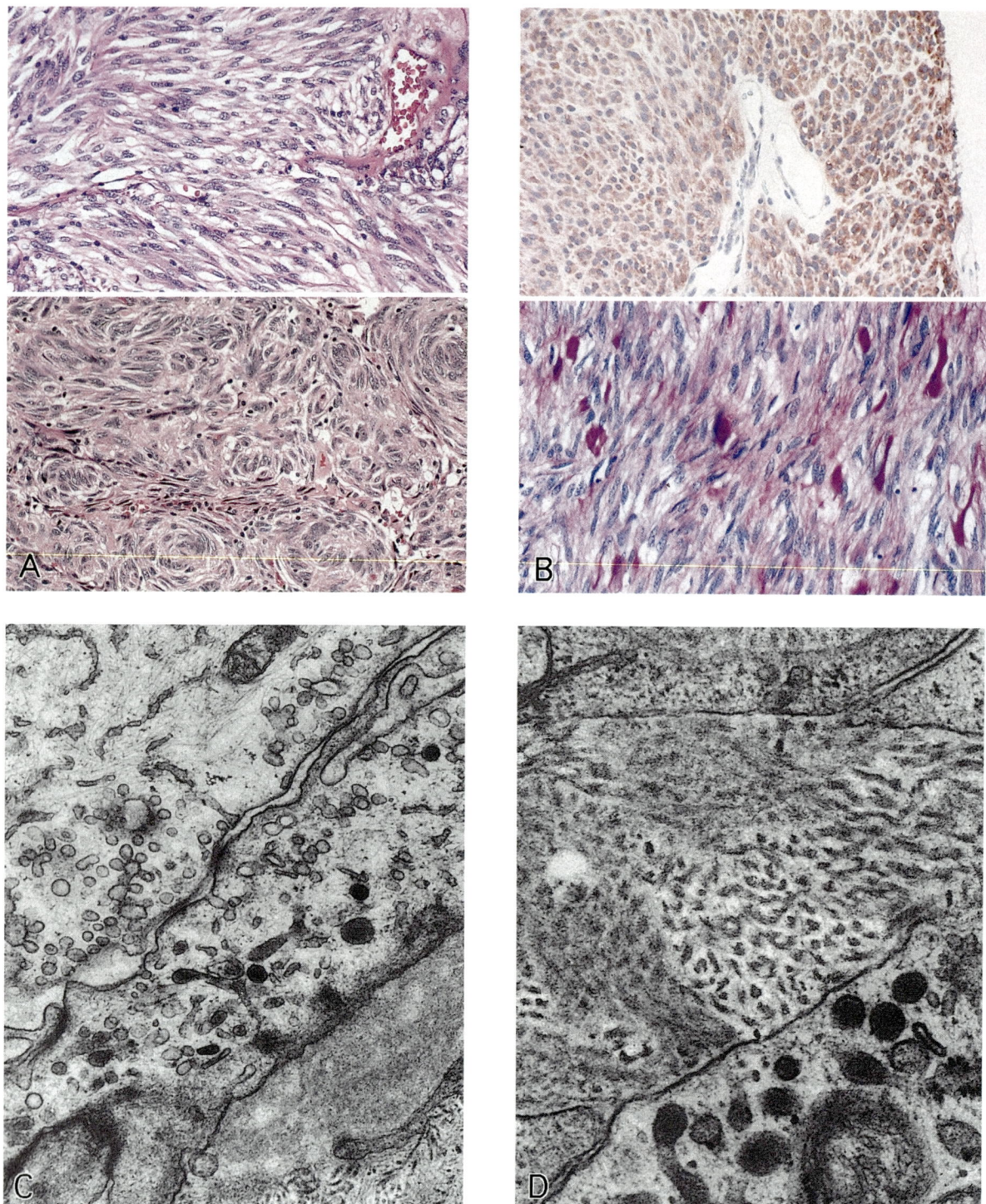

Figure 13-20
GASTROINTESTINAL STROMAL TUMOR IN NF1

Such lesions are frequently of the gastrointestinal autonomic nerve tumor (GANT) type, arise in muscularis propria, and occupy the subserosa. Their histologic pattern varies considerably (A). Immunoreactivity for CD117 is characteristic (B, top) as are skeinoid fibers which are PAS positive (B, bottom). Ultrastructurally, neurite-like cytoplasmic processes contain variable numbers of fine filaments, vesicles, and dense core neurosecretory-type granules (C, X23,900). Note the skeinoid fibers in the extracellular space (D, X48,300).

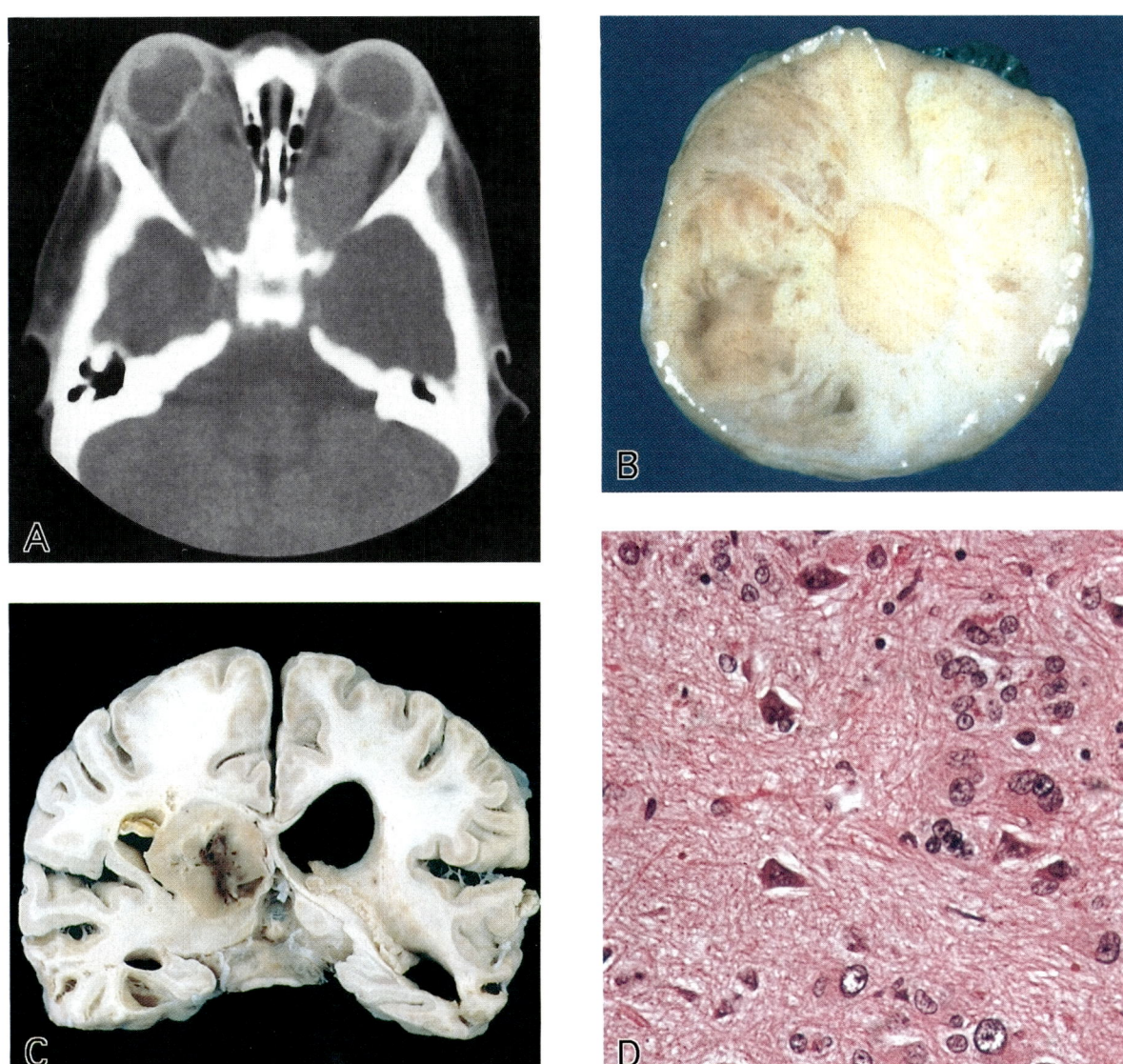

Figure 13-21
ASTROCYTOMAS IN NF1

Most common are "optic nerve gliomas," nearly always low-grade tumors of pilocytic type. Such lesions may be bilateral (A) and often involve both the optic nerve and fill its surrounding leptomeningeal space, a pattern typical of but not limited to patients with NF1 (B). Yet another favored location of pilocytic astrocytoma in NF1 is the thalamus (C). Glioneuronal hamartomas composed of dysmorphic neurons and astrocytes (D) are also seen. (Courtesy of Dr. L. Zimmerman, Washington, D.C.) (C,D: Figs. 3.495 and 3.498 from Okazaki H, Scheithauer BW. Atlas of neuropathology, 1988. With permission from the Mayo Foundation.)

vascular stenosis (fig. 13-23) (16) or the formation of aneurysms (41). Several examples of renovascular hypertension in patients with NF1 have been attributed to such intimal proliferation (11,25). Hypertrophic (obstructive) cardiomyopathy, also a hamartomatous lesion, is an uncommon feature of NF1.

NEUROFIBROMATOSIS 2 (NF2)

Also termed *central* or *bilateral acoustic neurofibromatosis,* NF2 is inherited in an autosomal dominant manner and exhibits a penetrance of almost 100 percent by age 60 (85a). Fifty percent of the cases represent new mutations (86). The

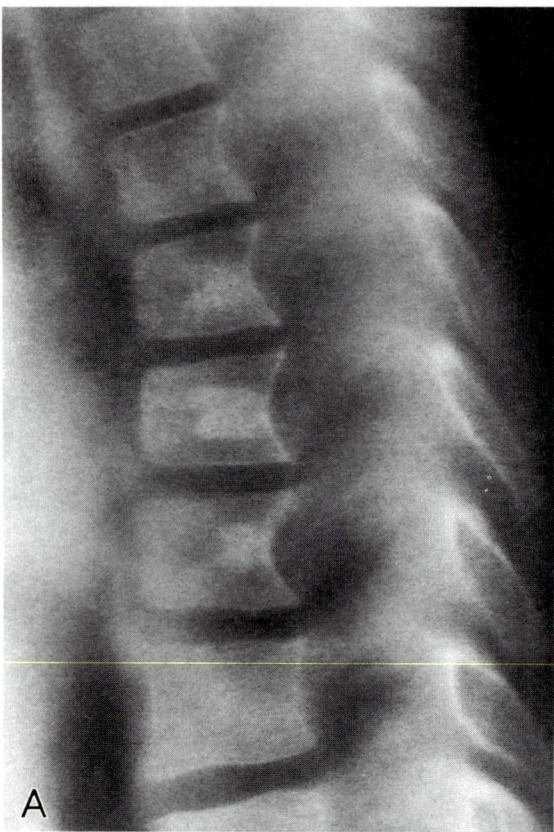

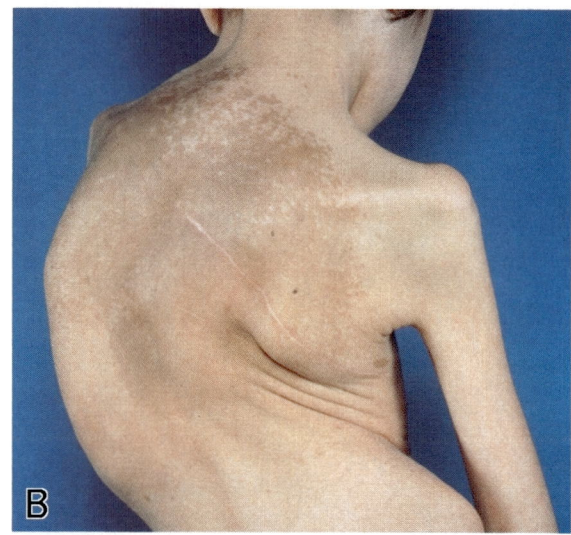

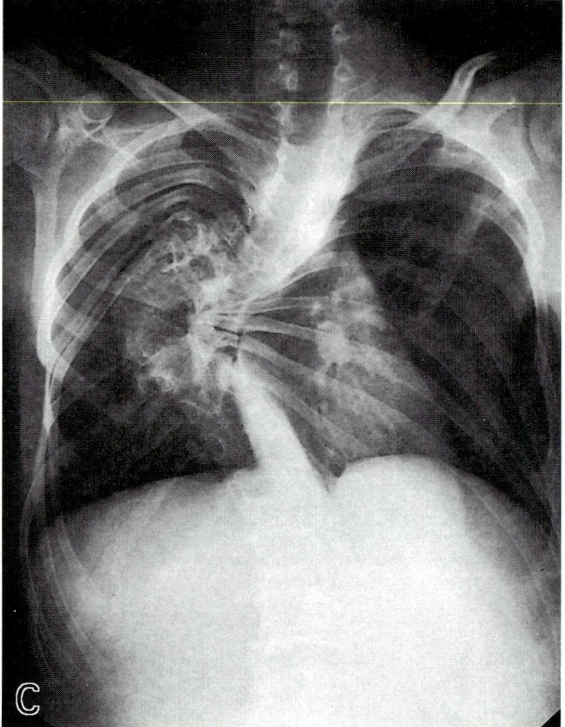

Figure 13-22
THE SPINE IN NF1
Abnormalities range from mild to marked. Scalloping of
vertebral bodies is here shown in association with widening
of the spinal canal (A). Kyphoscoliosis, a common manifestation of NF1 (B), is usually related to dysplasia of vertebral
bodies (C).

mutation underlying the condition is on chromosome 22 (100) and lies near the middle of its long
arm at 22q12 (99,105). The NF2 gene has been
cloned (99,105). It spans 110 kb of genomic DNA,
and encodes a member of the protein 4.1 family
termed merlin (schwannomin), the function of
which may be to mediate communication between the extracellular milieu and the cytoskeleton (94).

NF2 is less common than NF1 and shows a
population incidence of 1 in 40,000. Most patients
present in the second or third decade, but some
are "late onset" (85a). In many instances, it is a
far more devastating disease than NF1. A clinicopathologic comparison of both forms of neurofibromatosis is presented in Table 13-1. His-
torically (88a), a clinical diagnosis of NF2 was
made if a patient had either bilateral 8th cranial

nerve schwannomas or otherwise fulfilled the criteria listed in Table 13-3. Such criteria, however, are weighted toward familial cases and the presence of bilateral 8th cranial nerve schwannomas, tumors that may present years after the appearance of other tumors common in NF2. For this reason, Evans et al. (1992) (86) and Gutmann et al. (1997) (88a) suggested adoption of additional criteria for the diagnosis. Unlike in patients with NF1, café-au-lait spots, when present in NF2, are small and few in number (95). Furthermore, cutaneous neurofibromas are rare in NF2 (95); instead, patients develop multiple schwannomas (89). No Lisch nodules are noted, but posterior subcapsular cataracts occur in 60 to 80 percent of patients (84,97a).

The hallmark of NF2 is the occurrence of bilateral acoustic schwannomas (fig. 13-24) (83, 92), the symptoms of which appear at a wide range of ages only rarely before puberty (84). As previously noted, disease severity varies. These genotype-phenotype correlations are also reflected in age of onset (96a,101a). Since the tumors actually arise from the vestibular branch of the 8th cranial nerve, the recommended designation is *vestibular schwannoma* (86). Virtually all vestibular schwannomas are benign (83), but less than 1 percent invade bone. Although bilateral in most patients, they often present metachronously with years elapsing before the appearance of symptoms of the second tumor. Schwannomas in patients with NF2 affect sites similar to

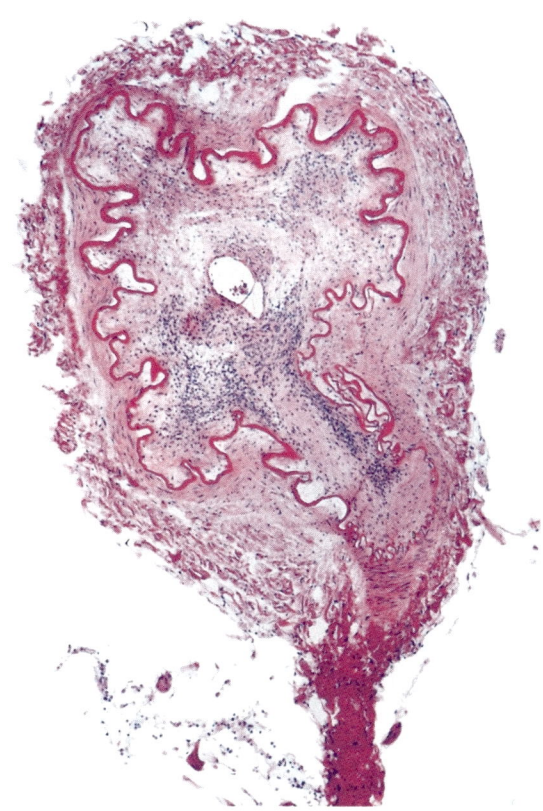

Figure 13-23
VASCULOPATHY IN NF1

This lesion, characterized by subintimal proliferation, mild inflammation, and partial attenuation of the media, was associated with cortical infarction of the temporal lobes. (Fig. 3.505 from Okazaki H, Scheithauer BW. Atlas of neuropathology, 1988. With permission from the Mayo Foundation.)

Table 13-3

DIAGNOSTIC CRITERIA FOR NEUROFIBROMATOSIS 2 (NF2)*

Individuals with the following clinical features have confirmed (definite) NF2:

Bilateral vestibular schwannomas (VS)
    or
Family history of NF2 (first-degree family relative
    plus
        1. Unilateral VS <30 years or
        2. Any 2 of the following: meningioma, glioma schwannoma, juvenile posterior subcapsular lenticular
           opacities/juvenile cortical cataract

Individuals with the following clinical features should be evaluated for NF (presumptive or probable NF2):

    Unilateral VS <30 years plus at least one of the following: meningiomas, glioma, schwannoma, juvenile
        posterior subcapsular lenticular opacities/juvenile cortical cataract

    Multiple meningiomas (2 or more) plus unilateral VS <30 years or one of the following: glioma, schwannoma,
        juvenile posterior subcapsular lenticular opacities/juvenile cortical cataract

*Table 2 from Gutmann MD, Aylsworth A, Carey JC, et al. The diagnostic evaluation and multidisciplinary management of neurofibromatosis 1 and neurofibromatosis 2. JAMA 1997;278:51–7.

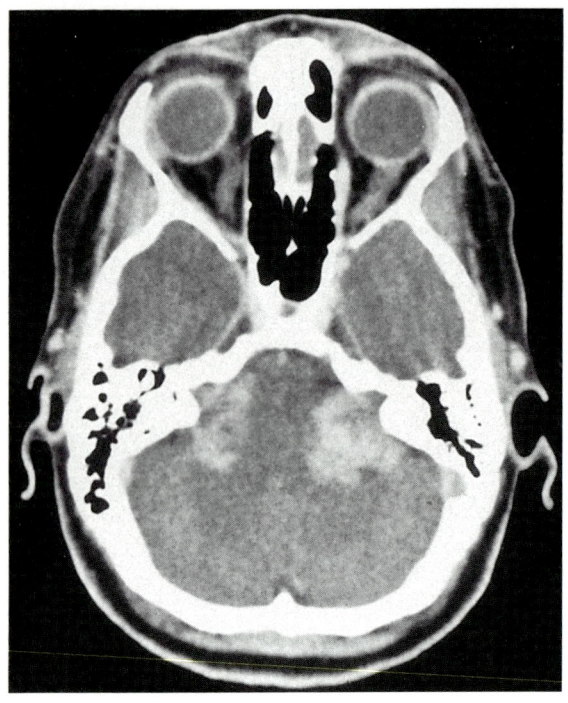

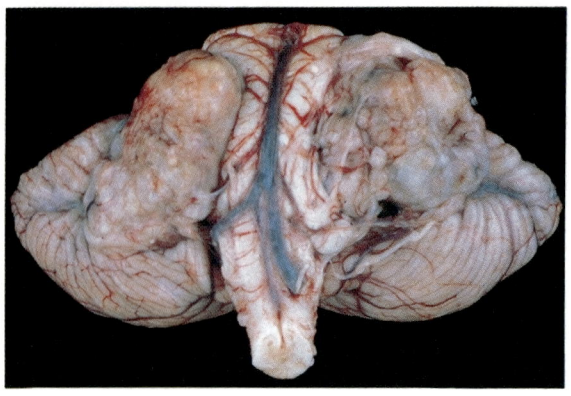

Figure 13-24
MULTIPLE SCHWANNOMAS IN NF2
Multiple schwannomas in NF2 include bilateral acoustic tumors, here shown on CT scan with contrast (left) and at autopsy (right), as well as multiple cranial or spinal nerve root schwannomas. (Top: Courtesy of Dr. P. C. Burger, Baltimore, MD.) (Bottom: Fig. 3.490 from Okazaki H, Scheithauer BW. Atlas of neuropathology, 1988. With permission from the Mayo Foundation.)

those of sporadic tumors, but may show several unusual features such as multifocality within a nerve (figs. 13-24, right, 13-25), a distinctly nodular microscopic growth pattern (103), an association with peritumoral arachnoidal cell proliferation (88), and the rare occurrence of a mixed schwannoma-meningioma phenotype (88). *Cutaneous schwannomas* occur in approximately 50 percent of NF2 patients; their prevalence and number vary with disease severity (95). Although some have a plexiform pattern of growth, neither plexiform neurofibroma nor plexiform schwannoma are considered components of NF2. On rare occasion, peripheral nerves show widespread nodular enlargement in the setting of a distal symmetric sensorimotor neuropathy (96,104). It is of note that the majority of sporadic schwannomas also show mutations in the NF2 gene (91).

Meningiomas frequently coexist with vestibular schwannoma and occur in a majority of patients. On occasion, multiple meningiomas are the only feature of NF2 (81). They arise early in life, are commonly multifocal, and sometimes assume the form of "meningiomatosis" in which diffuse or multifocal lesions involve both the cranial and spinal meninges (fig. 13-26). Nonetheless, multifocal meningiomas are not patho-

gnomonic of NF2. Studies of their distribution show that meningiomas occurring in NF2 are intracranial in 54 percent of cases, intracranial and intraspinal in 42 percent, and solely intraspinal in 4 percent (98). The fibrous variant of meningioma occurs with greater frequency in NF2 than among sporadic meningiomas. No increase in atypical or malignant meningiomas has been observed. As with schwannomas, sporadic meningiomas exhibit mutations of the NF2 gene, an occurrence highly associated with allelic loss of chromosome 22 (93,106). Also NF2 associated is meningoangiomatosis (90), a rare lesion in which meningothelial cells surrounding leptomeningeal and cortical vessels form single or multiple plaque-like lesions that literally replace a segment of cerebral cortex (fig. 13-27A,B). Some are associated with an overlying coarse calcification which often occupies a sulcus (fig. 13-27C). Similar calcifications may also occur in isolation and unassociated with NF2 (82).

Gliomas occur less commonly than acoustic schwannomas and meningiomas, and involve the spinal cord or, less frequently, the cerebrum or cerebellum. Seventy percent of these are ependymomas, which often present as multiple lesions with a predilection for the cervical and thoracic

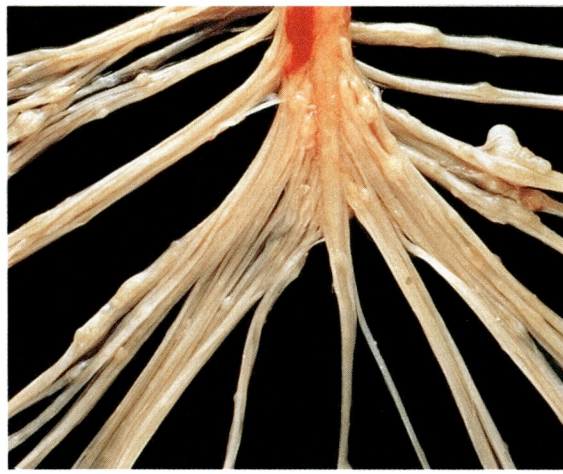

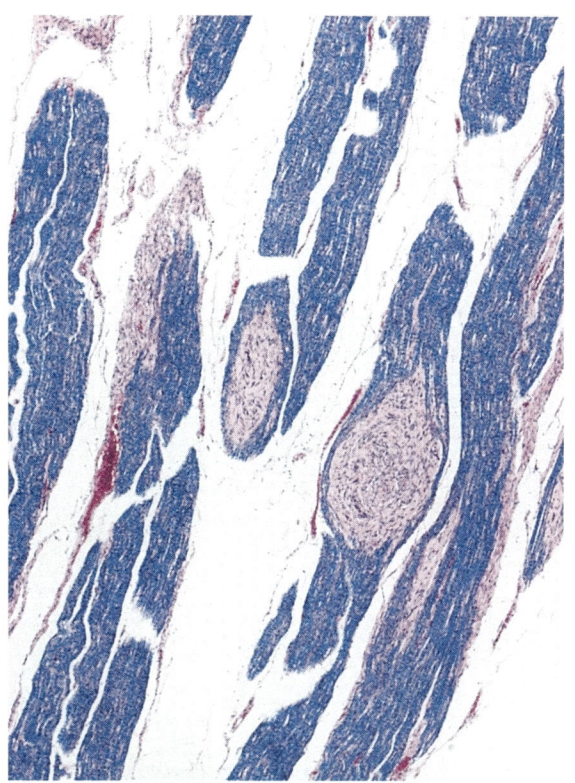

Figure 13-25

MULTIPLE SCHWANNOMAS IN NF2

Multiple cranial or spinal nerve root schwannomas shown arising in cauda equina nerve roots. (Right: H&E–Luxol-fast blue) (Above: Fig. 3.492 from Okazaki H, Scheithauer BW. Atlas of neuropathology, 1988. With permission from the Mayo Foundation. Right: Courtesy of Dr. P. C. Burger, Baltimore, MD.)

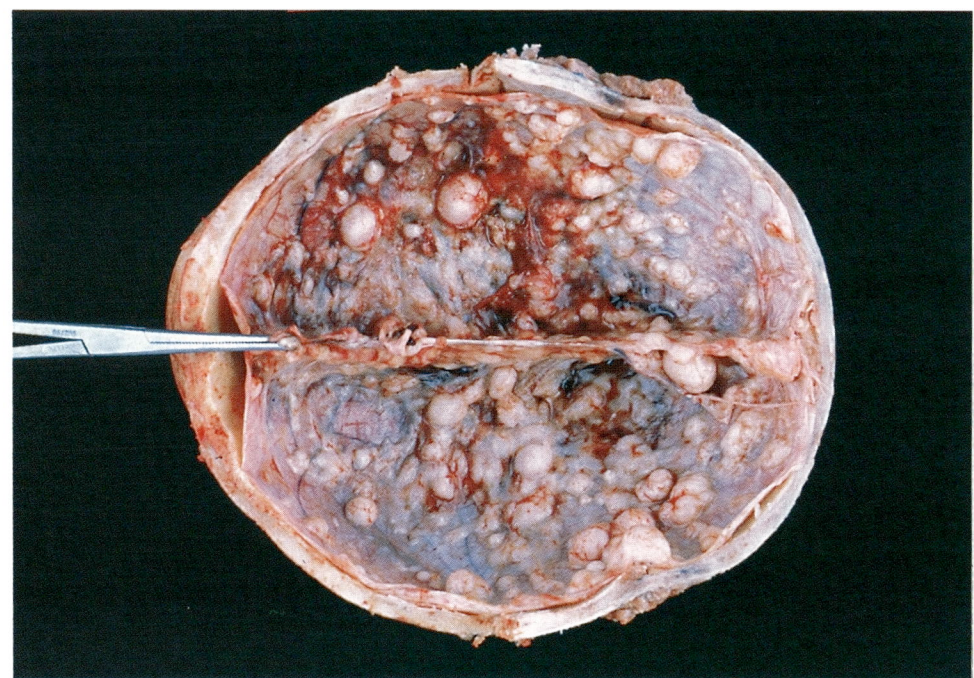

Figure 13-26

MULTIPLE MENINGIOMAS IN NF2

Such lesions sometimes cover the inner aspect of the dura. (Fig. 3.494 from Okazaki H, Scheithauer BW. Atlas of neuropathology, 1988. With permission from the Mayo Foundation.)

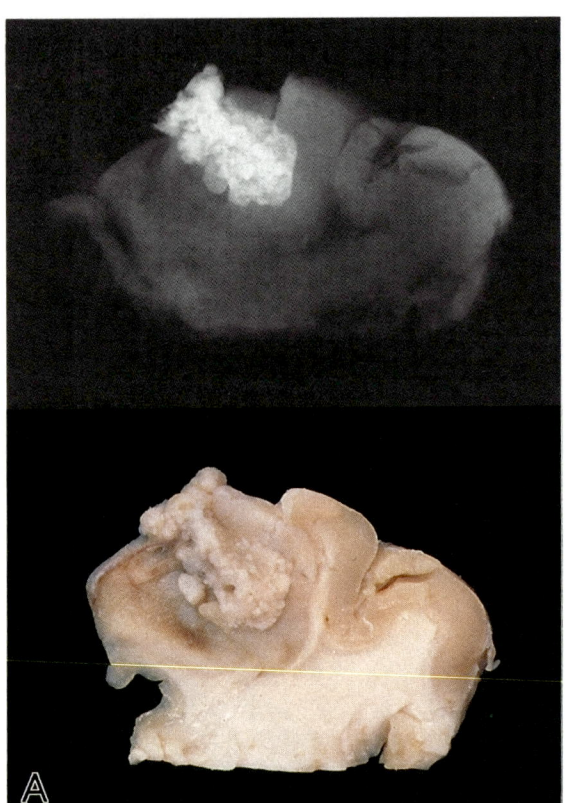

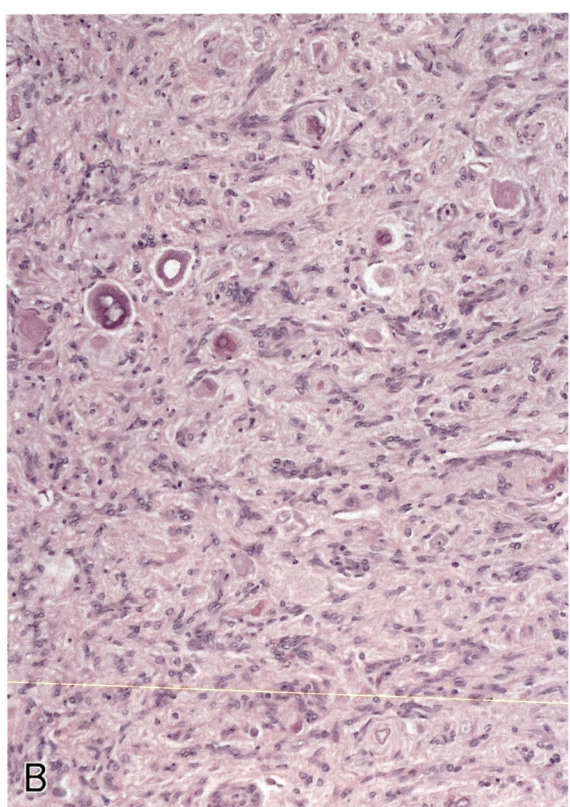

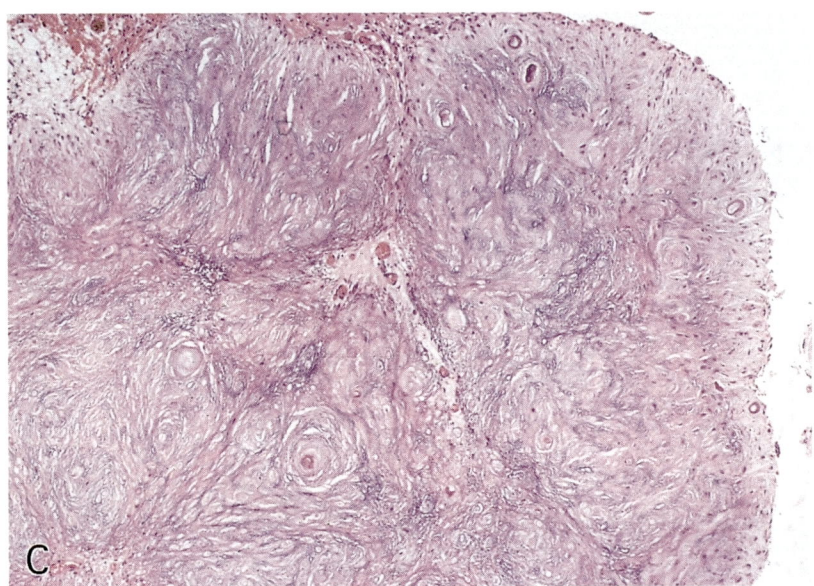

Figure 13-27
MENINGOANGIOMATOSIS

Although this example was not NF2 associated, such lesions do show a distinct association with that disorder. Fully formed, they consist of a firm pale cortical ribbon and an overlying leptomeningeal calcification (A). The cortex is largely replaced by arachnoidal cells associated with an increased vasculature (B). The often multinodular leptomeningeal calcification, which also may show osseous metaplasia, typically demonstrates peripheral hypercellularity (C). (A: Fig. 3.503 from Okazaki H, Scheithauer BW. Atlas of neuropathology, 1988. With permission from the Mayo Foundation.)

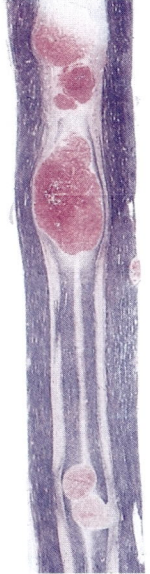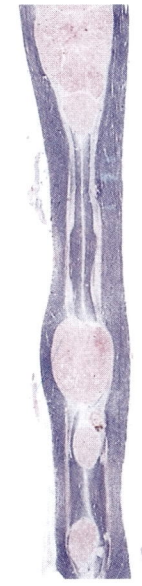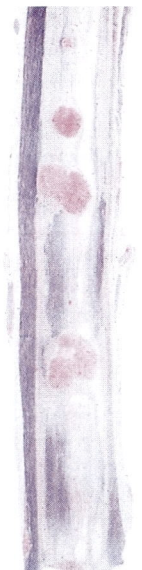

Figure 13-28
MULTIPLE SPINAL CORD
EPENDYMOMAS IN NF2
This whole mount longitudinal
section of the spinal cord shows tumors
forming numerous demarcated lesions
of varying size. (Fig. 3.497 from
Okazaki H, Scheithauer BW. Atlas of
neuropathology, 1988. With permission from the Mayo Foundation.)

spinal cord (fig. 13-28) (98). Ependymomas may involve the filum terminale, a site also prone to the development of multiple schwannomas. Pilocytic or diffuse fibrillary astrocytomas of optic nerve, brain stem, cerebellum, or cerebrum are far more commonly encountered in NF1. Patients with NF2 are also prone to develop dysplastic lesions of the CNS, albeit ones unassociated with mental retardation. These include multiple glial microhamartomas often affecting the cerebral cortex, cellular ependymal ectopias frequently involving the spinal cord, intramedullary schwannosis, and syringomyelia (97,101,108.) Such lesions are not considered preneoplastic. Other CNS lesions in NF2 include cerebral, cerebellar, periventricular, and choroid plexus calcifications (102).

The majority of patients with NF2 die from complications of the disorder (86). Some do so 2 to 3 years after the onset of symptoms, although the majority survive for longer periods, even into late middle age. There appear to be two distinct clinical presentations. The type described by Wishart (109) is characterized by early onset

multiple tumors in addition to bilateral vestibular schwannomas, and a rapid disease course (85,86). In the Gardner-Frazier type (87), the onset is late, the course is more protracted, and there are only bilateral vestibular schwannomas (85,86). A 1971 study of 55 members of an NF2 kindred with bilateral acoustic schwannomas (110) found that 71 percent of the 38 patients in whom a cause of death was known died of bilateral acoustic schwannomas. Death was variously due to impingement of the tumor upon the brain stem, elevated intracranial pressure, or to complications of surgery. Given the advances made in neurosurgical techniques, fewer patients today die as a result of acoustic schwannomas. The second major cause of death, and currently the most difficult to treat, is spinal ependymoma, which usually occurs in the cervical and thoracic levels. Slowly progressive growth of these often multiple tumors leads to destruction of the spinal tracts that innervate the respiratory system.

REFERENCES

Neurofibromatosis 1

1. Ajuriaguerra J de, David M, Haguenau F. Gliose meningo-cerebelleuse et maladie de Recklinghausen. Revue Neurologique 1955;93:645–55.

2. Akesson HO, Axelsson R, Sameulsson B. Neurofibromatosis in monozygotic twins: a case report. Acta Geneticae Medicae et Gemellelogiae 1983;32:245–9.

3. Barker D, Wright E, Nguyen K, et al. Gene for von Recklinghausen's neurofibromatosis is in the pericentrometric region of chromosome 17. Science 1987;236:1100–2.

4. Baumgarten HG, Holstein AF, Owman CH. Auerbach's plexus of mammals and man: electron microscopic identification of three different types of neuronal processes in myenteric ganglia of the large intestine from rhesus monkeys, guinea-pigs and man. Z Zellforsch 1970;106:376–97.

5. Blatt J, Jaffe R, Deutsch M, Adkins JC. Neurofibromatosis and childhood tumors. Cancer 1986;57:1225–9.

6. Borit A, Richardson EP Jr. The biological and clinical behavior of pilocytic astrocytomas of the optic pathways. Brain 1982;105:161–87.

6a.Cheng L, Scheithauer BW, Leibovich BC, Romani DM, Cheville JC, Bostwick DG. Neurofibroma of the urinary bladder. Am J Surg Pathol (in press).

7. Chutorian A. Panel on diagnosis and natural history of optic nerve glioma. In: Optic gliomas in neurofibromatosis. Conference Series Volume 2. New York: The National Neurofibromatosis Foundation, Inc., 1989:55–62.

8. Crowe FW, Schull WJ, Neel JV. A clinical, pathological, and genetic study of multiple neurofibromatosis. Springfield, Illinois: Charles C. Thomas, 1956.

9. Davis FA. Primary tumors of the optic nerve (a phenomenon of Recklinghausen's disease). A clinical and pathologic study with a report of four cases and review of the literature. Arch Ophthalmol 1940;23:735–821.

10. Dayal Y, Talberg KA, Nunnemacher G, DeLellis RA, Wolfe HJ. Duodenal carcinoids in patients with and without neurofibromatosis. A comparative study. Am J Surg Pathol 1986;10:348–57.

11. Elias DL, Ricketts RR, Smith RB III. Renovascular hypertension complicating neurofibromatosis. Am Surg 1985;51:97–106.

12. Erlandson RA, Klimstra DS, Woodruff JM. Subclassification of gastrointestinal stromal tumors based on evaluation by electron microscopy and immunohistochemistry. Ultrastruct Pathol 1996;20:373–93.

13. Fairbank J. Orthopaedic manifestations of neurofibromatosis. In: Huson SM, Hughes RA, eds. The neurofibromatosis: a pathogenetic and clinical overview. London: Chapman and Hall, 1994:275–304.

14. Feyrter F. Uber die vasculare neurofibromatose, nach utersuchlungen am menschlichen magendarmschlauch. Virchow Arch [A] 1949;317:221–65.

15. Fialkow PJ, Sagebiel RW, Gartler SM, Rimoin DL. Multiple cell origin of hereditary neurofibromas. N Engl J Med 1971;284:298–300.

16. Finley JL, Dabbs DJ. Renal vascular smooth muscle proliferation in neurofibromatosis. Hum Pathol 1988;19:107–10.

17. Friedman JM, Fialkow PJ, Greene CL, Weinberg WN. Probable clonal origin or neurofibrosarcoma in a patient with hereditary neurofibromatosis. JNCI 1982;69:1289–92.

18. Fuller CE, Williams GT. Gastrointestinal manifestations of type 1 neurofibromatosis (von Recklinghausen's disease). Histopathology 1991;19:1–11.

19. Gennatas CS, Exarhakos G, Kondi-Pafiti A, et al. Malignant schwannoma of the stomach in a patient with neurofibromatosis. Eur J Surg Oncol 1988;14:261–4.

20. Ghrist TD. Gastrointestinal involvement in neurofibromatosis. Arch Intern Med 1963;112:357–62.

21. Greene JF Jr, Fitzwater JE, Burgess J. Arterial lesions associated with neurofibromatosis. Am J Clin Pathol 1974;62:481–7.

22. Gutmann DH, Collins FS. Neurofibromatosis type 1. Beyond positional cloning. Arch Neurol 1993;50:1185–93.

22a.Gutmann DH, Aylsworth A, Carey JC, et al. The diagnostic evaluation and multidisciplinary management of neurofibromatosis 1 and neurofibromatosis 2. JAMA 1997;278:71–7.

23. Halliday AL, Sobel RA, Martuza RL. Benign spinal nerve sheath tumors: their occurrence sporadically and in neurofibromatosis types 1 and 2. J Neurosurg 1991;74:248–53.

24. Halling KC, Scheithauer BW, Halling AC, et al. p53 expression in neurofibroma and malignant peripheral nerve sheath tumor. An immunohistochemical study of sporadic and NF1-associated tumors. Am J Clin Pathol 1996;106:282–8.

25. Halpern M, Curranio G. Vascular lesions causing hypertension in neurofibromatosis. N Engl J Med 1965;273:248–52.

26. Herrera GA, DeMoraes HP, Grizzle WE, Han SG. Malignant small bowel neoplasm of enteric plexus derivation (plexosarcoma). Light and electron microscopic study confirming the origin of the neoplasm. Dig Dis Sci 1984;29:275–84.

26a.Hirota S, Isozaki K, Mariyama Y, et al. Gain-of-function mutations of c-kit in human gastrointestinal stromal tumors. Science 1998;279:577–80.

27. Hochberg FH, DaSilva AB, Galdabini J, Ricardson EP Jr. Gastrointestinal involvement in von Recklinghausen's neurofibromatosis. Neurology 1974;24:1144–51.

28. Hunt JC, Pugh DG. Skeletal lesions in neurofibromatosis. Radiology 1961;76:1–19.

29. Huson SM, Harper PS, Compston DA. Von Recklinghausen neurofibromatosis. A clinical and population study in Southeast Wales. Brain 1988;111:1355–81.

30. Ilgren EB, Kinnier-Wilson LM, Stiller CA. Gliomas in neurofibromatosis: a series of 89 cases with evidence of enhanced malignancy in associated cerebellar astrocytomas. Pathol Ann 1985;20:331–58.

31. Jimbow K, Szabo G, Fitzpatrick TB. Ultrastructure of giant pigmented granules (macromelanosomes) in the cutaneous pigmented macules of neurofibromatosis. J Invest Dermatol 1973;61:300–9.

31a.Kindblom LG, Remotti HE, Aldenborg F, Meis-Kindlblom JM. Gastrointestinal pacemaker cell tumor (GIPACT): gastrointestinal stromal tumors show phenotypic characteristics of the interstitial cells of Cajal. Am J Pathol 1998;152:1259–69.

32. Lauwers GY, Erlandson RA, Casper ES, Brennan MF, Woodruff JM. Gastrointestinal autonomic nerve tumors. A clinicopathological, immunohistochemical, and ultrastructural study of 12 cases. Am J Surg Pathol 1993;17:887–97.

33. Levy D, Khatib R. Intestinal neurofibromatosis with malignant degeneration: report of a case. Dis Colon Rectum 1960;3:140–4.

34. Lewis RA. Ocular features of neurofibromatosis. In: Rubinstein AE, Korf BR, eds. Neurofibromatosis. A handbook for patients, families, and health care professionals. New York: Thieme, 1990:80–7.

35. Lewis RA, Gerson LP, Axelson KA, Riccardi VM, Whitford RP. Von Recklinghausen's neurofibromatosis. II. Incidence of optic gliomata. Ophthalmology 1984;91:929–35.

36. Lisch K. Uber Beteiligung der Augen, Insbesondere das Vorkommen von Irisnotchen bei der Neurofibromatose (Recklinghausen). Z Augenheilkende 1937;93:137–43.

37. Louis DN, von Deimling A. Hereditary tumor syndromes of the nervous system: overview and rare syndromes. Brain Pathol 1995;5:145–51.

38. Ludwig J, Wester S, Elston AC. Evidence of neurofibromatosis and chronic myelogenous leukemia in a liver biopsy specimen [Letter]. J Clin Gastroenterol 1993;16:265–7.

39. Lund AM, Skovby F. Optic gliomas in children with neurofibromatosis type 1. Eur J Pediatr 1991;150:835–8.

40. MacEwen GD. Orthopedic aspects of neurofibromatosis. In: Rubenstein AE, Korf BR, eds. Neurofibromatosis. A handbook for patients, families, and health care professionals. New York: Thieme, 1990:125–41.

41. Malecha MJ, Rubin R. Aneurysms of the carotid arteries associated with von Recklinghausen's neurofibromatosis. Path Res Pract 1992;188:145–7.

42. Manuelidis EE, Solitare GB. Glioblastoma multiforme. In: Minckler J, ed. Pathology of the nervous system. Vol. 2. New York: McGraw-Hill, 1971:2026–71.

43. Menon AG, Anderson KM, Riccardi VM, et al. Chromosome 17p deletions and p53 gene mutations associated with the formation of malignant neurofibrosarcoma in von Recklinghausen neurofibromatosis. Proc Natl Acad Sci 1990;87:5435–9.

44. Min KW. Myenteric plexomas and pheochromocytomas in neurofibromatosis type-1 [Abstract]. Mod Pathol 1997;10:60A.

45. Min KW, Balaton A. Small intestinal stromal tumors with skeinoid fibers in neurofibromatosis. Report of 4 cases with ultrastructural study of tissue retrieved from paraffin blocks. Ultrastruct Pathol 1993;17:307–14.

46. Morier P, Merot Y, Paccaud D, Beck D, Frenk E. Juvenile chronic myelogenous leukemia, juvenile xanthogranulomas, and neurofibromatosis. Case report and review of the literature. J Am Acad Dermatol 1990;22:962–5.

47. Nakagawa H, Hori S, Sato S, Fitzpatrick TB, Martuza RL. The nature and origin of the melanin macroglobule. J Invest Dermatol 1984;83:134–9.

48. Nevin S. Gliomatosis cerebri. Brain 1938;61:170–91.

49. Parry DM, MacCollin MM, Kaiser-Kupfer MI, et al. Germ-line mutations in the neurofibromatosis 2 gene: correlations with disease severity and retinal abnormalities. Am J Hum Genet 1996;59:529–39.

50. Partin JS, Lane BP, Partin JC, Edelstein LR, Priebe CJ Jr. Plexiform neurofibromatosis of the liver and mesentery in a child. Hepatology 1990;12:559–64.

51. Pleasure J, Geller SA. Neurofibromatosis in infancy presenting with congenital stridor. Am J Dis Child 1967;113:390–3.

52. Pung S, Hirsch EF. Plexiform neurofibromatosis of the heart and neck. Arch Pathol 1955;59:341–6.

53. Rawlings CE III, Wilkins RH, Cook WA, Burger PC. Segmental neurofibromatosis. Neurosurgery 1987;20:946–9.

54. Reubi F. Les vaisseux et les glandes endocrines dans la neurofibromatose: Le syndrome sympathi cotonique dans la maladie de Recklinghausen. Schweiz Ztschr f Path u Bakt 1944;7:168–236.

55. Riccardi VM. Neurofibromatosis. Phenotype, natural history, and pathogenesis. 2nd ed. Baltimore: The Johns Hopkins University Press, 1992.

56. Riccardi VM. Von Recklinghausen neurofibromatosis. N Engl J Med 1981;305:1617–27.

57. Riccardi VM, Lewis RA. Penetrance of von Recklinghausen neurofibromatosis: a distinction between predecessors and descendants. Am J Hum Genet 1988;42:284–9.

58. Rubinstein LJ. The malformative central nervous system lesions in the central and peripheral forms of neurofibromatosis. Ann NY Acad Sciences 1986;486:14–29.

59. Russell DS, Rubinstein LJ. Pathology of tumours of the nervous system. 5th ed. Baltimore: Williams & Wilkins, 1989:769–84.

59a. Ruttledge MH, Andermann AA, Phelan CM, et al. Type of mutation in the neurofibromatosis type 2 gene (NF2) frequently determines severity of disease. Am J Hum Genet 1996;59:331–42.

60. Sakaguchi N, Sano K, Ito M, Baba T, Fukuzawa M, Hotchi M. A case of von Recklinghausen's disease with bilateral pheochromocytoma—malignant peripheral nerve sheath tumors of the adrenal and gastrointestinal autonomic nerve tumors. Am J Surg Pathol 1996;20:889–97.

61. Salyer WR, Salyer DC. The vascular lesions of neurofibromatosis. Angiology 1974;25:510–9.

62. Schaldenbrand JD, Appelman HD. Solitary solid stromal gastrointestinal tumors in von Recklinghausen's disease with minimal smooth muscle differentiation. Hum Pathol 1984;15:229–32.

63. Scheithauer BW, Nora FE, Le Chago J, Wick MR, Crawford BG, Weiland LH. Duodenal gangliocytic paraganglioma. Clinicopathologic and immunohistochemical study of 11 cases. Am J Clin Pathol 1986;86:559–65.

64. Schneider M, Obringer AC, Zackai E, Meadows AT. Childhood neurofibromatosis: risk factors for malignant disease. Cancer Genet Cytogenet 1986;21:347–54.

65. Seizinger BR, Rouleau GA, Ozelius LJ, et al. Genetic linkage of von Recklinghausen's neurofibromatosis to the nerve growth factor receptor gene. Cell 1987;49:589–94.

66. Skuse GR, Kosciolek BA, Rowley PT. The neurofibroma in von Recklinghausen neurofibromatosis has a unicellular origin. Am J Hum Genet 1991;49:600–7.

67. Stephens M, Williams GT, Jasani B, Williams ED. Synchronous duodenal neuroendocrine tumors in von Recklinghausen's disease—a case report of coexisting gangliocytic paraganglioma and somatostatin-rich granular carcinoid. Histopathology 1987;11:1331–40.

68. Tong AK, Fitzpatrick TB. The skin in neurofibromatosis. In: Rubinstein AE, Korf BR, eds. Neurofibromatosis. A handbook for patients, families, and health care professionals. New York: Thieme, 1990:88–98.

69. Van de Meulen J. Orbital neurofibromatosis. Clin Plast Surg 1987;14:123–35.

70. Verhest A, Heimann R, Verschraegen J, Vamos E, Hecht F. Hereditary intestinal neurofibromatosis. II. Translocation between chromosomes 12 and 14. Neurofibromatosis 1988;1:33–6.

71. Virchow RL. Die Kraukhafte Geschwülste: Dreissig Vorlesungen, gehalted wahrend des Wintersemesters 1862-1863 on the Universitat 3u Berlin. Berlin, A. Hirschwald, 1863:1.

72. Viskochil D, Buchberg AM, Xu G, et al. Deletions and a translocation interrupt a cloned gene at the neurofibromatosis type 1 locus. Cell 1990;62:187–92.

73. von Deimling A, Krone W, Menon AG. Neurofibromatosis type 1: pathology, clinical features and molecular genetics. Brain Pathol 1995;5:153–62.

74. Walker AE. Astrocytosis arachnoideae cerebelli. A rare manifestation of von Recklinghausen's neurofibromatosis. Arch Neurol Psychiatry 1941;45:520–32.

75. Walker P, Dvorak AM. Gastrointestinal autonomic nerve (GAN) tumor. Ultrastructural evidence for a newly recognized entity. Arch Pathol Lab Med 1986;110:309–16.

76. Wallace MR, Marchuk DA, Andersen LB, et al. Type 1 neurofibromatosis gene: identification of a large transcript disrupted in three NF-1 patients. Science 1990;249:181–6.

77. Walsh NM, Bodurtha A. Auerbach's myenteric plexus. A possible site or origin for gastrointestinal stromal tumors in von Recklinghausen's neurofibromatosis. Arch Pathol Lab Med 1990;114:522–5.

78. Wiestler OD, Radner H. Pathology of neurofibromatosis 1 and 2. In: Huson SM, Hughes RA, eds. The neurofibromatoses: a pathogenetic and clinical overview. London: Chapman and Hall, 1994:139–55.

79. Worster-Drought C, Carnegie-Dickson WE, McMenemey WH. Multiple meningeal and perineurial tumors with analogous changes in the glia and ependyma (neurofibroblastomatosis). With report of two cases. Brain 1937;60:85–117.

80. Zvulunov A, Barak Y, Metzker A. Juvenile xanthogranuloma, neurofibromatosis, and juvenile chronic myelogenous leukemia. World statistical analysis. Arch Dermatol 1995;131:904–8.

Neurofibromatosis 2

81. Battersby RD, Ironside JW, Maltby EL. Inherited multiple schwannomas: a clinical, pathological and cytogenetic study of an affected family. J Neurol Neurosurg Psychiatry 1986;49:362–8.

82. Bertoni F, Unni KK, Dahlin DC, Beabout JW, Onofrio BM. Calcifying pseudoneoplasms of the neural axis. J Neurosurg 1990;72:42–8.

83. Eldridge R. Central neurofibromatosis with bilateral acoustic neuroma. Adv Neurol 1981;29:57–65.

84. Eldridge R. Neurofibromatosis type 1. In: Rubenstein AE, Korf BR, eds. Neurofibromatosis. A handbook for patients, families, and health care professionals. New York: Thieme, 1990:29–39.

85. Eldridge R, Parry DM, Kaiser-Kupfer MI. Clinical heterogeneity and natural history based on 39 individuals in 9 families and 16 sporadic cases. Proceedings of the Eighth International Congress on Human Genetics. Am J Hum Genet 1991;49:133.

85a. Evans DG, Bourn D, Wallace A, Ramsden RT, Mitchell JD, Strachan T. Diagnostic issues in a family with late onset type 2 neurofibromatosis. J Med Genet 195;32:470–4.

86. Evans DG, Huson SM, Donnai D, et al. A clinical study of type 2 neurofibromatosis. Q J Medical Essay 1992;84:603–18.

87. Gardner WJ, Frazier CH. Bilateral acoustic neurofibromas. A clinical study and field survey of a family of five generations with bilateral deafness in 38 members. Arch Neurol Psychiatr 1930;23:266–302.

88. Geddes JF, Sutcliffe JC, King TT. Mixed cranial nerve sheath tumors: their occurrence sporadically and in neurofibromatosis types 1 and 2. Clin Neuropathol 1995;14:310–3.

88a. Gutmann DH, Aylsworth A, Carey JC, et al. The diagnostic evaluation and multidisciplinary management of neurofibromatosis 1 and neurofibromatosis 2. JAMA 1997;278:71–7.

89. Halliday AL, Sobel RA, Martuza RL. Benign spinal nerve sheath tumors: their occurrence sporadically and in neurofibromatosis types 1 and 2. J Neurosurg 1991;74:248–53.

90. Halper J, Scheithauer BW, Okazaki H, Laws ER Jr. Meningo-angiomatosis: a report of six cases with special reference to the occurrence of neurofibrillary tangles. J Neuropathol Exp Neurol 1986;45:426–46.

91. Jacoby LB, MacCollin M, Louis DN, et al. Exon scanning for mutation in the NF-2 gene in schwannomas. Hum Mole Genet 1994;3:413–9.

92. Kanter WR, Eldridge R, Fabricant R, Allen JC, Koerber T. Central neurofibromatosis with bilateral acoustic neuroma. Genetic, clincial and biochemical distinctions from peripheral neurofibromatosis. Neurology 1980;30:851–9.

93. Lekanne Deprez RH, Bianchi AB, Groen NA, Seizinger BR, Hagemeijer A, van Drunen E. Frequent NF-2 gene transcript mutations in sporadic meningiomas and vestibular schwannomas. Am J Hum Genet 1994;54:1022–9.

94. Louis DN, Ramesh V, Gusella JF. Neuropathology and molecular genetics of neurofibromatosis 2 and related tumors. Brain Pathol 1995;5:163–72.

95. Mautner VF, Lindenau M, Baser ME, Kuwe L, Gottschalk J. Skin abnormalities in neurofibromatosis 2. Arch Dermatol 1997;133:1539–43.

96. Ohnishi A, Nada O. Ultrastructure of the onion bulb-like lamellated structure observed in a sural nerve in a case of von Recklinghausen's disease. Acta Neuropathol (Berl) 1972;20:258–63.

96a. Parry DM, MacCollin MM, Kaiser-Kupfer MI, et al. Germ-line mutations in the neurofibromatosis 2 gene: correlations with disease severity and retinal abnormalities. Am J Hum Genet 1996;59:529–39.

97. Poser CM. The relationship between syringomyelia and neoplasm. Springfield, IL: Charles C. Thomas, 1956.

97a. Ragge NK, Baser ME, Klein J, et al. Ocular abnormalities in neurofibromatosis 2. Am J Ophthalmol 1995;120:634–41.

98. Rodriguez HA, Berthong M. Multiple primary intercranial tumors in von Recklinghausen's neurofibromatosis. Arch Neurol 1966;14:467–75.

99. Rouleau GA, Merel P, Lutchman M, et al. Alteration in a new gene encoding a putative membrane-organizing protein causes neurofibromatosis type 2. Nature 1993;363:515–21.

100. Rouleau GA, Wertelecki W, Haines JL, et al. Genetic linkage of bilateral acoustic neurofibromatosis to a DNA marker on chromosome 22. Nature 1987;329:246–8.

101. Rubinstein LJ. The malformative central nervous system lesions in the central and peripheral forms of neurofibromatosis. A neuropathological study of 22 cases. Ann NY Acad Sciences 1986;486:14–29.

102. Ruttledge MH, Andermann AA, Phelan CM, et al. Type of mutation in the neurofibromatosis type 2 gene (NF2) frequently determines severity of disease. Am J Hum Genet 1996;59:331–42.

103. Short MP, Martuza RL, Huson SM. Neurofibromatous 2: clinical features, genetic counselling, and management issues. In: Huson SM, Hughes RA, eds. The neurofibromatosis: a pathogenetic and clinical overview. London: Chapman and Hall, 1994:414–44.

104. Sobel RA. Vestibular (acoustic) schwannomas: histologic features in neurofibromatosis 2 and in unilateral cases. J Neuropathol Exp Neurol 1993;52:106–13.

105. Thomas PK, King RH, Chiang TR, Scaravilli F, Sharma AK, Downie AW. Neurofibromatosis neuropathy. Muscle Nerve 1990;13:93–101.

106. Trofatter JA, MacCollin MM, Rutter JL, et al. A novel moesin-ezrin-radixin-like gene is a candidate for the neurofibromatosis 2 tumor suppressor. Cell 1993;72:791–800.

107. Wellenreuther R, Kraus JA, Lenartz D, Menon AG, Sehramm J, Louis DN. Analysis of the neurofibromatosis 2 gene reveals molecular variants of meningioma. Am J Pathol 1995;146:827–32.

108. Wiestler OD, von Siebenthal K, Schmitt HP, Feiden W, Kliehues P. Distribution and immunoreactivity of cerebral microhamartomas in bilateral acoustic neurofibromatosis (neurofibromatosis 2). Acta Neuropathol 1989;79:137–43.

109. Wishart JH. Case of tumours in the skull, dura mater, and brain. Edinburgh Med Surg J 1882;18:393–97.

110. Young DF, Eldridge R, Nager GT, Deland FH, McNew J. Hereditary bilateral acoustic (central neurofibromatosis). Birth Defects: Original Article Series, 1971;7:73–86.

INDEX*

---

*Numbers in boldface indicate table and figure pages.